W9-DIZ-599

E-Health Systems Quality and Reliability:
Models and Standards

Anastasius Moumtzoglou
European Society for Quality in Healthcare, Greece

Anastasia Kastania
Athens University of Economics and Business, Greece

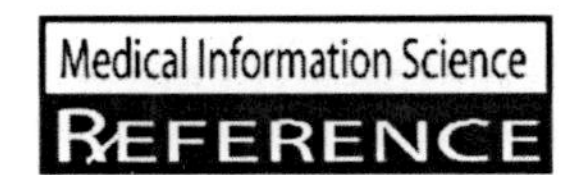

MEDICAL INFORMATION SCIENCE REFERENCE
Hershey · New York

Director of Editorial Content: Kristin Klinger
Director of Book Publications: Julia Mosemann
Acquisitions Editor: Lindsay Johnston
Development Editor: Dave DeRicco
Publishing Assistant: Jamie Snavely
Typesetter: Keith Glazewski
Production Editor: Jamie Snavely
Cover Design: Lisa Tosheff

Published in the United States of America by
Medical Information Science Reference (an imprint of IGI Global)
701 E. Chocolate Avenue
Hershey PA 17033
Tel: 717-533-8845
Fax: 717-533-8661
E-mail: cust@igi-global.com
Web site: http://www.igi-global.com

Library of Congress Cataloging-in-Publication Data

E-health systems quality and reliability : models and standards / Anastasius Moumtzoglou and Anastasia Kastania, editors.
p. ; cm.
Includes bibliographical references and index.
Summary: "This book addresses the reason, principles and functionality of health and health care systems and presents a novel framework for revealing, understanding and implementing appropriate management interventions leading to qualitative improvement"--Provided by publisher. ISBN 978-1-61692-843-8 (h/c) -- ISBN 978-1-61692-845-2 (ebook) 1. Information storage and retrieval systems--Medicine--Evaluation. 2. Health services administration--Information technology--Evaluation. 3. Management information systems--Data processing--Evaluation. 4. Medical records--Data processing--Evaluation. 5. Medical informatics--Evaluation. I. Moumtzoglou, Anastasius, 1959- II. Kastania, Anastasia, 1965- [DNLM: 1. Medical Informatics Applications. 2. Delivery of Health Care--
trends. 3. Quality Assurance, Health Care--methods. W 26.5 E337 2011]
R858.E28 2011
610.285--dc22
2010016323

British Cataloguing in Publication Data
A Cataloguing in Publication record for this book is available from the British Library.

Dedication

To Maria-Georgia Moumtzoglou
A polestar in the dark

A.M.

In memory of my father Nikolaos M. Kastanias

A. K.

Editorial Advisory Board

List of Reviewers

Table of Contents

Detailed Table of Contents

This chapter clarify that evidence-based medicine (EBM) refers to the careful consideration of all the available evidence when making decisions about the care of the individual patient. Moreover, they recognize that EBM still remains a complex and delicate process which needs Quality Assurance (QA).

This chapter provides a brief overview on some e-medicine resources and global definitions focused on the three main subjects of the healthcare quality – the patient, the costs and the evidence for quality. He also mentions sites that assist in the retrieval of information about methods for obtaining evidence along with the ways of measuring evidence validity.

This chapter provides some basic ideas on e-health safety and security, focusing on the provider perspective. They present one novel unpublished case and six cases from the Food and Drug Administration (FDA), Multi-Media Consumer Information, (FDA) Patient Safety News. Topics highlight fraud, impersonation of health care professionals, misuse of data and information, and backups.

The chapter points out those patient safety initiatives which have been launched in a number of countries, primarily focusing on problem identification, learning and improvement. However, so far there has been little emphasis on monitoring outcomes and surveillance of development of patient safety at the organizational and system level. They conclude that patient safety is a new field, which requires much more research-based documentation, and a comprehensive approach on a number of different measuring dimensions.

This chapter asserts that e-health communities can assist in maintaining a healthier life-style through ongoing interactions between community members. She presents a framework to evaluate e-health communities from a learning perspective, which covers different types of conversation topics, ways to respond and community awareness.

This chapter expects a new era for Telemedicine after the 2009 Prague Declaration. However, she argues that there are barriers, which include literacy, standard connectivity and quality control. Therefore, she addresses literacy regarding the type of standards in each topic of the Telemedicine Body of Knowledge.

This chapter reviews the mission of the American Telemedicine Association Standards and Guidelines Committee, and the process by which standards and guidelines documents are produced. They also report on the committee's progress in providing the telehealth community with standards and guidelines for the practicing medicine at a distance.

The chapter challenges the evidence on quality and reliability of telemedicine techniques. They describe the telepaediatric service in Queensland, Australia outlining some evidence for quality, reliability and sustainability.

The chapter reviews the reasons for the evaluation of e-health systems, the methods for designing an e-health evaluation and the main points that represent a successful evaluation procedure. She conducts an extensive literature search to encapsulate the dimensions of e-health quality assurance, and provide a conceptual framework for quality and reliability assessment.

Foreword

The E-Health Systems Quality and Reliability: Models and Standards edited by Anastasius Moumtzoglou and Anastasia Kastania provides a comprehensive insight into the E-Healthcare landscape. It is a daunting challenge to present the relevant concepts and networks of the e-transforming and e-learning healthcare community in the time of continuous rehearsal.

Already the chapters' titles are fascinatingly inviting, ranging from some general concepts models and features to the personalized e-health grids; covering the topics of both, individual user and patient – physician teamwork and all this within the context of education and research, evidence based practice, outcomes improvement, accountability and increasing the overall satisfaction of patients and professionals.

The list of authors team is very telling indeed: they are not only experts in the respective fields of knowledge but also have vast passion for education and a great heart for teaching and learning. I have been honored to work and collaborate with many of them.

The book is a powerful manual and a useful compendium that enables a breakthrough ride into E – Health - I wish you find it useful and also entertaining.

Basia Kutryba, President ESQH

Basia Kutryba *is President of the European Society for Quality in Healthcare (ESQH). The co-founder of the first quality institute in Eastern Europe and a Senior Adviser at National Centre for Quality Assessment in Health Care (NCQA) in Krakow, Poland. She has played the major role in the development of Polish national, JCAHO based accreditation system and in quality improvement initiatives in other ECC countries as well as in the Middle East. A co – chair of the Patient Safety and Quality of Healthcare EU Working Group and a Director of the WHO Collaborating Centre for Developing Quality and Safety in Health Systems in Krakow. She is the founding member of the Polish Society for Quality Promotion in Health Care (TPJ -1993) and its Honorary Secretary of the Board.*

Preface

A systematic collection of glimpses related to future healthcare, reveals at least two trends. One trend embodies increased uses of nanotechnology, individualized drugs, cell-based computing and microchip-enhanced brains. The other one relates to emerging e-health care provision services, like telemedicine. Notwithstanding the previously mentioned prospects, both healthcare professionals and patients remain increasingly dissatisfied as a result of unclear expectations and fundamentally different views with respect to the content of quality in healthcare and the reliability of systems and services. On the other hand, quality and reliability are thought to be measurable at least in specific domains. Thus, our knowledge on the subject could be compared with a fleeting glance. New ways of thinking should evolve based on what we actually know and those we do not understand. The safest way to achieve it is related with the juxtaposition of criticism and the existing body of knowledge. Thus, unilateral approaches, for example dealing only with continuous quality improvement or reliability assurance, do not work. Instead, a comprehensive analysis of the e-health and quality interaction should be applied.

In this context, we should mention that there are essentially three cumulative levels of quality, which include conformance quality, requirements quality, and quality of kind. However, the meaning of quality is constantly evolving. As a result, there are definitions, which describe the dimensions of access, choice, information, satisfaction, health improvement and continuity of care. Notwithstanding the abundance of definitions, the most prominent ones were put forward by Avedis Donabedian and the Institute of Medicine (IOM). Donabedian defined quality as 'the ability to achieve desirable objectives using legitimate means', and quality of care as 'that kind of care which is expected to maximize an inclusive measure of patient welfare, after one has taken account of the balance of expected gains and losses that attend the process of care in all its parts'. He also argued that we have to decide whether to enter monetary cost in the definition of quality, distinguishing between a 'maximalist' and an 'optimalist' statement of quality. The maximalist statement ignores monetary costs and defines the highest quality as the 'degree that can be expected to reach the greatest improvement in health'. In contrast, the optimalist statement of quality recommends avoiding expensive interventions that do not achieve a substantial improvement in health.

The Institute of Medicine, defined quality as 'the degree to which health services for individuals and populations increase the likelihood of desired health outcomes and are consistent with current professional knowledge'. The definition covers the dimensions of safety, equity, respect, patient centeredness, continuity, effectiveness, efficiency and timeliness. It is crucial to note that the focus narrows to the goal of improving health outcomes focusing from patients to individuals and populations. It also adds 'desired outcomes' to the definition so as to highlight the need to assess the perspective of the recipients of services, and 'consistent with current professional knowledge', which implies that we have to define the standards of the service.

Patient safety is increasingly being seen as an absolute path to quality. As a consequence, the patient safety debate is parallel to the established quality of health care initiatives. It is, therefore, essential to reiterate patient safety as a quality dimension. Safety refers to the reduction of risk and forms a key component of quality. According to the IOM, patient safety is 'freedom from accidental injury due to medical care, or medical errors', with medical error being defined as 'the failure of a planned action to be completed as intended or the use of a wrong plan to achieve an aim…[including] problems in practice, products, procedures, and systems'.

At the same time, patients seek more information about their condition and require an active role in the healthcare process. It is also increasingly likely to express their dissatisfaction if the quality of service does not meet their expectations. Therefore, patient empowerment is increasingly being seen as a vital component of a modern patient-centered health system. A patient-centered approach is defined by the Picker Institute Europe as:

- informing and involving patients, eliciting and respecting their preferences
- responding quickly, effectively and safely to patients' needs and wishes
- ensuring that patients are treated in a dignified and supportive manner
- delivering well coordinated and integrated care

There is evidence that patient-centered approaches increase patient and doctor satisfaction, reduce anxiety, and improve the quality of life. There also seems to be some evidence that patient-centered care is more efficient. Strengthening patient empowerment means that patients play a more active role in partnership with health professionals. This will help patients to benefit more from their healthcare and support professionals to better understand their patients.

Finally, systematic improvement of the quality of care is only possible when we educate physicians with the attitudes, knowledge and skills needed for continuous quality improvement. Unfortunately, we pay remarkably little attention to medical curricula and there are few exemplary teaching programs in this field.

On the other hand, there is a growing proportion of people aged 65 and over, and of people over 80 years old, which has dramatic consequences on health systems. Elderly people tend to use more health services as they are more prone to illness, and suffer from multiple conditions. As a result, we need new technologies, which improve disease prevention, shift healthcare from hospitals to primary care, and use electronic interactive tools for capturing and using patient feedback on the healthcare.

Unfortunately, the current strategy of many healthcare systems around the world is unsustainable. The efforts of healthcare professionals and the value of genomics, regenerative medicine, and information-based medicine cannot counteract the effect of globalization, consumerism, and demographic shifts. Therefore, health systems have to face a radical restructuring based on balancing different opinions of 'good value', consumer responsibility for personal health management, and an overall shift in the nature, mode, and means of care delivery.

E-health is an emerging field in the intersection of medical informatics, public health and business, referring to new electronic technologies, web-based transactions and advanced networks, and implies fundamental rethinking of healthcare processes based on electronic communication and computer based support. Currently, most e-health policies reflect technology driven decisions, focus on prescriptions, booking, diagnostic reports, and discharge summaries, while in the future will support clinical pathways, governance, and patient empowerment. E-health approach is mostly technology-cantered, product-based innovation and driven by the opportunities. Consequently, the health system is capable to cope with limited organizational problems.

There two basic definitions of reliability in the literature. The first relates to the probability that the system performs its functions in a specified time limit while the second relates with the 'reliability on demand', that is, the probability that the system, when invoked, successfully completes its mission. We could also define it as the probability that the software does not produce any system failure. The procedure involves the application of statistical distributions, like the exponential, gamma, Weibull, binomial, Poisson, normal, log normal, Bayes, and Markov distributions, on the previous failure data in order to predict the intended behavior of a system. The application of the previously mentioned distributions to the data of system failure avails the fitting of processes, which are based on maximum likelihood or least squares estimates. The effectiveness of the model involves chi-square or goodness-of-fit measures. Finally, we understand software reliability through the introduction of the fault, error, and failure hypothesis. Fault is a false statement in the software, and error an unexpected state of the system. An error might occur when an internal variable assumes an unexpected value. Finally, a failure relates to an error, which circulates up to the system output. It occurs, for example, when an output variable assumes an unexpected value.

'E-Health Systems Quality and Reliability: Models and Standards' addresses the reason, principles and functionality of health and health care systems and presents a novel framework for revealing, understanding and implementing appropriate management interventions leading to qualitative improvement. It also provides evidence on the quality and reliability of telemedicine and reviews standards and guidelines for practicing medicine at a distance. Finally, it presents an evaluation framework for e-health communities, analyzes e-health applications in e3Health, and exemplifies patient safety, and education in e-health.

As a result, it supports students understand the effect of new technologies on health systems, helps healthcare professionals better understand their patients, acts as an assistant for patients to derive more benefits from their healthcare, and encourages e-health systems designers and managers to ground everyday practice on quality principles.

In chapter 1, Aleš Bourek addresses the logic, principles and functionality of health and health care systems to present a framework for revealing, understanding and implementing appropriate and adequate management interventions leading to qualitative improvement in the specified areas. Medicine (healthcare) was traditionally considered an 'art'. However, it slowly, with the establishment of analytical methods of work, became 'science' and today it is usually classified as a 'service'. Therefore, profound understanding of what medicine truly is (art or science or service or a combination of these) is crucial for all processes leading to the improvement of quality of health care. However, any discipline, function or process of healthcare and health domains that requires information handling currently unattainable via the 'digital data flow' lies for the moment outside of the e-health and e-healthcare scope.

In chapter 2, Jana Zvárová and Ing. Karel Zvára describe how the scheme proposed by J.H. van Bemmel in 1984 can be used for classification of e-health applications. Apart from the electronic component of e-health applications, they consider two other features connected with health economics and environmental health. An excellent example of such a robust model is the Health Level 7 Reference information model (RIM, ISO/HL7 21731:2006). Finally, they argue that using the latest medical knowledge creates two novel families of e-health decision-support applications.

In chapter 3, Paola Di Giacomo states that e-health is a priority of the European i2010 initiative. She concludes that the attention towards electromechanical systems means the realization of tools of small dimensions, which have considerable advantages and greater diagnostic-therapeutic effectiveness. Therefore, an economic analysis has to take into consideration the use of biomedical technology, the study of alternatives, the choice of the economic evaluation method, and the identification and quantification of the costs and benefits.

In chapter 4, Susana Lorenzo, Gilberto Llinas, Jose J. Mira, and Emilio Ignacio probe into the impact of the Internet on some aspects of patient-centeredness. They write in support of the patient as a prudent actor who rationally decides where to go and what to do. However, they are prompt in stating that many patients are not familiar with the exact definition of e-health, and the terms associated with e-health. Nevertheless, patients might get a first opinion from the Internet. Therefore, websites should meet reliability and comprehensiveness requirements.

In chapter 5, Anastasius Moumtzoglou elucidates that people-centered health care represents a structural change in thinking, which encapsulates before anything else the consideration of the patient. The development of people-centered care might include a partnership approach based on equal footing, capacity-building and the expansion of organizational care. Its core values encompass empowerment, participation, family, community, and the elimination of any form of discrimination. As a result, they bestow people on shared decision-making not exclusively on issues of treatment but also for health care organization. On the other hand, a global e-health agreement is beginning to take shape on the involvement of stakeholders, the interoperability, and standards. Consequently, e-health can have a remarkable impact on people-centered care, despite the challenges of implementation and adoption.

In chapter 6, Stavros Archondakis, Aliki Stathopoulou, and Ioannis Sitaras analyze the guidelines concerning the use of laboratory information systems for medical records storage and retrieval. They affirm that post-examination procedures, such as authorization for release, reporting, and transmission of the results have a dramatic impact on laboratory quality improvement. Finally, they reveal their conclusion that cooperation between laboratory and hospital information system will be improved by the implementation of specific procedures concerning data replacement, recovery and updating.

In chapter 7, V.G. Stamatopoulos, G.E. Karagiannis, and B.R.M.Manning outline an approach which focuses on establishing and then using existing end-to-end care process pathways as early benchmarks against which to assess the effects of changes in clinical practice in response to new clinical knowledge inputs. The primary focus of this approach is to provide a practical means of validating improvement in best practice processes and performance standards as the basis of exemplary clinical governance. It also seeks to identify potential risks of adverse events and provide the basis for preventive measures. Finally, they argue that a pathway-linked knowledge service approach does not infringe on the professional autonomy.

In chapter 8, Ioannis Apostolakis, Periklis Valsamos, and Iraklis Varlamis clarify that evidence-based medicine (EBM) refers to the careful consideration of all the available evidence when making decisions about the care of the individual patient. Moreover, they recognize that EBM still remains a complex and delicate process which needs Quality Assurance (QA). Overall, they provide an introduction on the concepts of EBM, highlight the need for structured methodologies that will ensure the quality of the EBM process, and provide a critical overview of the existing methodologies in quality assurance of the evidence.

In chapter 9, Asen Atanasov provides a brief overview on some e-medicine resources and global definitions focused on the three main subjects of the healthcare quality – the patient, the costs and the evidence for quality. He also mentions sites that assist in the retrieval of information about methods for obtaining evidence along with the ways of measuring evidence validity. These sites provide information on implementing the ultimate evidence-based product – clinical guidelines for better medical practice and health service.

In chapter 10, Suzana Parente and Rui Loureiro provide some basic ideas on e-health safety and security, focusing on the provider perspective. They present one novel unpublished case and six cases from the Food and Drug Administration (FDA), Multi-Media Consumer Information, (FDA) Patient Safety News. Topics highlight fraud, impersonation of health care professionals, misuse of data and information, and backups.

In chapter 11, Solvejg Kristensen, Jan Mainz and Paul D. Bartels point out those patient safety initiatives, which have been launched in a number of countries, primarily focusing on problem identification, learning and improvement. However, so far there has been little emphasis on monitoring outcomes and surveillance of development of patient safety at the organizational and system level. They conclude that patient safety is a new field, which requires much more research-based documentation, and a comprehensive approach on a number of different measuring dimensions.

In chapter 12, Amar Gupta, Raymond Woosley, Igor Crk, and Surendra Sarnikar refer to an information technology architecture for enabling the monitoring of adverse drug events in an outpatient setting. The proposed system architecture enables the development of a web based drug effectiveness reporting and monitoring system that builds on previous studies, and demonstrates the feasibility of a system in which community pharmacists identify and report adverse drug events. They also specify the main technical requirements of such a monitoring and reporting system, identify the critical factors that affect the successful implementation and use of the system, and present information technology solutions that satisfy these requirements.

In chapter 13, Christopher L. Pate and Joyce E. Turner-Ferrier explore the concept of e-health as it relates to healthcare delivery, healthcare quality and education. They address these relationships by discussing and defining the concept of e-health, discussing fundamental linkages between e-health and quality-related healthcare outcomes, and highlighting key themes between health education, technology and quality.

In chapter 14, Shiu-chung Au and Amar Gupta illustrate a site, which is being developed for the field of Gastrointestinal Motility. The site augments the innovations of existing healthcare information sites with the intention of serving the diverse needs of lay people, medical students, and experts in the field. The site leverages the strengths of online textbooks, which have a high degree of organization, in conjunction with the strengths of online journal collections, which are more detailed and focused to build a knowledge base that can be easily updated but still provides reliable and high quality information to users. Gastrointestinal Motility Online uses automated methods to gather information from various heterogeneous data sources to create a coherent, cogent, and current knowledge base serving a diverse base of users.

In chapter 15, George Athanasiou, Nikos Maris, and Ioannis Apostolakis examine the structural transformation of the learning process, the paradigm shift of collaborative, and community learning, and the necessity of quality assurance of all learning assets. They provide a number of e-learning standards, a reference framework for the specification of quality approaches and an introduction on how the e-learning process can be founded on pedagogical standards. The novelty of their approach lies in the fact that it combines the merits of evaluation, self-support and collaboration for improving quality in learning, which makes it an appropriate solution for the highly volatile healthcare community.

In chapter 16, Åsa Smedberg asserts that e-health communities can assist in maintaining a healthier life-style through ongoing interactions between community members. However, whether these e-health communities actively promote learning depends on the ways they support community members reflect upon their habits, underlying reasons and motivational factors. Overall, she presents a framework to evaluate e-health communities from a learning perspective, which covers different types of conversation topics, ways to respond and community awareness.

In chapter 17, Ferrer-Roca expects a new era for Telemedicine after the 2009 Prague Declaration. However, she argues that there are barriers, which include literacy, standard connectivity and quality control. Therefore, she addresses literacy regarding the type of standards in each topic of the Telemedicine Body of Knowledge.

In chapter 18, Elizabeth A. Krupinski, Nina Antoniotti, and Anne Burdick review the mission of the American Telemedicine Association Standards and Guidelines Committee, and the process by which standards and guidelines documents are produced. They also report on the committee's progress in providing the telehealth community with standards and guidelines for the practicing medicine at a distance.

In chapter 19, Sisira Edirippulige, and Anthony C. Smith challenge the evidence on quality and reliability of telemedicine techniques. They describe the telepaediatric service in Queensland, Australia outlining some evidence for quality, reliability and sustainability.

In chapter 20, Anastasia Kastania reviews the reasons for the evaluation of e-health systems, the methods for designing an e-health evaluation and the main points that represent a successful evaluation procedure. She conducts an extensive literature search to encapsulate the dimensions of e-health quality assurance, and provide a conceptual framework for quality and reliability assessment.

In chapter 21, Anastasia Kastania and Sophia Kossida realize the potential of patient information management and medical decision support in an open and mobile medical environment. Therefore, they present an overview of personalized, mobile and Grid applications as well as evidence on quality issues of these fields. They conclude that the success of the information technology allows the biomedical researchers to capitalize in an eclectic selection of tools for resource allocation as well as ubiquitous and transparent distributed systems.

In chapter 22, Anastasius Moumtzoglou sketches a mental image of the future healthcare. He argues that the advancement of e-health in healthcare derives large quality and patient safety benefits. Moreover, advances in genomics, proteomics, and pharmaceuticals introduce new methods for unraveling the complex biochemical processes inside cells. Data mining detects patterns in data samples, and molecular imaging unites molecular biology and in vivo imaging. Finally, the field of microminiaturization enables biotechnologists to start packing their bulky sensing tools and medical simulation bridges the learning divide by representing certain key characteristics of a physical system.

Conclusively, 'E-Health Systems Quality and Reliability: Models and Standards' impacts both the field of quality and e-health contributing to the better understanding of their interaction. Specifically, the book opens new avenues for patient-centered medicine, enables the evidence-based patient choice, and cites examples to successful implementation. Moreover, it introduces novel approaches to improve the quality of health care, exemplifies the strategic evaluation of e-health systems, patient safety in e-health, people-centered care, personalized health, evidence-based medicine and reliability modeling.

Anastasius Moumtzoglou
European Society for Quality in Healthcare, Greece

Anastasia Kastania
Athens University of Economics and Business, Greece

Acknowledgment

We would like to thank the European Society for Quality in Healthcare (ESQH) for their support in promoting the call for chapters, the editorial advisory board for their invaluable advice, the reviewers for the care with which they reviewed the manuscripts and all the authors for their diverse and outstanding contributions to this book.

Anastasius Moumtzoglou
European Society for Quality in Healthcare, Greece

Anastasia Kastania
Athens University of Economics and Business, Greece

Chapter 1
General Principles and Logic of Quality Management in Health and Healthcare

Aleš Bourek
Masaryk University, Czech Republic

ABSTRACT

The following chapter addresses the logic, principles and functionality of health and health care systems to present a framework prerequisite for revealing, understanding and implementing appropriate and adequate management interventions leading to qualitative improvement in the specified areas.

INTRODUCTION

Although many parts of the word have witnessed in the last decades exponential growth in the area of technologies, surprisingly enough this growth does not reflect a similar growth in the perceived quality of life or well-being. Oddly enough pure technological growth does not produce happiness or joy. To a certain degree a similar situation, quite naturally as healthcare is a part of the real world, projects into the healthcare environment. Although many societies and many healthcare systems could potentially benefit from vast medical technological advancements, this alone does not assure high quality, safe, patient centered and humane care expected from the healthcare systems and the healthcare profession. Although there is always a risk in generalization, certain common principles from my point of view exist and if properly understood and applied could, as I would like to demonstrate, prime and initiate ways of improving the present state.

Our society, roughly from the year 1990, calls itself, the 'Information Society'. Although information is a valuable asset (an in health care environment we have plenty), alone it is useless as it allows only very basic decision making. Knowledge possession is a bit better, but knowledge is based on proper interpretation and understanding of the relations between the data / information subsets (this represents a complex issue, not only in healthcare, where typically many factors influence the interpretation of these relations). The variables we handle in the healthcare

DOI: 10.4018/978-1-61692-843-8.ch001

environment are at least as complex as those in the monetary sector, where the numbers handled represent one well defined and generally understood entity – money. Effects of misinterpretation of relations in the monetary sector are well felt world over in 2009. The healthcare sector is no better off (Kohn et. al., 2000).

Several near-term changes are likely to impact the overall environment in which healthcare providers and other stakeholders operate (Adams, 2006):

- Piecemeal, incremental approaches to healthcare change, sometimes with more results and unintended consequences.
- A struggle to seek a viable balance in public and private health care spending.
- An increasing portion of health related financial responsibility transfers to individual citizens.
- The emergence of new and nontraditional local and global competitors and collaborators in care delivery to meet changing stakeholder needs.
- Proliferation of health promotion and care delivery models and capabilities.

All stated may sound threatening; the truth may actually be even more alarming. At last, the health care professionals may be gaining some insight into reasons evoking uneasy feelings and distrust on the side of the patient community. In many areas, our knowledge of *what* (to do) is limited, but we are generally even worse off on the level of knowing *how* (to do it). Majority would agree that the most valuable part of a company or individual lies in its/his 'know-how'. This know-*how* may well be the under-performing part of the health care system.

If there is a challenge i.e. needed improvement of know-how of the health care environment (quality, efficiency, efficacy, safety, timeliness, patient centeredness…), there must be solutions. If our way of thinking created most of these challenges (sometimes politically incorrectly referred to as problems), then the same way of thinking, doing and attitudes have a low potential to provide solutions to these issues.

I am convinced, that the appropriate approach lies not in the knowledge of explicit facts, but in the understanding (and acceptance) of the following basic postulates, I have found independent on cultures to which the respective healthcare systems belong to. Only adequate understanding and proper definitions allow the use of all available tools, resources and processes (including those depending on the use of ICT) in the most efficient way, maximizing the benefits, understanding limitations and avoiding unnecessary risks.

BACKGROUND

Key Definitions

1. *Health care is a privilege* (granted to health care professionals) to serve their brothers and sisters in need.
2. *Health care is a science and skill* (often incorrectly named 'art'), requiring explicit, tacit and emotional information handling. Health and healthcare is *based on collaboration*. Resulting level of health and *healthcare quality is a function of communication*. The initial step lies in 'needs assessment'. Health and healthcare is a systemic issue requiring a systems and systematic approach. Reductionalist approaches are very limited in their contribution to the understanding of healthcare systems. The smallest functional unit / entity in health care is sometimes referred to as the 'healthcare microsystem'.
3. *A healthcare organization exhibits all attributes of a living organism* (has a memory, 'conscience – awareness', is responsible and accountable, and is able to reproduce. An organization **is** an organism. An organism is a self generating network of communications.

Seen from this point of view, the reason for reflection on 'E-health Systems Quality and Reliability: Models and Standards,' healthcare informatics and cybernetics in health care is meaningful.

4. *A normal organization is an organism that behaves naturally and the origin of this 'nature' lies in the 'genes' of this organism* (hence the need for 'Models and Standards' – standards = norms). *The skill of quality management is the introduction of the appropriate disturbances leading to better collaboration = symbiosis.* A quality manager may be looked upon as the 'vector of transfer' of the appropriate new pieces of genetic code into the existing genes of the organization and in such way aiding in the improvement of the genetic pool of this respective organism.

The following paragraphs will attempt to illuminate, provide basic insight and present supporting facts for the above framework. The comments will also seek to provide some examples of the potential of digitalization in health and healthcare, sometimes also referred to as e-health and e-healthcare.

HEALTH CARE IS A PRIVILEGE

The reason for considering healthcare service as a privilege of a certain subset of the human population (healthcare professionals) arises from the fact that, as opposed to other species, the human community behaves differently. Humans represent the only species, where one individual (genetically not belonging to the same family as another one) is capable of collaboration to such an extent as sacrificing one's life for another non-related individual. Humans inherently exhibit a high level of altruistic behavior. This behavior is observed in other species with a high order of specialization (for example ants or bees), but only if the individuals belong to the same family (they must be genetically strongly related). In order to survive as a species and due to the fact that not even the genetic family was sufficient to successfully assure the viability of the human newborn, non-related individuals were 'forced' into collaboration. As a driver / enabler for this process specific means of communication had to develop eventually leading to the human society as is known today (Koukolík, 2006). From my point of view, *there are two ways of looking at the role and importance of altruism in healthcare:*

1. Role and Effect of 'Reciprocal Altruism' and 'Game Theory' on Health Care Systems

The theory of reciprocal altruism, developed by Trivers (1971), is one attempt to explain the evolution of altruism among non-kin. The basic idea is straightforward: it may benefit an individual (sometimes seen also in animals) to behave altruistically towards another, if there is an expectation of the favor being returned in the future. ('If you scratch my back, I'll scratch yours'.). In compliance with this and with the 'game theory' some healthcare professionals provide health services not only 'for a profit', but because of their function in the health care system provides them with a payoff. Some rules must be observed. Game theory postulates, that a game is a formal description of a strategic situation. Game theory is the formal study of decision-making where several players must make choices that potentially affect the interests of the other players. A payoff, also called utility, is a number that indicates the desirability of an outcome from the point of view of a player, for whatever his reasons may be. When the outcome is random, payoffs are usually weighted with their probabilities. The expected payoff incorporates the player's attitude towards risk. A player is said to be rational if he seeks to play in a manner which maximizes his own payoff. It is often assumed that the rationality of all players is common knowledge (Theodore, 2001). The usual classical methods of game theory are based on several paradigms one of which postulates:

Players are individuals each one seeks only his own payoff (his own satisfaction), this being true also in coalitions (please read well, *a player is not seeking greatest gain / profit, but greatest payoff / satisfaction*). If he finds satisfaction in the fact that he helps his co-player, then he will act accordingly - but even in this case he will be satisfying his preferences. When collaboration is considered a player is willing to accept a treaty (settlement) that does not increase his payoff only if at the same time, it does not decrease it (this is the only acceptable sign of solidarity with co-players, which may lead to an increase in their individual payoffs).

This in healthcare translates into management methods based on *allocative efficiency* - At the end of the 1990s, a high-profile application of game theory was the design of auctions. Prominent game theorists were involved in the design of auctions for allocating rights to the use of bands of the electromagnetic spectrum to the mobile telecommunications industry. Most of these auctions were designed with the goal of allocating these resources more efficiently than traditional governmental practices, and additionally raised billions of dollars in the United States and Europe. The automation of strategic choices enhances the need, for these choices to be made efficiently, and to be robust against abuse. Game theory addresses these requirements and has a potential for a broader application in health and healthcare related issues.

2. Efficient Collaboration and Provision of Healthcare Services is Critically Dependent on Unselfish 'Psychological Altruists'

This is a specialized subset of the human population (usually possessing the altruistic genes). These healthcare professionals are privileged bearers of the 'right genotype - genes'. Ignorance in identifying these 'privileged' and our incapability of creating the appropriate environments leading to phenotypic expression of these genes may well be one of the factors hindering healthcare quality in many 'developed / industrial' societies. The reason for existence of such individuals was studied by Sober (Sober, 1998, Sober 1988). The authors argue that, even if we accept an evolutionary approach to human behavior, there is no particular reason to think that evolution would have made humans egoists rather than psychological altruists. On the contrary, it is quite possible that natural selection would have favored humans who genuinely do care about helping others, i.e. who are capable of 'real' or psychological altruism. Assume there is an evolutionary advantage associated with taking good care of one's children (a quite plausible idea). Then, parents who *really do* care about their children's' welfare, i.e. who are 'real' altruists, will have a higher inclusive fitness, hence spread more of their genes, than parents who only pretend to care, or who do not care. Evolution, therefore, may well facilitate 'real' or psychological altruism evolvement. Contrary to what is often thought, an evolutionary approach to human behavior does *not* imply that humans are likely to be motivated by self-interest alone. One strategy by which 'selfish genes' may increase their future representation is by causing humans to be *non*-selfish, in the psychological sense. Altruism and empathy also forms a binding relation between all health and healthcare stakeholders and organizations providing health related services. Meaningful exchange of signals (from the level of data to the level of information and knowledge) to their specifically targeted receptors (not all data and all information to everyone) forms the basis of organizational synergy. On a more generalized level, each organization builds its identity 'genome' on the basis of structured and coded information 'DNA' sometimes referred to in the medical environment as standards, guidelines or protocols of care. If we consider the healthcare environment as a space where games (as defined in the Game Theory) are played every day, better modeling of the social networks and their interactions in relation to health and healthcare is definitely another platform where the e-approach has a major potential in the future. It seems to me that existing inappropriate satisfaction of all stakeholders needs (the achievement of the best possible allocation efficiency and the ability to convince all stakeholders on the basis of facts that this allocation efficiency has been reached) is one of the reasons for health systems instability as seen today.

HEALTH CARE IS A SCIENCE AND SKILL BASED ON COLLABORATION

Medicine (healthcare) was traditionally considered an 'art' then gradually, with the introduction of scientific methods of work, it became 'science' and today it is often classified as a 'service' Profound understanding of what medicine really is (art or science or service or a mix of these) is extremely important for all processes leading to the improvement of quality of health care. Vague or incomplete definitions first of all prohibit meaningful discussions of issues relating to improvement, they also bear the risk that based on them, wrong conclusions will be reached and inappropriate measures undertaken. For this reason, it may be important to understand the original meaning of the word 'art' in this specific field of human activities, since there are many misconceptions and misinterpretations ranging as far back into history as the times of Pliny (Beagon, 1992). Pliny claims that the moral degeneracy on Rome is due more to medicine (*medicina*) than anything else. For Pliny, medicine is associated with the Greeks and condemned as an *ars* which constitutes an abuse of *ratio*. The first known manuscript containing the whole of the Ars medicinae dates from the beginning of the twelfth century and originated in the south of Italy. 'Ars Medicinae' is a collection of medical texts well documented for example in the Codex Gigas (Codex Gigas), mainly of Greek or Byzantine origin. The work addresses medical topics in both theoretical and practical terms. The last three medical treatises are devoted to practical medicine and were written by Constantine the African. All of these were adaptations of Arabic writings, which, in turn, were often based on classical texts by Hippocrates (c. 460-370 BC), the father of Greek medicine, or by Galen, a renowned Greek physician from Pergamum. Liber Pantegni (from the Greek pantechne, 'The whole art') was divided into a theoretical section, Theorica, and a practical one, Practica, each comprising ten books. It became the fundamental textbook for medical curriculum throughout the Middle Ages.

It may be deducted, that the concept of 'art' stems form the Latin translation of the original Greek τέχνη (techni)

The following interpretation is based on Wordnet (http://wordnet.princeton.edu/perl/webwn):

ART

[am. eng.] [α:rt] noun - τέχνη ***a superior skill that you can learn by study and practice and observation;*** *'the art of conversation'; 'it is quite an art'* *S: (n)* **art**, artistry, prowess *(a superior skill that you can learn by study and practice and observation) 'the art of conversation'; it is quite an art'* ***sister term*** *S: (n)* superior skill *(more than ordinary ability)* ***derivationally related form*** *W: (n)* artist *[Related to:* art*] (a person whose creative work shows sensitivity and imagination)*

Meticulous understanding and thorough definition of what health care is, is absolutely crucial for proper utilization of all e-health concepts. The area of e-health is intimately connected with ICT - information and communication technologies and with the 'digital'. Any area, function or process of the healthcare and health domains that require information handling currently unattainable via the 'digital data flow' lies for the moment outside of the e-health and e-healthcare scope.

Since practically all health and healthcare related issues contain and are influenced also by tacit and emotional information handling (sensitivity and imagination), the potential, limitations and risks of e-health and e-healthcare need to be thoroughly mapped and understood assuring the 'primum non nocere' ('do not harm') concept of quality care. The basic understanding of this approach will have to, in the long run influence the attitudes and activities of the lay and professional community in relation to health services. The generally requested attitude is somewhat „schizophrenic". All stakeholders should understand that they are required to be *progressive* (very proactive) in their quest for evidence based facts (relevant and up-to-date information) *and* extremely *conservative* in the application of the respective facts to the concrete individual situation. It does not need to be emphasized that the advantage of using ICT lies in its capability to gather, store, transmit and present large data volumes to specific subpopulations of the healthcare process stakeholders, but that exactly this capability of ICT bears a considerable risk of misinterpretation (since this data is not an input from the proprioceptors / senses of the decision-maker(s), it is mediated and medialised) and resulting inappropriate decision making. The right amount of conservatism was best voiced by Socrates (469-399 BC) 'True knowledge exists in knowing that you know nothing. And in knowing that you know nothing, that makes you the wisest of all'. Most of The today's e-health activities are based on the information provision. Information alone is not enough for decision-making. The first level enabling appropriate decision-making is the 'knowledge level' (the level of understanding relations between different information subsets).

Information alone is not enough! It serves as a basis of knowledge and concept construction. It may be used for - Learning >> Modeling / simulations => Decision- making (see Figure 1)

The potential of e-health and e-healthcare concepts lies in the capability of the technology infrastructure to provide timely data subsets (on-

Figure 1. Data, information, knowledge, concepts - relation to decision-making

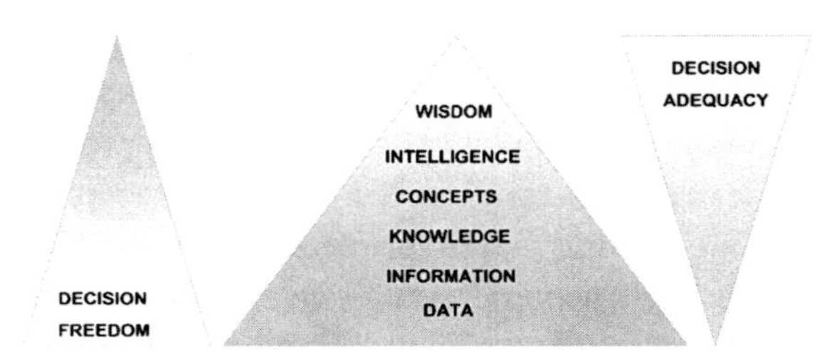

line, on-demand) and provide means for visualization of the relations eventually leading to the understanding of the challenge (issue, problem). Together with the use of the 'virtual digital environment' it enables us to model and produce possible and robust scenarios for their solution. The 'computer' or ICT infrastructure is no substitute for 'common sense', but it is an efficient tool to help us identify where common sense misleads us into 'illusions' (lies). ICT and e-health as of today must be approached, and handled as existing, available and necessary tools supplementing human senses, instincts and 'imagination', and providing the right mirror (reflection basis) for thinking pausing and reorientation (the iterative process of improving the quality of care). Observing, recording, visualization and interpretation of discontinuous fragments of the healthcare system present a potential threat for misinterpretation of the gathered facts. Reductionalist approaches are only very limited in their contribution to the understanding of healthcare systems. A more rewarding approach is to focus on smallest functional elements of the system rather than at individual systems stakeholders and their communities (traditionally physicians, nursing staff, administrative staff, patients and their families etc.).

Such elements are referred to as 'Clinical Microsystems' or in a broader sense could be referred to as '*Healthcare Microsystems*'. They may be defined as small groups of people continuously collaborating in the provision of care services

Figure 2. Healthcare microsystem schematically

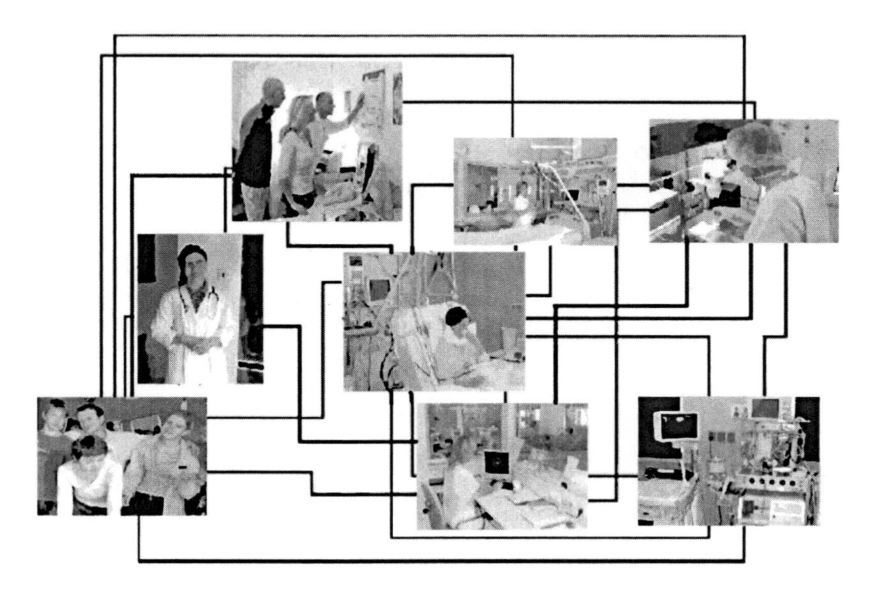

to patients and individuals (identifiable also by belonging to a certain subgroup of patients) who are receptors of this respective care. In the same manner as any complex adaptive system the 'microsystem' has to (1) perform the work, (2) satisfy the needs of the employees, (3) maintain its characteristics as a clinical / healthcare unit and (4) contribute to the specific larger organization. In short, the healthcare microsystems may be labeled as the 'space' where patients, their families and healthcare professional team meet.

A *Healthcare Microsystem* is composed of:

- a small population of patients
- a small population of doctors and nurses in other health care professionals
- interrelated and with a common goal and intentions
- with a certain amount of administrative support
- with a certain access to information and a background of information and ICT

Health care microsystems exhibit a high level of mutual dependencies of all its elements (parts). Mutual relations between healthcare professionals (nurses, doctors and other health care professionals) as well as the incorporation of the patient (client, healthcare service consumer - and his family) into the healing process are essential. *The necessity of incorporating the patient and his family into the team derives from the fact that effective teems are bound together by a common goal and vision and these goals reflect the subjective and objective needs of the ill* (Bourková, 2007) (See Figure 2).

The advantage of the e-environment lies in its capability of assuring unambiguous data sharing, data storage and retrieval, convergence of devices used for data handling (a single device like a cell phone instead of three specialized devices for sound and image capture and storage and a third device for data sharing) and especially in the area of data, information and knowledge representation (visualization). All of these areas are by now well established in healthcare and gradually introduced into the context of health, not only of healthcare management. To me there seems to be one area, which has generally been overlooked in relation to health and healthcare and that is the area of models, modeling and

Figure 3. Evolvement of collaboration in healthcare over time including possible projection

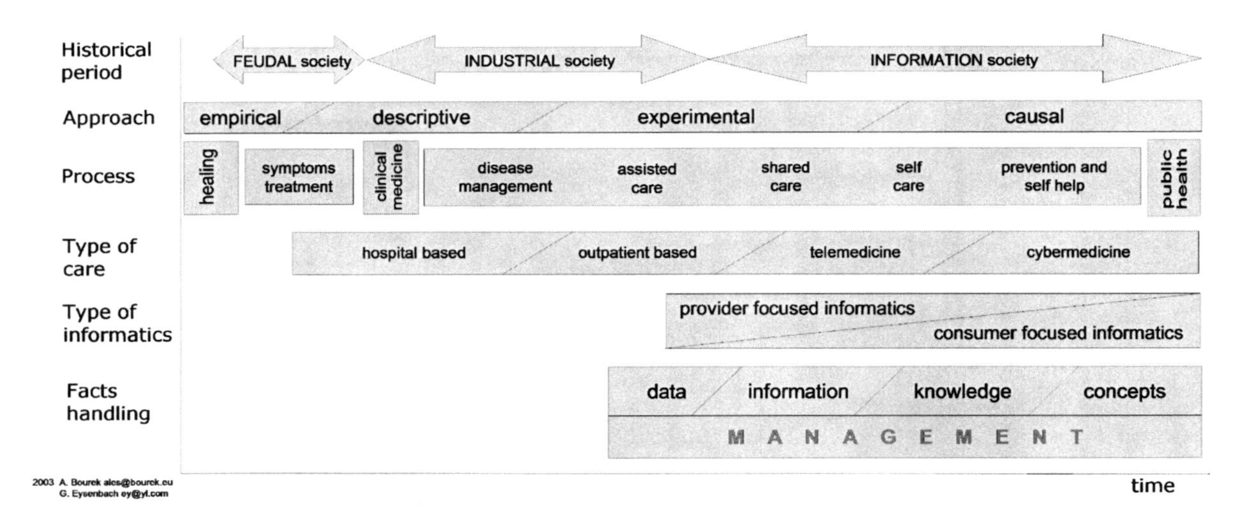

simulations. If we define the medical 'art' as a certain skill, than a decade ago the only way how to acquire this skill was mostly by practicing in real everyday situations. Whether it is tacit or explicit skills, we are slowly reaching a level where the e-environment allows repetitive pre-training with the advantage of a 'reset button'. In certain areas (robotic operation), there is practically no difference between the e-environment and the real environment. Certain diagnostic skills as well as communication skills may also be pre-trained through the use of digital technology (virtual patients all way up to the level of simulating virtual hospitals). All of this again with the advantage of resetting option and of course with the ability of recording and replaying a situations in the course of education of healthcare professionals as well as the patients and families themselves. The great benefit of the 'virtual' e-space is training without the possibility of 'harming a person'. The traditional health and healthcare training also allowed for corrections of inappropriate actions taken, but literally with 'leaving scars' on the body and soul of the involved stakeholders. For the future, it may be anticipated that simulation and virtual approaches will ultimately be targeted at the lay population, not only at professionals.

HEALTHCARE QUALITY IS A FUNCTION OF COMMUNICATION

Quality health care is a collaborative effort affected by means of an organization (through collaboration and competition). Individual-to-individual health-care was possible only in the 'healing' period of healthcare service provision. Information and communication technologies have their effect (Eysenbach, 2000) (See Figure 3).

Health and healthcare services were initially based on empiricism, on observation and transferring of the observation on to another 'similar' situation. During the empirical 'healing' period the individual healer, 'shaman', served the individual in need. The growing body of medical knowledge, as early as at the feudal age, evolved from pure treatment of symptoms to gradually addressing the underlying causes. This required a formalization of medical practice and formal training for health care service professionals. It also led to institutionalization and first hospitals appear on the scene. The imperative of collaboration requested formalization of communication and by receiving a common language (devised by Vesalius in the form of Latin anatomy nomenclature), medicine became a formalized science. At first, in the feudal age and early industrial age the science was predominantly descriptive and disease management and treatment oriented. The development of the society from the industrial age into the information age again strongly influenced the shift in health and healthcare service provision. Such development is schematically presented in Figure 1. The late industrial and early information age moved medical practice from the observational phase into the experimental phase. Large data volumes were initially produced and targeted at a professional community. The focal point of care gradually moves from hospital care to outpatient care. The impact of the information society and ICT gradually led to more and more data and information provision to the lay community and to the shift to 'assisted care' (patients and their families assist the professionals) and more and more to 'shared care' (where patients and their families share the care process and responsibilities with the professionals providing health and healthcare services). Today in many areas we see a shift to 'self care', where empowered healthcare service consumers are capable of self diagnosing and self management of certain health conditions. Finally, it may be expected with the appropriate provision of health and healthcare related knowledge (in an understandable format) to the general society that the society will react (with reasonable motivation and with access to meaningful knowledge) by self-care and in the best possible scenario by 'self prevention' attitudes and behaviors.

It seems to me that this way of understanding of the existing situation is receiving more attention lately. The increasing focus on value, the rising needs to activate responsible citizen, and the changing requirements of care delivery will force many care delivery organizations (CDO) to adopt and develop service delivery models with new and sharper strategic focus. Regardless of their choosing service delivery models CDOs will also require a core set of enhancement expanded strategic competencies (Adams, 2006):

- Empower and activate citizens
- Collaborate and integrate
- Innovate
- Optimize operational efficiencies
- Enable through ICT

Similar line of thinking from my point of view should form the main axis of e-health and the e-healthcare targets and activities. The potential of e-health lies in its capability of appropriate management of data, information, knowledge and concepts form the basis of decision support for professionals and the lay community. From this point of view, it is known that „shared opinions“ drive society: what we read, how we vote, and where we shop and how we handle health and healthcare issues are all heavily influenced by the choices of others. However, the cost in time and money to systematically share opinions remains high, while the actual performance history of opinion generators is often not tracked (Masumm 2002). This area is again open for e-health activities and their appropriate use. As has been already mentioned, the strength of the digital or e-environment lies in the unprecedented capability of data handling. This holds true also for communication and communication strategies. Since the underlying reason for all health related activities is 'staying alive', 'being physically and emotionally productive' and being 'reproductive' (again physically or mentally), introduction of more precise, accurate, timely means of communication (as a supplement to the already existing verbal and emotional communication) again has a great potential for the improvement of collaboration improvement. If we are able to witness the effect of voluntary synergy building in areas as diverse as the construction of the Wikipedia (and

Figure 4. Semantics of quality as seen by 'public' – British National Corpus (Infomap group, CSLI, Stanford University)

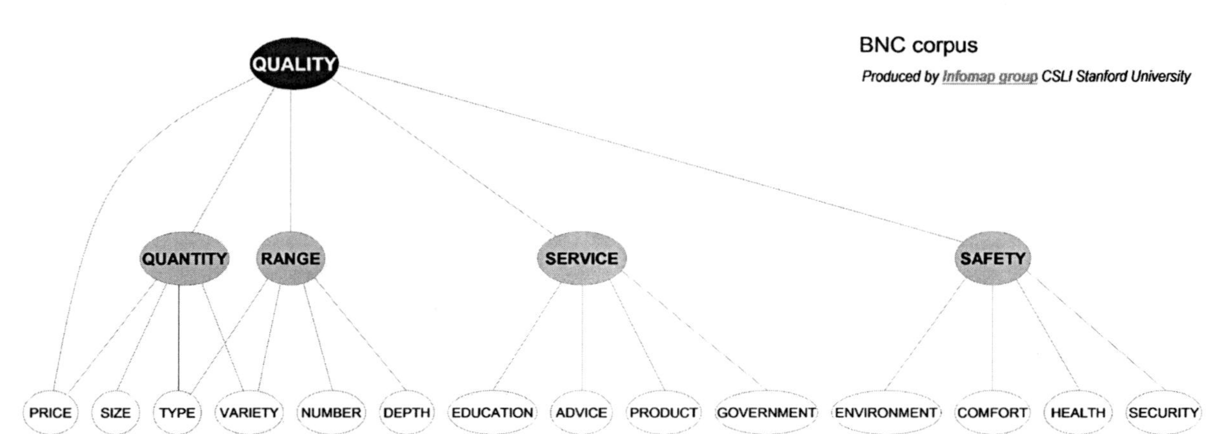

other 'Wikies') or networks such as the Facebook, it is obvious that the e-environment will be one of the major shaping factors of health and healthcare service provision of the future. Again it is extremely necessary to observe, identify and understand the possibilities limitations and risks of using ICT approaches in health which is traditionally considered as a sensitive area. The study of social interactions in the health arena has the potential to dramatically improve the quality of health care services provided (as we have often seen in other human service activities – banking, shopping, educational or leisure activities etc). Since health and healthcare is generally considered as an important issue, it is obvious that the most appropriate viewing position is through the eyes of the service receiver. In order to really serve, empathy of the service provider is crucial and often addressed at the level of needs assessment.

Needs Assessment: Fundamental Questions about Quality

- Who is the customer?
- What are the customer's needs and expectations?

Semantics of Quality

When considering the semantics of the word quality, different populations understand the meaning differently, or at least use a different vocabulary related to the quality concepts. The BNC (British National Corpus) based semantics are strikingly different from the OHSUMED (Medline based corpus) representation. Unless this is understood, quality health care management will always be biased towards one of the groups – professionals vs. general society (See Figure 4, Figure 5).

A thorough description and understanding of the environment where one is supposed to function forms the basis of rational, conscious and subconscious behavior. The rational and conscious behavior may be acquired through the process of learning, whereas the subconscious (automatic) behavior and actions are trained and developed by doing. The subconscious decision making and action also closely relates to the topic of 'art' in health care as has already been discussed. Both form an integrated part in the management of the health care system. Both must be acquired by those referred to as managers, leaders or educators. The theory of leadership forms a science of its own. The most shorthand form of understanding how a proper manager, leader or educator is

Figure 5. Semantics of quality as seen by 'health care professionals' – MEDLINE ® corpus (Infomap group, CSLI, Stanford University)

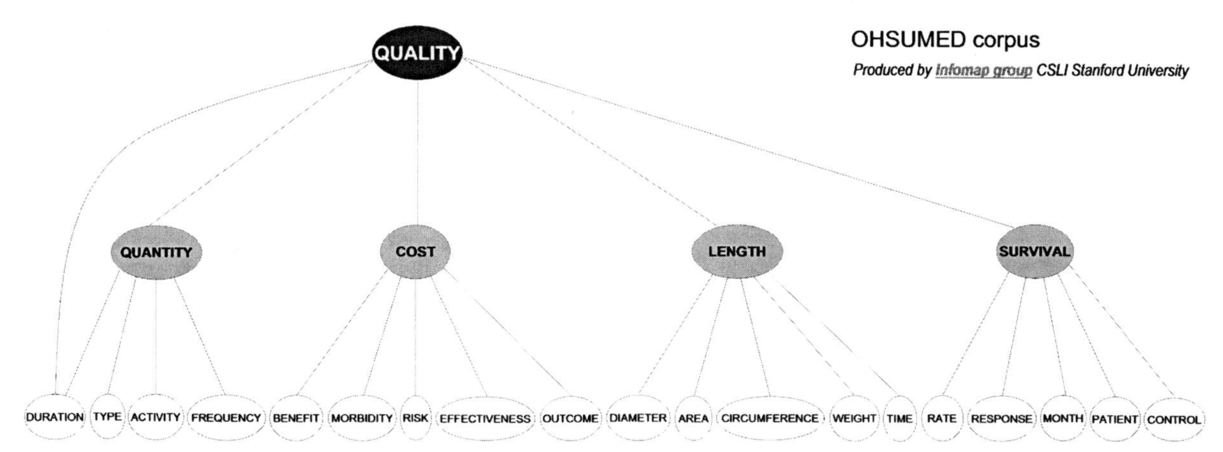

supposed to function can be derived from the word education (educatio /Latin/ - e duce /from a leader/ or e ductus /from a channel, duct/). A person who is supposed to take care of assets in order to multiply them must first of all have the capacity to manage (possess a high level of self awareness) himself in order to become a leader in the domain where he intends to operate. Not just a formally declared leader but the balanced personality with knowledge, willingness, skills and wisdom to serve. Such a harmonious / balanced authority will then be able to elegantly (with ease and simplicity) perform his tasks using numerous tools available on the 'management market'.

Systems Thinking

The whole issue of management is based on common sense and the ability of prediction of likely future evolution (forecasting) of the system, in our case the health care system, on each and respective systemic level - from the level of ambulatory and clinical micro-systems to the level of national, international and global health care systems – people of course form an integrated part of these systems. The human factor is essential to implement the process of bringing concepts into practice.

Forecasting tools can be didactically divided into two main subgroups: individual tools focused on quantity numbers or data and collective tools based on qualitative and unstructured information. Again only the 'balanced' use is capable of producing desirable outputs and outcomes. All scientific methods used for quality improvement in health care are based on knowledge and knowledge management; all require the systems thinking approach. Tools and methods relating to this approach have been well described by O'Connor and McDermott (O'Connor, 1997) (See Figure 6).

In addressing knowledge management, it is important to distinguish between 'data', 'information' and 'knowledge'. Data is discrete, unorganized facts; information is data that is organized into groups or categories (is collated) and is capable of altering the individual's perception - allows elementary decision making; knowledge is familiarity, awareness or understanding gained through experience or study. "Because knowledge is intuitive it is difficult to structure, can be hard to capture on machines and presents a challenge to its transfer. Knowledge is pragmatic as far as

Figure 6. Systems thinking representation

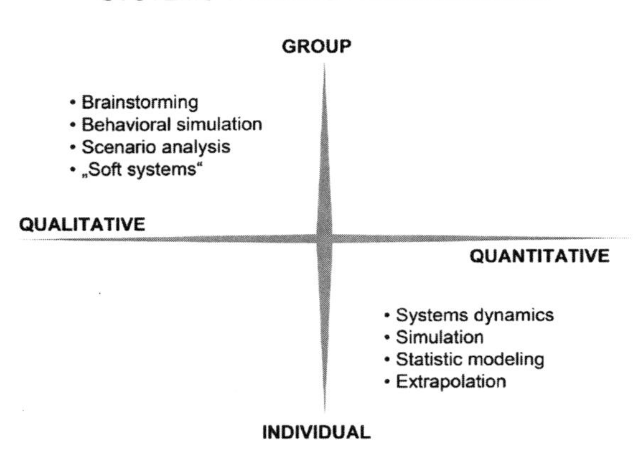

it enables someone to do something correctly, providing the potential for action. The application of knowledge is linked to continuous learning and refinement, and the development of awareness of the self and the potential of the self in action. The term 'knowledge management' was reportedly first used by Karl Wiig in 1986. Knowledge management can be considered as being composed of three processes: 'knowledge construction'; 'knowledge representation' and 'knowledge transfer' (Dixon, 2000).

Knowledge construction is the process by which knowledge is abstracted in the human mind and can take place 'after the event' (e.g. after-action reviews, evaluations) creating templates stored in several areas of the brain for future re-use.

Knowledge representation is the process by which knowledge is made explicit for others to learn from. It takes the 'implicit' or 'tacit' knowledge, derived from human abstraction, evaluating its usefulness for specific purposes, and making it 'explicit' in a variety of forms (e.g. textual reports, computer programs, guide books, web pages). Obviously it is difficult to store / archive tacit, emotional and social knowledge. From my personal point of view, probably the greatest leap in healthcare service training will be achieved through e-health approaches addressing this hard to store knowledge (virtuality, simulations, social networks etc.).

Knowledge transfer is the process by which knowledge is passed from a person or group to others. This usually requires the use of a suitable didactic or educational approach. Several categories exist (Serial Transfer - knowledge gained from doing a task in one context is re-used by the same team in another context. Near Transfer - explicit knowledge gained from doing a routine task is re-used by others for a similar task and context. Far Transfer – explicit and tacit knowledge gained from doing a non-routine task is made available to others performing the similar work in a different context. Strategic Transfer - collective knowledge of the organization is transferred to accomplish a strategic task that occurs infrequently but is critical for the whole organization. Expert Transfer – a team facing a technical question beyond the scope of its own knowledge seeks the expertise of others in the organization. Great care has to be taken especially in healthcare since all of these transfers are context sensitive and no mechanical application (transfer) of knowledge from other areas of human activities can be accepted without the involvement of professionals thoroughly understanding the healthcare environment.

A HEALTHCARE ORGANIZATION EXHIBITS ALL ATTRIBUTES OF A LIVING ORGANISM

A healthcare organization exhibits all attributes of a living organism. It has a memory, 'conscience – awareness', is responsible and accountable, and is able to reproduce. *An organizationisan organism.* A normal organization is an organism that behaves naturally and the origin of this 'nature' lies in the 'genes' of the organism, hence the need for 'Models and Standards' – standards = norms.

Genes are responsible for the, rather broad, 'coordinates' (limits, boundaries) in which the organism has the potential to develop. The surrounding environment determines how and to what extent this genetic potential will be expressed, which genes will be active and which inactive. The genetic background, to a certain extent, determines what the organism will favor in the environment where it exists. Apart from this it is necessary to take into account the effect of inestimable random events. The result of this interaction process (genes, environment, and random events) is the emergence of an individual entity unlike any other. The reason why each and every organization represents an individual entity although genetically at a certain period of their development they may have been identical lies in the iterative process of their development. Slightly different conditions at the time of each iteration (growth, replication) always lead to a slightly different phenotypic expression. After a large number of iterations, although genetically, practically identical, each organism (organization) becomes a distinct individual phenotypic entity. The similarity of two or more entities is best described and modeled by fractals. Such model representation demonstrates the resulting divergence of resulting organisms (fractals) and forms also the basis to understanding why no single management template is transferable between two, even though similar, organizations.

An organization has a memory, is viable and capable to reproduce and have offsprings.... It behaves like a living system and its functionality (serving brothers and sisters in need) is assured in the same way as by living systems - by sharing energy, and information with the surrounding environment, by behaving as an open system. A very concise way of formulating the above sums up to *'No code – no protocol – no life (no function, no relations, no reproduction)'* (Bourek, 2008).

Since health care organizations represent in principle a self-generating network of relations / communications (a system) (Capra, 2009), which to me exhibits (possesses) all the attributes of a living organism, the basic goals of a viable organization may be rationalized to be the same as the goal of all viable systems (organisms, individuals, organizations). This is manifested by processes designed to help the organism to live / survive, reproduce, leave a legacy and to love and be loved. In other words, every viable organism strives to 'win' (Welch, 2005) - although our perception of what this 'win' is may be totally different from one another or from one organization to another organization (what satisfies me or my organization, again a close link to the games theory).

Concept of Winning

To understand the concept of winning, the following should be considered. Winning from the point of above defined tasks is the ability to create or adapt. Winning is assured by means of collaborative competition; winning is not targeted at destroying the competitor but rather at achieving of symbiosis. We are not playing against our competitors, but rather we play with our competitors. (As a crude example, the following may be used: the organization called the human body does not win by killing all bacteria in the gastrointestinal tract, but by achieving a symbiosis - through identification of synergies providing benefits for all involved stakeholders). Playing games (going to the pains of exercising) with a flexible co-player (sparing partner) strengthens the organism / organization and improves its flexibility. Essential building blocks are represented by a synergic goal (vision) of all the entities forming the organization, by will (willingness, internal motivation), by identifying and applying the right strategy (decision) and doing that at the right time (tactics). Each and everyone of these essential building blocks requires a certain amount of energy and a certain amount of facts (timely reliable and valid data appropriately collated to produce information that gives a meaning to the facts – in-formation, giving the facts the form in order to allow their handling, in order to make the manageable). Information from this point of view represents a transmitted, received, processed and understood message that lowers the level of uncertainty of the recipient. The function of e-health and e-healthcare tools in this process is obvious. ICT equips organizations with the infrastructure, codes and protocols and if used in conjunction with valid facts (and not applied to illusions, gamed or manipulated data) has the potential to function as the 'information system' for organizations and their individual entities (for their specific receptors - as one with a biological thinking would say). If applied in an environment that disfavors the creation of illusions the resulting more timely and precise assurance of data and information flow may facilitate quality improvement (mainly on the level of accountability, responsibility and responsiveness) in the organization since all collaboration / competition is based on needs assessment (monitoring, evaluation).

A concise way of appropriate management within e-health and e-healthcare concepts could be based on following generic ideas published by Fritjof Capra (Capra, 2009).

You can never direct a social system; you can only disturb it. A living network chooses which disturbances to notice and how to respond. A message will get through to people in a community of practice when it is meaningful to them. The creativity and adaptability of life expresses itself through the spontaneous emergence of novelty at critical points of instability. Every human organization contains both designed and emergent structures. The challenge is to find the right balance between the creativity of emergence and the stability of design.

In addition to holding a clear vision, leadership involves facilitating the emergence of novelty by building and nurturing networks of communications; creating a learning culture in which questioning is encouraged and innovation is rewarded; creating a climate of trust and mutual support; and recognizing viable novelty when it emerges, while allowing the freedom to make mistakes.

On the managerial level, adherence to the above cited concepts requires the understanding and acceptance of the dynamics of a living organization (individual entity). In every organism, at all times, some entities (in the human organism we may refer to individual cells) are being replaced by new ones. After 50+ years of age, most of these individual entities have been replaced in me by new cells, still I am referred to as (and identified as) the entity (organization) called Aleš Bourek (or having a unique identifier code 570628/2164), even though most 'parts' of me have been replaced over time. The way how I function (serve my brothers and sisters in need) is essentially determined by the 'disturbances' I willingly and actively implemented in myself, that interacted with my inherited 'genome' in the environments (social networks, ecosystems) that I functioned in. Traditional approaches in biology may be reaching their limits. I am convinced that a higher level of understanding of the complex healthcare systems will be achieved using the concepts of semiotics and mainly biosemiotics and that these scientific disciplines together with other e-health and e-healthcare methodologies will assist in planning more appropriate strategies and tactics resulting in higher quality more efficient and more humane healthcare and health in general.

Semiotics

Semiotics, also called semiotic studies or semiology, is the study of sign processes (semiosis), or signification and communication, signs and symbols, both individually and grouped into sign systems. It includes the study of how meaning is constructed and understood. Semiotics is essentially a discipline studying everything that may be used for lying. If something may not be used to express a lie, it cannot be used to express the truth: in fact, it may not be used for speaking at all (Eco, 2004). From the point of view of semiotics, 'things' of this world are provided / given to us (or actually emerge) only by means of signs. There is no other approach for coming into close contact with things then through the interpretation of these signs - even though by patient comparison of signs, historically given relations and accents in the existing culture we are able to reach asymptotic vicinity of the nature of thus institutionalized 'things'. (Vesmír, 2009).

Biosemiotics (from Greek bios meaning 'life' and semeion meaning 'sign') is a science focusing on production, action and interpretation of signs in the domain of biology and works on integrating biology and semiotics. This leads to a shift in the occidental scientific view of life in showing that semiosis (sign process, including meaning and interpretation) is life's imminent feature. (Wikipedia, 2009). At the same time biosemiotics addresses some unsolved issues within the general study of sign processes (semiotics), such as the question about the origin of signification in the Universe. Signification (and sign) is studied in a very general sense. Not simply as transfer of information from one place to another (as in informatics), but as the generation of the very content and meaning of that information in human as well as non-human sign producers and sign receptors. Sign processes are thus taken as real, they are governed by regularities (habits, or natural rules) that can be discovered and explained. They are intrinsic in living nature and accessible only indirectly through other sign processes such as qualitative distinction methods. Human representation and understanding of these processes results in a separate (scientific) sign system distinct from the organisms' own sign processes. (Wikipedia, 2009).

One of the central characteristics of living systems is the highly organized character of their physical and chemical processes, partly based upon informational and molecular properties of what was defined in the 1960s as the genome. Complex self-organized living systems are also governed by formal and final causality. Formal in the sense of the downward causation from a whole structure (such as the organism) to its individual molecules, constraining their action but also providing them with functional meanings in relation to the whole metabolism. Final in the sense of the tendency to take habits and to generate future interpreters of the present sign actions. In these areas biosemiotics draw also upon the insights of fields like systems theory, theoretical biology and the study of complex self-organized systems (Wikipedia, 2009).

CONCLUSION

I personally find it striking to observe how much effort and financing our information society invests into activities like the cracking the human genetic code (by the way a lovely example of on-line collaboration / competition), how we are competent in gene sequencing and genome mapping in order to understand its functionality as opposed to our activities in healthcare organizations where we are hardly on the level of being able to measure and produce meaningful indicators (signals) and way off from using them correctly in most of the institutions or healthcare systems. It is amazing to see the level of knowledge we are using in applied computer science (virtualization of processes and resources, distributed computing, appropriate coding, exactly defined protocols) and at the same time still use and rely on traditional, almost medieval, approaches when it comes to generically the same issues in the health and healthcare environment. With the advent of the information society, striving to reach the level of the knowledge society it is only to be wished that enough attention will be given to sensitive application and cultivation of some of the already identified approaches and methodologies also in the area of human health and healthcare.

It needs to be understood, that a manager (even when he is involved in the birth of an organization) is not the one that creates a living organism from nonliving 'material'. The organization receives its life from the living elements (all individuals engaged in the communities of practice). A proper quality management system and the right management is a skill best expressed by *a competence to help the organism / (healthcare) organization to win (in the sense as defined in this article). The issue of quality is then reduced to conscientious introduction of the appropriate 'disturbances' (tactics and strategies) to increase the viability and desired functionality of the system and 'risk management' principles to address the issue of (healthcare) safety.* The achieved level of understanding (how meaningful are these disturbances to the 'communities of practice' or 'health care microsystems') is accountable for the response to one of the toughest questions we personally and our organizations get asked every day '*how do you do?*'. In principle, these people are asking us 'how do you manage?' The understanding and adherence to general principles related to the management of systems as a bonus provides a very personal benefit. When performed well it allows, when being asked by someone 'how do you do' to answer 'I am doing very well, thank you'. If this is becomes true for all participants of a healthcare community of practice, then the highest possible level of healthcare service is being approached.

REFERENCES

Adams, J., Edgar, L., & Mounib, A. P. (2006). Healthcare 2015: Win-win or lose-lose? *IBM Institute for business value,* Retrieved May 10, 2009, from http://www.ibm.com/healthcare/hc2015

Beagon, M. (1992). *Roman Nature: The Thought of Pliny the Elder. Oxford Classical Monographs.* Oxford, UK: Clarendon Press.

Bourek, A., Tůma, P., & Bourková, A. (2008, July). *Indicators as signals for assuring living and healthy health care organizations.* Paper presented at the WHO Vienna Public Healthcare Conference Performance Assessment in Healthcare Delivery PATH II, Vienna, Austria.

Bourková, A., & Bourek, A. (2007). Týmová spolupráce – Techniky týmové spolupráce, process týmové spolupráce, definice pojmu teamwork, zavádění týmové spolupráce do zdravotnického prostředí, klinické protokoly . In Forýtková, L., & Bourek, A. (Eds.), *Programy kvality a standardy léčebných postupů* (pp. 1–12). Praha, Czech Republic: Verlag-Dashofer.

Capra, F. (n.d.). *Management.* Retrieved May 4, 2009, from http://www.fritjofcapra.net/management.html

Codex Gigas. ff. 240r-243v. Retrieved February 7, 2009, from http://www.kb.se/codex-gigas/eng/Browse-the-Manuscript/Ars-medicinae/

Dixon, N. (2000). *Common Knowledge: How companies thrive by sharing what they know.* Boston: Harvard Business School Press.

Eco, U. (2004). *Theory of semiotics.*

Eysenbach, G. (2000). Consumer health informatics. *BMJ (Clinical Research Ed.), 320,* 1713–1716. doi:10.1136/bmj.320.7251.1713

Kohn, L. T., Corrigan, J. M., & Donaldson, M. S. (Eds.). (2000). *To err is human: building a safer health system.* Washington, DC: National Academy Press.

Konference Biosémiotiků (anouncement). (n.d.). *Vesmír, 88*(139), 343.

Koukolík, F. (2006). *Sociální mozek.* Praha, Czech Republic: Karolinum.

Lanktree, C., & Briere, J. (1991, January). *Early data on the Trauma Symptom Checklist for Children (TSC-C).* Paper presented at the meeting of the American Professional Society on the Abuse of Children, San Diego, CA.

Masum, H. (2002). TOOL: The Open Opinion Layer. *First Monday, 7*(7). Retrieved June 28, 2003 fromhttp://firstmonday.org/issues/issue7_7/masum/index.html

O'Connor, J., & McDermott, I. (1997). *The Art of Systems Thinking*. San Francisco: Thorsons.

Theodore, L., & Turocy, B. (2001). *Texas A&M University London School of Economics*. CDAM Research Report LSE-CDAM-2001-09.

Trivers, R. L. (1971). The Evolution of Reciprocal Altruism. *The Quarterly Review of Biology*, *46*, 35–57. doi:10.1086/406755

Chapter 2
e_3Health: Three Main Features of Modern Healthcare

Jana Zvárová
Institute of Computer Science of the Academy of Sciences of the Czech Republic, The Czech Republic

Karel Zvára
EuroMISE s.r.o., The Czech Republic

ABSTRACT

The chapter studies e-health applications in the frame of the broader concept of the e_3Health. It shows how the scheme proposed by J.H. van Bemmel in 1984 can be used for classification of e-health applications. Apart from the electronic feature of e-health applications, the authors discuss two other features connected with health economics and environmental health. In addition, two areas of e-health applications (electronic health record and clinical guidelines) with concrete examples from the point of view of the e_3Health concept are discussed.

INTRODUCTION

The main role of the e-health is to provide an easy transmission and communication of information in healthcare in forms of data or knowledge (Zvárová, 2009a). During the 58th World Health Assembly held in Geneva in May 2005, the Ministers of Health of the 192 member states of the United Nations approved the so called *e-health* Resolution (Healy, 2007) that officially recognizes the added value of the information and communication technologies for health purposes. E-health technologies opened the doorway to a new type of medical services where healthcare professionals are able to utilize them fully for prevention and management of diseases, lifelong learning and communication with colleagues and patients. Moreover, education and use of *e-health* technologies can help to change a passive attitude of patients against their diseases towards a proactive attitude of informed citizens for managing their own health. E-health concept has been the main topic of many books, papers in journals and presentations at conferences, e.g. (Iakovidis, 2004), (Demiris, 2004), (Blobel, 2008), (Andersen, 2008). New information and communication technologies (ICT) make possible to describe in a structured and unique way patient state, given procedures and the use of structured

DOI: 10.4018/978-1-61692-843-8.ch002

information for statistics and examination of quality of healthcare services. For example, new tools make possible to transfer a structured electronic health record to the point of care, even in case that the transfer is provided at the point of care abroad. However, medical data can be extremely complicated due to the abundance of clinical terminology, as well as the structural complexity in the formation of the presented information. Thus, this information must be presented in a standardized format in order to ensure that the data is universally understood and organized. In order to achieve this, all healthcare information must be sent in a specialized healthcare language. The language that has been developed to overcome these obstacles is HL7 (HL7, 2009). We will discuss in more details several examples of e-health applications developed thanks to new ICT, e.g. structured electronic healthcare documentation, data standards and EHR, medical concepts modeling, formalized knowledge and clinical guidelines. In this chapter, we discuss e-health in the context of the broader e_3Health concept.

BACKGROUND

e_3Health CONCEPT

Nowadays healthcare systems in Europe and other economically developed countries are going through the process of a significant transmission. From the central controlled healthcare, they are going to process controlled or shared healthcare with the aim to reach personalized healthcare. As soon as we place a patient or a citizen in the center of a healthcare system, the system will reflect its individual needs, expectations and wishes. However, such healthcare systems should have three main features that correspond to an electronic view, economics view and environmental view.

We introduce the concept e_3Health that is harmonizing interrelationship among all three main features of the modern healthcare, i.e. electronic, economic and environmental (Figure 1) for all ICT tools and service in healthcare.

Figure 1. e_3Health features

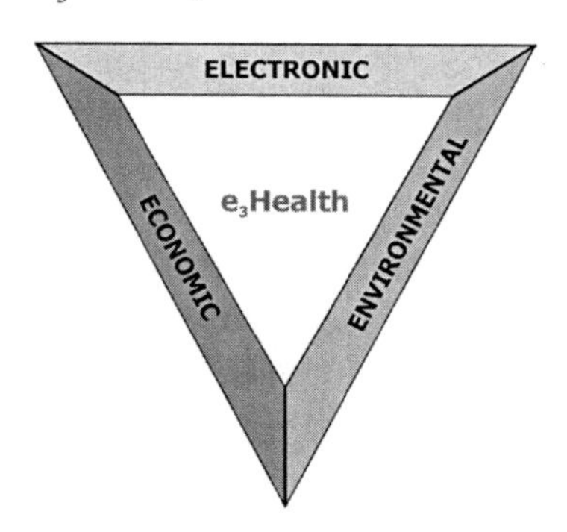

e3Health: Information and Communication Technologies View

Electronic health (e-health) is the first main feature of the modern healthcare. We understand e-health according to a rather broad definition of the European Commission (e-health, 2009). E-health is described as the application of information and communication technologies (ICT) across the entire range of functions that affect the healthcare sector. E-health represents the interaction between patients and health/service providers, institution-to-institution transmission of data, or peer-to-peer communication between patients and/or health professionals. E-health tools play an important role in improving the health of citizens. If the e-health tools and services are used appropriately, they may provide better and more efficient healthcare services for all people. Examples include health information networks, electronic health records, telemedicine services, wearable and portable systems which communicate, health portals, and many other ICT-based tools assisting disease prevention, diagnosis, treatment, health monitoring and lifestyle management. For this reason, the research in biomedical and healthcare informatics is the prerequisite for the development of e-health applications.

E-health applications can be evaluated according to different levels of complexity, e.g. by the scheme proposed by J.H. van Bemmel (Van Bemmel, 1984). J.H. van Bemmel´s scheme is also published in the book (Van Bemmel, 1997) and used to be available on the Internet. The scheme can serve for structuring ICT applications in healthcare into six levels. Each level contains different types of ICT applications with, from bottom to top, increasing complexity and a growing human involvement. According to this scheme we could assign each e-health application to one level of complexity. Level 1 *"Communication and telematics"* is the lowest level of complexity. On the lowest level of complexity, data enter the computers for information processing, are coded, transmitted, decoded and presented to users or other processing systems. E-health applications on level 1 are providing simple telematic applications. Therefore, e-health applications are transferring and share information in the form of data and knowledge on different levels of complexity. Level 2 "*Storage and Retrieval*" is extended with CT technologies offering storage and retrieval of data. Databases of patient data are used in hospitals, clinical departments and primary care practices, but databases in healthcare can be also used to control the stock of goods necessary to run the institution. Nowadays, medical imaging systems deliver pictures in a digital form, and communication systems (PACS) are more used in healthcare. Databases in healthcare often store knowledge offered by different classification systems and nomenclature, e.g. *Systematized Nomenclature of Medicine - Clinical Terms* (SNOMED CT) is a comprehensive clinical terminology (SNOMED, 2009), originally created by the College of American Pathologists and, as of April 2007, owned, maintained, and distributed by the International Health Terminology Standards Development Organization (IHTSDO), a non-for-profit association in Denmark. The purpose of the *Logical Observation Identifiers Names and Codes* (LOINC) classification system (LOINC, 2009) is to facilitate the exchange and pooling of clinical results for clinical care, outcomes management, and research by providing a set of universal codes and names to identify laboratory and other clinical observations or the *International Classification of Diseases* (ICD) that provides a public global standard to organize and classify information about diseases and related health problems (ICD, 2009). The use of ICTs on level 3 *"Processing and Automation"* is much more dependent on people because the design of e-health applications at this level requires much more knowledge that is specific to healthcare. Level 4 "*Diagnosis and Decision Making*" requires enough human knowledge and experience that should be incorporated in e-health applications. The e-health applications at this level are supporting diagnosis and decision/making in healthcare, and the methodology of the support should be fully justified. Level 5 "*Treatment and Control"* covers e-health applications, which involve humans, while the therapeutic and control processes are complex. E-health applications on level 5 need to use formalized medical knowledge, advanced information, and communication technologies. Level 6 "*Research and development*" reflects the creative human tasks in the development of new methods during research.

It is a long road from research in biomedical and healthcare informatics to implementation in e-health applications. However, we have reached real maturity of many e-health applications that can be placed in the health market.

e_3Health: The Economics View

The common views on economics use the distinction between microeconomics and macroeconomics. *Macroeconomics* studies the behavior of an economy as a whole and addresses issues of policies (fiscal, monetary), unemployment etc. *Microeconomics* studies the behavior of individuals, especially merits of their decision-making. The microeconomic view of healthcare may help to identify and understand reasons of unhealthy behavior. This view may also help to find an appropriate model of healthcare funding. The neoclassical theory formerly viewed personal and household behavior as a way of searching for delights and enjoyments. Later the view on household microeconomic behavior changed. It is commonly viewed as a manifestation of preferences no matter what they are based on. Both views assume finality and exogenous character of recipient's benefit. The finality of benefit means that the rational decision-making is aimed to achieve a benefit with no influence to subsequent economic processes. The exogenous character of a benefit means that the mode of operation of the economic system has no influence on the process of achieving a benefit. The real economic system consumption surely contains a considerable amount of consumption with substantive influence on future economic processes (Valenčík, 2003). The consumption of education usually influences abilities of the subject and therefore influences its ability of future production and subsequent consumption. The consumption of healthcare services and the subject's lifestyle influences the future health state of the subject and therefore influences its abilities to produce. Building and maintenance of social contacts surely influences the relationships among subjects within the group defined by interpersonal relationships. The productive aspect of consumption may be represented in a way hinted by Milton Friedman (Friedman, 1967). No matter if households consume or save they are building their portfolios of actives and they usually behave the way to maximize their future income (Valenčík, 2003). Healthcare is one of major industries in the human society. The accessibility of healthcare is not only a matter of available technologies but is also a subject of social and political processes. The main political issue of healthcare is the interrelationship between coequality and efficiency. Current theories believe that the relation between coequality and efficiency is substitutive (Stiglitz, 2000).

Health Economics studies resources on pharmacoeconomics, outcomes research, and managed care, value in medicine, health-related quality of life, performance assessment, and quality of care. *Economic feature* in a modern healthcare offers solutions that can bring enormous savings. If properly deployed, it could contribute to the transformation of the health sector and change substantially business models of healthcare facilities. Limits on resources – both in budgetary and staffing terms – weigh constantly on healthcare providers. E-health tools and services enable more efficient organization of resources and care provision leading to greater productivity. Therefore, economic feature in healthcare means an optimal allocation of restricted sources both human and financial.

e_3Health: The Environmental View

Environmental health in the narrow sense addresses all the physical, chemical, and biological factors external to a person, and all the related factors impacting behaviors. It encompasses the assessment and control of those environmental factors that can potentially affect health. It is targeted towards preventing disease and creating health-supportive environments (WHO, 2009). *Environmental health in the broad sense* covers also all environmental factors developed in the society that belong to legal, social and cultural environment that can potentially affect health. Further we use the term environmental health in the broad sense. We assume that the concept of the environmental health in the broad sense will play a very important role in future. Similarly as epidemiology in its origin focused on communicable diseases only, the changing distribution of diseases in population changed the focus of the epidemiology to non-communicable diseases. The use of information and communication technologies in healthcare is strongly dependent on the legal, social and cultural status of the society. Therefore, e-health applications have to consider differences in culture, language, geographic position, healthcare system, legislative and social environment and other characteristics as age, sex and other features specifying the target population.

Examples of $e_3$health Applications

Further we show two examples of e_3Health applications developed in the Czech Republic concerning electronic health record and clinical guidelines. We will discuss them in the context of three views of the e_3Health concept, i.e. electronic, economic and environmental and we will classify them according to J.H. van Bemmel scheme.

Structured Electronic Health Record in Dentistry

The information technology in healthcare consists of persistent information storage and messaging. This can be clearly illustrated by two standards by one standardizing body: the HL7 v2/v3 messaging and the HL7 Clinical Document Architecture (CDA). While CDA focuses on storing persistent information, its entirety, integrity and security, the messaging focuses on communicating between parties. In this chapter, we will focus on persistent information storage, information usability across different domains and application of economic and environmental views on *electronic health record.* The basic prerequisites for storing structured healthcare information are the existence of an appropriate conceptual model, the means of information storage and the availability of a tool for transferring the information into the information storage. The most problematic part is often the availability of an appropriate conceptual model. The reason is that easily usable straightforward models are usually tributary to the domain. It is awkward to use such models in other domains because doing so usually requires beforehand knowledge of the domain for which the model has originally been created. Therefore, special interdisciplinary tools are often created (using knowledge of more than one domain, e.g. healthcare and economics). Such problem is often seen in the domain of healthcare. General practitioners, physicians with different specialties, researchers in the field of healthcare and other stakeholders usually have different needs for the level of detail. Therefore, the level of detail and robustness of a particular conceptual model must adhere to its intended use.

Local, national and purely healthcare models often adhere to the principle of "usability-first", producing bottom-up models. This helps to quickly develop tools and gather from structured documentation fast. On the other hand, such models become obsolete fast when a need for communication outside the domain or outside the region emerges because the induction is always much more difficult than deduction. Robust concept models have the advantage of being able to hold almost any information within the broad domain. The disadvantage of such models is that it is not straightforward to use them in most cases. Since this robust approach produces broader models than traditional bottom-up models, simple "usability-first" models may be usually simple derived from broad model using deductive approach. Since the concepts of the world are usually somehow more related than the conceptual model of the scientist, it is highly unlikely that anyone would be able to create a conceptual model that would

- be stable forever,
- allow direct mapping (deriving) of directly usable models and
- provide a base for storing information that would be universally understood.

The robust and at the same time usable approach is a compromise between the two approaches. A good example of such a robust model is the Health Level 7 Reference information model (RIM, ISO/HL7 21731:2006). The reference model specifies very robust model of classes with predefined allowed relationships and uses internal and external vocabularies (classification systems) to specify the semantics (the meaning). Domain information models are derived from the RIM. The same approach may be used for mapping (deriving) RIM to other relevant existing information models (e.g. information models of specific clinical information systems). The main key for interoperability is to preserve the semantics of data converted. There are several classification systems that serve this need, e.g. SNOMED CT, LOINC and ICD.

The e_3Health concept states that there is also economic and environmental aspect of healthcare. Even the medical-only electronic health record contains economic information. It contains information on subject's (patient's) behavior, information about the prescribed treatment (which itself is an economic process bearing its costs and a potential for revenue in the form of improving subject's health). Also, the treatment contains information the prescribing physician had to take into account because the treatment reflects not only the desired change of the patient's health but also information on patient's adherence to the therapy, cost constraints and availability of treatment options. Environmental aspects are included not only in patient's anamnesis (e.g. living environment, type of work, social status) but also as a part of the prescribed treatment (residues of drugs prescribed will become part of the living environment, prescribing job change will affect other people).

New requirements to efficiently collect data in healthcare are based on an electronic health record, where information is stored in a structured form. Data entry into the EHR systems during examination of a patient should be supported by user-friendly interfaces. For the field of dental medicine, we developed a graphical component called DentCross. This component is fully interactive. A dentist can choose among about 60 different actions, treatment procedures or tooth parameters that are displayed graphically and in a well-organized manner. Further the DentCross component was supported by automatic speech recognition and connected with the structured electronic health record (Zvárová, 2009b; Zvárová, 2008). The synergy of the voice control and the graphical representation of data make hand-busy activities in the dental practice easier, quicker and more comfortable (Dostálová, 2008). This can result in a better quality of data stored in a structured form in the EHR for dentistry. Moreover, structured information in EHRs can highly support decision-making processes and telemedical applications. Till now the dental health data for more than 100 patients were collected using EHR with the DentCross component in University Hospital in Prague-Motol. We assigned this e-health application to the level 2 of J.H. van Bemmel scheme. There is dental knowledge incorporated in EHR for both gathering data as well as their classification.

Formalized Electronic Clinical Guidelines

Evidence Based Medicine has been proposed as the most significant intellectual advance in the process of clinical decision-making. It is questionable though if real evidence is achieved today, as observation of patients is limited in time and in scope, i.e. patients tend to be observed under a single angle depending on the prevalent pathology they suffer from. Effectiveness and undesired effects of treatments, correlation between treatments received and pathologies developed at a later stage, etc., to be really "demonstrated", would require instead a comprehensive analysis of vast amounts of data about large numbers of individuals followed during a time long enough for correlations to appear. Using the new medical knowledge in addition to existing knowledge will create two innovative families of *e-health decision-support applications* to help both clinicians and health authorities to act according to practical evidence. This means, of course, different things for the two groups of users. A first family of *e-health decision-support applications* will support *clinicians* in their diagnostic, therapeutic and prognostic activities; acting in an "intelligent" way: they can explore the medical knowledge base and the electronic health records of the specific patient whom the clinician is consulting, and issue suggestions, warnings or alarms. This family of e-health applications will rely on multiple sources of codified medical knowledge. These sources are "traditional" (e.g. current clinical guidelines and existing clinical databases which could be linked to EHR systems) and "new" (medical knowledge extracted using methods of knowledge discovery in databases (Shapiro, 1991)). A second family of *e-health decision-support applications* will assist health authorities in their healthcare planning activity. They will be geared to provide answers to questions concerning the most suitable mix of healthcare resources. They are required to assist a given population on the basis of the likely evolution of their healthcare needs. The difficulties and failures of clinical decision-making in everyday practice are largely failures in *knowledge coupling*, due to the over-reliance on the unaided human mind to recall and organize all the relevant details. These are not, specifically and essentially, failures of the medical knowledge reasoning once it is presented completely and in a highly organized form within the framework of the patient's total and unique situation. Medicine is the area, where decision-support systems can rely on two basic types of medical knowledge (Van Bemmel, 1997): *scientific knowledge* (based on results of biomedical research) and *empirical knowledge* (based on experience gathered from diagnostic and treatment processes). Both types of knowledge are described in textbooks and other publications. Scientific knowledge in particular is taught at medical faculties in universities. Scientific "know how" knowledge is of a cognitive type, i.e. it helps to recognize the basis of biological processes, relationships among patho-physiological conditions and symptoms of diseases. Clinical experience is concentrated in medical documentation, and it can be stored in medical database. This empirical "know why" knowledge helps physicians to recognize a disease from observed features of a patient. In practice, physicians use both these types of knowledge. In most common cases, physicians have sufficient scientific and empirical knowledge not to need decision support systems. However, there are situations when decision support systems are desirable. This is likely to be more and more the case in the future because of the rapid increase of medical knowledge which makes impossible for an individual doctor to be informed of the latest developments even in a narrow domain of medicine.

Different methodologies are used to formalize the reasoning processes using gathered data and knowledge. However, formalization and structuring of medical data and knowledge is not easy. Even admitting that all scientific and empirical knowledge is stored in computers, decision-support systems can only propose decisions based on our current knowledge of the decision making process. Nowadays e-health decision-support applications are often focused on specific tasks such as the generation *of alerts and reminders* when a particular combination of events occurs. In *therapy planning and evaluation* they can either look for inconsistencies, errors and omissions in an existing treatment plan, or can be used to suggest a treatment based upon a patient's specific condition and accepted treatment guidelines. E-health decision-support applications often use the knowledge gathered by experts gathered in medical societies in the form of clinical guidelines written in conventional free text form. Unfortunately, finding knowledge in free text may be difficult. The need to create computer interpretable representation of medical knowledge contained in clinical guidelines is the need for any e-health application using clinical guidelines. Many knowledge representing languages has been introduced. The Arden Syntax (Peleg, 2001) is perhaps the best known representing language, but there are many other related languages suc-

Figure 2. Process of construction, coding and use of GLIKREM

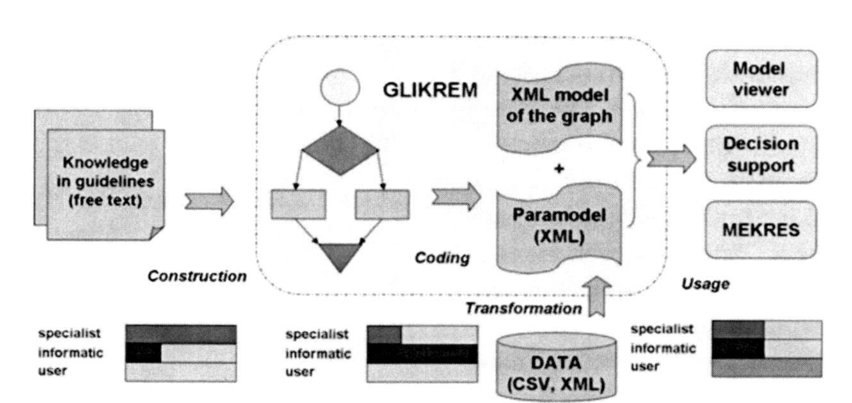

cessfully introduced for representing medical knowledge, such as Asbru (Shahar, 1998), EON (Tu, 1999), GUIDE (Quaglini, 2001), PRODIGY (Johnson, 2000), PROforma (Fox, 2006), GLIF (Ohno-Machado, 1998) etc. The most recent GLIF specification is the GLIF3.5.

GLIF was selected as the model for representing the Computerized Clinical Guidelines in SAPHIRE (Laleci, 2009). The SAPHIRE system continuously monitors the patients through dedicated agents and supports the healthcare professionals through an intelligent decision support system. GLIF was also selected for guideline the knowledge representation system GLIKREM. GLIKREM contains some changes and extensions of the definition and implementation of the original GLIF model. The GLIKREM is described in detail in (Buchtela, 2009), e.g. its construction, implementation in XML (*eXtensible Markup Language*), a realization of the data interface and the use of GLIKREM in Medical Knowledge Representation System (MEKRES) (Buchtela, 2008).

We specified our own XML scheme for representation of graphic model and developed a graphical editor for construction of the graphical model and its translation into XML. The whole model consists of a sequence of XML elements, which represent steps of the graphic model. The XML syntax of the model contains elements for the description of attributes of model steps, elements for graphical symbols of steps and elements for the decision support. We used GLIKREM to formalize medical knowledge from more than 30 clinical guidelines mainly for the use in cardiology and general practice and added formalized medical knowledge to electronic guideline presented as the free text only. That way, we developed a new form of clinical guidelines, that we call *formalized electronic clinical guidelines*. Judging formalized electronic clinical guidelines from the e_3Health point of view, we can draw the following conclusions. The human involvement is medical knowledge formalization is very high. Therefore, formalized electronic clinical guidelines belong to e-health application that can be assigned to the level 4 of J.H. van Bemmel´s scheme. There is a large potential of formalized electronic clinical guidelines to enhance the quality of clinical decision-making, reduce the number of medical errors and save human and financial resources. However, the use of formalized electronic clinical guidelines is also highly dependent on factors of legal, social and ethical environment.

CONCLUSION

New information and communication technologies have the potential to revolutionize healthcare and health systems and contribute to their future sustainability (EC, 2007). E-health applications can improve prevention of illness, delivery of treatment and support a shift from hospital care to prevention and primary care. The above mentioned application "Structured Electronic Health Record in Dentristry" is in a pilot use in University Hospital in Motol in Prague in Czech and English languages. Future research focus is on enhancement of this e-health application and its enlargement to more languages. The second e-health application "Formalized Electronic Clinical Guidelines" is validated in the field of cardiology in cooperation with University Hospital in Prague 2 and with Municipal Hospital in Čáslav. The research is focused on utilization of formalized electronic clinical guidelines in medical practice and evaluation of the adherence to guidelines.

The e_3Health concept shows that e-health applications considering economic and environmental factors can help to provide better care, lower costs in healthcare and support patient mobility and safety. This holistic approach to e-health applications can show the true benefits of e-health and make healthcare better.

ACKNOWLEDGMENT

The work was supported by the Centre of Biomedical Informatics, project no.1M06014 of MŠMT ČR.

REFERENCES

Andersen, S. K., Klein, G. O., Schulz, S., Aarts, J., & Mazzoleni, M. C. (Eds.). (2008). *eHealth Beyond the Horizon – Get IT There. Proceedings of MIE2008*. Amsterdam: IOS Press.

Blobel, B., Pharow, P., & Nerlich, M. (Eds.). (2008). *eHealth: Combining Health Telematics, Telemedicine, Biomedical Engineering and Bioinformatics to the Edge. Global Experts Summit Textbook*. Amsterdam: IOS Press.

Buchtela, D., Peleška, J., Veselý, A., & Zvárová, J. (2008). Medical Knowledge Representation System . In Andersen, S. K. (Eds.), *eHealth Beyond the Horizon-Get It There* (pp. 377–382). Amsterdam: IOS Press.

Buchtela, D., Peleška, J., Veselý, A., Zvárová, J., & Zvolský, M. (2009). Guideline Knowledge Representation Model. *European Journal for Biomedical Informatics*. Retrieved April 28, 2009, from http://www.ejbi.eu/

Commission of the European Communities. (2007). *Together for Health: A Strategic Approach for the EU 2008-2013*. White Paper 23.10.2007. Brussels: Author.

Demiris, G. (Ed.). (2004). *eHealth: Current Static and Future Trends*. Amsterdam: IOS Press.

Dostálová, T., Seydlová, M., Zvárová, J., Hanzlíček, P., & Nagy, M. (2007). Computer-Supported Treatment of Patients with the TMF Parafunction. In B. Blobel, P. Pharow, J. Zvarova, & D. Polez (Eds.), *eHealth: Combining Health Telematics, Telemedicine, Biomedical Engineering and Bioinformatics to the Edge* (pp. 171-178). Berlin: CEHR Conference Proceedings 2007, AKA. ehealth(AT) ec.europa.eu. (2009). *Europe's Information Society. Thematic Portal*. Retrieved July 21, 2009, from http://ec.europa.eu/information_society/activities/health/whatis_ehealth/index_en.htm

Fox, J., Patkar, V., & Thomson, R. (2006). Decision Support for Healthcare: the PROforma evidence base. *Informatics in Primary Care*, *14*, 49.

Friedman, M. (1967). *A Theory of Consumption Function*. Princeton, NJ: Princeton University Press.

Health Level Seven, Inc. (2009). *Health Level Seven*. Retrieved July 21, 2009, from http://www.hl7.org/

Healy, J. C. (2007). The WHO eHealth resolution - eHealth for all by 2015? *Methods of Information in Medicine*, *46*, 2–5.

Iakovidis, I., Wilson, P., & Healy, J. C. (Eds.). (2004). *eHealth: Current Situation and Examples of Implemented and Beneficial eHealth Applications*. Amsterdam: IOS Press.

Johnson, P. D., Tu, S. W., Booth, N., Sugden, B., & Purves, I. N. (2000). *Using scenarios in chronic disease management guidelines for primary care* (pp. 389–393). Proc. AMIA Annu. Fall Symp.

Laleci, G. B., Dogac, A., et al. (2009). *SAPHIRE: A Multi-Agent System for Remote Healthcare Monitoring through Computerized Clinical Guidelines*. Retrieved April 28, 2009, from http://www.srdc.metu.edu.tr/webpage/projects/saphire/

National Institutes of Health. (2009). *SNOMED Clinical Terms®*. Retrieved July 21, 2009, from http://www.nlm.nih.gov/research/umls/Snomed/snomed_main.html

Ohno-Machado, L., Gennari, J. H., Murphy, S. N., Jain, N. L., Tu, S. W., & Oliver, D. (1998). The GuideLine Interchange Format: A model for representing guidelines. *Journal of the American Medical Informatics Association*, 357–372.

Peleg, M., Ogunyemi, O., Tu, S., et al. (2001). Using features of Arden Syntax with object-oriented medical data models for guideline modeling. In *Proc AMIA Symp*. (pp. 523-7).

Quaglini, S., Stefanelli, M., Lanzola, G., Caporusso, V., & Panzarasa, S. (2001). Flexible guideline-based patient careflow systems. *Artificial Intelligence in Medicine*, *22*, 65–80. doi:10.1016/S0933-3657(00)00100-7

Regenstrief Institute, Inc. (2009). *Logical Observation Identifiers Names and Codes*. Retrieved July 21, 2009, from http://loinc.org/

Shahar, Y., Miksch, S., & Johnson, P. (1998). The Asgaard Project: a task-specific Framework for the application and critiquing of time-oriented clinical guidelines. *Artificial Intelligence in Medicine*, *14*, 29–51. doi:10.1016/S0933-3657(98)00015-3

Shapiro, G. T., & Frawley, W. J. (Eds.). (1991). *Knowledge Discovery in Databases*. San Francisco: AAAI/MIT Press.

Stiglitz, J. (2000). *Economics of the Public Sector*. New York: W. W. Norton & Co Inc.

Tu, S. W., & Musen, M. A. (1999). *A flexible approach to guideline modeling* (pp. 420–424). Proc. AMIA Symp.

Valenčík, R. (2003). *Theory of a productive consumption (Teorie produktivní spotřeby)*. Praha, Czech Republic: Vysoká škola finanční a správní o.p.s.

Van Bemmel, J. H. (1984). The structure of medical informatics. *Medical Informatics*, *9*, 175–180. doi:10.3109/14639238409015187

Van Bemmel, J. H., & Musen, M. A. (Eds.). (1997). *Handbook of Medical Informatics*. Heidelberg, Germany: Springer.

WHO. (2009). *Environmental health*. Retrieved July 21, 2009, from http://www.who.int/topics/environmental_health/en/

WHO. (2009). *International Classification of Diseases (ICD)*. Retrieved July 21, 2009, from http://www.who.int/classifications/icd/en/

Zvárová, J., Dostálová, T., Hanzlíček, P., Teuberová, Z., Nagy, M., & Pieš, M. (2008). Electronic health record for forensic dentistry. *Methods of Information in Medicine*, *47*, 8–13.

Zvárová, J., Hanzlíček, P., Nagy, M., Přečková, P., Zvára, K., & Seidl, L. (2009). Biomedical Informatics Research for Individualized Life-Long Shared Healthcare. *Biocybernetis and Biomedical Engineering*, *29*(2), 31–41.

Zvárová, J., Veselý, A., & Vajda, I. (2009). Data, Information and Knowledge . In Berka, P., Rauch, J., & Zighed, D. A. (Eds.), *Data Mining and Medical Knowledge Management: Cases and Applications* (pp. 1–36). Hershey, PA: Medical Information Science.

Chapter 3
The European Perspective of E-Health and a Framework for its Economic Evaluation

Paola Di Giacomo
University of Udine, Italy

ABSTRACT

E-health is a priority of the European i2010 initiative, which aims to provide safe and interoperable information systems for patients and health professionals throughout Europe. Moreover, the use of electronic storing and transmission of data to patients is increasing while through the deployment of e-health applications, health care is improved in terms of waiting time for patients. The concentration results from the cumulative incidence of chronic-degenerative pathologies, the greater utilization of biomedical technologies, and the increased health services demand. Finally, the interest towards electromechanical systems means the realization of tools of small dimensions, which have tremendous advantages thanks to their invasivity and greater diagnostic-therapeutic effectiveness. Therefore, an economic analysis has to take into consideration the use of biomedical technology, the analysis of alternatives, the selection of the economic evaluation technique, and the identification and quantification of the costs and benefits.

INTRODUCTION

Innovation is essential to improve accessibility, effectiveness and efficiency of healthcare delivery. E-health promises these improvements, provided we comply with fundamental requirements with respect to quality and safety. E-health must be implemented thoughtfully to provide the maximum advantage of the innovation. However, there exists no structured framework of the basic requirements of quality and safety issues. This often hampers development, implementation and usage. Therefore, a framework of quality and safety requirements must evolve to support and encourage innovation.

The analysis of an innovation, which contributes to quality, safety and efficiency, leads to an evaluation process, which should be followed to assess an e-health application. The issue of minimum requirements is a political one while

DOI: 10.4018/978-1-61692-843-8.ch003

the requirements themselves are the subject of research. Furthermore, one problem in addressing this issue is the mere fact that e-health is under development and that it can assume various forms and sizes. It is, therefore, hardly likely to formulate all requirements in advance. For each service offered to the market, it is anticipated that different aspects will have to be assessed while a rigorous program of requirements will make innovation difficult.

It is worthwhile mentioning that e-health is a priority of the European i2010 initiative, which aims to provide safe and interoperable information systems for patients and health professionals throughout Europe. Based on a pan-European survey on electronic services in healthcare, 87% of general practitioners use a computer and 48% have a broadband connection. Moreover, the use of electronic storing and transmission of data to patients is increasing while through the deployment of e-health applications, health care is improved in terms of waiting time for patients. There is, however, considerable space for improvement since ICT assists many aspects of the doctor-patient relationship. This includes remote monitoring services (used in Sweden, the Netherlands and Iceland), electronic prescriptions (used by only 6% of EU general practitioners, and only three Member States, which include Denmark, Netherlands and Sweden), and medical care, practiced by only 1% of general practitioners, with the highest percentage in the Netherlands (5%). The survey also shows that e-health services are used where the broadband Internet use is widespread. In Denmark, for example, where the penetration of broadband Internet is the highest in Europe, 60% of doctors are currently exchanging emails with patients. On the contrary, the EU average is stuck at 4%. Overall, despite considerable progress, there are still notable differences between different countries. The main barriers to adoption of new technologies in health care include the lack of training and technical support. To encourage the routine use of ICT in health care and accelerate the adoption of appropriate strategies at the country level, the Commission adopted an action plan for e-health, under the title 'Lead Market Europe' (Commission of the European Communities, 2007).

The analysis aimed at the cost-benefit of the patient treatment, an essential part of the quality evaluation, is widely documented in healthcare literature. The focus results from the cumulative incidence of chronic-degenerative pathologies, the greater utilization of biomedical technologies, and the increased health services demand. The method is based on the formulation of testable criteria and standard values with respect to the particular parts of the service. Therefore, it can determine the criteria, which are not met, leading to a provisional acceptance of the e-health application.

Methods of comparative analysis, like the cost-benefit approach have to be adapted to the various aspects of the healthcare process, in order to determine the advantage of a traditional model of care with respect to an integrated one, which is based on new computer science technologies. Among the new methods of book keeping that operate in this direction, the most widely used is the Activity Based Costing (ABC). ABC is a method of imputation of the costs incurred by the activities of the cost centers. Therefore, every re-engineering decision can be isolated, and estimated in relation to the cost that it incurs.

In this chapter, we will provide an overview of the European strategy in e-health, the research programs and initiatives of the European Union, as well as a framework for the economic evaluation of e-health applications (Drummond et al., 2005; Scrivens, 1997; Hughes & Humphrey, 1990).

BACKGROUND

Commissioner for Health and Consumer Protection Markos Kyprianou said: 'e-health can improve health care. Even more important, it is possible to reduce medical errors and save lives.

We need a partnership between the ministers of health, technology providers, patient associations and NGOs to realize the full potential of e-health in Europe'.

'The EU-US e-health is important because there are large economic areas with the same characteristics, such as the aging population. We need to coordinate the development of standards and interoperability in this area,' said the General Director of the Commission for Information Society, Fabio Colasanti. He also clarified that the technology itself is not enough. It needs to be accompanied by an appropriate legal environment and education of health professionals, said Frans de Bruin of the EU Directorate General for Information Society:

'The e-health should no longer be a subject of specific conferences, but simply the normal way of doing health care,' said Petra Wilson, Director for the public health sector and Cisco Internet Business Solutions Group. 'We need to give incentives to doctors to encourage them to adopt and use technology.' Peter Langkafel of SAP agrees that the incentive of physicians is important, stressing that it is not enough: 'You have to demonstrate value and a business case for e-health - a better quality of care and patient safety, as well as improved use of resources in health care (human resources, processes). The business case must be presented with the cost-benefit analysis'.

'Why should not patients have the same type of service in health care such as in the banking sector? (...) Patients should contact their health care providers and start putting pressure on them claiming greater use of technology', said Baldur Johnsen, Hewlett Packard Director of Development of health services in the e-health market. .

'The one devoted to health is the segment with the highest growth rate in our society,' according to Charles Scatchard, Vice-president of health sciences at Oracle, '... and we also know that all new health technologies need a period of 17 years to finally be usable'. 'The e-health helps to overcome the obstacles related to the distance of the organization and the delivery of health services and is, therefore, an important tool for both rural and urban areas. The development of these technologies contributes to the development of a global economic region, attracting firms specializing in this area and the creation of new employment opportunities, 'said Agneta Granström, Advisor of Norrbotten. 'We must begin with the strengthening of cooperation between hospitals and between other sectors of health care across Europe. We do not need a single system, the same for everyone, but interoperable systems. Both universities and companies should fully appreciate the enormous potential of e-health and provide the necessary tools along with the regions that should work for the development of e-health', he added. The Group of Pharmacists of the European Union (PGEU) calls the national and European authorities to help pharmacists to understand the advantages and opportunities of the greater use of data from the Internet and the development of e-health applications. PGEU promotes the development of European standards and the certification of P2P applications, including the necessary standards for the electronic transmission of prescriptions. The standards should help all stakeholders to expand existing services and draw medical attention to the security of the Internet applications. Finally, in 2007, the European Data Protection Statement approved a working document that discusses the legal requirements and application parameters for the structure and management of a national system of electronic health records. The document is open for public consultation to solicit contributions and comments.

THE EUROPEAN STRATEGY IN E-HEALTH

'E-health' implies e-health applications of Information and Communication Technologies (ICT) for health, which encompass hospital doctors, patients and social security data processing. The goal is to improve the quality, access and efficiency of health services for all. In the EU, e-health plays a key role in the strategy for action on innovation, which was launched in 1999. A series of action plans followed in 2002 and in 2005(*e*Europe 2005: An information society for all). The Action Plan i2010 - A European Information Society for growth and employment, was followed by the Communication 'Preparing Europe's digital future i2010: Mid-Term Review' in April 2008. Regional networks of health, electronic health records, primary care and deployment of electronic health cards have contributed to the rise of e-health, which has the potential to become the third largest industry, after the pharmaceutical industry and the medical imaging. In particular, for the period 2006-2009, Member States and the Commission promoted interoperability and encouraged greater standardization. They then set the target to establish the basis of European E-health services by the end of 2009.

The key stages included:

December 2005: E-health stakeholder's group meets for the first time. The group is an organization that brings together the leading European actors involved in the standardization (such as CEN - European Committee for Standardization, CEN / ISSS - Information Society Standardization System, CENELEC - Comité Européen de Normalization Electrotechnique, ETSI - European Telecommunications Standards Institute), industry associations, and user groups.

June 2006: the Assembly of European Regions (AER) is organizing an international conference and presents a session on the e-health (Thematic Dossier of the Assembly of European Regions).

June 2006: The Commission for Health Information Technology adopted a new strategy (ICT for Health and 2010, 'Transforming the European healthcare landscape: Towards a strategy for ICT for Health') to promote the transformation of the European health systems. The strategy argues that in order to meet the challenges of aging, Europe needs a new model of health care, which should be based on prevention and people-centeredness.

The approach involves the E-health Action Plan and includes research under the Seventh Framework Program for Science and Research. The strategy is also in line with the communication of the new framework of i2010 (i2010 Annual Information Society Report 2007), which promotes the application of ICT to improve social inclusion, public services and quality of life.

October 2006: The results of the study on the impact e-health are published (economic benefits of the e-health implementation in several European sites).

April 2007: Conference and exhibition on e-health

April 2007: A report argued that Member States have made considerable progress in implementing the strategy for e-health, but had failed to establish educational and socioeconomic guidelines for matters falling under their responsibility.

May 2007: Workshop on e-health, which was organized by the European Commission and the U.S. Department of Health & Human Services, in collaboration with the European-American Business Council. The main issues included the health practices which were supported by information technology, interoperability, certification and improvement of patient safety

July 2007: Presentation of a draft recommendation on interoperability

December 2007: The Task Force on e-health publishes a report on Accelerating the Development of the E-health Market in Europe.

December 2007: Publication of a kick-off study by the EU Commission on financing e-health. The Commission adopts a Communication on the action guide for the European market ('A lead market initiative for Europe'), with e-health as one of the top six markets.

April 2008: A study provides an overview on e-health emerging markets regulation and a report on the use of ICT among general practitioners in Europe.

May 2008: The EU Portorož Declaration on the e-health is adopted. It reaffirms the need to share experiences and collaborations carried out in Europe, and the terms of interoperability for cross-border care.

June 2008: Two European pilot projects are launched to check the European cooperation in the use of data relating to emergencies and prescriptions.

In 2008, the Commission issued a Recommendation on cross-border e-health systems. By the end of the year, the Commission had also planned to publish a Communication on telemedicine and innovative ICT solutions for the management of chronic diseases.

It is worthwhile mentioning that the Action Plan for 2004-2010 focused on three priority areas:

- Dealing with common challenges and creating an appropriate framework to support e-health, such as the interoperability of health information systems, the electronic health records, and patient and staff mobility
- Accelerating the implementation of the of e-health use in the areas of health education and disease prevention, and promoting the use of electronic health cards
- linking state efforts in monitoring, benchmarking and dissemination of best practices

European E-Health Research Projects

The EU is supporting research in e-health for nearly two decades. The technologies developed in hundreds of successful projects have helped to improve health care provision in many different fields. Research on e-health is a priority in the Seventh Framework Program, which is valid until 2013. The Seventh Framework Program for Research (presented in the Decision of December 18, 2006) will continue to this direction until 2013, with a total budget more than 50 billion euros. It aims to create an 'intelligent environment' in which the state of health of each individual can be monitored and managed continuously. The key points of the program on e-health are the following:

- Personal Health Systems (PHS)
- Patient Safety (PS)
- Software tools, which help health professionals to find the available information each time they have to draw conclusions.
- Virtual Physiological Human (VPH) Framework

Multidisciplinary networks of researchers in the field of bioinformatics, genomics and neuroinformatics, which create a new generation of e-health systems.

Research Projects

Bepro

Enabling Best Practices for Oncology (IST-2000-25252 BP)
The project focused on a multinational network of oncology and assessed the effectiveness of oncology services. The project involved three phases: establishment, medical evaluation, and assessment. The results were disseminated to the most influential European medical communities and, in some cases, to standardization bodies.

Diaffoot

Remote Monitoring of Diabetic Foot (IST-2001-TR 33281)
Diabetes mellitus is a growing problem in European countries with a high impact both on the quality of life of millions of citizens, and the financial situation of national health systems. The technical objective of the project was to test the use of a remote system, capable of measuring data on clients and sending data to the hospital for further analysis and monitoring of patients

with diabetes mellitus. Another objective was to compare current procedures and techniques in order to redefine the protocol for the treatment of diabetes mellitus and propose an operational procedure.

E-Scope

Digital Microscopy for Diagnostics and Data Integration in the Hospital (IST-2001-33294 BP)
The last decade, the technology of a pathology diagnosis takes advantage of multimedia systems, which include standards for images (DICOM Visible Light), electronic forms of reporting, storage systems and support procedures for accreditation and certification. The project, therefore, aimed to prepare a digital microscopy to effectively integrate the standard for medical imaging, storage and communication. The digital microscopy could then allow the integration of PACS (Picture Archiving and Communication System), HIS (Hospital Information System) and information available in hospitals.

Ihelp

Electronic Remote Operating Room (IST-2001-33269 BP)
The project Ihelp analyzed the state of art of e-health platforms and investigated the methodology for establishing best practices for online support, 24 hours, anywhere in the world, with the latest systems in neurosurgery. The project aimed to ensure the proper use of the new technologies by the surgeons and the drastic reduction of complications. The service is integrated with treatment systems already in use for the operations of neurosurgery.

Prideh

Privacy in Data Management for E-Health (IST-2001-TR 32647)
Technologies for securing privacy, using encryption methods, are complex. Prideh takes advantage of the experience gained from its partners (Custodix as a supplier and as Wren's) for the implementation of services in the pharmaceutical and health industries.

Reshen

Security in Regional Networks of Health (IST-2000-25354 BP)
The project aimed at the demonstration of best practices in health care information exchange. The goal was to develop a business case for information security in health care and highlight the best practices, which ensure communication and information exchange between all participants (providers of health care services, end users).

Screen-Trial

Regional Secure Healthcare Networks (IST-2001-TR 33439)
Millions of women perform a mammography screening in Europe. The new technologies of digital mammography and Soft-Copy Reading (SCR) will have an impact on radiology and the quality of service. SCR allows the use of computer-aided detection, as well as the use of digital images and digital communications. SCR is the key to the integration of screening programs in the e-health while it will accelerate the adoption of a SCR system, which was developed in the Screen project.

Spirit Priming

The Virtuous Spiral for Healthcare: Implementing an Open Source Approach to Accelerate the Uptake of Best Practice and Improvement, Regional Healthcare Network Solutions (IST-2000-26162 BP)

Spirit is a pioneering initiative, which accelerates the adoption of regional health network solutions. The project aimed to establish best practices in Open Source Business software for health care. This will enable the implementation, use and dissemination of regional networks for health. The project created a partnership between the worldwide community of software developers and healthcare professionals to share, enhance, and create innovative solutions for health care.

Stemnet

Information Technology for the Transplantation of Stem Cells (IST-2000-26117 BP)

The project aimed to demonstrate best practices in a network database of stem cells donors. The project facilitates the sharing of best European practices, including standards, the best laboratory practices, and quality control procedures. This translates into greater efficiency and quality, reducing waiting time and cost.

Woman

European Network of Services for the Health of Women (IST-2001-TR 32672)

Woman II, a project funded by the EC in 1998-2000, has created an innovative approach for the protection of women's health, with the combination of a Web portal and the Electronic Patient Record (EPR). The multilingual portal provides access to women and professionals with respect to women's health information. The project's objective was to increase the number of Web sites, in order to create a European network working for the collection and compilation of data, and promote the use of the Web portal among citizens and experts. The work ahead is adaptation, personalization and improvement of the results of Woman.

The Economic Evaluation of E-Health

Health care expenditures are increasing in the industrialized countries (Scrivens, 1997; Hughes & Humphrey, 1990; Ranci Ortigiosa, 2000). Therefore, European countries spend, in the health sector, 8-10% and the U.S.A 15% of their Gross Domestic Product. The interest towards electromechanical systems (MEMs - Micro-Electro-Mechanical to you Systems) means the realization of tools of small dimensions, which have remarkable advantages thanks to their invasivity and greater diagnostic-therapeutic effectiveness. Moreover, telemedicine requires a methodology, which analyzes its potential effects, taking into account the different actors of the health industry. Therefore, an economic evaluation has to take into consideration the following aspects/variables (Gerhardus, 2003; Luke et al., 2004; Zuckerman & Coile, 2003):

- Use of biomedical technology: The perspective of evaluation is limited to a single service or is extended to the entire health system. Therefore, it is necessary to assess the effects of change, estimating the total economic impact. That way, we estimate the cost of the changes, produced from the new technology, on the entire health system;
- Identification of the point of view: The financial resources for the patient admission are usually provided by a public system. However, although the main reference is the entire society it is necessary to identify the gains and losses of the single groups.
- Analysis of the alternatives: The scarce resources make choice necessary. Therefore, we have to compare the new and existing technology.

- Selection of the economic evaluation technique: Levels of different sophistication exist in the economic analysis, all deriving from the approach cost-benefits (cost analysis, cost minimization, cost-effectiveness, cost-utility, cost-benefits) that differ essentially because of the different ways they estimate benefits. However, the technique of evaluation is tied to the question we must answer.
- Identification and quantification of the costs and benefits: The studies reported in the literature do not show the same amplitude and variety of costs and benefits. For example, the capital costs are often omitted while the complexity in quantifying benefits is increasing. Normally, for the economic evaluation we use market prices or proxies, which are referred as prices, and we have to take into account the different aspects of outcome evaluation comparing the existing and the new model (Walston & Bogue, 1999; Coile, 2000; Bolon, 1997).

CONCLUSION

Healthcare supply and the public health concept are being modified according to new standards. Nevertheless, although the budget constraints, e-health represents an interesting opportunity for the exchange, integration and sharing of information among health care providers and patients (Grimson et al., 2001; Maceratini et al., 1995; Leisch et al., 1997).

REFERENCES

Bolon, D. S. (1997). Organizational citizenship behavior among hospital employees: a multidimensional analysis involving job satisfaction and organizational commitment. *Hospital & Health Services Administration*, *42*(2), 221–241.

Coile, R. (2000). E-health: Reinventing healthcare in the information age. *Journal of Healthcare Management*, *45*(3), 206–210.

Commission of the European Communities. (2007). *A lead market initiative for Europe*. Brussels: Commission of the European Communities.

Drummond, M., Sculpher, M., Torrance, G., O'Brien, B., & Stoddart, G. (2005). *Methods for the Economic Evaluation of Health Care Programmes*. Oxford, UK: Oxford University Press.

Gerhardus, D. (2003). Robot-Assisted Surgery: The Future Is Here. *Journal of Healthcare Management*, *48*(4), 242–251.

Grimson, J., Stephens, G., Jung, B., Grimson, W., Berry, D., & Pardon, S. (2001). Sharing Health-Care Records over the Internet. *IEEE Internet Computing*, *5*(3), 49–58. doi:10.1109/4236.935177

Hughes, J., & Humphrey, C. (1990). *Medical Audit in General Practice: Practice Guide to the literature*. London: King's Fund Centre.

Leisch, E., Sartzetakis, S., Tsiknakis, M., & Orphanoudakis, S. C. (1997). A framework for the integration of distributed autonomous healthcare information systems. *Informatics for Health & Social Care*, *22*(4), 325–335. doi:10.3109/14639239709010904

Luke, R., Walston, S., & Plummer, P. (2004). *Healthcare strategy: in pursuit of competitive advantage*. Chicago, IL: Health Administration Press.

Maceratini, R., Rafanelli, M., & Ricci, F. L. (1995). Virtual Hospitalization: reality or utopia? *Medinfo*, *2*, 1482–1486.

Ranci Ortigiosa, E. (2000). *La valutazione di qualità nei servizi sanitari*. Milano, Italy: Franco Angeli Edizioni.

Scrivens, E. (1997). *Accreditamento dei servizi sanitari: Esperienze internazionali a confronto*. Torino, Italy: Centro Scientifico Editore.

Walston, S. L., & Bogue, R. J. (1999). The effects of reengineering: Fad or competitive factor? *Journal of Healthcare Management*, *44*(6), 456–474.

Zuckerman, A., & Coile, R. (2003). *Competing on Excellence: Healthcare Strategies for a Consumer-Driven Market*. Chicago, IL: Health Administration Press.

Chapter 4
E-Health:
A New Framework for the Patient-Physician Relationship

Susana Lorenzo
Hospital Universitario Fundación Alcorcón, Spain

Gilberto Llinas
Miguel Hernandez University, Spain

Jose J. Mira
Miguel Hernandez University, Spain

Emilio Ignacio
Universidad de Cadiz, Spain

ABSTRACT

E-health does not only imply technological progress but also a new framework for improving citizens' health. E-health has many strong points, which include clinical applications, and training devices. Health websites have a tremendous impact, as they increase accessibility to health information. Therefore, they encourage patients in becoming a prudent actor who decides where to go and what to do. However, many patients are not familiar with the precise meaning of e-health, which varies with the context in which the term is used. Moreover, they are not familiar with terms associated with e-health. Nevertheless, the Internet might contribute towards patient-centeredness, as patients might get their first opinion from the Internet. However, websites should meet reliability and comprehensiveness requirements.

INTRODUCTION

Patient-centeredness argues that healthcare professionals have to be responsive to patient preferences and needs. On the other hand, patients should be a prudent actor who decides where to go and what to do in a sensible manner (Kaisser, 2000; Rong-Huang, 2003). As a result, patients need e-health technologies, which improve accessibility of information. First cited by Mitchell in 1999, according to Jadad in 2005, e-health implies clinical appliances, professional training devices, accessibility of information (including hospital outcome information), and education (Eysenbach, 2001; Richardson, 2003; Carrasco,

DOI: 10.4018/978-1-61692-843-8.ch004

2002; Suarez et al., 2005; SEIS, 2008). However, patients are not familiar with terms associated with e-health (e-mail, e-commerce), and as with most neologisms, the precise meaning of e-health varies with the context in which the term is used. Nevertheless, the internet might contribute towards patient-centeredness (Pallares, 2000) as patients might get their first opinion from the Internet, and then go to visit their doctor. In a study conducted among arthritis patients (Hay, 2008), 87.5% of them looked for information before attending the consultation. Moreover, the use of e-mail by doctors and patients improves communication (Car & Sheikh, 2004). Therefore, it is likely that its use by doctors and patients will gradually increase, given the fact that its adoption rates are low (Lorenzo & Mira, 2004). For example, Leong et al. (2005) found that the number of messages is lower than the number of emails.

On the other hand, doctors can respond to the more 'Internet informed' patient in three ways. In the first scenario, the relationship between the health professional and the patient becomes health professional-centered. In this scenario, health professionals may think that their medical authority is threatened by the information the patient brings. Therefore, they might respond defensively, asserting their 'expert opinion'. They will also use a brief consultation to quickly and authoritatively steer the patient towards their choice of action. The second scenario involves the collaboration between the health professional and patient. After all, many patients not only have the time, but also the incentive to search for information about their health problems. As they are usually only interested in one condition, their search is mostly focused (McMullan, 2006). In this scenario, health professionals (not only doctors, but also nurses, psychologists, therapists, etc.) argue that they do not have the time to search for every clinical condition. However, they do have the expertise to analyze the information and assess the relevance to the patient (Lorenzo, 2008). In the third scenario, the health professional recommends websites and guides patients to reliable and accurate information. However, it then becomes crucial for the health professional not only to understand the information, but also where to get it on the Internet. As it is difficult to keep track of all the information that is on the Internet, health professionals should know about reliable repositories of health information and medical links. Jadad (2005) suggested that e-patients and doctors share websites and medical office equipment is organized so both can look up the Internet during the consultation. As a result, we have an intruder in the consultation room or the clinic. Study findings point out that (1) patients have no problem with the use of a computer in the consultation room; and (2) doctors are willing to use a system that they feel it derives benefits for patient care (Aydin et al., 2004).

The perspectives of patients and health professionals are remarkably different and will evolve as time goes by (Ortendahl, 2008). Doctors will acknowledge the number of patients visiting health web sites (Schwartz et al., 2006) although some of them do not consider it suitable (Murray et al., 2003). However, using the Internet or the so-called Dr. Google, as a first opinion, can be problematic because of misinformation or misinterpretation of information. As a result, there is a series of recommendations to check for reliable websites either for professionals (Bravo & Merino, 2001; Louro González & González Guitián, 2001) or patients (Gutierrez & Blanco, 2001). Websites should meet reliability and comprehensiveness requirements (Pandolfini et al., 2002) while the search styles should be taken into account when designing health websites (Eysenbach & Köhler, 2002).

Therefore, the perspective of the chapter is to examine initiatives, which might assist patients in searching for scientific information in an effective and reasonable way (Leaffer & Gonda, 2000).

BACKGROUND

The advantage of the Internet is that it is widely available (home, work, libraries), convenient (24 h a day), cheap and anonymous. It can improve patients' understanding of their medical condition and self-care, thus reducing unnecessary visits to doctors and the burden on the health system. There is also a strong correlation between the Internet use and patients' health behavior resulting in a patient-centered interaction between the health professional and patient. Health information is one of the most commonly sought topics on the Internet. According to a Reuters study, 53% of the Americans search the Internet for health information (Reuters, 2003). Moreover, the Euro barometer study in 2003 showed that 43% of the EU citizens believe that the web is a convenient way to collect information. Overall, there are several studies, which highlight the positive impact of the web on the doctor-patient relationship. However, most of the studies conclude that doctors believe that their authority is challenged, and, as a result, they are skeptic or feel threatened (Anderson et al., 2003). They are also worried about the accuracy of the information, the probability of inappropriate self-diagnosis, and the future demand for unavailable treatments (Hart et al., 2004). They argue that they do not have enough time to respond to patients' questions. Moreover, they cannot surf the web to check what their patients may be viewing (McMullan, 2006; Sullivan, & Wyatt, 2005). Websites can be a valuable source of information for patients, and healthcare professionals on any disease -either acute or chronic. A recent European Union (EU) Euro barometer survey on online health information, found that health professionals are still, by far, the main source of health information (45.3% of EU health population). Television (19.8%) and newspapers (7.4%) follow. Nevertheless, on average, nearly a quarter of the Europeans (23%) use the Internet to get health information. However, the percentage varies with the country (40% in Denmark and the Netherlands and 15% or fewer in Greece, Spain and Portugal). Finally, 41.5% of the people within the EU consider the Internet a convenient way of getting health information (Eysenbach & Köhler, 2004). However, this data vary day by day. The Spanish Statistical Institute showed that 40% of the web visits are related to health (INE, 2003) while similar results have been found in other countries (MITC, 2007; Ferguson & Frydman, 2004). In Canada, a third of patients use the web for getting health information while one third discuss results with their doctor (Underhill & Mkeown, 2008). In the US, 80% of the Internet users, accounting for eight million of adults per day, search for health information (Fox, 2006).

Most of e-patients highlight the fact that poorly designed applications can harm patients (Eysenbach & Köhler, 2002). They also think that when you search the web, you can find top validity pages next to others with lapses or errors (Jadad & Gagliardi, 1998; Eysenbach & Köhler, 2002; Mira et al., 2004). Excellent or good websites represent less than 30% of the existing ones and many of them (about 70%) can be considered fair or bad (Ferguson & Frydman, 2004). This fact instigated periodical reviews of the website quality (Rancaño et al., 2003).

Nonetheless, these results should not deceive us. More than 75% of e-patients believe that they find what they are trying to find (Murray et al., 2003). A survey conducted in 2000 concluded that 55% of individuals with Internet access have used the Web to find health or medical information (Pew Internet, 2000). Moreover, several studies suggest that more than 95% of consumers use search engines when they 'hunt' for specific, health-related, questions (Eysenbach & Köhler, 2004). For instance, if we use the two of the most popular search engines (Google & Yahoo) to find information on diabetes and hypertension, results are enormous. Using Google, the most commonly used search engine (64.1% of the e-health searchers) in Spain (INE, 2003), in about 1-second, the search string on diabetes finds approximately

70.100.000 websites and the search string on hypertension almost 3.000.000 websites. On the other hand, Yahoo returns 297.000.000 websites on diabetes and 6.750.000 on hypertension.

Quality of Health Websites

The Internet can be used in many ways (Mira et al., 2004). It can provide information about health and illness, health education, chats and debates (among patients or professional people or both) or spread medical news. Moreover, patients can share experiences, and get information about their illness or therapeutic methods. Unfortunately, not everything that glitters is gold. Impicciatore and others (1997) published one of the first published studies on the reliability of health websites in 1997. They analyzed websites that provided general information on treating a child with fever. After reviewing 41 websites, which encompassed considerable recommendation variability, they concluded that only 28 of them included a definition of child fever, 36 stressed the convenience of calling the doctor, 26 mentioned the appropriate body temperature, and 31 mentioned that proper treatment was paracetamol. Moreover, Wyatt (1997) described the advantages of the Internet and the aspects that should be reviewed to find out a website's content credibility.

The Internet provides an easily accessible means to communicate both accurate and unreliable health information, so it has the potential to assist but also to put the healthcare provision at risk. (Kunst et al., 2002; Bessell et al., 2002; Ávila de Tomás et al., 2001). Therefore, the World Health Organization (WHO), the European Union, Germany, France, the UK and Spain, among others, support strategies to improve the quality of health information on the Internet. Moreover, observatories, user guides (for example DISCERN), filters, checklists, codes of conduct, quality labels -such as HON- and third-party certifications have been created to 'wipe out' inaccurate or controversial information on the Web. In Spain, we have undertaken several initiatives (Mayer et al., 2004). For example, EU is financing the MedIEQ project, to analyze websites in six different languages (Ansani et al., 2005).

Content comprehensiveness, in other words, if the texts have been prepared in accordance to the targeted population (legibility analysis), has been analyzed in several studies (Navarro et al., 2002; Rubiera et al., 2004; Graber et al., 1999; D'Alessandro et al., 2001; Jaffery & Becker, 2004; Friedman et al., 2004). PageRank from Google and, above all, DISCERN have showed their usefulness to assess the scientific quality of a website (Griffiths & Christensen, 2005). A scale measuring the quality of a health center website has been developed in Spain (Mira et al., 2006); it uses a legibility and accessibility analysis divided in 73 elements.

Recently, a new educational model and a tool to assess information on the Internet has been designed and tested with consumers. The new model replaces the "traditional" static questionnaire/checklist/ rating approach with a dynamic, process-oriented approach, which highlights three steps the consumers should follow when navigating the Internet (Eysenbach & Thomson, 2007). The so-called FA4CT results in three phases: (1) Finding Answers and Comparing information from different sources, (2) Checking Sources Credibility, and (3) Checking Reputation. The FA4CT model is a reliable, valid, and usable approach for consumers, which might be the basis for more sophisticated tools or portals, which automate the evaluation according to the FA4CT algorithm. Moreover, the Medication Website Assessment Tool (MWAT) checks the completeness, accuracy, format, reliability, and readability of the information. The US Department of Health and Human Services Steering Committee 'action plan' endorsed these categories for evaluating and improving the usefulness of written medical information for printed documents (Thomson & Graydon, 2009).

Table 1. Recommendations for Internet users that visit health information web sites

1. The first web page might not be the best choice.
2. Not all the information on the Internet is reliable. Your GP knows best.
3. When surfing the Web, check to see whether the page is updated regularly.
4. Information should be distinguished from banners by checking the site's information source.
5. Try to identify if the sites are based on opinion or evidence. Check to see whether research has been conducted during the last five years.
6. Do not be influenced by the web's design, since images are not as important as content.
7. Do not assume that technical language provides better information.
8. When searching for a treatment, keep in mind that each patient may have a different therapeutic profile.
9. Pay attention to outcome information, information about the patient's profile, possible complications and adverse events.
10. Think twice before revealing personal and clinical data to websites.

Overall, when we refer to reliable websites, the following characteristics are cited (Louro González & González Guitián, 2001):

- periodical updating
- published sources
- reliable sources
- accessibility of unskilled surfers
- references
- unbiased information about treatments and their effectiveness

Solutions and Recommendations

The usefulness of health websites is undeniable. A study conducted in Spain (Mira et al., 2008), confirmed that Internet users resort to the same search engines for medical information and information about other topics. In the US, it is common for the Internet users (2/3) to resort to popular search engines (Google, Yahoo, etc.) to find health-related web pages.

However, despite the fact that health information has beneficial effects on consumer empowerment (between 36% and 55% of Internet users access online health information); it might also become frightening if surfers have to:

- check for the quality of the information (Pealer & Dorman, 1997; Kim et al., 1999; Curro et al., 2004)
- analyze the website content (validity and truthfulness), authorship (credibility, objectivity), purpose (tell or persuade), accessibility, simplicity.

A few simple recommendations (Table 1) can keep e-patients away from trouble.

FUTURE RESEARCH DIRECTIONS

Health literacy is crucial to patient empowerment. If individuals do not have the capacity to understand basic health information, they will not be able to look after themselves effectively. However, there has been little research into the prevalence of health illiteracy. Despite various initiatives to improve the quality and availability of health information, studies suggest that patients want more information than they currently receive.

The Internet has become an indispensable source of health information, but a 'digital divide' has been widely documented, with access and use more prevalent among younger, more affluent and more advantaged groups. Websites can improve knowledge and studies have demonstrated high user satisfaction and beneficial effects on self efficacy and health behavior. There is also some evidence of greater health benefit for disadvantaged groups when they overcome access barriers.

On the other hand, there are concerns about the accessibility, quality, readability, reliability and usefulness of electronic health information. Moreover, harm arising from unreliable websites may be under-reported. Therefore, there is a clear need for more research into the prevalence of low health literacy, on making information available, and on discovering the interests of e-patients. In addition, we have to examine the effect of a second opinion through the Internet. Finally, patients need training on using databases, like Medline. At the same time, we have to educate handicapped persons and elderly patients in surfing health websites.

CONCLUSION

ICT influence in daily activities is undeniable. Its success is transforming our society. Fast Internet access is already creating opportunities for online communication. Health professionals, policy makers, managers, and patients have to acquire different skills to use these electronic communication tools efficiently. Young generations use and take more advantage of these technologies. Therefore, the use of the Internet, as a health information source, will increase exponentially in the future. However, new clinical skills are not enough. Even if doctors and nurses become proficient in using modern communication technology, we have to address their fears about the internet's impact on their workload, income, personal liability, and quality of life. Developing on-line systems for empowering citizens to access health knowledge, for either information or education, is urgent.

REFERENCES

Anderson, J. G., Rainey, M., & Eysenbach, G. (2003). The impact of cyberHealthcare on the physician-patient relationship. *Journal of Medical Systems*, *27*, 67–84. doi:10.1023/A:1021061229743

Ansani, N. T., Vogt, M., & Henderson, B. A., McKaVeney, T. P., Weber, R. J., Smith, R. B., Burda, M., Kwoh, C. K., Osial, T. A., & Starz, T. (2005). Quality of arthritis information on the Internet. *American Journal of Health-System Pharmacy*, *62*, 1184–1189.

Ávila de Tomás, J. F., Portillo Boyero, B. E., & Pajares Izquierdo, J. M. (2001). Calidad en la información biomédica existente en Internet. *Atencion Primaria*, *28*, 674–679.

Aydin, C., Anderson, J., Rosen, P., Felitti, V. J., & Weng, H. (2004). *Computers in the Consulting Room: A Case Study of Clinician and Patient Perspectives.* In JG. Anderson & CE. Aydin (Eds.), *Evaluating the Organizational Impact of Healthcare Information Systems, Second Edition*, (pp.225-47).

Bessell, T., McDonald, S., Silagy, Ch., Anderson, J., & Hiller, J., & Sansom, Ll. (2002). Do Internet interventions for consumers cause more harm than good? A systematic review. *Health Expectations*, *5*, 28–37. doi:10.1046/j.1369-6513.2002.00156.x

Bravo, J., & Merino, M. (2001). Pediatría e Internet. *Atencion Primaria*, *27*, 574–578.

Car, J., & Sheikh, A. (2004). E-mail consultations in health care: scope and effectiveness. *British Medical Journal*, *329*, 435–438. doi:10.1136/bmj.329.7463.435

Carrasco, G. (2002). Medicina basada en la evidencia "electrónica" (e-MBE): metodología, ventajas y limitaciones. *Revista Calidad Asistencial*, *17*, 113–125.

Curro, V., Buonuomo, P. S., Onesimo, R., de Rose, P., Vituzzi, A., di Tanna, G. L., & D'Atri, A. (2004). A quality evaluation methodology of health web-pages for non-professionals. *Medical Informatics and the Internet in Medicine*, *29*, 95–107. doi:10.1080/14639230410001684396

D'Alessandro, D. M., Kingsley, P., & Johnson-West, J. (2001). The readability of pediatric patient education materials on the World Wide Web. *Archives of Pediatrics & Adolescent Medicine*, *155*, 807–812.

Eysenbach, G. (2001). What is e-health? *Journal of Medical Internet Research*, *3*, E20. doi:10.2196/jmir.3.2.e20

Eysenbach, G., & Köhler C. (2002). Does the internet harm health? Database of adverse events related to the internet has been set up. *British Medical Journal*, 324-239. Retrieved September 23, 2008 from 10.1136/bmj.324.7337.573.

Eysenbach, G., & Köhler, C. (2002). How do consumers search for and appraise health information on the world wide web? Qualitative study using focus groups, usability tests, and in-depth interviews. *British Medical Journal*, *324*, 573–577. doi:10.1136/bmj.324.7337.573

Eysenbach, G., & Köhler, C. (2004). Health-Related Searches on the Internet. *Journal of the American Medical Association*, *291*, 2946. doi:10.1001/jama.291.24.2946

Eysenbach, G., & Thomson, M. (2007). The FA4CT Algorithm: A New Model and Tool for Consumers to Assess and Filter Health Information on the Internet. Studies in Health Technology and Informatics.In Klaus A. Kuhn, James R. Warren, Tze-Yun Leong, (Eds.), MEDINFO 2007 - *Proceedings of the 12th World Congress on Health (Medical) Informatics – Building Sustainable Health Systems. (vol.* 129).

Eysenbach, G., Powell, J., Kuss, O., & Sa, E. R. (2002). Empirical studies assessing the quality of health information for consumers on the World Wide Web: a systematic review. *Journal of the American Medical Association*, *287*, 2691–2700. doi:10.1001/jama.287.20.2691

Ferguson, T., & Frydman, G. (2004). The first generation of e-patients. *British Medical Journal*, *328*, 1148–1149. doi:10.1136/bmj.328.7449.1148

Fox, S. Online Health Search 2006. Pew Internet & American Life Project. Retrieved October 23, 2008 from http://www.pewinternet.org/PPF/r/190/report_display.asp

Friedman, D. B., Hoffman-Goetz, L., & Arocha, J. F. (2004). Readability of cancer information on the internet. *Cancer Education*, *19*, 117–122. doi:10.1207/s15430154jce1902_13

Graber, M. A., Roller, C. M., & Kaeble, B. (1999). Readability levels of patient education material on the world wide web. *The Journal of Family Practice*, *48*, 58–61.

Griffiths, K., & Christensen, H. (2005). Websites quality indicators for consumers. *Journal of Medical Internet Research*, *7*, e55. doi:10.2196/jmir.7.5.e55

Gutiérrez, U., & Blanco, A. (2001). Información para pacientes en español en Internet. *Atencion Primaria*, *28*, 283–288.

Hart, A., Henwood, F., & Wyatt, S. (2004). The role of the Internet in patient–practitioner relationships: findings from a qualitative research study. *Journal of Medical Internet Research*, *6*, 36. doi:10.2196/jmir.6.3.e36

Hay, M. C., Cadigan, R. J., Khanna, D., Strathmann, C., Lieber, E., & Altman, R. (2008). Prepared patients: internet information seeking by new rheumatology patients. *Arthritis and Rheumatism*, *59*, 575–582. doi:10.1002/art.23533

HONcode. Retrieved November 25, 2008 from: http://www.hon.ch/HONcode/Conduct.html http://www.communities.gov.uk/publications/communities/understandingdigitalexclusion

Impicciatore, P., Pandolfini, C., Casella, N., & Bonati, M. (1997). Reliability of health information for the public on the world wide wed: systematic survey of advice on managing fever in children at home. *British Medical Journal*, *314*, 1875–1879.

Instituto Nacional de Estadística (INE). (2003). Encuesta sobre equipamiento y uso de tecnologías de información y comunicación en las viviendas. Datos preliminares. Segundo trimestre de 2003. Press note. Retrieved October 11, 2005 from: http://www.ine.es/prensa/np1203.htm.

Jadad, A. (2005). What will it take to bring the internet into the consulting room? We cannot remain oblivious to our patients' expectations. *Journal of General Internal Medicine*, *20*, 787–788. doi:10.1111/j.1525-1497.2005.051359.x

Jadad, A. R., & Delamothe, T. (2003). From electronic gadgets to better health: where is the knowledge? *British Medical Journal*, *327*, 300–301. doi:10.1136/bmj.327.7410.300

Jadad, A., & Gagliardi, A. (1998). Rating health information on the Internet. Navigating to knowledge or to Babel? *Journal of the American Medical Association*, *279*, 611–614. doi:10.1001/jama.279.8.611

Jaffery, J. B., & Becker, B. N. (2004). Evaluation of e-Health web sites for patients with chronic kidney disease. *American Journal of Kidney Diseases*, *44*, 71–76. doi:10.1053/j.ajkd.2004.03.025

Kaisser, J. P. (2000). Patients, physicians, and the Internet. *Health Affairs (Project Hope)*, *19*, 115–123. doi:10.1377/hlthaff.19.6.115

Kim, P., Eng, T. R., Deering, M. J., & Maxfield, A. (1999). Published criteria for evaluating health related web sites [review]. *British Medical Journal*, *318*, 647–649.

Kunst, H., Groot, D., Latthe, P., & Khan, K. (2002). Accuracy of information on apparently credible websites: survey of five common health topics. *British Medical Journal*, *324*, 581–582. doi:10.1136/bmj.324.7337.581

Leaffer, T., & Gonda, B. (2000). The Internet: an underutilized tool in patient education. *Computers in Nursing*, *18*, 47–52.

Leong, S., Gingrich, D., Lewis, P., Mauger, D., & George, J. (2005). Enhancing doctor-patient communication using email: a pilot study. *Journal of the American Board of Family Medicine*, *18*, 180–188. doi:10.3122/jabfm.18.3.180

Lorenzo, S. (2008). Toward new approaches to quality. The patient as coprotagonist. *Gaceta Sanitaria,* 22(Supl 1), 186-91.

Lorenzo, S., & Mira, J. J. (2004). Are Spanish physicians ready to take advantage of the Internet? *World Hospitals and Health Services*, *40*, 31–35.

Louro González, A., & González Guitián, C. (2001). Portales sanitarios para la atención primaria. *Atencion Primaria*, *27*, 346–350.

Mayer, M. A., Leis, A., & Ruiz, P. (2004). Navegando por Internet: los sellos de calidad y la web semántica pueden ser un camino para encontrar el oro que reluce. *Atencion Primaria*, *34*, 383. doi:10.1157/13067780

McMullan, M. (2006). Patients using the Internet to obtain health information: How this affects the patient–health professional relationship. *Patient Education and Counseling*, *63*, 24–28. doi:10.1016/j.pec.2005.10.006

MedIEQ. Retrieved November 25, 2008 from: http://www.medieq.org/about

Medscape, L. L. C. Retrieved February 22 2009, from http://www.medscape.com/pages/features/hospitalcompare/hospitalcompare

MITC. Ministerio de Industria, Turismo y Comercio. Estudio sobre Actividades realizadas en Internet 2007. Red.es. Retrieved October 23, 2008 from: http://observatorio.red.es/estudios/documentos/actividades_internet_2007.pdf

Mira, J. J., Pérez-Jover, V., & Lorenzo, S. (2004). Navegando en Internet en busca de información sanitaria: no es oro todo lo que reluce.... *Atencion Primaria*, *33*, 391–399. doi:10.1157/13060754

Mira, J. J., Llinás, G., Tomás, O., & Pérez-Jover, V. (2006). Quality of websites in Spanish public hospitals. *Medical Informatics and the Internet in Medicine*, *31*, 23–44. doi:10.1080/14639230500519940

Mira, J. J., Llinás, G., & Perez Jover, V. (2008). Habits of Internet users and usefulness of websites in Spanish for health education. *World Hospitals and Health Services*, *44*, 30–35.

Mitchell, J. (1999). *From telehealth to e-health: the unstoppable rise of e-health*. Canberra, Australia: National Office for the Information Technology.

Murray, E., Lo, B., Pollack, L., Donelan, K., Catania, J., Lee, K., et al. (2003). The impact of health information on the internet on health care and the physician-patient relationship: national U.S. survey among 1,050 U.S. physicians. *Journal of Medical Internet Research,* 5:e17. Retrieved April 21 2009, from: http://www.jmir.org/2003/3/e17

Murray, E., Lo, B., Pollack, L., Donelan, K., Catania, J., & White, M. (2003). The impact of health information on the Internet on the physician-patient relationship. *Archives of Internal Medicine*, *163*, 1727–1734. doi:10.1001/archinte.163.14.1727

Navarro-Royo, C., Monteagudo-Piqueras, O., Rodríguez-Suárez, L., Valentín-López, B., & García-Caballero, J. (2002). Legibilidad de los documentos de consentimiento informado del Hospital La Paz. *Revista de Calidad Asistencial*, *17*, 331–336.

New York State Department of Health. Retrieved February 22 2009, from: http://hospitals.nyhealth.gov/

Ortendahl, M. (2008). Different time perspectives of the doctor and the patient reduce quality in health care. *Quality Management in Health Care*, *17*, 136–139.

Pallarés, A. (2000). Las nuevas tecnologías de la información desde la perspectiva de los ciudadanos: la paradoja de Internet. *Revista de Calidad Asistencial*, *15*, 221–222.

Pandolfini, Ch., & Bonati, M. (2002). Follow up of quality of public oriented health information on the world wide web: systematic re-evaluation. *British Medical Journal*, *324*, 582–583. doi:10.1136/bmj.324.7337.582

Pealer, L. N., & Dorman, S. M. (1997). Evaluating health-related Web sites. *The Journal of School Health*, *67*, 232–235. doi:10.1111/j.1746-1561.1997.tb06311.x

Pew Internet and American Life Project. The Online Health Care Revolution: How the Web Helps Americans Take Better Care of Themselves. November 26, 2000. Retrieved November 23, 2008 from: http://www.pewinternet.org.

Rancaño, I., Rodrigo, J. A., Villa, R., Abdelsater, M., Díaz, R., & Alvarez, D. (2003). Evaluación de las páginas web en lengua española útiles para el médico de atención primaria. *Atencion Primaria*, *31*, 575–584. doi:10.1157/13048143

Reuters. (2003) Consumer-targeted internet investment: online strategies to improve patient care and product positioning. Reuters Business Insight Report; May.

Richardson, R. (2003). eHealth for Europe. *Studies in Health Technology and Informatics*, *96*, 151–156.

Rong-Huang, Q. (2003). Creating informed consumers and achieving shared decisions making. *Family Physician*, *32*, 335–341.

Rubiera, G., Arbizu, R., Alzueta, A., Agúndez, J. J., & Riera, J. J. (2004). La legibilidad de los documentos de consentimiento informado en los hospitales de Asturias. *Gaceta Sanitaria*, *18*, 153–158. doi:10.1157/13059288

Schwartz, K. L., Roe, T., Northrup, J., Meza, J., Seifeldin, R., & Neale, A. V. (2006). Family medicine patients' use of the Internet for health information: a MetroNet study. *Journal of the American Board of Family Medicine*, *19*, 39–45. doi:10.3122/jabfm.19.1.39

SEIS. Sistema de Información Esencial en Terapéutica y Salud. Retrieved October 23, 2008 from: http://www.icf.uab.es/informacion/Papyrus/

SEMFYC. Sociedad Española de Medicina Familiar y Comunitaria. Informatización en la Atención Primaria. Documento nº 13. Retrieved October 13, 2008 from: http://www.semfyc.es/es/actividades/publicaciones/documentos-semfyc/docum013.html.

Suárez, J., Beltrán, C., Molina, T., & Navarro, P. (2005). Receta electrónica: de la utopía a la realidad. *Atencion Primaria*, *35*, 451–459. doi:10.1157/13075469

Sullivan, F., & Wyatt, J. (2005). Is a consultation needed? *British Medical Journal*, *331*, 625–627. doi:10.1136/bmj.331.7517.625

Thompson, A. E., & Graydon, S. L. (2009). Patient oriented methotrexate information sites on the Internet: A review of completeness, accuracy, format, reliability, credibility, and readability. *The Journal of Rheumatology*, *36*, 41–49.

Underhill, C., & Mkeown, L. (2008). Getting a second opinion: health information and the Internet. *Health Reports*, *19*, 65–69.

Wyatt, J. (1997). Commentary: Measuring quality and impact of the world wide web. *British Medical Journal*, *314*, 1879–1881.

Chapter 5
E-Health: A Bridge to People-Centered Health Care

Anastasius Moumtzoglou
Hellenic Society for Quality & Safety in Healthcare & European Society for Quality in Healthcare, Greece

ABSTRACT

People-centered health care represents a structural change in thinking, which encapsulates before anything else the consideration of the patient. The development of people-centered care might include a partnership approach based on equal footing, capacity-building and the expansion of organizational care. Its central values encompass empowerment, participation, family, community, and the abolition of any kind of discrimination. As a result, they bestow people on shared decision-making not exclusively on issues of treatment but also for health care organization. On the other hand, a global e-health agreement is beginning to take shape on the engagement of stakeholders, the interoperability, and standards. Consequently, e-health can have a significant impact on people-centered care, despite the challenges of implementation and adoption.

INTRODUCTION

Health systems have reached a historic turning point. Changing population health patterns and outcomes shift the disease burden; higher levels of education, increased availability of information and access to goods and services alter expectations of health care delivery; patient satisfaction, patient safety, responsiveness of care are major issues, and patient-centeredness is a global issue.

DOI: 10.4018/978-1-61692-843-8.ch005

However, the current health care is becoming overly biomedical-oriented, technology-driven, doctor-dominated, and market-oriented. Changing health needs, community expectations, ageing populations, rise of chronic conditions; increased literacy and purchasing power, superior information technology and access to information lead to increasing consumerism. Weaknesses in medical education, which concentrates on body systems and disease conditions and pays less attention to social context, psychosocial and cultural issues, ethics, interpersonal communication and relational skills fragments provision. Low health literacy means limited availability of pertinent information and weaknesses in quality systems less responsiveness. There are also gaps in health policy – financing incentives; workforce production, distribution and regulation; weaknesses in primary care and in continuity of care, and clamor for more responsible and accountable health care governance. Consequently, health systems provide insufficient opportunities for consumer input and feedback and little reporting to the community.

People-centered health care represents a substantial change in thinking, which encapsulates the foremost consideration of patient and covers patient-centered care (WHO, 2007). It stems its origin from the human rights campaign and has a protracted history in research, clinical practice and medical education. The fundamental values of people-centered care encompass empowerment, participation, family, community, and the abolition of any kind of discrimination. People have the right and duty to shared decision-making not only on issues of treatment but also for health care planning and implementation. Health systems should serve individuals, families and communities in humane and holistic ways in all settings and at every opportunity.

Nevertheless, we have not satisfactorily enunciated the concept at the health system level. Some of the reasons for the gap between vision and practice might include:

- The evidence demonstrates that there are significant gaps in what we know about how to raise standards of health literacy (Coulter & Ellins, 2006).
- Implementation of innovations, which improve shared decision-making (Coulter & Ellins, 2006).
- Barriers which include lack of knowledge and skills, concerns about time and negative attitudes among clinicians (Billings 2004, Graham et al., 2003).
- We need to understand how to enhance safety improvement through patient involvement, and we are not entirely aware of the effect of patient feedback, provider choice, complaints, and advocacy systems.
- 'Accountability' is a term of many nuances (Savage & Morre, 2004) and open to various interpretations (Mander 1995; Ferlie et al., 1996). Lewis and Batey (1982) make a practical distinction between structural accountability (disclosure) and accountability as an internalized predisposition (the willingness to assume responsibility for the outcomes of professional actions). Tingle (1995) argued that the various definitions of accountability are just starting points, while McSherry and Pearce (2002) state that accountability for health care professionals bears on changing practice. Therefore, to be truly accountable, practitioners need to check that their practice is evidence-based, efficient and effective.
- Quality improvement systems seem to be effective with regard to the implementation of selected patient-centeredness strategies, but they seem to be inadequate to ensure their widespread implementation (Groene et al., 2009).

On the other hand, empirical research has identified e-health behaviors, which include the decline in expert authority, pervasiveness of health information on the Internet and empowerment (Donelly et al., 2008). The findings demonstrate a decline in expert authority with ensuing implications for health management. Thus, the perspective of the chapter is to examine the prospects of e-health to the realization of people-centered care.

BACKGROUND

Eysenbach (2001) defined e-health as 'an emerging field in the intersection of medical informatics, public health and business, referring to health services and information delivered or enhanced through the Internet and related technologies. In a broader sense, the term characterizes not only a technical development, but also a state-of-mind, a way of thinking, an attitude, and a commitment for networked, global thinking, to improve health care locally, regionally, and worldwide by using information and communication technology'. We might also characterize e-health as the tools that accelerate the processing, transfer and sharing of information between citizens, patients, and health professional (Wilson, 2005). These tools include health information websites, electronic health records, booking systems, digital image capture and sharing systems, bio-data sensors and captors or any other of the extensive collection of applications that exist. Overall, e-health means new electronic technologies, web-based transactions and advanced networks, and implies fundamental rethinking of healthcare processes based on electronic communication and computer based support (Blumenthal & Glaser, 2007). However, e-health does not imply a particular application, as we commonly describe it as comprising four pillars (Richardson et al., 2004):

- Clinical applications, which include teleconsultations, and clinical decision-making support software
- E-dissemination of healthcare professional education
- Public health information, which focuses on improving health literacy
- Lifetime health records, which involve recording and usage of information on various levels

Currently, most e-health policies reflect technology driven decisions, focus on prescriptions, booking, diagnostic reports, and discharge summaries, while in the future will support clinical pathways, governance, and patient empowerment (Rossi Mori, 2008). E-health approach is mostly technology-cantered, product-based innovation and driven by the opportunities. Therefore, the health system is capable to cope with limited organizational problems, while e-health requires large-scale programs, which are pervasive and accelerated. As a result, we should return to the healthcare policies and put them in the center. Brailler and Thompson (2004) defined Health Information Technology (HIT) as the information processing, which involves hardware, software, integrated technologies and deals with the storage, retrieval, sharing, use of health care information, data, knowledge for communication and decision making. However, HIT faces a terminology problem with the existence of many differing and even conflicting definitions (The National Alliance for Health Information Technology, 2008). There are common elements among some of the definitions, but there are also areas of significant divergence. Similar problems occur with the network terms.

The full adoption and implementation of HIT requires that the public realizes the usefulness of HIT and seems to require access to electronic health information for providers and patients. This lifestyle change is contingent on a shared understanding of what constitutes HIT. Eliminating the confusion around terminology will present the following benefits:

- Individuals will comprehend IT concepts
- Policy makers use common terms for policy evaluation
- Effective contracting between HIT vendors and customers

People-centered care encompasses the subsequent elements and principles (WHO, 2007):

- Culture of care and communication
- Responsible, responsive and accountable services and institutions
- Supportive health care environments

The domains of people-centered health care include (1) individuals, families, and communities (2) health practitioners (3) health care organizations and (4) health systems. The first domain involves (WHO, 2007):

- Health literacy
- Communication and negotiation skills
- Self-management and self-care
- The voluntary sector, community-based organizations and professional organizations
- Social infrastructure that supports community involvement in health services organization and facilitates greater collaboration between regional governments and communities
- Community leaders who promote and encourage community participation in health service delivery

The domain of health practitioners requires (WHO, 2007):

- Capacity for holistic and compassionate care
- Commitment to quality, safe and ethical services

The domain of health care organizations implies (WHO, 2007):

- Conducive and comfortable environment for people receiving and providing health care
- Efficient and effective coordination of care
- Multidisciplinary care systems
- Multidisciplinary care teams
- Integration of patient education, family involvement, self-management and counseling into health care
- Standards and incentives for safe, quality and ethical services
- Introduction and strengthening models of care
- Leadership capacity of health services managers

Finally, the domain of health systems suggests (WHO, 2007):

- Development and strengthening of primary care and the primary care workforce
- Putting in place economic incentives that induce positive provider behavior and enhance access and financial risk protection for the entire population
- Establishing a stronger evidence base on ways to achieve superior health outcomes
- Ensuring rational technology use
- Strengthening the monitoring of professional standards
- Setting up public accountability measures for the organization, delivery and financing of health services
- Keeping an eye on and addressing patient and community concerns about health care quality
- Assisting persons who have experienced adverse events in the health system
- Ensuring protection of patient information

People-centered care is an umbrella term, which encapsulates patient-centered care. Patient-centered care is a problematic concept and its interpretation depends on the circumstances in which we use it. Grin (1994) defines patient-centered care as 'a collaborative effort consisting of patients; patients' relatives; friends, doctors and other health professionals; achieved through a broad system of patient education. Patients and the health care professionals collaborate as a team, share knowledge and work toward the common goals of optimal healing and recovery'. Laine and Davidoff (1996) define patient-centered care, as the health care that is closely congruent with and responsive to patients' wants, needs and preferences. Mallett (1996) considers patient-centered care as placing patients at the center of the system of care and developing quality services that revolve around them. Johnston & Cooper (1997) argue that it represents a construct that advocates simplifying the care at the bedside in the acute care setting by focusing on the expected outcomes for the patient rather than the diversity of tasks of each department. Mead and Bower (2002) mention five essential dimensions of patient-centeredness:

- A focus on illness rather than disease
- A focus on the specific individual's experience of the illness
- Sharing authority and responsibility so that the patient is an active participant rather than a passive recipient of care
- A therapeutic relationship between doctor and patient; and the doctor's, as well as the patient's, passionate responses and experiences being part of that alliance or relationship

For the Institute of Medicine (IOM) patient-centered is responsive to individual patient predispositions, needs, values; patient values guide all clinical decisions (IOM, 2001). The US Federal Agency for Healthcare Research and Quality (AHRQ) defines it as the health care that establishes a partnership among practitioners, patients and their families (when appropriate) to ensure that decisions respect patients' wants, needs and preferences and solicit patients' input on the education and support they need to reach decisions and participate in their own care (AHRQ, 2001). Lewin, Skea, Entwiste, and Dick (2001) perceive patient-centered interventions as those where providers share consultation, decision and management with patients. The Picker Institute (2004) defines patient-centered care as 'informing and involving patients, eliciting and respecting their preferences; responding quickly, effectively and safely to patients' needs and wishes; ensuring that we treat patients in a dignified and compassionate; delivering well-coordinated and integrated care'. Cronin (2004) identified the following concepts that appeared in different definitions of patient-centered care:

- Education/shared knowledge
- Involvement of relatives and friends
- Collaboration/team management
- Holistic/sensitive to non-medical or mental issues
- Respect for patient's needs and wants
- Free flow/accessibility of information

Conspicuously missing in the definitions are (IAPO, 2007):

- Patients' rights
- Patients' responsibilities
- Evidence-based care
- Patient safety
- Public health

E-Health and People-Centered Care

Cost reduction and cost savings is the standard measure of e-health value. However, as e-health matures, it is clear that this is just one side to the added value suggestion.

Citizen-Patient Empowerment

Kilbridge (2002) suggested that twelve information technology applications, which involve the management of health care information, empower patients: (1) technologies which allow access to general and specific health care information (2) technologies capable to conduct data entry and tracking of personal self-management data. The applications included:

- Personal Health Records

A Personal Health Record (PHR) retains patient-specific health information for future direct access by the patient. Some enable the patient to develop and refine the record, while others are consumer portals into provider-maintained electronic medical records (EMRs). The PHR contributes to patient empowerment by granting patients access to their medical record and permitting them to review and, modify that information (Halamka et al., 2007; Hess et al., 2007; Kupchunas, 2007; Lee et al., 2007; Morales Rodriguez et al., 2007; Nelson, 2007; Pagliari et al., 2007; Smith & Barefield, 2007).

- Patient Access to Hospital Information Systems

A subcategory of the personal health record is a technology that permits outpatients to gain access to their laboratory test results, imaging study reports, etc. through online access to hospital information systems. In general, these sites permit only selected patients to access the system; they restrict access to some categories of data; and they construct information/referral resources to answer patients' questions and manage their concerns. In addition, all such sites must have robust security approaches and well-defined policies and procedures safeguarding the privacy of patient data.

- Patient Access to General Health Information

Electronic access to health care topics is primarily accomplished through the Internet. Public availability of medical information on the Internet can help patients develop a better understanding of their illness and treatment options. Having such information can empower patients in discussing treatment with providers and in fact alter the balance of power in the provider-patient relationship.

- Electronic Medical Records (EMRs)

Although there is not a consensus about the definition (Jha et al., 2008), EMRs can reduce various types of errors through clinical decision support functions. Important features of modern EMRs include drug-drug and drug-food interaction checks, allergy checks, standard drug dosage, patient education information, recurring alerts, track referrals and test results. The more sophisticated EMRs support reliability because they provide clinical decision support functions, particularly the capacity to encourage adherence to guidelines in diagnosis, treatment, and prescribing.

- Pre-Visit Intake

These applications allow patients to do a self-assessment and build a health profile for presentation to their physician. The tools guide patients through an "interview" to gather a comprehensive medical history and contribute to the accuracy and completeness of the patient history.

- Inter-Hospital Data Sharing

Central to these schemes is the capacity for remote access to hospital clinical data, from departmental systems (laboratory, radiology, etc.) or from a central clinical data repository. The technologies are either Internet-based or rely upon secure dial-up connections and increase efficiency in various ways. Patient data are available more quickly than is possible when reliant on access to copies of paper records; data on a patient may actually be accessible to a referral center before the patient arrives.

- Information for Physicians to Manage Patient Populations

These technologies assist providers in tracking and managing populations of patients, according to clinical practice guidelines. The most advanced approaches incorporate the population management application into an EMR. They assist with the patient population management tracking anticipated needs of patients and systematize the approach to the tracking and care of substantial numbers of patients.

- Patient-Physician Electronic Messaging

Electronic message exchange between patient and physician can occur in diverse circumstances and through a variety of technology applications. The asynchronous nature of electronic messaging allows patients and physicians to easily contact each other, while its self-limited nature of electronic messaging helps control the scope of the exchange. Patients appreciate the improved access to the physician and physicians the improved efficiency. Electronic messaging is a self-documenting improvement over the phone contact (Anand et al., 2005; Car & Sheikh, 2004; Kleiner et al., 2002; Leong et al., 2005; Stalberg et al., 2008).

- Patient Access to Tailored Medical Information, Online Data Entry, and Tracking

These applications address patients' medical condition in the context of their personal clinical data. They include online "disease management" applications, use online data-entry and the results can be made accessible to physicians to assist them in patient monitoring. These technologies support patient self-care as well as provider monitoring and support of care between office visits.

- Online Scheduling

Online Scheduling provides patients the means to connect with a practice over the Internet and schedule appointments. In most instances, practices manage online scheduling by accepting patient requests for appointment times. The practice administrator then examines the schedule and responds to the request with a confirmation. The technology improves the physician-patient relationship by facilitating access to care, reducing the duration and inconvenience of the standard appointment scheduling process.

- Computer-Assisted Telephone Triage and Assistance

Various models of call center technology improve communications between patients and their caregivers. The staff of the most advanced centers includes trained customer service representatives (CSRs) and advice nurses. The latter are competent to provide a range of service, including appointment booking, prescription refills, dispensing medical advice (guided by protocols), and provider messaging. Computer-telephony integration assist CSRs and advice nurses, while online advice protocols, appointment guidelines, scheduling and registration systems are also accessible to assist the patient. They represent a more expedient form of communication with the provider.

- Online Access to Provider Performance Data

Governments, regulatory bodies, and private companies offer free online access to physician and hospital performance or quality data.

Further evidence about people-centered care and e-health we can find in patient-focused interventions. The advancement of information technology provided alternative methods for making health information accessible to consumers. Through the Internet, patients receive health information, advice, and form virtual health communities and advocacy groups. Research shows an improvement of health awareness and high user satisfaction, evidence of greater benefit for under-served people and beneficial impact on health behavior (Gaston et al., 2005; Murray et al., 2005; Santo et al., 2005; Wofford et al., 2005). Moreover, low literacy initiatives include interactive computer systems but show disparate results for knowledge and comprehension; some evidence of improved satisfaction; no change in the rates of utilization, and some evidence of improved health-care behaviors (Gerber et al., 2005; Griffiths et al., 2005; Harmsen et al., 2005;

Holmes-Rovner et al., 2005). The mass media reach sizeable sections of the population through interactive mass media applications. The evidence shows effectiveness in awareness raising and some impact on utilization (Marcus & Crane, 1998; Sowden & Arblaster, 2000; Grilli et al., 2002; Black et al., 2002; Stone et al., 2002). Patient decision aids (O'Connor et al., 2004) use computer programs, interactive videos, and websites. Their effects include increased uptake of screening and some improvement of health status (Briss et al., 2004; Evans et al., 2005). Computer-based self-management education shows improved knowledge, enhanced social support, reduced therapist time, and improved health behavior and outcomes (Kaltenhaler et al., 2002; Murray et al., 2004). Moreover, technological developments are enabling patients to have greater involvement and autonomy in care. This includes devices for home self-monitoring of health status, and diagnostic kits for self-testing. However, the health outcomes of self-monitoring are at least equivalent to regular care (Coster et al., 2000; Fitzmaurice et al., 2002; Fahey et al., 2006; Siebenhofer et al., 2003; Cappuccio et al., 2004; Farmer et al., 2005; McManus et al., 2005; Welschen et al., 2005; Heneghan et al., 2006; Jansen, 2006). Facilitating patient access to personal medical information improves patient involvement (Drury et al., 2000; Warner et al., 2000; Williams et al., 2001; Cornbleet et al., 2002; Lecouturier et al., 2002; Currell & Urquhart, 2003; Lester et al., 2003; Scott et al., 2003; Brown & Smith, 2004; Koh et al., 2005; Liddell et al., 2004; Ross et al., 2004). New communication technologies are creating alternative means for the delivery of health information and advice, which may help to reduce the demand for face-to-face consultations in general practice, acute care, accident, and emergency(). Among various telemedicine applications, digital imaging technology can remotely link patients and health professionals for the purpose of distance consultations. Replacing the conventional face-to-face consultation are two alternative methods of tele-consultation: (1) asynchronous consultations using store-and-forward technology (2) real-time consultations using videoconferencing facilities.

Health Professionals-Health Authorities Support

Furukawa, Raghu, Spaulding, and Vinze (2008) classified health information technology (HIT) applications as prescribing, dispensing and administrative. Prescribing applications included: (1) electronic medical records (EMR) (2) clinical decision support (CDS) (3) computerized physician order entry (CPOE). Dispensing applications included: (1) bar-coding at medication dispensing (BarD) (2) robot for medication dispensing (ROBOT) (3) automated dispensing machines (ADM). Administrative applications included: (1) medication administration records (EMAR) (2) bar-coding at medication administration (BarA) (3) electronic Health Record (EHR) (4) computerized provider (physician) order entry (CPOE).

Clinical decision support systems (CDSS) are intelligent systems, which assist healthcare professionals with decision making tasks. Knowledge-based CDSS consist of the knowledge base, the inference engine, and the communication mechanism, while non-knowledge-based CDSS have the capacity to learn. CDSS could run with an electronic patient record or alert clinical data show significant changes in a patient's condition. The benefits from CDSS are reduction in medication errors, change of prescribing behavior, compliance with clinical guidelines and pathways, and time released for patient care (Kawamoto et al., 2005; Berner et al., 2007). Automated dispensing machines (ADMs) support the logistic systems(Colen et al., 2006) and may stand alone or be integrated within decentralized machines. In addition, to electronic prescribing, a bar code scheme prevents a quarter of medication errors (IOM, 2006; Poon et al., 2006) but bar coding in medication administration creates new paths for adverse events (Patterson et al., 2002).Computerized provider order entry (CPOE) can reduce medication errors and adverse events but can also be the cause of error as there is evidence that it may contribute to some types of adverse events and medical errors (Campbell et al., 2007, Bradley; Steltenkamp, & Hite, 2006; Bates, 2005a; Bates, Leape, Cullen, & Laird, 1998; Bates; 2005b; Koppel et al., 2005). These reported adverse events raised the terms of technological iatrogenesis (Palmieri, 2007) and e-iatrogenic (Weiner, 2007) with the first to describe the process and the second the individual error. Sources for these errors include prescriber and staff inexperience, shortcuts or default selections and interaction of work flow by irrelevant or frequent warnings.

The Commission of the European Communities (2004) argued that e-health tools and applications can provide access to electronic health records, support diagnosis by non-invasive systems, assist surgeons in planning clinical interventions, and radiologists access images at any place. Moreover, it can serve not only health practitioners but also all the employees employed in the health sector, and contribute to a safer working environment. E-health systems can also empower managers by spreading leading practices and helping to limit inefficient and inappropriate treatment. Most importantly, e-health clearly holds potential for improving the quality of care and developing of clinical-effectiveness research. As the cost of health care services escalates, clinical-effectiveness research can help stakeholders make cost-effective clinical and coverage decisions (Davenport, 2007). A really compelling argument for promoting the adoption of e-health is its promise in improving healthcare processes.

One of the advantages of pairing process improvement and adoption of e-health is that this partnership sidesteps the risk that we will simply digitize inefficient processes of care (Davenport, 2007). Value maximization and waste elimination involves identification of the value stream, and elimination of non-value-added steps (IHI, 2005). If the U.S. properly implements e-health will enjoy (RAND, 2006):

- Efficiency savings amounting to $77 billion or more annually
- Double savings from health and safety benefits

Finally, Chaudhry, Wang, Wu, Maglione, Mojica, Roth, Morton, and Shekelle (2006) demonstrated the efficacy of health information technologies in improving quality and efficiency.

FUTURE RESEARCH DIRECTIONS

The evidence review demonstrates that there are substantial gaps in what we know about the relationship of people-centered care and e-health. Therefore, there is a need for continued research of possible e-health interventions in the following areas of people-centered care:

- The effect of interventions for improving health information quality
- The barriers of shared decision-making and the strategies on overcoming them
- The cost-effectiveness of self-care interventions
- The feasibility of self-care interventions in standard care
- The efforts on training patients to develop practical skills and the self-confidence for managing their health problems
- The ways in which we can enhance the safety improvement through patient involvement
- The factors, which influence patients' willingness and ability to be involved in the safety of their care
- The issues and settings where patient involvement is most achievable
- The patients' experience and views of medical errors/adverse events

- The effectiveness of current patient-focused initiatives for safety improvement
- The barriers to patient-focused patient safety initiatives
- The organizational changes, which will create a patient-oriented patient safety culture
- The most effective techniques in encouraging and supporting patients to openly raise safety concerns
- The evaluation of walk-in centers and specialist outreach clinics
- The impact of patient-focused access interventions on regional health economies
- The impact of patient feedback, provider choice, complaints, and advocacy systems

On the other hand, new medical technologies and the tendency towards technological convergence are blurring the traditional demarcation between regulatory frameworks. Therefore, we have to impose new regulations to ensure patient safety (Cerchiari, 2007), promote commitment and leadership of health authorities for the e-health implementation and enable interoperability of e-health systems.

CONCLUSION

E-health has a great potential to empower citizens, patients, and healthcare professionals. It can also offer governments a way to cope with increasing demand for healthcare services, and reshape the expectations of health care delivery, making it people-centered. We might not realize how to plan in detail our course, but we know the coordinates of this goal and some of the landmarks along the route.

REFERENCES

Agency for Healthcare Research and Quality and National Institute of Mental Health. (2001). *Patient-centered care: customizing care to meet patients' needs*. Retrieved April 24, 2009, from http://grants.nih.gov/grants/guide/pa-files/PA-01-124.html.

Anand, S., Feldman, M., Geller, D., Bisbee, A., & Bauchner, H. (2005). A content analysis of e-mail communication between primary care providers and parents. *Pediatrics*, *115*, 1283–1288. doi:10.1542/peds.2004-1297

Bates, D. (2005a). Computerized Physician Order entry and medication errors: finding a balance. *Journal of Biomedical Informatics*, *38*(4), 250–261. doi:10.1016/j.jbi.2005.05.003

Bates, D. W. (2005b). Physicians and ambulatory electronic health records. *Health Affairs*, *24*(5), 1180–1189. doi:10.1377/hlthaff.24.5.1180

Bates, D. W., Leape, L. L., Cullen, D. J., & Laird, N. (1998). Effect of computerized physician order entry and a team intervention on prevention of serious medical errors. *Journal of the American Medical Association*, *280*, 1311–1316. doi:10.1001/jama.280.15.1311

Berner, E. (Ed.). (2007). *Clinical Decision Support Systems: Theory & Practice*. New York, NY: Springer. doi:10.1007/978-0-387-38319-4

Billings, J. (2004). Promoting the dissemination of decision aids: an odyssey in a dysfunctional health care financing system. *Health Affairs*, (Supplement Web Exclusive), 128–132.

Black, M. E., Yamada, J., & Mann, V. (2002). A systematic literature review of the effectiveness of community-based strategies to increase cervical cancer screening. *Canadian Journal of Public Health*, *93*(5), 386–393.

Blumenthal, D., & Glaser, J. (2007). Information Technology Comes to Medicine. *The New England Journal of Medicine, 356*(24), 2527–2534. doi:10.1056/NEJMhpr066212

Bradley, V. M., Steltenkamp, C. L., & Hite, K. B. (2006). Evaluation of reported medication errors before and after implementation of computerized practitioner order entry. *Journal of Healthcare Information Management, 20*(4), 46–53.

Briss, P, Rimer, B, Reilley, B, Coates, RC, Lee, NC, Mullen, P, Corso, P, Hutchinson, AB, Hiatt, R, Kerner, J, George, P, White, C, Gandhi, N, Saraiya, M, Breslow, R, Isham, G, Teutsch, SM, Hinman, AR, & Lawrence, R, & Task Force on Community Preventive Services. (2004). Promoting informed decisions about cancer screening in communities and healthcare systems. *American Journal of Preventive Medicine, 26*(1), 67–80. doi:10.1016/j.amepre.2003.09.012

Brown, H. C., & Smith, H. J. (2004). Giving women their own case notes to carry during pregnancy. *Cochrane Database of Systematic Reviews, CD002856*(2). doi:10.1002/14651858.CD002856.pub2

Campbell, H. S., Phaneuf, M. R., & Deane, K. (2004). Cancer peer support programs - do they work? *Patient Education and Counseling, 55*, 3–15. doi:10.1016/j.pec.2003.10.001

Cappuccio, F. P., Kerry, S. M., Forbes, L., & Donald, A. (2004). Blood pressure control by home monitoring: metaanalysis of randomised trials. *British Medical Journal, 329*(7458), 145. doi:10.1136/bmj.38121.684410.AE

Car, J., & Sheikh, A. (2004). Email consultations in health care: 2—acceptability and safe application. *British Medical Journal, 329*, 439–442. doi:10.1136/bmj.329.7463.439

Cerchiairi, D. (2007). Revolutionising patient care – medical technology of the future. Thought-provoking ideas for policymaking. In Health First Europe (Ed), *2050: A Health Odyssey* (pp. 24-27). Brussels: Health First Europe.

Chaudhry, B., Wang, J., Wu, S., Maglione, M., Mojica, W., & Roth, E. (2006). Systematic Review: Impact of Health Information Technology on Quality, Efficiency, and Costs of Medical Care. *Annals of Internal Medicine, 144*, E12–W18.

Colen, H., Neuenschwander, M., Neef, C., Krabbendam, K. (2006). Using Automated Dispensing Machines to improve medication safety. *Journal of the European Association of Hospital Pharmacists, 12*(5), 71-73-1.

Commission of the European Communities. (2004). e-Health - making healthcare better for European citizens: An action plan for a European e-Health Area. Brussels: Commission of the European Communities.

Cornbleet, MA, Campbell, P, Murray, S, Stevenson, M, & Bond, S, & Joint Working Party of the Scottish Partnership Agency for Palliative and Cancer Care and National Council for Hospice and Specialist Palliative Care Services. (2002). Patient-held records in cancer and palliative care: a randomized, prospective trial. *Palliative Medicine, 16*(3), 205–212. doi:10.1191/0269216302pm541oa

Coster, S., Gulliford, M. C., Seed, P. T., Powrie, J. K., & Swaminathan, R. (2000). Monitoring blood glucose control in diabetes mellitus: a systematic review. *Health Technology Assessment, 4*(12).

Coulter, A., & Ellins, J. (2006). *Patient-focused interventions: A review of the evidence*. London: The Health Foundation.

Cronin, C. (2004). *Patient-Centered Care: An overview of Definitions and Concepts*. Washington, DC: National Health Council.

Currell, R., & Urquhart, C. (2003). Nursing record systems: effects on nursing practice and health care outcomes. *Cochrane Database of Systematic Reviews, CD002099*(3). doi:10.1002/14651858.CD002099

Davenport, K. (2007). Navigating American Health Care: How Information Technology Can Foster Health Care Improvement. Center for American Progress, Retrieved April 24, 2009, from www. americanprogress.com

Donelly, L., & Shaw, R., & van der Akker. (2008). eHealth as a challenge to 'expert' power: a focus group study of internet use for health information and management. *Journal of the Royal Society of Medicine, 101*, 501-506. Drury, M., Yudkin, P., Harcourt, J., Fitzpatrick, R., Jones, L., Alcock, C. & Minton, M. (2000). Patients with cancer holding their own records: a randomised controlled trial. *The British Journal of General Practice, 50*(451), 105–110.

Evans, R., Edwards, A., Brett, J., Bradburn, M., Watson, E., Austoker, J., & Elwyn, G. (2005). Reduction in uptake of PSA tests following decision aids: systematic review of current aids and their evaluations. *Patient Education and Counseling, 58*(1), 13–26. doi:10.1016/j.pec.2004.06.009

Eysenbach, G. (2001). What is e-health? *Journal of Medical Internet Research, 3*(2), e20. doi:10.2196/jmir.3.2.e20

Fahey, T., Schroeder, K., Ebrahim, S., & Glynn, L.(2006). Interventions used to improve control of blood pressure in patients with hypertension. *Cochrane.Database.of SystematicReviews*, CD005182 (1).

Farmer, A., Gibson, OJ., Tarassenko, L., & Neil A. (2005). A systematic review of telemedicine interventions to support blood glucose self-monitoring in diabetes. *Diabetic medicine:A journal of the British Diabetic Association, 22* (10), 1372-1378.

Ferlie, E., Pettigre, A., Ashburner, L., & Fitzgerald, L. (1996). *The New Public Management in Action*. Oxford: Oxford University Press.

Fitzmaurice, D., Murray, E., Gee, K., Allan, T., & Hobbs, F. (2002). A randomised controlled trial of patient self management of oral anticoagulation treatment compared with primary care management. *Journal of Clinical Pathology, 55*(11), 845–849. doi:10.1136/jcp.55.11.845

Furukawa, M. F., Raghu, T. S., Spaulding, T. J., & Vinze, A. (2008). Adoption of Health Information Technology for Medication Safety in U.S. Hospitals, 2006. *Health Affairs, 27*(3), 865–875. doi:10.1377/hlthaff.27.3.865

Gaston, C. M., & Mitchell, G. (2005). Information giving and decision-making in patients with advanced cancer: A systematic review. *Social Science & Medicine, 61*(10), 2252–2264. doi:10.1016/j.socscimed.2005.04.015

Gerber, B. S., Brodsky, I. G., Lawless, K. A., Smolin, L. I., Arozullah, A. M., & Smith, E. V. (2005). Implementation and evaluation of a low-literacy diabetes education computer multimedia application. *Diabetes Care, 28*(7), 1574–1580. doi:10.2337/diacare.28.7.1574

Graham, I. D., Logan, J., O'Connor, A., Weeks, K. E., Aaron, S., & Cranney, A. (2003). A qualitative study of physicians' perceptions of three decision aids. *Patient Education and Counseling, 50*, 279–283. doi:10.1016/S0738-3991(03)00050-8

Griffiths, C., Motlib, J., Azad, A., Ramsay, J., Eldridge, S., & Feder, G. (2005). Randomised controlled trial of a lay-led self-management programme for Bangladeshi patients with chronic disease. *The British Journal of General Practice, 55*, 831–837.

Grilli, R., Ramsay, C., & Minozzi, S. (2002). Mass media interventions: effects on health services utilisation. *Cochrane.Database.of Systematic Reviews*, CD000389 (1).

Grin, O. W. (1994). Patient-centered care: Empowering Patients to Achieve Real Health Care Reform. *Michigan Medicine*, *93*, 25–29.

Groene, O., Lombarts, M., Klazinga, N., Alonso, J., Thompson, A., & Sunol, M. (2009). Is patient-centredness in European hospitals related to existing quality improvement strategies? Analysis of a cross-sectional survey (MARQuIS study). *Quality & Safety in Health Care*, *18*(Supplement I), i44–i50. doi:10.1136/qshc.2008.029397

Halamka, J. D., Mandl, K. D., & Tang, P. C. (2008). Early experiences with personal health records. *Journal of the American Medical Informatics Association*, *15*(1), 1–7. doi:10.1197/jamia.M2562

Harmsen, H., Bernsen, R., Meeuwesen, L., Thomas, S., Dorrenboom, G., Pinto, D., & Bruijnzeels, M. (2005). The effect of educational intervention on intercultural communication: results of a randomised controlled trial. *The British Journal of General Practice*, *55*(514), 343–350.

Healthcare, R. A. N. D. (2006). *Health Information Technology: Can HIT Lower Costs and Improve Quality?*Santa Monica, CA: RAND Corporation.

Heneghan, C. J., Glasziou, P. P., & Perera, R. (2006). Reminder packaging for improving adherence to self-administered long-term medications. *Cochrane Database of Systematic Reviews, (1),* CD005025. Hess, R., Bryce, C., Paone, S., Fischer, G., McTigue, K., Olshansky, E., Zickmund, S., Fitzgerald, K., & Siminerio, L. (2007). Exploring challenges and potentials of personal health records in diabetes self-management: implementation and initial assessment. *Telemedicine and e-health, 13* (5), 509–18. Holmes-Rovner, M., Stableford, S., Fagerlin, A., Wei, J., Dunn, R., Ohene-Frempong, J., Blake, K., & Rovner, D. (2005). Evidence-based patient choice: a prostate cancer decision aid in plain language. *BMC Medical Informatics and Decision Making*, *5*(1), 16.

Institute for Health Improvement. (2005). *Going Lean in Health Care*. Cambridge, MA: Institute for Health Improvement.

Institute of Medicine. (2001). *Crossing the Quality Chasm: A new health system for the 21st century*. Washington, DC: National Academy Press.

Institute of Medicine. (2006). *Preventing Medication Errors*. Washington, DC: The National Academies Press.

International Alliance of Patients' Organizations. (2007). *What is Patient-Centred Healthcare? A Review of Definitions and Principles*. London: International Alliance of Patients' Organizations.

Jansen, J. P. (2006). Self-monitoring of glucose in type 2 diabetes mellitus: a Bayesian meta-analysis of direct and indirect comparisons. *Current Medical Research and Opinion*, *22*(4), 671–681. doi:10.1185/030079906X96308

Jha, A. K., Doolan, D., Grandt, D., Scott, T., & Bates, D. W. (2008). The use of health information technology in seven nations. *International Journal of Medical Informatics*, *77*(12), 848–854. doi:10.1016/j.ijmedinf.2008.06.007

Johnston, C. L., & Cooper, P. K. (1997). Patient-Focused Care. What is it? *Holistic Nursing Practice*, *11*, 1–7.

Kaltenthaler, E., Shackley, P., Stevens, K., Beverley, C., Parry, G., & Chilcott, J. (2002). A systematic review and economic evaluation of computerised cognitive behaviour therapy for depression and anxiety. *Health Technology Assessment*, *6*(22), 1–89.

Kawamoto, K., Houlihan, C., Andrew Balas, E., & Lobach, D. (2005). Improving clinical practice using clinical decision support systems: a systematic review of trials to identify features critical to success. *British Medical Journal*, *330*, 765. doi:10.1136/bmj.38398.500764.8F

Kilbridge, P. (2002). *Crossing the Chasm with Information Technology: Bridging the Quality Gap in Health Care*. CA: California HealthCare Foundation.

Kleiner, K., Akers, R., Burke, B., & Werner, E. (2002). Parent and Physician Attitudes Regarding Electronic Communication in Pediatric Practices. *Pediatrics*, *109*, 740–744. doi:10.1542/peds.109.5.740

Koh, G., Budge, D., Butow, P., Renison, B., & Woodgate, P. G. (2005). Audio recordings of consultations with doctors for parents of critically sick babies. *Cochrane Database of Systematic Reviews*, (1): CD004502.

Koppel, R., Metlay, J., Cohen, A., Abaluck, B., Russell Localio, A., Kimmel, S., & Strom, B. (2005). Role of Computerized Physician Order Entry Systems in Facilitating Medication Errors. *Journal of the American Medical Association*, *293*(10), 1197–1203. doi:10.1001/jama.293.10.1197

Kupchunas, W. R. (2007). Personal health record: new opportunity for patient education. *Orthopedic Nursing*, *26*(3), 185–191. doi:10.1097/01.NOR.0000276971.86937.c4

Laine, C., & Davidoff, F. (1996). Patient-centered medicine. A professional evolution. *Journal of the American Medical Association*, *275*(2), 152–156. doi:10.1001/jama.275.2.152

Lecouturier, J., Crack, L., Mannix, K., Hall, R. H., & Bond, S. (2002). Evaluation of a patient-held record for patients with cancer. *European Journal of Cancer Care*, *11*(2), 114–121. doi:10.1046/j.1365-2354.2002.00301.x

Lee, M., Delaney, C., & Moorhead, S. (2007). Building a personal health record from a nursing perspective. *International Journal of Medical Informatics*, *76*(Supplement 2), S308–S316. doi:10.1016/j.ijmedinf.2007.05.010

Leong, S., Gingrich, D., Lewis, P., Mauger, D., & George, J. (2005). Enhancing Doctor-Patient Communication Using Email: A Pilot Study. *The Journal of the American Board of Family Practice*, *18*(3), 180–188. doi:10.3122/jabfm.18.3.180

Lester, H., Allan, T., Wilson, S., Jowett, S., & Roberts, L. (2003). A cluster randomised controlled trial of patient-held medical records for people with schizophrenia receiving shared care. *The British Journal of General Practice*, *53*(488), 197–203.

Lewin, S. A., Skea, Z. C., Entwistle, V., Zwarenstein, M., & Dick, J. (2001). Interventions for providers to promote a patient-centred approach in clinical consultations. *Cochrane Database of Systematic Reviews*, (4): CD003267.

Lewis, F., & Batey, M. (1982). Clarifying autonomy and accountability. Part 2. *The Journal of Nursing Administration*, 10–15.

Liddell, C., Brown, T., Johnston, D., Coates, V., & Mallett, J. (2004). Giving patients an audiotape of their GP consultation: a randomised controlled trial. *The British Journal of General Practice*, *54*(506), 667–672.

Mallett, J. (1996). Sense of Direction. *Nursing Times*, *92*, 40–42.

Mander, R. (1995). Where does the buck stop? In Watson, R. (Ed.), *Accountability in midwifery* (pp. 95–106). London: Chapman and Hall.

Marcus, A. C., & Crane, L. A. (1998). A review of cervical cancer screening intervention research: implications for public health programs and future research. *Preventive Medicine*, *27*(1), 13–31. doi:10.1006/pmed.1997.0251

McManus, R. J., Mant, J., Roalfe, A., Oakes, R. A., Bryan, S., Pattison, H. M., & Hobbs, F. D. (2005). Targets and self monitoring in hypertension: randomised controlled trial and cost effectiveness analysis. *British Medical Journal*, *331*(7515), 493. doi:10.1136/bmj.38558.393669.E0

McSherry, R., & Pearce, P. (Eds.). (2002). *Clinical Governance: A Guide to Implementation for Health Care Professionals*. Oxford: Blackwell Science.

Mead, N., & Bower, P. (2002). Patient-centred consultations and outcomes in primary care: a review of the literature. *Patient Education and Counseling*, *48*, 51–61. doi:10.1016/S0738-3991(02)00099-X

Morales Rodriguez, M., Casper, G., & Brennan, P. F. (2007). Patient-centered design. The potential of user-centered design in personal health records. *Journal of American Health Information Management Association*, *78*(4), 44–46.

Murray, E., Burns, J., See Tai, S., Lai, R., & Nazareth, I. (2005). Interactive Health Communication Applications for people with chronic disease. *Cochrane Database of Systematic Reviews*, CD004274 (4).

Murray, E., Fitzmaurice, D., McCahon, D., Fuller, C., & Sandhur, H. (2004). Training for patients in a randomised controlled trial of self management of warfarin treatment. *British Medical Journal*, *328*(7437), 437–438. doi:10.1136/bmj.328.7437.437

Nelson, R. (2007). The personal health record. *American Journal of Nursing, 107 (9),* 27–8. O'Connor, A., Llewellyn-Thomas, H., & Barry Flood, A. (2004). Modifying unwarranted variations in health care: shared decision making using patient decision aids. *Health Affairs (Project Hope)*, (Supplement Web Exclusive), VAR63–VAR72.

Pagliari, C., Detmer, D., & Singleton, P. (2007). Potential of electronic personal health records. *British Medical Journal*, *335*(7615), 330–333. doi:10.1136/bmj.39279.482963.AD

Palmieri, P., Peterson, L., & Ford, E. (2007). Technological iatrogenesis: New risks force heightened management awareness. *Journal of Healthcare Risk Management*, *27*(4), 19–24. doi:10.1002/jhrm.5600270405

Patterson, E. S., Cook, R. I., & Render, M. L. (2002). Improving patient safety by identifying side effects from introducing bar coding in medication administration. *Journal of the American Medical Informatics Association*, *9*(5), 540–553. doi:10.1197/jamia.M1061

Picker Institute. (2004). *Patient-Centered Care 2015: Scenarios, Vision, Goals & Next Steps*. Camden, Maine: The Picker Institute.

Poon, E. G., Cina, J. L., Churchill, W., Patel, N., Featherstone, E., & Rothschild, J. M. (2006). Medication dispensing errors and potential adverse drug events before and after implementing bar code technology in the pharmacy. *Annals of Internal Medicine*, *145*(6), 426–434.

Richardson, R., Schug, S., Bywater, M., & Lloyd-Williams, D. (2004). *Development of eHealth in Europe: Position Paper*. Brussels: European Health Telematics Association.

Ross, S. E., Moore, L. A., Earnest, M. A., Wittevrongel, L., & Lin, C. T. (2004). Providing a web-based online medical record with electronic communication capabilities to patients with congestive heart failure: randomized trial. *Journal of Medical Internet Research*, *6*(2), e12. doi:10.2196/jmir.6.2.e12

Rossi Mori, A. (2008*). eHealth deployment roadmap and roll-out planning: Guiding design principles*. Paper presented at the eHealth Planning and Management Symposium, Copenhagen, Denmark.

Santo, A., Laizner, A. M., & Shohet, L. (2005). Exploring the value of audiotapes for health literacy: a systematic review. *Patient Education and Counseling*, *58*(3), 235–243. doi:10.1016/j.pec.2004.07.001

Savage, J., & Morre, L. (2004). *Intrpreting Accountability: An ethnographic study of practice nurses, accountability and multidisciplinary team decision-making in the context of clinical governance*. London: RCN Institute.

Scott, J. T., Harmsen, M., Prictor, M. J., Entwistle, V. A., Sowden, A. J., & Watt, I. (2003). Recordings or summaries of consultations for people with cancer. *Cochrane. Database.of Systematic Reviews*, *2*, CD001539.

Siebenhofer, A., Berghold, A., & Sawicki, P. T. (2004). Systematic review of studies of self-management of oral anticoagulation. *Thrombosis and Haemostasis, 91* (2), 225-232. Smith, SP., Barefield, AC. (2007). Patients meet technology: the newest in patient-centered care initiatives. *The Health Care Manager*, *26*(4), 354–362.

Sowden, A. J., & Arblaster, L. (2000). Mass media interventions for preventing smoking in young people. *Cochrane.Database.ofSystematic. Reviews*, *2*, CD001006.

Stalberg, P., Yeh, M., Ketteridge, G., Delbridge, H., & Delbridge, L. (2008). E-mail Access and Improved Communication Between Patient and Surgeon. *Archives of Surgery*, *143*(2), 164–169. doi:10.1001/archsurg.2007.31

Stone, E. G., Morton, S. C., Hulscher, M. E., Maglione, M. A., Roth, E. A., & Grimshaw, J. M. (2002). Interventions that increase use of adult immunization and cancer screening services: a meta-analysis. *Annals of Internal Medicine*, *136*(9), 641–651.

The National Alliance for Health Information Technology. (2008). *Defining Key Health Information Technology Terms*. Washington, DC: Department of Health & Human Services.

Thompson, A. (2004). Moving beyond the rhetoric of citizen involvement: Strategies for enablement. *Eurohealth*, *9*(4), 5–8.

Tingle, J. (1995). The legal accountability of the nurse . In Watson, R. (Ed.), *Accountability in Nursing Practice* (pp. 163–176). London: Chapman and Hall.

Warner, J. P., King, M., Blizard, R., McClenahan, Z., & Tang, S. (2000). Patient-held shared care records for individuals with mental illness. Randomised controlled evaluation. *The British Journal of Psychiatry*, *177*, 319–324. doi:10.1192/bjp.177.4.319

Weiner, J., Kfuri, T., Chan, K., & Fowles, J. (2007). "e-Iatrogenesis": The Most Critical Unintended Consequence of CPOE and other HIT. *Journal of the American Medical Informatics Association*, *14*(3), 387–388. doi:10.1197/jamia.M2338

Welschen, L. M., Bloemendal, E., Nijpels, G., Dekker, J. M., Heine, R. J., Stalman, W. A., & Bouter, L. M. (2005). Self-monitoring of blood glucose in patients with type 2 diabetes who are not using insulin. *Cochrane.Database.of Systematic.Reviews,* (2), CD005060.

Williams, J., Cheung, W., Chetwynd, N., Cohen, D., El-Sharkawi, S., & Finlay, I. (2001). Pragmatic randomised trial to evaluate the use of patient held records for the continuing care of patients with cancer. *Quality in Health Care*, *10*(3), 159–165. doi:10.1136/qhc.0100159..

Wilson, P. (2005). *E-health - Building on Strength to Provide Better Healthcare Anytime Anywhere.* Paper presented at the eHealth 2005 Conference, Tromsø, Norway.

Wofford, J., Smith, E., & Miller, D. (2005). The multimedia computer for office-based patient education: a systematic review. *Patient Education and Counseling*, *59*(2), 148–157. doi:10.1016/j.pec.2004.10.011

World Health Organization. (2007). *People-Centred Health Care: A Policy Framework.* Geneva: World Health Organization.

ADDITIONAL READING

Chen, C., Garrido, T., Chock, D., Okawa, G., & Liang, L. (2009). The Kaiser Permanente Electronic Health Record: Transforming and Streamlining Modalities of Care . *Health Affairs (Project Hope)*, *28*, 323–333. doi:10.1377/hlthaff.28.2.323

Dentzer, S. (2009). Health Information Technology: On The Fast Track At Last? *Health Affairs (Project Hope)*, *28*, 320–321. doi:10.1377/hlthaff.28.2.320

Frampton, S., & Charmel, P. (2009). *Putting Patients First: Best Practices in Patient-Centered Care*. San Francisco: Jossey-Bass.

Frisse, M. (2009). Health Information Technology: One Step at a Time. *Health Affairs (Project Hope)*, *28*, 379–384. doi:10.1377/hlthaff.28.2.w379

Gerber, T. (2009). Health Information Technology: Dispatches from the Revolution . *Health Affairs (Project Hope)*, *28*, 390–391. doi:10.1377/hlthaff.28.2.w390

Grossman, J., Zayas-Cabán, T., & Kemper, N. (2009). Information Gap: Can Health Insurer Personal Health Records Meet Patients' and Physicians' Needs? *Health Affairs (Project Hope)*, *28*, 377–389. doi:10.1377/hlthaff.28.2.377

Halamka, J. (2009). Making Smart Investments In Health Information Technology: Core Principles. *Health Affairs (Project Hope)*, *28*, 385–389. doi:10.1377/hlthaff.28.2.w385

Hillestad, R., Bigelow, J., Bower, A., Girosi, F., Meili, R., Scoville, R., & Taylor, R. (2009). Can Electronic Medical Record Systems Transform Health Care? Potential Health Benefits, Savings, and Costs. *Health Affairs (Project Hope)*, *24*, 1103–1117. doi:10.1377/hlthaff.24.5.1103

Kahn, J., Aulakh, V., & Bosworth, A. (2009). What It Takes: Characteristics Of The Ideal Personal Health Record. *Health Affairs (Project Hope)*, *28*, 369–376. doi:10.1377/hlthaff.28.2.369

Miller, R., & Sim, I. (2004). Physicians' Use of Electronic Medical Records: Barriers and Solutions. *Health Affairs (Project Hope)*, *23*, 116–126. doi:10.1377/hlthaff.23.2.116

Mostashari, F., Tripathi, M., & Kendall, M. (2009). A Tale of Two Large Community Electronic Health Record Extension Projects. *Health Affairs (Project Hope)*, *28*, 345–356. doi:10.1377/hlthaff.28.2.345

Parente, S., & McCullough, J. (2009). Health Information Technology and Patient Safety: Evidence From Panel Data. *Health Affairs (Project Hope)*, *28*, 357–360. doi:10.1377/hlthaff.28.2.357

Chapter 6
ISO 15189:2007: Implementation in a Laboratory Information System

Stavros Archondakis
401 Athens Army Hospital, Greece

Aliki Stathopoulou
Hellenic Accreditation System, Greece

Ioannis Sitaras
Hellenic Accreditation System, Greece

ABSTRACT

ISO 15189:2007 constitutes an international certification standard, based upon ISO/IEC 17025 and ISO 9001, which can be used by medical laboratories wishing to improve their quality standards. The requirements of this standard form a group of general guidelines that will help laboratories establish and enhance their quality systems. Although direct references to the use of computer systems are made in only 7 cases, through the mandatory section of the ISO 15189:2007, many more clauses of the standard include indirect references to electronic medical records handling. The chapter analyzes the guidelines concerning the use of laboratory information systems for medical records storage and retrieval. Furthermore, the authors discuss challenging difficulties that may be detected during implementation of ISO 15189:2007 in the field of electronic laboratory medical records.

INTRODUCTION

During the last decades, medical data deriving from the analysis of patient samples was stored in medical laboratories and was provided to physicians manually (Brerider-Jr-McNai, 1996). Manual processing of medical information during specimen collection, order entry, results entry and results reporting was presenting many significant problems with crucial impact to patient care. The absence of an integrated laboratory information system was making medical data transfer slow and possibly ineffective while results inquiry, quality control and results correction a time and money spending process (Kubono, 2004).

DOI: 10.4018/978-1-61692-843-8.ch006

Over the last years, informatics and computer sciences have changed dramatically the practice of clinical laboratory professionals. The wide implementation of laboratory information systems became a necessity dictated by the need of real-time results and the increasing role of laboratory medicine in therapeutic decisions (Georgiou & Westbrook, 2007).

Laboratory information systems have been implemented in many medical laboratories wishing to improve their quality standards. A laboratory information system (LIS) is a valuable tool for medical professionals in order to manage complex processes, ensure regulatory compliance, promote collaboration between departments of the same or different laboratories, deliver detailed reports, and develop the laboratory networking capabilities. The result is better data management and sharing between the laboratory and its clients (either laboratories or clinicians) (Brerider-Jr-McNai, 1996).

However, LIS implementation in the everyday laboratory workflow may present specific problems, concerning medical data storage, protection and retrieval, as well as improper use of hardware and software. Medical data stored in computer systems may be lost or changed by unauthorized personnel. Therefore, specific measures should be followed in order to protect the laboratory information system, and solve the problems that may be encountered (Brerider-Jr-McNai, 1996).

ISO 15189:2007 is a powerful tool for diminishing dramatically all unsuspected errors or problems that may be encountered during LIS use.ISO 15189:2007 requirements for laboratory information systems suggest the implementation of specific measures concerning environmental conditions, system security, data entry control, medical reports, data retrieval and storage, and finally system's hardware and software maintenance (Kubono, 2004).

The objective of the chapter is to emphasize on the necessity of adopting specific policies concerning electronic laboratory records storage and retrieval. Furthermore, we intend to discuss all challenging difficulties that may be detected during implementation of ISO 15189:2007 in the field of electronic laboratory medical records. Finally, we give clear and comprehensive guidance to all members of the medical community, wishing to overcome bureaucratic or technical problems in this field.

BACKGROUND

Laboratory automation has been propelled during the last 10 year by the advantages of greater productivity, lower cost and the capacity of integration with modern instrumental equipment, which connect to a laboratory intranet (Westbrook et al., 2008; Vacata et al., 2007). Laboratory information systems provide better functionality through automation in parts of the inspection procedures, permitting the lab to achieve maximum efficiency (Westbrook et al., 2008; Vacata et al, 2007). Laboratory information systems also improve service to physicians and other stakeholders and ultimately reduce the probability of human errors. It is widely accepted that error-prone activities can be substantially reduced, but not eliminated. However, information technology systems can provide reasonable, accurate, and reliable standardized procedures of quality control for the assessment procedure as well as sophisticated quality indices for all the control system of the medical laboratory (Westbrook et al., 2008; Vacata et al., 2007). Medical laboratory computers may be used in many ways. They may be used for preparing and administering the management handbook and standard operation procedures, for personnel training, for providing and archiving documents via intranet. The laboratory computers may also be used for creating customer databases, for evaluating test results, for connecting via the Internet with external sources of information and for contacting with customers, or as a typewriter. A computing system contains at least one computer, some peripheral devices and some software products. Moreover, computing systems operating parameters require custom verification and validation.

Verification is the confirmation that specified requirements have been fulfilled. Computing system monitoring, user acceptance testing, and code reviews are some verification tools. Validation is the confirmation that the requirements for the specific use are fulfilled. Electronic records contain any combination of digital data that is created, modified, archived, or distributed by a computer system. Electronic records must be protected from exposure to accidental or malicious alteration or destruction (record security).

Computing systems may be open or closed. In closed computing systems, individuals responsible for the content of the electronic records control access to medical archives. On the contrary, in open computing systems, people not responsible for the content of the electronic records (Vacata et al., 2007) control access to medical archives.

The computing systems software may be used for testing, calibration and sampling purposes (testing software) or for managing document control (document software) (Westbrook et al, 2008; Vacata et al., 2007). The integrity of electronic records must be checked periodically (file integrity check), while the computing system must be tested periodically in order to determine if it meets specific requirements (acceptance test). Finally, according to the European Federation of National Associations of Measurement (2006), the software of the laboratory computing system must be tested in such a way that the internal workings of the item being tested are known (white-box testing) or unknown by the tester (black-box testing).

The ISO 15189:2007 requirements cover all aspects of the laboratory activities, including the laboratory information system (LIS) (Vacata et al., 2007; Westbrook et al., 2008). Annex B of ISO 15189:2007 suggests specific measures for the protection of laboratory electronic records (Vacata et al., 2007; Westbrook et al., 2008). The essence of this annex is still informative, and the implementation of its requirements remains non-mandatory for the time being (Vacata et al., 2007; Westbrook et al., 2008). Still, the measures proposed in annex B of ISO 15189: 2007 comprise a valuable tool for quality improvement in the field of electronic documentation of medical records. It is worthwhile mentioning that the ISO 15189:2007 requirements do not apply to desk top calculators, small programmable technical computers, computers used only for word processing or spreadsheets by one single user, or microprocessors integrated in assessment instruments (Kubono, 2004; Westbrook et al., 2008).

THE IMPLEMENTATION OF ISO 15189:2007 IN LABORATORY INFORMATION SYSTEMS

The ISO 15189:2007 requirements for quality and competence concerning the electronic medical data constitute a set of general guidelines that will help each laboratory to establish and develop its quality system (Kubono, 2004; Kubono, 2007). The procedures that will eventually be implemented by each laboratory during the development of an acceptable quality system may differ according to its specific needs and limitations (Kubono, 2004; Kubono, 2007). Meanwhile, the efforts of the medical community continuously aim at the creation of a secure electronic environment for medical data management, storage, retrieval and updating as well as decision support and quality control mechanisms (Kubono, 2004; Kubono, 2007). Although direct references to the use of computer systems are made in only 7 cases, through the mandatory section of the ISO 15189:2007, many more clauses of the standard include indirect references to electronic medical records handling (Kubono, 2004; Kubono, 2007). According to clause 3.5, the capability of the laboratory is affected by the information resources available for the tests in question. Post-test procedures, such as authorization for release, reporting, and transmission of the results have a dramatic impact on laboratory quality improvement (clause 3.10). Therefore, specific policies and procedures must ensure the protection of confidential information (clause 4.1.5 c). Moreover, adequate laboratory personnel must be trained regarding the LIS (clause 4.1.5 g, and. adequate communication processes carried out by the LIS should be established (clauses 4.1.6 and 4.2.1). Written policies related to LIS should be described in the laboratory quality manual (clause 4.2.4 f, g, r, w), while controlled documents may be maintained in electronic media. Procedures and policies for controlling all types of documents should be defined. This definition might apply to a LIS for the controlling of documents as well (clause 4.3.1). Furthermore, specific procedures should be established for describing documents control and changes in computerized systems (clause 4.3.2 h).

Requirements referring to the selection of hardware, software and services for maintenance, troubleshooting, update, peripherals and consumables (for example storage devices) have to be documented (clause 4.6). Concerning LIS, the laboratory has to evaluate suppliers of critical equipment, consumables and services and maintain records for this evaluation and approval (clause 4.6). LIS should be able to halt results of nonconforming work, recall already released nonconforming tests, define the authority or the resumption of examinations, record and review root causes of non-conformity incidents (clauses 4.9, 4.10, 4.11). Systematic monitoring of the laboratory contribution to patient care through quality indicators should include the use of LIS (clause 4.12). In case the laboratory chooses to or has to (subject to legal requirements) implement electronic media for the storage of quality and technical data, its facilities have to be suitable in order to prevent loss, deterioration or unauthorized access (clause 4.13.2). LIS may be used for the maintenance of personnel records, while special care has to be taken for authorized access to records of exposure to occupational hazards and records of immunization status (clause 5.1.2). The confidentiality of information regarding patients has to be safeguarded also from external risks, coming from the LIS and its external communication (web, remote access and other options) (clause 5.1.13). Environmental conditions (temperature, electrical supply, electromagnetic interference, Wi-Fi should have to be taken into consideration in case of the existence of an integrated LIS system (clause 5.2.5). The use of the LIS for the implementation of internal communication as well as the efficiency of the message transfer has to be documented (clause 5.2.8), and space and conditions appropriate for the storage of electronic media and relevant LIS equipment have to be provided (clause 5.2.9).

In clause 5.3 (except 5.3.11 and 5.3.14) general requirements for laboratory equipment are given. Those requirements include:

a. use of energy and future disposal (environmental care)
b. qualification of hardware and software equipment during installation
c. regular performance verification through established requirements
d. labeling of equipment
e. record keeping
f. operation by authorized personnel
g. check of non-conformity work because of defected equipment

In clause 5.3.11, reference is made to:

a. validation of software
b. procedures for protection of data integrity
c. proper maintenance and proper conditions for LIS equipment
d. protection for unauthorized alteration of software

Protection of equipment from adjustments or invalidation of test results should be provided (clause 5.3.14) The use of electronic request form and the way the request is communicated to the laboratory should be selected after discussion with the laboratory clients (clause 5.4.1). All primary samples should be recorded by the LIS (clause 5.4.7), and the use of electronic manuals for the documentation of working procedures are acceptable at the workstations. Use of intranet web pages could be examined as an alternative to a card files system for use as a quick reference option at the work station (clause 5.5.3) Use of electronic signature or a traceable system of authorization through the LIS should be examined where possible (clause 5.8.3). The way and the time reported results would be stored in a LIS system should be carefully selected in order to assure prompt retrieval as well conformity with legal requirements (clause 5.8.6). LIS and electronic media could be used for immediate notification of "alert" or "critical" results (clause 5.8.7). The issue of alteration of reports, availability of the original report, and traceability at the alteration, time and responsible person is referred in clause 5.8.15 of the standard. Many options are provided through a LIS system and document control software, and requirements for the organization of revised reports and file keeping system are given in clause 5.8.16.

The ISO 15189: 2007 requirements for electronic archives are concerning environmental conditions, procedures in use, system's electronic security, hardware and software integrity and system's maintenance. Environmental requirements for the implementation of a high quality electronic medical database include proper maintenance of computer facilities, accessibility to firefighting equipment, dependable protection of wires and cables, provision of an uninterruptible power supply and protection from unauthorized access (Vacata et al, 2007; Kubono, 2007).

Procedural requirements for the implementation of a high quality electronic medical database cover the acquisition of an electronic procedure manual, available to all computer users and the implementation of specific procedures aiming at the protection of electronic data from any damage caused by hardware or software failure (Vacata et al., 2007; Kubono, 2007).

System's electronic security from unauthorized personnel alterations is of paramount importance and has to be ensured by implementing strict policies concerning authorization for entering, changing or editing electronic medical records. Medical data integrity must be continuously monitored for any errors during transmission and storage process. Specific procedures for reviewing all automatic calculations as well as the data entered in the laboratory information system must be implemented, in order to ensure electronic medical data's integrity (Vacata et al., 2007; Kubono, 2007).

Specific procedures must ensure that electronic medical data will be easily retrievable by all authorized personnel. Parameters such as footnotes, interpretative comments and uncertainty of a given measurement must be easily reproducible as part of the electronic medical report, offering the clinician the chance to interpret, with precision, laboratory medical data. The specific needs of each laboratory will determine the time, during which medical data will remain electronically retrievable (Vacata et al., 2007; Kubono, 2007).

Hardware and software requirements for the implementation of a high quality electronic medical database cover the acquisition of a complete record of all preventive actions concerning computer maintenance (Vacata et al., 2007).

Every back-up must be followed by systematic verification of the software integrity. All mistakes detected during back-up have to be documented and a corrective action must restore the system's proper function., while every modification of the system hardware and software must be documented and verified (Vacata et al., 2007; Kubono, 2007). Authorized personnel must verify that all programs run properly after first installation or any documented modification, and all serious computer malfunctions must be reported to an authorized laboratory's member, responsible for the proper use of medical laboratory's electronic records (Vacata et al., 2007; Kubono, 2007). System's maintenance must be scheduled in such a way that it will not interrupt patient-care service. Documented procedures for handling computer's shutdown and restart will ensure medical data's integrity (Vacata et al., 2007; Kubono, 2007). Cooperation between laboratory and hospital information system will be improved by the implementation of specific procedures concerning data replacement, recovery and updating. All computer problems, such as unexpected shutdown, downtime or breakdown must be fully documented and a corrective action must be taken in order to avoid these problems in the future (Vacata et al., 2007; Kubono, 2007).

Issues, Controversies, Problems

Medical data that is stored and retrieved from a laboratory information system contains valuable information that needs to remain confidential. The widespread use of computers makes access to classified documents easier than ever. The use of electronic signature in medical reports may diminish bureaucratic problems but, on the other hand, makes the laboratory information system more vulnerable. The laboratory management has to implement specific policies that will protect medical data from unauthorized access but will not endanger cooperation between medical and laboratory information systems (Shen & Yang, 2001; Vacata et al., 2007).

Laboratory personnel training in informatics is necessary for ensuring efficient function of the laboratory information system. The laboratory management has to plan personnel training in such a way that the laboratory main function will not be put in danger (Shen & Yang, 2001; Vacata et al., 2007). Poor hardware maintenance or improper use by inadequately trained personnel may cause a laboratory information system failure. Laboratory reports may be lost or deteriorated due to malignant software (virus programs), while LIS hardware may be damaged by adverse environmental conditions, such as heat, humidity or a possible fire, due to the vulnerability of wires and cables to unfavorable environmental conditions (Vacata et al., 2007; Westbrook et al., 2008). Finally, medical data stored only in electronic mediums may be easily lost due to a system's unexpected failure (Vacata et al., 2007). All these possible threats of a laboratory information system require the implementation of specific measures and policies that may have considerable economic impact, or may even prove non-affordable. The laboratory management is responsible for making an economic plan, after taking into account the specific laboratory resources and needs (Shen & Yang, 2001; Westbrook et al., 2008).

Solutions and Recommendations

Before new software or hardware is introduced in a laboratory, the risk connected with such an introduction should be assessed (Vacata et al., 2007). A risk assessment should include identification of possible events, which may result in non-compliance, estimation of their likelihood, identification of their consequences, and ways of avoiding them, costs, drawbacks, and benefits (Vacata et al., 2007). Good knowledge of computer software and hardware details is also essential for maintenance, troubleshooting and update. Medical laboratory personnel have to be periodically trained to the use of new computer facilities and new software products. Their training may be extremely difficult. Therefore, the laboratory director has to encourage these training sessions and continuously motivate its personnel (Pearlman et al., 2001; Westbrook et al., 2008).

Moreover, we have to take into account that computer facilities maintenance is of paramount importance in the workflow of a medical laboratory. Therefore, the laboratory personnel should take specific measures for protecting the hardware (Markin et al., 2000; Sciacovelli et al., 2007).

These measures should be documented in specific procedures, including:

- the way a computer should be turned off
- the way data should be stored
- the way the top and rear of the PC monitor should be kept clean and clear of debris
- the way to avoid excessive heating of the computer facilities
- the way to clean the inner surfaces of the PC
- how often hard disks should be scanned and defragmented
- how many MBs should be kept free in the hard disk
- the way peripherals should be plugged or unplugged from the computer
- how many programs should load up when the computer starts
- what firewall program should be used in case the computer facilities are connected to the Internet
- how often and what type of virus checker should be used
- what programs should be installed
- how often should the antivirus programs be updated
- how often should the Internet cache be emptied
- how often should unnecessary files be cleaned up from the hard drives

The hardware should also be fully protected from any actual damages, and especially fire (Markin et al., 2000; Sciacovelli et al., 2007; Vacata et al., 2007). The measures should be documented in specific procedures, and might include:

- smoke alarms installation and periodical testing
- flammable items storage and use
- storage and use of heating sources
- control of electrical wires
- installation of fire extinguishers

Wires and cables of the computer facilities should also be fully protected. Procedures might include:

- identification and maintenance of underground cables
- cables maintenance
- record keeping to determine the position of underground cables
- looping, linking and servicing connections
- maps or computer databases for all cable installations

The provision of an uninterruptible power supply will protect the computer from crashing during power outages, or from low and high voltage occurrences (Markin et al., 2000; Sciacovelli et al., 2007). A UPS is much better than a surge protector and can save the laboratory computer facilities from virtually any type of power failure.

Medical records and computer facilities should also be well protected from unauthorized access (Markin et al., 2000; Sciacovelli et al., 2007). The laboratory should establish guidelines for the protection of medical data from unauthorized access, which should:

- protect all laboratory data and information
- analyze access methods based on standards
- use the standard application methods wherever possible
- designate individuals responsible for the integrity of specific data sets
- restrict access to data and information to authorized individuals only
- restrict writing, updating, and deleting data

The laboratory should also obtain a complete record of all preventive actions concerning computer maintenance (Markin et al., 2000; Sciacovelli et al., 2007). Hardware preventive maintenance is the best way to dramatically reduce all factors threatening or shortening computer's life. The laboratory should implement specific procedures referring to many issues, such as:

- excessive heat prevention
- dust removal
- magnetism, radiated electromagnetic interference and static electricity prevention
- power surges, incorrect line voltage, and power outages handling
- water and corrosive agents prevention

Finally, software preventive maintenance is achieved by using anti-virus applications, defragmentation software and testing utility programs (Markin et al., 2000; Sciacovelli et al., 2007). The laboratory should/must implement specific procedures referring to many issues, such as:

- computers cleaning and defragmenting
- periodical virus check
- back-up, followed by systematic verification of the software's integrity. All mistakes detected during back-up should be documented, and a corrective action should restore the system's proper function.
- every modification of the system hardware and software should be documented and verified. Authorized personnel should verify that all programs run properly after the first installation or any documented modification.
- all serious computer malfunctions should be reported to an authorized laboratory's member
- system's maintenance should be scheduled in such a way that it will not interrupt patient-care service
- documented procedures for handling computer's shutdown and restart
- implementation of specific procedures concerning data replacement, recovery and updating
- all computer problems, such as unexpected shutdown, downtime or degradation should be fully documented
- a corrective action must be taken in order to avoid these problems in the future

FUTURE RESEARCH DIRECTIONS

The use of ISO 15189:2007 requirements in electronic data storage and retrieval is expanding, and many informative clauses of the standard are expected to become normative in the near future. A net of accredited laboratories is globally expanding (Pearlman et al., 2001; Kubono 2007). Many more countries will incorporate ISO 15189 requirements in their national or local regulations. Medical laboratories that will develop the most innovative and up to date procedures for electronic medical reporting and storage will become referral laboratories for their countries or regions (Okada 2002; Murai 2002; Kubono 2007).

All laboratories notices concerning the implementation of the ISO 15189:2007 are collected by an international working group, which is responsible for the revision of the standards, when necessary. Problems that might be reported to this international working group are examined and suitable solutions will be incorporated in the standard's future editions or in specific guidelines (Okada 2002; Murai 2002; Kubono 2007).

CONCLUSION

The standard ISO 15189:2007 includes direct and indirect references to the requirements concerning the implementation of laboratory information systems in medical laboratories. These requirements constitute a powerful tool for medical laboratories wishing to improve the quality of their laboratory information system because they diminish dramatically the possibility of human error or unexpected hardware or software failure.

Laboratories should only specify the procedures to be followed according to their needs.

REFERENCES

Brerider-Jr-McNai, P. (1996). User requirements on the future laboratory information systems. *Computer Methods and Programs in Biomedicine*, *50*(2), 87–93. doi:10.1016/0169-2607(96)01738-Q

Georgiou, A., & Westbrook, J. I. (2007). Computerized order entry systems and pathology services — a synthesis of the evidence. *The Clinical Biochemist. Reviews / Australian Association of Clinical Biochemists*, *27*, 79–87.

Kubono, K. (2004). Quality management system in the medical laboratory--ISO15189 and laboratory accreditation. *Rinsho Byori*, *2*(3), 274–278.

Kubono, K. (2007). Outline of the revision of ISO 15189 and accreditation of medical laboratory for specified health checkup. *Rinsho Byori*, *55*(11), 1029–1036.

Markin, R. S., & Whalen, S. A. (2000). Laboratory automation: trajectory, technology, and tactics. *Clinical Chemistry*, *46*, 764–771.

Murai, T. (2002). Future outlook for LAS, LIS. *Rinsho Byori*, *50*(7), 698–701.

Okada, M. (2002). Future of laboratory informatics. *Rinsho Byori*, *50*(7), 691–693.

Pearlman, E., Wolfert, M., & Miele, R. (2001). Utilization management and information technology: adapting to the new era. *Clinical Leadership & Management Review*, *15*(2), 85–88.

Sciacovelli, L., Secchiero, S., Zardo, L., D'Osualdo, A., & Plebani, M. (2007). Risk management in laboratory medicine: quality assurance programs and professional competence. *Clinical Chemistry and Laboratory Medicine*, *45*, 756–765. doi:10.1515/CCLM.2007.165

Shen, Z., & Yang, Z. (2001). The Problems and Strategy relevant to the Quality Management of Clinical Laboratories. *Clinical Chemistry and Laboratory Medicine*, *39*(12), 1216–1218. doi:10.1515/CCLM.2001.194

Vacata, V., Jahns-Streubel, G., Baldus, M., & Wood, W. G. (2007). Practical solution for control of the pre-analytical phase in decentralized clinical laboratories for meeting the requirements of the medical laboratory accreditation standard DIN EN ISO 15189. *Clinical Laboratory*, *53*, 211–215.

Westbrook, J. I., Georgiou, A., & Rob, M. I. (2008). Computerized order entry systems: sustained impact on laboratory efficiency and mortality rates? *Studies in Health Technology and Informatics*, *136*, 345–350.

Chapter 7
Safe Implementation of Research into Healthcare Practice through a Care Process Pathways Based Adaptation of Electronic Patient Records

V. G. Stamatopoulos
Biomedical Research Foundation of the Academy of Athens, Greece & Technological Educational Institute of Chalkida, Greece

G. E. Karagiannis
Royal Brompton & Harefield NHS Trust, UK

B. R. M. Manning
University of Westminster, UK

ABSTRACT

Concern has been expressed over the lack of evidence of the effective transfer of new research findings, guidelines and protocols into front-line clinical use. This book chapter outlines an approach which focuses on establishing and then using existing end-to-end care process pathways as initial benchmarks against which to evaluate the effects of changes in clinical practice in response to new clinical knowledge inputs. Whilst the prime focus of this approach is to provide a robust means of validating improvement in best practice processes and performance standards as the basis of good clinical governance, it will also seek to identify potential risks of adverse events and provide the basis for preventive measures, further backed-up by training within the relevant specialist domains. The objective is to close this loop by monitoring incremental change in care processes through a rolling analysis of input to Electronic Patient Record integrated into the clinical governance process. A pathway-linked knowledge service approach that could radically simplify and speed up the record updating process that supports and does not impinge on the professional autonomy.

DOI: 10.4018/978-1-61692-843-8.ch007

INTRODUCTION

Despite the introduction of multi-disciplinary team working, the healthcare professions still maintain much of their traditional 'silo' centric approach to knowledge exchange across their specialist domain boundaries (Pirnejad, Bal, Stoop, & Berg, 2007). Whilst Continuing Professional Development requirements should ensure that appropriately validated new knowledge is properly disseminated within these domains, and clinical decision quality is improved, procedures to confirm its adoption in practice and quality improvement are missing. There also tends to be little in the way of formalised interdisciplinary exchanges, reinforcing the 'silo' effects. Currently this effect is fairly well mitigated by clinical management use of procedures, guidelines and recommended best practice processes and pathways to establish performance standards as the basis of good governance. However, problems and adverse events have been shown by forensic studies to arise out of variability at the detailed level and in particular where there are hidden or unrecognised interdependencies between treatment practices by different professions, as well as at the interface of different healthcare settings (Kohn, 2001).

Healthcare providers also exhibit the same 'silo' approach displayed as by their constituent professions, due to the need for all organisations to set boundaries that clearly delineate the limits of operations with obvious implications in continuity of care (Pirnejad et al., 2007). The unfortunate consequence for patients is that their end-to-end care process threads its way across these domain boundaries with resultant changes both in organisations and professionals in responsible for their treatment.

The overall effect is that there is a lack of clarity of the likely sequence of events involved in resolving or ameliorating the patient's presenting conditions, especially when new procedures and guidelines are adapted. The prevailing culture appears to consider that it is pointless to have to have even an approximate plan of action in view of the innate variability in the progression of either the illness concerned or its treatment. However, this is tantamount to saying that in other potentially hazardous domains, the use of navigation charts and flight plans are unnecessary, as they will not be followed to the letter – which is patently wrong and would be highly unsafe!

The key issue is that whilst such charts fulfil the need for the point of reference for decision making in these domains, their use is noticeably absent in the clinical domain. This defect is even more evident in the context of the complete cross-border 'patient journey' from one end of the overall process to the other. This transit not only crosses primary, hospital and community care organisational boundaries, but also many treatment stages, which may well be 'fenced-in' within departmental sub-domains settings, as shown in Figure 1.

Figure 1. The cross border patient journey through the different healthcare settings

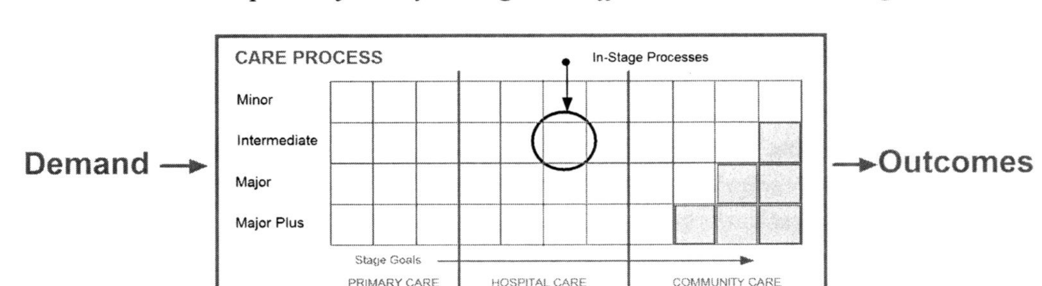

These stage boundary conditions involve achievement of target organisational or treatment outcome goals that act as 'gateways' to the next stage. These could be organisational transfers from Intensive Care Unit (ITU) – to High Dependency Unit (HDU) – towards; or clinical assessment – diagnosis – treatment outcomes/s – discharge
– community needs assessment – community care.

Case complexity adds a further dimension in the level of treatment complexity in in-stage processes required. These follow the same pattern of minor, intermediate, major, and major plus sets used in surgery. These severity sets act as further domains, where transfers are driven by the level of care response required by changes in the patient's condition.

Finally, implementation of new knowledge in the form of new recommendations/guidelines/procedures may complicate matters even further as it requires a number of steps to translate the knowledge contained in guideline text into a computable format and to integrate the information into clinical workflow (Shiffman, Michel, Essaihi, & Thornquist, 2004).

BACKGROUND

Care Process Pathways (CPP)

High-level care pathways (Manning, 2003) are generally used to identify all the major steps across the spectrum of complexity that are potentially involved in the treatment of a given condition, such as shown below in Figure 2 for Acute Myeloblastic Leukaemia (Schey, 2001), including latest evidence based guidelines.

Figure 2. Acute Myeloblastic Leukaemia care pathways

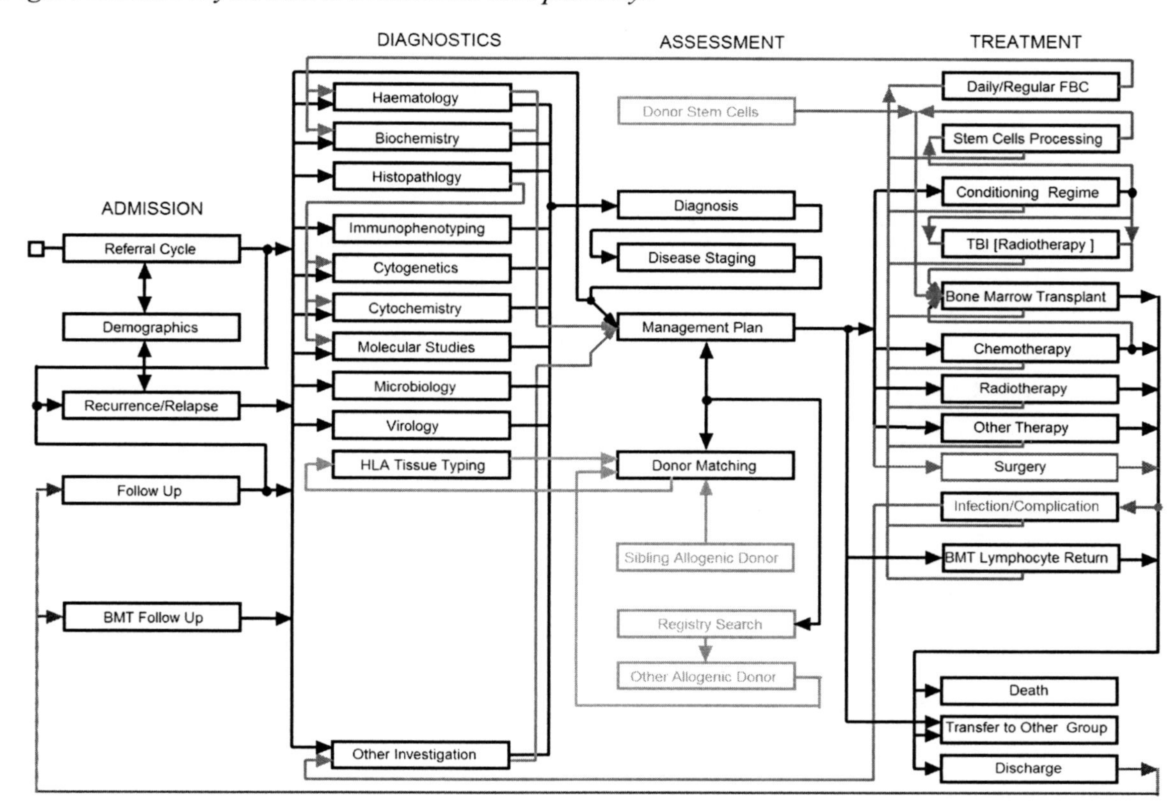

Whilst one of the more complicated conditions to diagnose and treat, it illustrates at high-level only just how wide a variety of routes the 'patient journey' treatment sequence may take. Whilst this provides the starting point for gathering statistical data to support clinical governance and control procedures, it is not sufficient to provide the necessary insights into actual routes taken – both formal and experience-led - or the decision criteria used.

As ever the 'devil is in the detail', and emphasises the need to map formal in-stage processes at various levels of detail, dependent on the level of case complexity and the options available. This will provide a sound foundation on which to tackle the problem of coping with experience-led process variability that invariably occurs in decision-making. Tacit knowledge derived from years of professional activity invariably leads to idiosyncratic process evolution around the formal norm, which generally remains hidden and yet contributes to variations in clinical outcomes.

The complexity of potential formal treatment options is well illustrated by the chemotherapy/bone marrow transplant CPP options shown below in Figure 3 for Acute Myeloblastic Leukaemia (Schey, 2001). Here the four main routes each have major variability in-built in the initial two stages with 'switch-out/over' decision points where complete remission has not been achieved.

Whilst the potential for dosage variability is immediately obvious from the first route shown below in Figure 3, it also demonstrates the potential to attach and index knowledge to a process map. This knowledge-indexing approach (McKeon Stosuy, Manning, & Layzell, 2005), together with appropriate version release controls would be central to providing the latest validated clinical information to support decision-taking directly to those in the 'front-line' of service delivery.

However, provision of such information alone will not ensure that it is used appropriately or at all. Its adoption into the everyday clinical working culture is ultimately dependent on delivering real, clinically desired benefits to professional practice and to resultant patient outcomes. As a result, evidence of its latent worth and subsequent delivered value is essential to secure a successful transformation in attitude and uptake by all the professions concerned. This evidence can only be gathered through much improved detailed knowledge of the current processes in use together with their limitations, deficiencies and attendant risks of errors or error producing conditions. The key to this lies in integrating a widely acceptable feedback mechanism that makes negligible downside impact on clinical activities, and does not adversely affect or limit the use of professional judgement and experience

Electronic Health Record implementation of Care Process Pathways

This can be achieved through an adaptation of the way the Electronic Patient Record (EPR) is created. The proposed approach centres on the use of well-structured CPP maps as a means of semi-automatically logging events into the EHR.

Its aim is to use the relevant pathway step together with the knowledge indexed to it as a means of updating the record. The essence of the approach is that updating would either entail adopting the recommended action and uploading its 'as is', adapting it to suit the circumstances, or choosing an alternative approach - effectively ignoring the recommendation - and entering the action taken as per current practice.

Automatically categorising all record updates in terms of the three types of action taken: adopted; adapted; or ignored, would provide a direct profile of the clinician's responses to newly available knowledge. More importantly it could radically reduce record input workloads, provided the pathway correctly reflected the bulk of current practice, whilst not constraining or impacting professional autonomy.

Figure 3. Chemotherapy/bone marrow transplant care process pathway options and potential for dosage variability

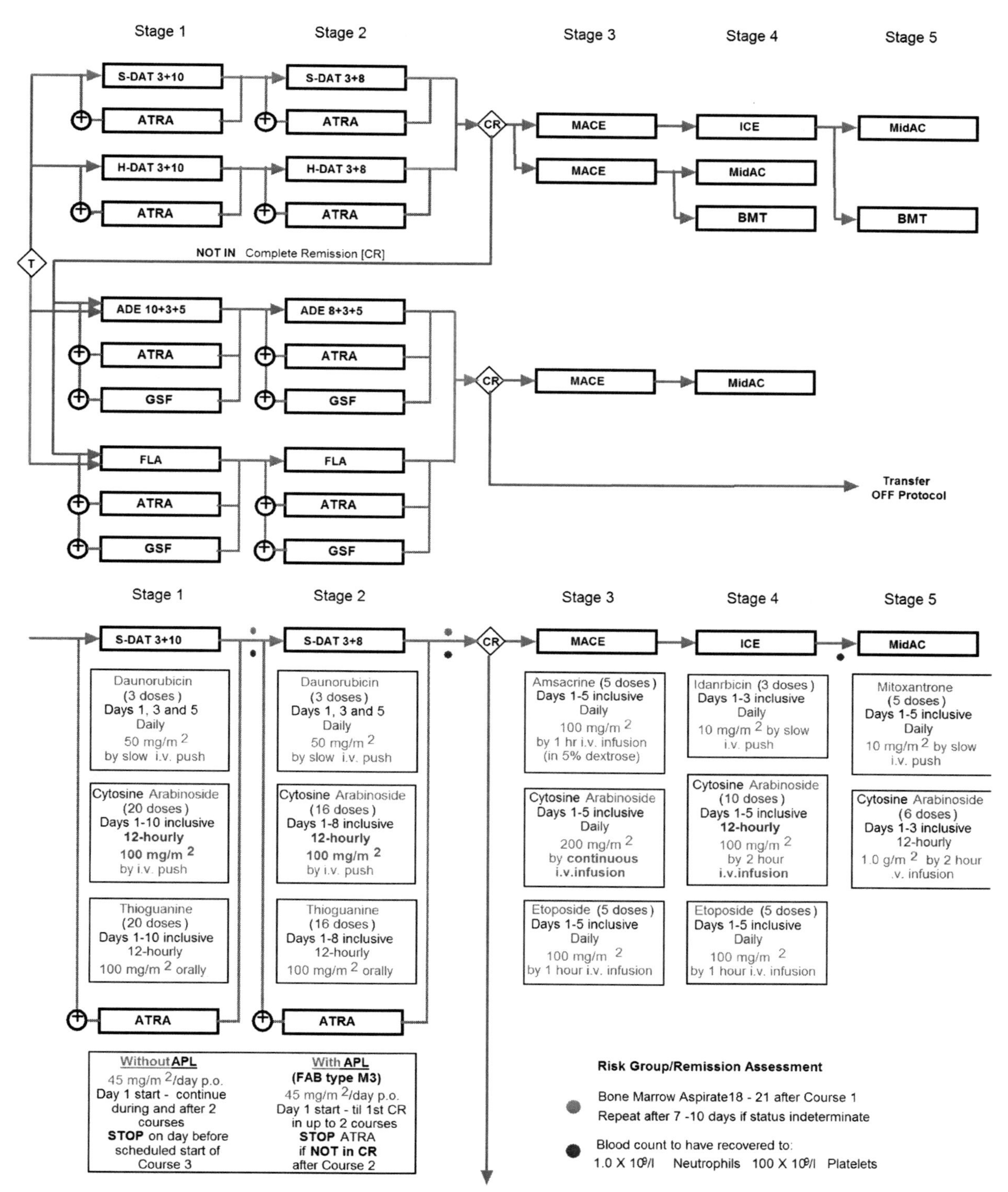

Combating Adverse Events

The introduction of the proposed CPP approach would provide much greater transparency not only in governance terms, but also provide the basis for early identification of potential hazards and latent exposure to adverse event risks. The risk of accidents or other incidents almost invariably result from a combination of clinical error producing conditions and/or violations of guidelines/procedures together with unidentified points of failure in defence mechanisms. These are frequently compounded by a chain of unforeseen events that are often set in motion by a mixture of corporate and clinical cultural stresses.

However, another major contributory factor that lies behind this problem is the general lack of any clear visibility either of the processes and their interaction with the resources that enable them to proceed. This is particularly surprising when compared with sectors, where high stress-levels and threats to life are inherent, all base their risk management defence procedures on process-based modelling and analysis. As healthcare is centrally reliant on experienced clinical human resources to deliver its care delivery processes, it almost inevitable that most adverse events stem from errors and omissions in the various supply chain processes and their interaction.

Care delivery is naturally the core process enabled in turn by other sets of supply chains. Whilst the series of alternative routes, discussed earlier, outline the broad treatment process, they in turn are likely to involve a mixture of inter-related parallel processes carried out by care professionals from different disciplines. Even though they may be operating as part of a multidisciplinary team, a combination of the lack of a shared interdisciplinary pathway plans, plus the professional 'silo' effect can result in a serious disconnect between the activity streams.

At best, this may result in wasted effort; at worst it may negate the work of the other professions involved and trigger an adverse event. The key to avoiding these circumstances lies in identifying these points of interdependence and putting in place procedures to obviate or mitigate such potential disconnects. Since the trigger for most adverse events result from human errors, often made under stressful circumstances, minimising and mitigating their effects, is paramount. Whilst the deployment of appropriately skilled and experienced clinicians, is central to enabling consistent high quality care to be delivered, ensuring that continuously evolving new clinical knowledge is absorbed into their working culture is vital.

The success of the 'rolling' change process is ultimately determined by a well-balanced input from three main supply chains. Whilst subtly delivered professional development through effective knowledge transfer contributing to the growth of individual clinician's expertise is central to this, so is a controlled exposure to situations that help build up their experiential knowledge.

The second chain delivers a supporting framework to this development through the provision of guidelines and procedures, which provide the control mechanism needed to ensure best practice consistency. However, at present this control process suffers from lack of day-to-day visibility of performance quality; no point of reference to identify significant deviations from currently evolving norms; little or no basis for timely, proactive identification of treats or triggers of adverse events; and of necessity, reliance on post-event preventative action.

The final chain is more amorphous in that it delivers a wide range of different types of information – and by definition knowledge – in a variety of forms, ranging from the readily understandable though to the highly complex, difficult to assimilate and potentially error producing. Almost more importantly, there are relatively few controls in place to ensure validity of content, or reduce latent ambiguities in its presentation.

Whilst reducing the error potential both within these individual chains and where they join to interact at the point of delivery of care is a decidedly

Figure 4. Changes in clinical practice as a result of the dissemination and take-up of new knowledge as seen in changes to care processes

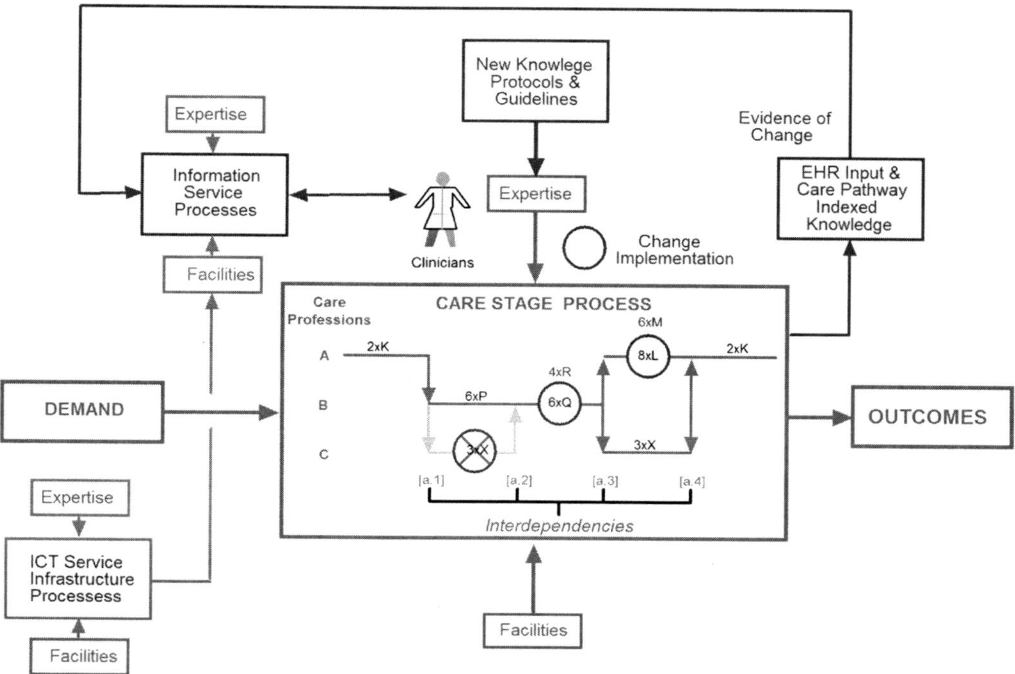

non-trivial task, much can be achieved through the development of process mapping and monitoring techniques proposed earlier. The emergence of a far clearer picture of clinical practice processes will in turn provide the basis for identifying potential adverse event triggers and putting in preventive measures.

Care Process Change Cycle

The impact of changes in clinical practice as a result of the dissemination and take-up of new knowledge inputs will be seen in changes to care processes, as shown above in Figure 4 for a typical care stage. Evidence of this will be derived jointly from regular checks for changes in process practice from that of the opening benchmarks, and from analysis of adaptations or alternative 'off pathway' treatments found in EHR updates.

As distinct changes in the patterns of treatment practice, are established – and confirmed as valid improvements by the expert medical panel – process pathways will be up-issued under conventional version control. Similarly revisions to the knowledge base are reflected in the clinical content, indexed to the relevant steps in the CPP.

Implementing AND Managing Change

Human nature inherently abhors change, especially if it is imposed. The remedy is to engage all sides in identifying the defects and discrepancies of the 'As Is' situation together with the benefits carefully managed change could deliver and resulting in a benefits 'roadmap'. Exploiting the full potential of newly available clinical knowledge requires the combination of process mapping methodology together with supporting

Figure 5. Effects of process change assembly as dimensions in a relational database structure

BASIC QUANTITATIVE MEASURES

Aggregation Hierarchy	BENCHMARK			Variance/Period		
	Stages	Steps	AECs	Stages	Steps	AECs
All	xxx	xxx	xxx	vvv	vvv	vvv
Country	xxx	xxx	xxx	vvv	vvv	vvv
Hospital	xxx	xxx	xxx	vvv	vvv	vvv
Specialty	xxx	xxx	xxx	vvv	vvv	vvv
Diagnosis	xxx	xxx	xxx	vvv	vvv	vvv
Consultant 1	xxx	xxx	xxx	vvv	vvv	vvv
....	xxx	xxx	xxx	vvv	vvv	vvv
Consultant n	xxx	xxx	xxx	vvv	vvv	vvv

BASIC QUALITATIVE MEASURES

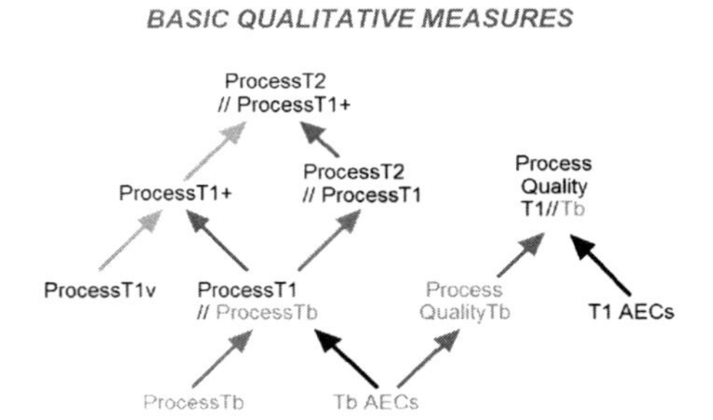

technology to deliver the operational environment needed to enable changes in clinical practice to take place. However, for it to take root the benefits must be seen by all to substantially outweigh any perceived risks and disadvantages.

Whilst the motivational issues are central to securing commitment and on-going involvement of users to their developmental programmes, they are equally relevant to service providers both at the individual professional as well as at all levels throughout their organisations. However, from the service provider perspective this needs to take full account of the additional influencing factors (benefit, value, cost, risk) and their inter-actions. Inevitably service costs will tend to be the dominant issue, followed closely by its relationship to perceived deliverable benefits. The problem that this poses is that by polarising interest on these two factors alone it is all too easy to lose sight of the more subjective aspects of risk and value.

Ignoring these two latter elements can all too easily destabilise any consensus for change and with it any chance of achieving anything approaching an optimal solution. In particular, value tends to be wrongly equated to cost incurred, rather than as the expected or actual return on the investment made. This difficulty usually arises out of the subjective nature of value, especially when viewed from different standpoints and often associated entrenched positions.

Viewed as an inter-related whole, rather than as two sets of dissociated of pairs, suggests a far more subtle judgement criteria should generally be considered – balancing each aspect in turn against the three others in the combined set. Testing this from the various perspectives involved in such a complex and multifaceted problem area as outlined above, would add considerable insight into the options available.

Measuring Change

In general terms, measurement splits broadly between quantitative and qualitative aspects of the issue under study – albeit sometimes using an intermediate approach either ranking selected qualitative criteria or by scoring them against an agreed subjective scale.

Where the effects of process change are concerned its effects can be measured in part by counting the number of given attributes and specific effects. These can be collected, and the results assembled into one or more aggregation hierarchies – as dimensions in a relational database structure, as shown Figure 5 in simplistic tabular form.

This would allow the effects of change to be assessed as variances – typically as changes in the number of stages and steps in comparison with those of the initial benchmark within a defined period. Similarly, occurrence of actual or prevented adverse events – as indicated by the triggering Adverse Events Countermeasure [AECs] - can be monitored.

Figure 6. Radar plot methodology for assessment of the impacts of changes in clinical practice

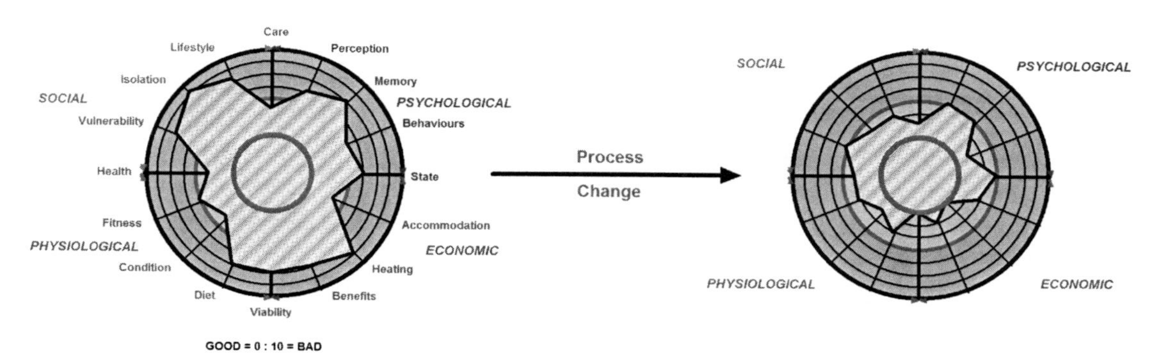

One of the limitations of any purely quantitative analytical approach is that the numbers alone invariably lead to a point where qualitative interpretation and perceptive input or reasoning is needed to add value and insight into the results obtained.

A useful bridge between these tabular and purely textual domains is a range of Cognitive Mapping techniques – shown in simplistic outline form above right. The essence of the approach is to breakdown the mass of qualitative input into short concept statements in the form – ideally as polar arguments framed as "this rather than that" and expressed as x // y. However of necessity this is often unipolar where a particular aspect is dominant.

These are then linked as consequential or reasoned chains to capture the essence of the knowledge obtained. This is illustrated above in terms of aspects of the starting benchmark conditions – Process Tb; Tb AECs; Process Quality Tb – in reality an extended set of concepts surrounding these focal topics. These typically then focus on the effects of change that centre around the node - Process T1// Process Tb and its evolution through variants such as Process T1v to Process T1+, etc.

The source of this qualitative information will be derived as a by-product of the proposed simplification of the EHR updating process. These changes in practice will be evident where decisions to adopt a process step in a newly authorised option will be a positive confirmation of it acceptance.

As significant changes in clinical practices, as a result of new knowledge are regulated by ethical committees or similar bodies, their authorisation procedures should ensure that current clinical process maps are updated though an appropriate change control process. A similar procedure would be followed under local clinical governance control in response to frequently used process adoptions.

Whilst an assessment of the quality of clinical decision-making must remain in the hands of experts from the clinical professions concerned, the provision of evidence of the effects of change will be available as outputs from this study. Where a qualitative assessment of the relative worth of the impacts of changes in clinical practice is required, the "radar plot" methodology (Benton & Manning, 2006), shown in Figure 6 can be used.

This uses a radial set of multiple assessment criteria with a common scale range. The area enclosed by linking the initial settings gives an immediate view of the scale and segmentation of the deficits. Regular re-assessment plots reveal progress made towards an end goal as a result of any change process.

Whilst the example used, demonstrates the principle in terms of an elderly patient's presenting circumstances and subsequent improvement as a result of multi-agency care, its applicability

Figure 7. Schematic diagram of pathways for adverse event risk sources/countermeasures

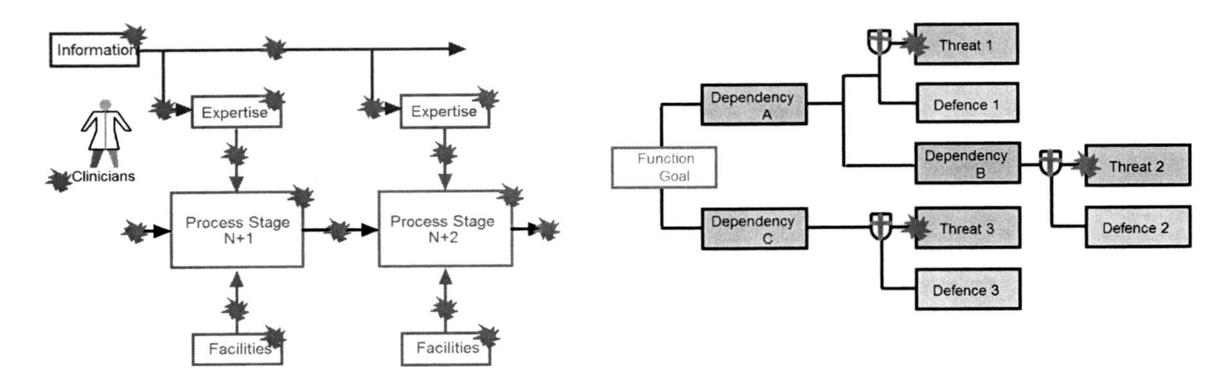

to a wide range of applications is evident. Its application to the impact of knowledge enabled process change merely requires the definition and agreement on an appropriate set of assessment criteria and any required segmentation. Although its implementation would primarily be based on case group governance reviews, it has the potential to be a semi-automatic derivative of the proposed EHR updating process.

Identifying Risk Potential

Inevitably, potential risk is spread throughout any care process, both within and between interacting elements (Vincent, Taylor-Adams, & Stanhope, 1998). No individual element is risk-free – a clinician can inadvertently be carrying a transmittable infection; a process stage can fail; information may be incomplete or wrong. Equally interaction between them can be equally risk-prone.

A rigorous in-depth risk assessment review of the complete end-to-end process sequence that covers every element, their actual and potential interactions, and all supply chains – e.g sterile supplies, information – is essential. However, although risk management techniques are now an integral part of healthcare service provision, little attempt has been made to map in detail all aspects involved in service delivery – no doubt due in particular to the inherent complexity and variability in treating each diagnostic condition.

Once the clinical process has been mapped, it provides the ideal basis for assessing the likely sources of risk threatening the achievement, the functional goals of each step along the pathway, as shown above right in Figure 7.

This centres on identifying the key dependencies, whose failure would prevent or seriously disable achievement of each functional goal. This in turn leads to identifying threats and their damage potential and probability of occurrence. Blocking or mitigating these effects leads directly to the design and implementation of appropriate countermeasures.

Once countermeasures are in place as part of a clinical risk reduction strategy, the triggering of any defence process will provide an indication of the occurrence – and hopefully prevention of an adverse event. Whilst each of these 'attacks' will obviously need to be investigated and followed up by any necessary additional countermeasures, the trigger action can provide a measurable indicator of Adverse Event Countermeasure response.

Educational Aspects

Whilst one of the main thrusts of this approach is acquiring knowledge and its addition to the knowledge base, which in turn is indexed to each of the relevant steps in the pathway, it can also be the basis of a web-based e-Learning Service. The focus of this would be to 'drip-feed' information to frontline clinical staff as part of their Continued Professional Development training. The process would be built upon a Clinical Decision Support Service.

Its aim will be to deliver a sequence of modular 'bite-sized' packages using a limited-access web service. These would be assembled using well-proven e-Learning methodologies set in the context of a careful assessment of the prevailing clinical cultures and motivational issues to ensure acceptance as a valued aid, rather than an imposed inconvenience. Of necessity, its output would have to be validated by an independent expert panel not only in terms of content, but also as fitness to fulfil training needs.

Technical Solution Description and Customisation Technology

As mentioned earlier, an Electronic Health Record should be implemented with the use of well-structured CPP maps as a means of semi-automatically logging events into the EHR. Its aim is to use the relevant pathway step together with the knowledge indexed to it as a means of updating the record. The essence of the approach is that updating would either entail adopting the recommended action and uploading its 'as is', adapting it to suit the circumstances, or choosing an alternative approach - effectively ignoring the recommendation - and entering the action taken as per current practice.

Automatically categorising all record updates in terms of the three types of action taken, viz: adopted; adapted; or ignored, would provide a direct profile of the clinician's responses to newly available knowledge. More importantly it could radically reduce record input workloads, provided the pathway correctly reflected the bulk of current practice, whilst not constraining or impacting professional autonomy.

Advance that Care Process Pathways Would Bring Beyond the State of the Art

To date Integrated Clinical Pathways based projects have almost invariably been focused on gaining a high-level view of the optimal process sequence, often centred on establishing management information datasets. This has not been helped by the lack of any generic process mapping standard, which has led to a profusion of different and highly idiosyncratic approaches

The proposed CPP mapping approach is in part derived from initial ISO TC215 and CEN TC251 Working Group activities on Strategic Architecture development, coupled with that for Security and Safety. Its ultimate objective would be to form the basis of a generic standard within the ISO 9000 set, which could be supplemented if necessary by healthcare specific guidelines as in the case of ISO 27799.

The integration of Clinical Knowledge access with CPP is novel – as is the application of dependency modelling and mapping techniques to Clinical Risk Management. Similarly, the potential simplification and reduction in clinical administrative effort inherent in the 'adopt, adapt or alternative' approach to updating the EHR is a further innovative feature.

Whilst analysis of EHR updates will inevitably involve a variety of knowledge acquisition methods dependent of facilities available at each of the hospital sites, the long term aim would be to access relevant information, under appropriate security controls from a back-up service. Such an approach would ultimately be based on access to pseudonymised information from a dynamic archive running as a back-up to the main EHR, as currently under discussion within ISO and CEN.

The use of e-learning methods appears to be somewhat novel as means to disseminate new

Figure 8. Conceptual overview of the main elements of the proposed CPP approach

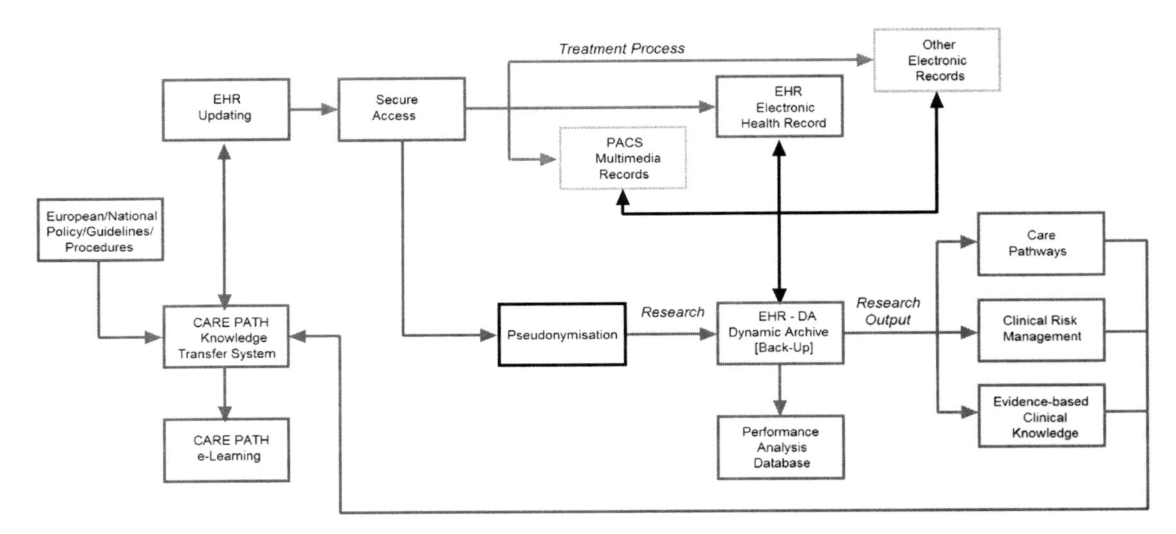

clinical knowledge especially in the context of Continuing Professional Development, although it has been pioneered in other environments. However, the proposed 'drip-feed' of mini, or even micro modules designed specially to meet clinical interests and provided as an interactive web service is likely to be an attractive innovation – as well as a training aid to support the introduction of CPP.

The technical infrastructure, although new to the healthcare environment, should be constructed from as set of inter-operable software applications that have been used to provide similar functionality, albeit in different economic sectors.

Overall this approach combines a number of novel concepts which will not only provide a robust methodology to track the successful dissemination and usage of new knowledge, but also develop a radically new approach both to giving easy access to clinical knowledge and simplifying clinical reporting routines.

CONCLUSION

The primary focus of the proposed CPP methodology is to track the transfer of newly validated evidence-based clinical knowledge through to its application in frontline application, and to determine the degree and timescales involved in its incorporation into mainstream treatment, together with its effects on outcome quality.

Basing the approach on a detailed analysis of the CPP, their variability and the knowledge used in clinical decision-making should provide a sound platform from which to establish an adverse event risk management system. Moreover, the innovative combination of several analytical tools and techniques will not only provide insights and actions to counter adverse events and improve quality of care delivery, but also establish the basis for enhanced clinical decision support systems development to underpin this.

Inherent in this approach is the use of these systems to provide data for clinical governance and comparative analysis to local and international benchmarks. The development of adverse event countermeasure triggers will aim to initiate timely preventive action and contribute to enhancing patient safety.

In addition to providing the basis for providing rapid frontline access to newly validated evidence-based clinical knowledge, a further aim will be to develop sets of easily absorbed incremental e-learning packages that can be accessible via controlled-access web services not only to clinicians but also to support self-management of disease by patients where appropriate.

REFERENCES

Benton, S., & Manning, B. R. M. (2006). Assistive Technology - Behaviourally Assisted . In Bos, L., Roa, L., Yogesan, K., O'Connell, B., Marsh, A., & Blobel, B. (Eds.), *Medical and Care Compunetics* (*Vol. 3*, pp. 7–14). Amsterdam: IOS Press.

Kohn, L. T. (2001). The Institute of Medicine report on medical error: Overview and implications for pharmacy. *American Journal of Health-System Pharmacy*, *58*(1), 63–66.

Manning, B. R. M. (2003). Clinical Process Maps as an indexing link to knowledge and Records. In *Healthcare Digital Libraries Workshop, 7th European Conference on Research and Advanced Technology for Digital Libraries*, Trondheim, Norway.

McKeon Stosuy, M., Manning, B. R. M., & Layzell, B. R. (2005). *E-care co-ordination: An inclusive community-wide holistic approach*. Boston: Springer.

Pirnejad, H., Bal, R., Stoop, A. P., & Berg, M. (2007). Infrastructures to support integrated care: connecting across institutional and professional boundaries: Inter-organisational communication networks in healthcare: centralised versus decentralised approaches. *International Journal of Integrated Care*, *7*, 14.

Schey, S. (2001). *Guidelines for Haemo-oncology Treatment Processes* [Internal Document]. London: Guys and St Thomas' Hospitals NHS Trust.

Shiffman, R. N., Michel, G., Essaihi, A., & Thornquist, E. (2004). Bridging the Guideline Implementation Gap: A Systematic, Document-Centered Approach to Guideline Implementation. *Journal of the American Medical Informatics Association*, *11*(5), 418–426. doi:10.1197/jamia.M1444

Vincent, C., Taylor-Adams, S., & Stanhope, N. (1998). Framework for analysing risk and safety in clinical medicine. *British Medical Journal*, *316*, 1154–1157.

Chapter 8
Quality Assurance in Evidence-Based Medicine

Ioannis Apostolakis
National School of Public Health, Greece

Periklis Valsamos
Greek Ministry of Health and Social Solidarity, Greece

Iraklis Varlamis
Harokopio University of Athens, Greece

ABSTRACT

Evidence-based medicine (EBM) refers to the careful examination of all the available evidence when making decisions about the care of the individual patient. It assumes that well known medical practices and solutions are combined with the patient's preferences and necessities in order to provide the most appropriate solution per case. The abundance of medical information in the web, the expansion of Semantic Web and the evolution of search services allowed the easier retrieval of scientific articles. Although the available infrastructure exists and continuously improves in performance, EBM still remains a complicated and sensitive process of high importance and has a need for Quality Assurance (QA). The purpose of this chapter is twofold: first, to provide an introduction on the concepts of Evidence-based Medicine, and second, to stress the necessity for structured methodologies that will assure the quality of the EBM process and ameliorate the final recommendations therapy. Since evidences are the building blocks of EBM, we capitalize on their quality and provide a critical overview of the existing methodologies in Quality Assurance of evidences.

INTRODUCTION

Evidence-Based medicine (EBM) can be thought of as the careful, explicit and reasonable use of patient related evidence (e.g. preferences, special needs etc.) in order to facilitate doctors in the selection of the most appropriate medical solution per case. It assumes the integration of individual clinical expertise with the best available external clinical evidence from systematic research (Sackett, 2003).

Tons of scientific journals, articles, patient guidelines and other related information are produced every day from scientific bodies and

DOI: 10.4018/978-1-61692-843-8.ch008

research centers. The development of the Internet and other related technologies made sharing, distribution, searching and retrieval of scientific information easier than ever.

Clinicians can use the scientific databases available on the Internet (PUBMED, Medline etc) or the general purpose search engines in order to retrieve information quickly and effectively. Moreover, apart from these "pull services, modern tools (RSS, mailing lists etc) can "push" selected information to their subscribers. Also, the development of mobile technologies and wireless networks made the distribution of knowledge at the point of care easier than ever. A clinician can use a smart phone or a PDA to retrieve information at the point of care, or in other words "on the move".

Although significant progress is made in the area of the distribution, retrieval and searching of information, less is done in the area of its quality assurance. Consequently, the increase in information quantity had not an analogous impact in the quality of medical decisions. As a result the clinician is "left alone" to perform a time consuming, costly and error-prone process: the filtering and evaluation of the available information.

Truly, not the entire flood of provided knowledge is valid or useful for patient care. The study of Lundberg (Lundberg, 1992) on 100.000 scientific journals revealed that only 150 of those publications reported the 90% of all major scientific advances and less than 1,000 journals attained the 80% of the citations noted by Science Citation Index. The need to identify relevant information and to critically evaluate the scientific methodology and conclusions of the available information is obvious.

The purpose of this chapter is bifold. Initially, a short introduction in the concepts of evidence based medicine is given. This short introduction will provide the necessary definitions of EBM in order to avoid common misunderstandings and incorrect interpretations of the concept. Moreover, the importance of EBM for everyday clinical practice will be stressed.

In the following section we emphasize on the need for structured methodologies for the quality assurance and strength of recommendations. We focus on the problems that arise in the absence of a methodology, which assures the quality and relevance of provided information. Finally, we provide a critical review of existing methodologies in this field. The purpose of this presentation is to examine the proposed solutions for the quality assurance of the provided evidence as well as the provision of some suggestions.

BACKGROUND

Evidence-Based Medicine (EBM)

Clinicians in their everyday medical practice confront an overwhelming number of patients. In each medical session made, several questions arise concerning the proper prognosis, diagnosis and treatment. Moreover the differences between each individual patient case require the questions to be specialized according to the patient's medical condition, history and personal preferences. Truly, the selection of the "proper" treatment for each patient depends not only on scientific evidence but also from personal factors such as quality, personal beliefs and preferences of the patient.

Unfortunately, usually the decisions made by the clinicians are not supported by the suitable knowledge. The heavy workload and the absence of appropriate decision making tools hinder the clinicians from the careful processing of the available information and the selection of the most appropriate solution per incident. The lack of trustworthy and up to date information, make things even worse. As a result, the clinician is frequently left alone and her decisions are not adequately supported. Obviously, it is not practical for individual clinicians and patients to make these judgments unaided. In this context, Evidence Based Medicine (EBM) can be of great help for the clinicians, providing the best possible evidence at the point of clinical care.

EBM employs scientific and engineering tools and techniques in order to collect medical evidence process them and apply results in medical practice. These tools comprise meta-analysis of medical literature, risk-benefit analysis, randomized controlled trials (RCTs) etc. EBM assesses the quality of evidence and evaluates the risks and benefits of various treatments. The Centre for Evidence Based Medicine defines EBM as the "conscientious, explicit and judicious use of current best evidence in making decisions about the care of individual patients" (Sackett, 2003). In other words evidence-based medicine integrates individual clinical expertise with the best available external clinical evidence from systematic research.

The algorithm for the practice of evidence-based medicine can be summarized in the following steps:

- **Define of the problem:** The first and most important step of the whole process. A misjudgment in the identification of the problem can disorient the clinician, lead to irrelevant questioning and consequently to wrong conclusions and actions. On the other side, the proper definition of the problem area can narrow the search space of the relevant literature and facilitate the clinician.
- **Select the appropriate clinical questions:** As previously, the accuracy of the clinical questions is crucial. An irrelevant or badly formed question will result to an unrelated or meaningless answer and a useless fact.
- **Track and appraise the best evidences:** Clinicians must search and utilize the most relevant available resources that answer the clinical questions, bearing in mind to gather both qualitative and quantitative evidences, which properly answer the questions. The quality of the selected information must be assessed, taking into account the validity of study results and their relevance to the questions.
- **Estimate the clinical importance of the evidence and the clinical applicability of any recommendation or conclusion:** In this step information is evaluated according to its relevance and applicability to the patient's problem. All evidences that are not applicable in a real clinical environment must be considered as a secondary source of information. Clinicians must compare the characteristics of their patient to those of the patients in the clinical study and verify that the study covered all important aspects of the patient's problem.
- **Integrate the evidence, the clinical expertise and the patient preferences and apply results to the clinical practice:** In cooperation with the patient, the clinician discusses the gathered evidence and suggested treatments.
- **Summarize and cache records for future reference:** An optional but highly recommended step in the process that maintains a "memory" for the system and builds useful knowledge base for the future.

Evidence based medicine is connected with some common misinterpretations, which should be carefully examined and avoided. A common misconception is that evidence-based medicine does not take into account clinical experience. This belief is wrong since signs and symptoms form the basis for the questions asked and guide the literature search. Moreover, evidence based medicine tries to support and back-up the clinician in her decision making process. Another wrong belief is that basic investigation and path physiology is not important for EBM. In contrast to this belief, the process of clinical problem solving followed by EBM has as a basic prerequisite a good understanding of pathophysiology. Finally, the faulty perception that Evidence-based medicine ignores standard aspects of clinical training such as the physical examination is contradicted from the fact that Evidence-based practice considers the physical conditions of the patient while evaluating the evidence and also before applying treatment to the patient.

In conclusion, it is important to stress the factors that influence the adoption and implementation of the EBM (Freeman & Sweeney, 2001):

- **Clinician's experiences and personal beliefs**: The way the evidence is adopted and implemented is influenced by the doctor's experiences as well as her formed personal beliefs.
- **Clinician-Patient relationship:** The way the evidence is implemented is largely affected by the developed doctor-patient relationship, as well as by the specialized characteristics and beliefs of the patient.
- **Level of care provision:** The attitude towards evidence based medicine is different between clinicians of primary and secondary care.
- **Emotional-Psychological Factors:** EBM is not a "pure" intellectual process from which knowledge from studies and medical journals is transferred to the clinical practice. It involves also and an emotional part for both doctors and patients. Doctor's sometimes feel anxiety for the appliance of the new evidence or on the contrary may be neglecting it if the patient seems unwilling to follow new kinds of treatments. On the other hand, patients sometimes "jump" to new evidence and feel anxious to use them.
- **Developed Habits:** In some occasions, both patients and doctors are unwilling to follow new treatments and medications.

Quality Assurance of Medical Evidence

As already stated, the most important factor in the practice of EBM is to assure the quality of the evidence employed for supporting the medical decisions. In this context, it is crucial for the clinicians to follow a structured methodology and with the use of scientific tools to be able to evaluate the quality of evidence. In other words, it is necessary to reach the highest level of objectiveness during the evaluation of the validity, suitability, appropriateness, of the evidence used.

Before examining the methods for Quality Assurance of EBM, it is necessary to present the most widely employed techniques in EBM. These techniques originate from science, engineering and statistics and their results are the evidence for the Evidence based Medicine.

Randomized controlled trials (RCTs) are scientific experiments that evaluate the effectiveness of healthcare services and technologies over a population sample. The process assumes that a different solution is selected randomly from the set of available solutions and is applied to each test subject, thus eliminating causality and bias. RCTs can be *open*, *blind* or *double-blind*, depending on what degree the patient and the doctor are aware of the treatment. In an open trial the patient knows the full details of the treatment and a placebo effect is possible. Similarly in a blind process, it is possible that the treatment aware clinician can give hints to the patient about important treatment-related details, thus influencing the objectiveness of the study. On the contrary, in a double-blind trial the clinician is not informed on the treatment selected per case and as a result she is unable to affect the patient. In all cases, the administrator of the experiment is aware of all treatment allocations to patient-doctor pairs and thus is responsible to integrate the clinical results. The advantage of randomized controlled trials is that patients are not examined in isolation but rather in groups (*control groups*). In this way, it is possible to compare results of different treatment methods, to evaluate them in reference to the group characteristics and to get valuable knowledge. The knowledge drawn from RCTs comprises clues on the effectiveness of the treatment, its side effects, the parameters that affect the treatment performance and is valuable for the decision making problem of treatment selection.

The randomness of assignments and the continuous monitoring of the trial results are necessary in order to avoid skewing of the results over the population groups. More specifically, a *randomization procedure* will generate a random and unpredictable sequence of allocations to patient groups at equal probabilities and the *allocation concealment* will guarantee that the group assignment of patients will not be revealed to the study investigators prior to definitively allocating them to their respective groups.

In **risk-benefit analysis** the risk of a decision and its expected benefits are put in the balance. In the sensitive case of patient care, the investigator must assure that the amount of benefit clearly outweighs the amount of risk. Those studies that have a clearly favorable risk-benefit ratio and guarantee not to harm the patient, may be considered ethical.

Meta-analysis is performed on the results of several studies that address a set of related research hypotheses. The results of the different studies are first aligned and then combined thus creating a fictional research output on a larger sample. The aggregated results have extended coverage and control and offer more powerful estimates of the true effect size than those derived in a single study under a given single set of assumptions and conditions. The meta-analysis on a group of studies can allow more accurate data analysis.

Clinical trials evaluate the safety and efficacy of new drugs, remedies or medical devices. They refer to products that have been already tested for quality and non-clinical safety. They comprise small scale pilot studies in the first step followed by larger scale studies when the initial results are positive in terms of safety and efficacy. They can vary in size from a single center in one country to multicenter trials in multiple countries. The medical products in a clinical trial are evaluated either individually or in comparison to existing products and the currently prescribed treatment.

Case-control studies originate from epidemiology and aim in locating the factors that affect a medical condition. They are performed on a set of subjects with similar properties and compare the *positive* (i.e. cases) and *negative* subjects (i.e. controls) in order to identify the minor differences that may affect their difference in condition. Case control studies examine the history of subjects and in order to locate past exposure to suspect factors that reasons their current condition. Although, they are easily applicable and require limited resources, they lack of large scale design and randomness. As a consequence, their conclusions are useful but cannot be widely applied in all medical cases. However, they can be employed in a preprocessing step for quickly and inexpensively identifying risk factors, and can be followed by a more profound analysis with more "credible" and comprehensive studies (e.g. randomized controlled studies). Moreover, they can be repeated over different population samples and fed as an input to a meta-analysis process.

Cohort or **panel studies** are widely employed in social sciences. They examine groups of people who are linked in some way, have experienced the same significant life event or share a common characteristic within a defined period in the past (e.g. birth, disease, leave school, lose their job, exposure to a drug, etc.) and compare their current behavior in a subject of interest (e.g. smoking). The analysis of cohort related information can tell us what circumstances in early life are associated with the population's characteristics in later life and allow us to find what encourages the development in particular directions and what can impede it. Similarly in medicine, a cohort study attempts to uncover the suspected association between cause and disease; the negation of a hypothesis is refuted thus strengthening the confidence in the initial hypothesis. For this reason, the cohort should be identified and monitored a long time before and at least a short period after the appearance of the disease under investigation. The frequency of disease incidents, their severity, the geographical and temporal dispersion are some of the facts that should be evaluated in the results of a cohort study. Conducting a cohort study has a significant cost in time, people and money and thus it is a technique that should be utilized sparingly. Moreover, cohort studies are sensitive to erosion and are take a lot of time in order to generate useful data. Nevertheless, long-term cohort studies produce results of high quality, substantially superior to those of other techniques and are considered the "gold standard" in observational epidemiology. Less expensive research techniques can be employed to prepare the ground for a cohort study and further experimental trials can be utilized to maintain validity of the conclusions.

Cross-sectional studies refer to the concurrent observation of population subsets that expose significant differences in independent variables, such as IQ and memory. The subjects belong to different age groups and are examined at a single point in time. Cross-sectional research takes a 'slice' of its target group and bases its overall finding on the views or behaviours of those targeted, assuming them to be typical of the whole group.

Apart from the aforementioned techniques, evidence can be based on expert opinions (consensus practice guideline), or on literature review and do not include a systematic search.

In order to maximize the profit from combining evidence from medical research in the process of medical decision, Evidence based Medicine requests that the quality of resulting evidence is assessed. For the evaluation of evidence, several characteristics are examined:

- **Disease and Patient-Oriented Outcomes:** Outcomes that reflect the patient health status (e.g. blood sugar, blood pressure etc) and relate to the quality of life of the patients (i.e. the help them live longer an/ or better lives) are of higher interest.
- **Research Evidence:** Evidence that is provided from original research is valuable but should be considered with care.
- **Level of Evidence:** It is tightly connected to the validity and structure of the study that produced the evidence. It is used for the results of individual studies but applies well on evidence that stem from multiple studies.
- **Strength of a recommendation:** Indicates the extent to which the conformance to this recommendation will do more good than harm. The strength (or grade) of a recommendation is based on a body of evidence (usually more than one study). Thus, in order to determine the strength of recommendation we take into account: the study that produced the evidence, the type of outcomes measured, the consistency and coherence of the evidence and the expected benefits, harms and costs.

SYSTEMS FOR QUALITY ASSURANCE OF EVIDENCE

The efficiency of Evidence-based Medicine is strongly connected to the appropriateness and quality of medical evidence. The multitude of research techniques and the abundance of evidence make it impossible for a doctor to become aware of all the related evidence and moreover to evaluate each one of them. As a result several efforts have been made in order to standardize and automate the quality assurance process for medical evidence and several systems have been developed in order to justify the quality of evidence.

One of the first efforts was made in 1979 by the ***Canadian Task Force on Periodic Health Examination (1979)*** and resulted to a classification of the evidence produced by the different research methods. More specifically, evidence supported by Randomized Controlled Trials (RCTs) was classified as Level I (good), evidence supported by cohort and case control studies was classified as Level II (fair), and finally, evidence provided by expert's opinion was classified as Level III (poor). Consequently, the strength of recommendation was directly associated with the level of evidence that supported it. For example, a recommendation that was supported by Level I evidence was classified as a "strong" recommendation. The main advantage of this early system was its simplicity, which made it easy to understand and apply. On the other hand, there were many drawbacks, such as that it was based on many implicit judgments about the quality of randomized controlled trials.

Several systems, which have been developed since then attempted to provide alternative classifications and rate the evidence strength. The most important approaches are presented in the following.

U.S. Preventive Services Task Force (USPSTF) System

The U.S. Preventive Services Task Force (USPSTF) was established in 1984 aiming to provide a systematic review of medical evidence. Based on the Canadian Task Force System they presented their own grading system for the quality evidence and the strength of recommendation. As far as it concerns the quality of evidence they rated separately the individual study and the body of evidence and the service as a whole.

The classification of individual studies contained three main levels and several sublevels. More specifically:

- Level I referred to studies that contained at least one properly designed randomized controlled trial
- Level II comprised well-designed studies from one or more research groups. Controlled trials without randomization were at the top of this level; cohort or case-control analytic studies followed; multiple time series with or without intervention and exceptional results in uncontrolled trials concluded this level.
- Level III comprised the opinions of expert committees, the statements of respected authorities which were based on clinical experience and descriptive studies.

For the assessment of the body of evidence three criteria have been proposed, which refer to: the internal validity, the external validity, and coherence (i.e. consistency among studies and with other supporting evidence).

Finally, a three-point scale has been employed for rating the overall quality of the evidence. The levels were:

- **Good:** For consistent results from studies of high quality. Such evidence demonstrates high applicability, direct and clinically important positive effects on the population.
- **Fair:** For evidence that demonstrates clinically important positive effects, but is limited by the number, quality or consistency of the individual studies. Such evidence can be easily generalized to routine practice.
- **Poor:** For those results that do not demonstrate positive effects on health outcomes. Such evidence is based on a limited number of poorly designed studies, which lack of important health outcomes.

At last, the quality of a medical service based on evidence is depicted to the strength of the produced recommendation. For this reason, a 5-level rating scale has been suggested:

- **"A"** was accredited to services, which are based on good evidence and will potentially improve health outcomes. The output of these services must be provided to eligible patients since their benefits substantially prevail over harms.

- **"B"** was used for services that evidently improve health outcomes. Their benefits outweigh harms and thus it is advisable to be provided to eligible patients.
- **"C"** refers to those services that can improve some health outcomes, but whose balance of benefits and harms is too close and thus cannot be a general recommendation. The decision is left to each individual patient and should take her preferences in account.
- **"D"** applies to services that are not recommended for use in asymptomatic patients. Usually, evidence shows that these services are ineffective and their harms outweigh the benefits.
- **"I"** applies to the services for which we have insufficient evidence and we are unable to recommend for or against their use.

The main strength of the system presented by USPSTF is that it provides a clear and direct linkage between quality of evidence and strength of recommendation. Moreover, it is more complete than the classification of the Canadian Task Force on Periodic Health Examination, since it takes into account other elements of evidence apart from the study design and it weighs benefits and harms. However, it has several limitations, since it is not adaptable to prognostic/diagnostic questions and it cannot provide recommendations in the absence of good evidence. Finally, the assessments do not always adjust for the individual patient values.

Oxford Centre for Evidence-Based Medicine (OCEBM) System

The Oxford Centre for Evidence-based Medicine (OCEBM) developed another set of Levels of Evidence and Grades of Recommendation, which was based on the grading system provided by the Canadian Task Force on the Periodic Health Examination (Ball, Sackett, Phillips, Straus & Haynes, 1998). OCEBM defines four main axes namely "therapy/aetiology", "prognosis", "diagnosis" and "economic analysis", which correspond to the broad type of clinical question. Each axe is divided into 5 broad levels of evidence ranging from 1 (least potential bias) to 5 (most potential bias), which mainly take into account the quality of design of each specific study. Additional factors estimate the outcome assessment ("minus" in case of imprecise result) and clinical sensibility (e.g. "appropriate spectrum" of patients).

Based on the level of evidence, OCEBM defines grades of recommendation strength (or grade of recommendation), which intrinsically is a mapping of levels of evidence to grades as follows:

- **Grade A** corresponds to Evidence Level 1 and comprises studies supported by randomized controlled trials, cohort studies, clinical decision rules validated in different populations etc.
- **Grade B** corresponds to Evidence Levels 2 and 3 and comprises studies such as consistent retrospective cohort, exploratory cohort, ecological studies etc.
- **Grade C** is for case-series studies and maps to evidence Level 3.
- **Grade D** comprises evidence based on experts' opinion, physiology, bench research or first principles etc.

The main advantages of the OCEBM system are the detailed classification of studies according to the level of evidence and the horizontal partitioning in the four axes that relate to diagnosis, aetiology, prognosis and economic analysis. However, the high level of detail may seem difficult for inexperienced users to follow. The main disadvantage of the system is the way the translation of levels of evidence to grades of recommendations is made. Thus, no assessment is given of the clinical importance of the outcomes. Moreover, no balancing of benefits and harms is given. Finally, no assessment of the applicability of the studies is given.

American College of Chest Physicians (ACCP) System

The Consensus Conferences on Antithrombotic Therapy of the American College of Chest Physicians (ACCP) has developed guidelines to help clinicians make antithrombotic treatment decisions in average patients (Guyatt et al., 2001).

The Levels (quality of evidence) in the ACCP system are categorized as follows:

- **Grade A:** Randomized controlled trials (RCTs) with consistent results.
- **Grade B:** Randomized trials with inconsistent results, or with major methodological weaknesses
- **Grade C:** observational studies and generalization from randomized trials in one group of patients to a different group

In the ACCP system, the strength of recommendations is directly connected to the level of evidence.). The uncertainty associated with this trade-off will determine the strength of recommendations. The strength of the recommendation is denoted first using Grade 1 for strong and Grade 2 for weak recommendations. In this context, if experts believe that benefits outweigh risks then they will make a Grade 1 (strong) recommendation. On the opposite, if they are less sure they will make a Grade 2 recommendation. The grade is followed by the letter which denotes the quality of the evidence level (A, B and C), thus creating the following possible categories: 1A, 1B, 1C, 2A, 2B, and 2C.

The main advantage of the ACCP system is its simplicity. By simply checking the numeric grade the clinician can easily see if it is either a strong or weak recommendation. On the other hand, evaluating disease prognosis is not practicable with this approach. Moreover, this approach has been used little outside the antithrombotic therapy area.

Scottish Intercollegiate Guidelines Network (SIGN) System

The Scottish Intercollegiate Guidelines Network (SIGN) established in 1993 to develop evidence-based clinical guidelines for the National Health Service in Scotland (Harbour & Miller, 2001). The guidelines produced cover a wide range of healthcare professionals and clinical areas.

The quality of evidence is assessed using levels of evidence categorized from 1++ (least likely to be biased) to 4 (most likely to be biased). Studies are evaluated using critical appraisal checklists. These checklists have been originally designed in the Method for Evaluating Research and Guidelines evidence (MERGE) and are completed by clinicians of different background and degrees of expertise. Based on the qualitative assessment of answers to this checklist, we are able to define the evidence's quality level. Different questions are used to appraise the different types of study.

The strength of recommendations is graded using a scale from A to D. The grade of recommendation is drawn from the level of evidence and clinical judgement. The later includes the size and consistency of the body of evidence, its applicability, clinical impact and generalisability.

The main advantages of the SIGN system are its simplicity, and its potential to discriminate between study design requirements for different clinical questions. On the other hand, there are disadvantages too. The grades of recommendation have and unstructured formation. The "considered judgement" has many areas to be considered. Assimilation of the other factors is not well described. Finally, there is no way of assessing or challenging these considerations.

Australian National Health and Medical Research Council (ANHMRC) System

The Australian National Health and Medical Research Council (ANHMRC) provides a framework for evaluating the strength of evidence across several dimensions (National Health and Medical Research Council, 2000), which relate to the type, size and randomness of the study.

First, the level of evidence depicts the quality of the study design and the scale is as follows:

- Level I: Contains evidence obtained from a systematic combined review of all relevant randomized controlled trials
- Level II: Is limited into evidence obtained from at least one properly-designed randomized controlled trial
- Level III: Has three sublevels comprising evidence obtained from well-designed pseudorandomised controlled trials, comparative studies with concurrent controls and allocation not randomized and comparative studies with historical control respectively.
- Level IV: Contains evidence obtained from case series.

Second, the quality of the evidence is assessed using methods that measure the bias of the study and its effects on the results. For each study type, standard quality assessment methods have been developed.

Third, the statistical precision of the evidence is assessed. In this context, the magnitude of the P-value and the precision of the estimate of the treatment effect are important. Similarly, the *size* of the treatment effect (i.e. the distance from the null value) is assessed as an indicator of the evidence usability.

Last but not least, the system evaluates the relevance of evidence as a measure of appropriateness of the outcomes to the specific case. The importance for the patient, the duration of effects and the applicability of the study findings to different settings and patient groups are examined.

Each recommendation is accompanied with a checklist that summarises the data and classifies it according to the dimensions of evidence strength (level of evidence, quality of evidence, statistical precision,. relevance and size of treatment). The checklist summarizes the results from the synthesis of the available evidence. Opposite to other systems, there is no single strength of recommendation climax.

The main advantage of the ANHMRC system is the multidimensional evaluation of the strength of evidence. In this manner, it allows clinicians to focus on the dimensions that are more important to them and to combine more than one dimension by applying weights to each one of them, according to their interest. On the other hand, the absence of a single classification system for the strength of recommendations is one of the major drawbacks of the system. Moreover the system does not evaluate fully the applicability of the results to individual patients, but covers them in a separate guide. Finally benefits, harms and costs are not integrated in the process.

U.S. Task Force on Community Preventive Services (USTFCPS)

The *Guide to Community Preventive Services* (*Community Guide*) is being developed by the non-federal Task Force on Community Preventive Services (Task Force) and is supported by the U.S. Center for Disease Control and Prevention (CDC) and others (Truman et al., 2000).

USTFCPS provides systematic reviews and evidence-based recommendations that can be applied on population-level and not on single patients. Consequently, the evaluation of population-based interventions differs from that of individually-oriented clinical care interventions, which was the subject of all the aforementioned systems. The systematic reviews are conducted by various teams of researchers. The effectiveness and quality of each individual study is assessed, the results are extracted and analyzed. To give an example, randomized controlled trial (RCT) is less critical in population-based research than it is in a clinical research. More specifically, it is not always ethical or feasible, may have limited internal validity, or may have serious threats to external validity.

The body of evidence is characterized as strong, sufficient or insufficient using as criteria the strength of their design and execution, the number of available studies and the size and consistency of reported results. The suitability of study design is based on characteristics that protect against potential threats to validity. Finally, the quality of the study is affected by the execution details, such as: the population of the study and the descriptions of intervention, the population sampling, the exposure and outcome measurement, the data analysis method employed, the interpretation of results (including follow-up, bias, and confounding), etc.

The result of this analysis is to characterize a study for having good, fair, or limited quality of execution. Decision is based on the number of limitations noted, with values close to 0 for good execution and 5 for limited execution performance. The latter studies are not used to support recommendations. Sufficient or strong evidence can be based either on a small number of studies with better execution and more suitable design or a larger number of studies with less suitable design or weaker execution.

Consistency of results is defined as being generally consistent in direction and size based on the opinion of the Task Force. *Effect sizes* are defined to be large, intermediate or small based on the opinion of the Task Force. In general, larger effect sizes (e.g., absolute or relative risks) are considered to represent stronger evidence of effectiveness than smaller effects. *Expert opinion* can be applied by the Task Force when other evidence is not available. The strength of evidence is related directly to the strength of recommendations.

One of the main advantages of the Community Guide is that it allows the participation of people from different backgrounds and perspectives and thus helps minimizing institutional and individual bias. Moreover, it supports the decision making process with different kinds of evidence (e.g. effectiveness, economic evaluations, etc.) and takes into account many factors (e.g., study design, study execution, numbers of studies, etc.) when assessing the process effectiveness. Its main disadvantage is the high complexity. Furthermore, it is demanding in time, resources and expertise and strongly dependent on the Task Force opinions.

Grade Working Group System

The Grade Working Group takes in account more dimensions than just the quality of medical evidence. It performs data extrapolation, thus allowing research outcomes to be employed in situations that significantly differ from that of the original study. Thus, the quality of evidence used to support a clinical decision is a combination of the quality of research data and the clinical 'directness' of the data (Atkins, Best & Briss, 2004).

Although these systems have several differences their aim remains practical the same: Guide clinicians and users in the selection of the most valid and trustworthy evidence.

CRITICISM OF METHODOLOGIES

It is obvious that the lack of a concrete methodology for evidence quality assurance has several drawbacks and creates many problems. Firstly, there is no "common ground" for the evaluation of evidence quality, resulting in controversial opinions and complicating the decision process for the clinician. Secondly, without the justification and documentation provided by these methodologies the usage of the evidence and its results may be wrong. Any scientific results apply to several conditions and populations which must be taken into account before its application. Also, the compliance with such structured methodologies provides a common ground-common language for the way in which evidence should be evaluated enabling knowledge transfer between the clinician and healthcare organizations.

The factors that can lower our confidence about the quality of evidence (Guyatt et al., 2008) comprise of:

- The limitations of the study such as lack of blinding, no report of outcomes etc.
- The incapability to justify the causes of variability.
- The indirect comparison of population samples, methodologies, therapies etc.
- The small size of the sample and the wide confidence intervals.

On the contrary, several factors can increase our confidence about the quality of evidence:

- The magnitude of the effect and the absence of bias. Observational studies for example give low-quality evidence due to the large number of unknown parameters that could not be measured. However, they are based on larger population sample and are more resistant to bias. Thus, the evidence is stronger.
- If all plausible confounding would decrease the magnitude of effect, this increases the quality of the evidence, since we can be more confident that an effect is at least as large as the estimate and may be even larger.

Methodologies and tools used in EBM usually use statistical inference methods in order to generalize the study outcomes and make them applicable to a particular population/sample. The factors related with each individual patient are numerous and consequently the complexity and uncertainty in the projection of results is a great obstacle that should be handled with skepticism (Atkins, 2008). In many cases the knowledge retrieved from clinical research cannot answer the primary question of what is best for the particular case of the patient at hand. Although EBM is not meant to replace clinical practice and examination it can ideally act as a complement.

In a similar manner, the projection of studies results to different populations or time periods should remain in question. Also, the variations of the quality of studies complicate the generalization of results. Moreover, in some medical cases (such as surgeries) the randomized controlled trials can be considered as unethical. Also, historically, certain groups are been under-researched. This lack of available research affects the quality of evidence and does not allow the generalization of results (Rogers, 2004).

Randomized controlled trials are useful for examining therapies effectiveness for controlled medical conditions ("normal situations"), but for complex patient situations the effect of each treatment is difficult to be evaluated. As a result, some studies conclude in results of small significance. Moreover, RCTs give evidence of high quality but are rather expensive. Since research is strongly depended on the available funds, several areas of research receive less interest than others. For example pharmaceutical companies, traditionally fund studies that investigate the efficiency and safety of drugs, but this is not common for the majority of studies. Another obstacle is that not all studies are published and consequently are not accessible to everyone. This results in leaving important parts of the available evidence out of the literature, and makes them useless for EBM (Friedman & Richter, 2004). Finally, the results reported in a clinical trial or study may be higher compared to those of the real clinical practice due to closer patient monitoring during trials.

CONCLUSION

The chapter provides an introduction to the main concepts of Evidence Based Medicine giving emphasis on the evaluation of the quality of evidence. The main aim of EBM is to provide a different paradigm in the everyday clinical practice, which defines documentation of medical decisions, justification and comparative analysis of evidence and leads to less error-prone and more qualitative medical treatment. Due to the high variability of the human factor, attention should be taken for the proper evaluation of the provided evidence. In this context, we have presented the main methodologies from literature that attempt to standardize the ways the evidence is evaluated. The details, advantages and disadvantages of each methodology have been detailed thus providing the ground for the compliance and homogenization of these systems in the future. Our next step is to examine the available semantic technologies such as ontologies and other knowledge representation models, which can be employed for proper defining the quality assessment systems and systematically incorporate them into the evidence based medicine paradigm.

REFERENCES

Atkins, D. (2008). *The limits of evidence based medicine.* Retrieved January 15, 2009, from http://www.dbskeptic.com/2008/08/17/the-limits-of-evidence-based-medicine/

Atkins, D., Best, D., & Briss, P. A. (2004). Grading quality of evidence and strength of recommendations. *British Medical Journal, 328*(7454), 1490. doi:10.1136/bmj.328.7454.1490

Ball, C., Sackett, D., Phillips, B., Straus, S., & Haynes, B. (1998). *Levels of evidence and grades of recommendations*. Retrieved January 17, 2009, from http://www.cebm.net/levels_of_evidence.asp

Canadian Task Force. (1979). Canadian Task Force on the Periodic Health Examination: The periodic health examination. *Canadian Medical Association Journal, 121*, 1193–1254.

Freeman, A. C., & Sweeney, K. (2001). Why General Practitioners Do Not Implement Evidence: Guidelines for Reading Literature Reviews. *British Medical Journal, 323*(7321), 1100–1104. doi:10.1136/bmj.323.7321.1100

Friedman, L. S., & Richter, E. D. (2004). *Relationship between conflicts of interest and research results*. Retrieved January 18, 2009, from http://www.ncbi.nlm.nih.gov/entrez/query.fcgi?cmd=Retrieve&db=pubmed&dopt=Abstract&list_uids=14748860&itool=iconabstr

Guyatt, G. H., Oxman, A. D., Kunz, R., Vist, G. E., Falck-Ytter, Y., & Schunemann, H. J.Grade Working Group. (2008). What is 'quality of evidence' and why is it important to clinicians? *British Medical Journal, 336*(1), 995–998. doi:10.1136/bmj.39490.551019.BE

Guyatt, G. H., Schünemann, H., Cook, D., Pauker, S., Sinclair, J., Bucher, H., & Jaeschke, R. (2001). Grades of recommendation for antithrombotic agents. *Chest, 119*(1), 3S–7S. doi:10.1378/chest.119.1_suppl.3S

Harbour, R., & Miller, J. (2001). A new system for grading recommendations in evidence based guidelines. *British Medical Journal, 323*(1), 334–336. doi:10.1136/bmj.323.7308.334

Lundberg, G. D. (1992). Perspective from the editor of JAMA. *The JAMA Bulletin of the Medical Library Association, 80*(2), 110–114.

National Health and Medical Research Council. (2000). *How to use the evidence: assessment and application of scientific evidence*. Retrieved January 18, 2009, from http://www.nhmrc.gov.au/publications/synopses/cp65syn.htm

Rogers, W. A. (2004). Evidence based medicine and justice: a framework for looking at the impact of EBM upon vulnerable or disadvantaged groups. *Journal of Medical Ethics*, *30*(1), 141–145. doi:10.1136/jme.2003.007062

Sackett, D. (2003). Evidence-based medicine. What is it and what it isn't. *The Origins and Aspirations of ACP Journal Club.* Retrieved January 20, 2009, from http://www.minervation.com/cebm/ebmisisnt.html

Truman, B. I., Smith-Akin, C. K., & Hinman, A. R. (2000). Developing the Guide to Community Preventive Services--overview and rationale. The Task Force on Community Preventive Services. *American Journal of Preventive Medicine*, *18*(1), 18–26. doi:10.1016/S0749-3797(99)00124-5

Chapter 9
Quality and Reliability Aspects in Evidence Based E-Medicine

Asen Atanasov
Medical University Hospital "St. George", Bulgaria

ABSTRACT

This chapter is a brief survey on some e-medicine resources and international definitions focused on the three main subjects of the healthcare quality – the patient, the costs and the evidence for quality. The patients can find in e-medicine everything that they need, but often without data on the supporting evidence. The medical professionals can learn where to find e-information on cost, quality and patient safety, and, more importantly, how to distinguish claims from evidence by applying the principles of evidence based medicine. The goal is to spread and popularize the knowledge in this field with an emphasis on how one can find, assess and utilize the best present evidence for more effective healthcare. The sites discussed below could assist in the retrieval of information about methods for obtaining evidence along with the ways of measuring evidence strength and limitations. These sites also provide information on implementing the ultimate evidence-based product – clinical guidelines for better medical practice and health service.

INTRODUCTION

The international consensus document (CLSI, HS1-A2, 2004) emphasized that the top in the hierarchy of healthcare quality is the undivided of complete customer satisfaction at minimal cost and highest quality. The customer, who might be unsatisfied by healthcare quality or other reasons, may prefer to search the Internet for some alternative sources of health information. Looking for a solution to her/his own problem amongst hundreds of thousands of Web sites, she/he might find exactly what is needed in "minimal cost" but sometimes with unknown quality. The health professionals can also find scientific basis for continuous education along with answers of almost all practical problems of their patients.

DOI: 10.4018/978-1-61692-843-8.ch009

However, information about the evidence strength and quality is not always available.

This chapter shortly considers the three main subjects of total quality in healthcare - customer, cost, and evidence for quality, in the context of e-medicine. The goal is more people to obtain knowledge in this field and use properly the best present evidence. The patient can find in e-medicine everything that she/he needs, but often without data on the supporting evidence. The medical professionals can be assisted to decide what kind of e-resources they are interested in and how they can learn more about evidence in medicine. The information concerning the achievement of basic medical science, specific regulations, laws, accreditation and healthcare audits remains beyond the scope of the chapter.

BACKGROUND

A lot of e-medical information can be easily obtained through Internet and Wikipedia. Its usefulness, however, depends on the users' willingness, behavior, knowledge and skills to distinguish a claim from actual evidence, and to users' ability to use properly e-medical information. Although for some regions the access to e-resources might be a problem, Bratislava Declaration clearly outlined as a priority the validity and quality of electronic health information, education and training (UEMS, 2007).

THE CUSTOMER

Most of us have been, are, or will be patients. The patient, a suffering human being, becomes "customer", one of the numerous external and internal customers of the healthcare system (other patients, suppliers, institutions, factories, agencies, hospitals, doctors, nurses, pharmacists, technicians, and all other staff engaged in healthcare). As a customer, the patient is told that his/her welfare is paramount for the healthcare system. Thus, the patient-customer expects the best quality of help or, in other words, service. Being a customer and receiving service, the patient obtains the opportunity to actively assist the medical staff regarding his/her personal health. The result, however, is that the customer evaluates the health service rather than his/her health behavior.

However, customer's "satisfaction" with the quality of health service might be far away from the "evidence for quality". Satisfaction is very subjective and cannot be objectively measured hence it is not the best end point for healthcare evaluation. Most patients today are well informed, but some prefer illusions in place of reality. People are not always able to make a clear distinction between personal satisfaction and healthy life style.

The best health strategy for the society is not be the best approach for a single person. Any healthcare system needs money and can be easily destroyed by growing expectations of uncertain nature in an environment of limited and often badly managed resources. An organized group of active, even aggressive, patients might politically impose disproportional distribution of funds that otherwise might be spent more effectively for the advantage of more patients. Attractive new technologies, diagnostic instruments, tools and devices, new curative approaches and therapeutic drugs are often subject of commercial rather than medical interest.

In such a complicated situation, the healthcare customers are looking at the Internet for health information because they want to obtain dependable service, communicate online with their physicians, talk for their health problems, receive interpretation for their laboratory or instrumental records and medications, or arrange an appointment. They are ready to browse pay-for-performance programs in which recognized physicians are committed to providing quality care and service. Such e-Medicine and e-Prescribing sources need support for delivering high quality and efficient healthcare focused on the physician as the core of the network. Improvement of the customer's experience with a physician's knowledge contains the providers' medical costs.

The providers of medical advice directly use the technology and should be accountable for patient care. Moreover,, the providers should guarantee service and system quality together with the quality of information for the ultimate consumer of e-healthcare – the patient (LeRouge, & al, 2004).

Another cash service is online clinical conferencing. It offers consultations on many clinical cases. The patient tells his/her medical history and answers clinical questionnaires, including data of physical examination, laboratory findings, medication, and other relevant topics. The patient receives third party comments, and expert opinion about diagnosis, medication, or other questions in sites like [http://www.thirdspace.org], [Clinical Conferences Online.mht], and [e-medicine.com] which are continuously updated.

Web-based health services, such as [WebMD], also provide health information, including symptom checklists, pharmacy information, blogs of physicians with specific topics, and a place to store personal medical information. [WebMD], the Magazine is a patient-directed publication distributed bimonthly to physician waiting rooms in the USA. Similar health-related sites include [MediCineNet] - an online media publishing company; [Medscape] - a professional portal with 30 medical specialty areas which offers up-to-date information for physicians and other healthcare professionals; [RxList] – providing detailed pharmaceutical information on generic and name-brand drugs. The web site formerly known as [eMedicine.com], created for physicians and healthcare professionals, is now [eMedicineHealth] - a consumer site offering similar information to that of [WebMD]. Most are last modified February 2009.

Another useful site is MedHelp [http://www.medhelp.org/]. It delivers the opportunity for online discussion on different healthcare topics by a partnership with medical professionals from hospitals and medical research institutions. The site offers several forums of contacts - "Ask an Expert" for users' questions, "Health Communities" for questions, comments, responses and support from other users, and "International Forums" on topics including addiction, allergy, cancer, cosmetic surgery, dental, and various other topics.

The site Med-e-Tel [http://www.medetel.lu/index.php] comprises e-health, Telemedicine and Health ICT as tools for service to medical and nurse practitioners, patients, healthcare institutions and governments. The site offers broad information on markets, various research and experience, and appears to be a gathering place, for education, networking and business aimed at a worldwide audience with diverse professional backgrounds.

Another site destined for professionals is eMedicine - a separate medical website that provides regular clinical challenges comprising of a short case history accompanied by a visual cue in the form of a radiograph, ECG or photo, along with the clinical resolution for each case. The customer can click on one of the cases listed in the index, after which will leave the Global Family Doctor website and go to the eMedicine website [http://www.globalfamilydoctor.com/education/emedicine/eMedicine.asp]. eMedicine offers also a series of clinical problems in an interactive format with CME credit available after completion.

E-medicine related sites are continuously updated and offer enormous information useful for everybody. For example, if one is concerned by healthy life styles, he or she may find information about which are the benefits of physical exercise, how to avoid undesirable events, how to incorporate exercise in customer lifestyle, how to succeed with weight control, what to do for a healthy pregnancy and post-natal care. Another example is the Journal Bandolier Extra, [www.ebandolier.com]. The top ten eMedicine Case Studies can be seen in recently updated [http://www.who.is/whois-net/ip-address/emedcine.net/].

One analysis of American Sociological Association [http://www.asanet.org] showed that the users should be capable of evaluating the quality of e-health information since the information might be inaccurate or out of date. The users also have to distinguish between commercial advertising and appropriate health information, and recognize potential conflicts of interest. The abundance of health information permits customers to assume more responsibility for their own health care, and, therefore, patients should be included in developing standardized quality assurance systems for online health information [http://www.emedicine.com/med/].

An important support of the patient needs is so cold Bratislava Declaration on e-Medicine. It was published by the Council of European Union of Medical Specialists (UEMS) on October 13th 2007. [www.uems.net]. The Declaration establishes that there is existing potential for improvement of e-medicine in the context of quality and the manner in which the patient' care is provided. The priority of quality over the cost-efficiencies is advocated, and the electronic development, recording, transfer, and storage of medical data are accepted as useful and inevitable. The Declaration also recognizes the need of support for (1) further progress in the accessibility of medical information; (2) developing higher standards in medical qualification and specialisation; (3) promotion of improvements in the well-being and healthcare of persons. The Council of EUMS also emphasizes that the misuse of e-Medicine could damage persons, communities and countries, and can become a risk to the security of data, patient confidentiality, the medical ethics, and the law. "The principles of a patient's privacy and confidentiality must be respected, and only patients have the right voluntarily to decide to have their data held in storage" – the Declaration says. In the context of the electronic recording, transfer and storage of medical information, the Council will make an effort, through registration and validation procedures, to implement, promote, develop and control future development of the fields

- respect for the security and privacy of persons, and the rights and laws governing these;
- respect for medical ethical principles;
- the validity of electronic health information;
- the quality of electronic medical education and training (UEMS, 2007).

Patients' values and preferences are important and might differ markedly from those of physicians.

COSTS

It is always useful to keep cost in mind, especially in times of financial crisis. An analysis of the first generation e-health companies showed that some of them lost billions in value during the early 2000 and failed to build a profitable business. Four most important factors in predicting the success or failure of an Internet healthcare company are identified - compelling value, unambiguous revenue model, competitive barriers, and organizational structure for cost control. Companies that make certain that they meet all or most of these factors, will have a better chance for success with a unique and valuable product and disciplined spending. Three factors introduce more challenges (Itagaki, & al, 2002).

Some companies have a more impressive array of e-health properties that allow them to offer a bulk of services, earn enough revenue, and continue operating successfully. However, today's economic situation introduces a great deal of uncertainty into their future. The success depends on the stability of users' interest and how long their cash reserves will last.

Few industries can sustain the rapid economic downturn. However, despite the people less income, some medical supply industries continue to grow. An example is Total e-Medical - a physician-supervised supplier of diabetic testing materials, durable medical equipment, respiratory care, and arthritis and pain management products. The company realizes unprecedented growth of revenue, hired new employees in the past months, and intends to continue its workforce expansion [www.totalemedical.com], last updated 13.02.2009.

On February 16, 2009 it was announced that as much as $21 billion in the economic stimulus package is designated for IT for medical records in the USA. The funds will help health care providers to implement such IT systems, which are expensive and difficult to deploy. About $3 billion will be directed to help health care providers buy IT systems while an additional $18 billion would be covering for additional Medicare and Medicaid payments to health care providers who use technology to improve patient care. Hospitals could receive up to $1.5 million while physicians would qualify for about $40,000 over several years. The hope is that the potential for e-health to improve medical care remains excellent. This is important because the improvement can produce savings for healthcare and profits for enterprising start-ups. The prospect that any person might have his/her personal e-medical record would be a realistic goal (Kolbasuk, & McGree, 2009).

The e-medicine needs governmental support to improve the delivery of healthcare services to the elderly and poor customers. It is estimated that e-medicine or telemedicine can reduce about 60% of the on-site care cost by using e-mail, faxes and telephone consultations to link patients with health-care providers. It also improves access to health-delivery services in rural areas with shortages of doctors and hospitals. Instead, some insurance agencies reimburse only "face-to-face consultations" – an expensive type of communication between patient and the doctor. Telemedicine was proven especially effective in Norway where even the installation of costly equipment turned out to be cheaper than flying doctors into remote regions [http://www.emedicine.com/med/].

The described events concern costs of e-health and e-medical information. However, the decisions about costs of the real health care are much more complicated and concern large parts of the society. Health professionals, especially governmental experts, should be familiar with economical analyses which allow objective choice between different health interventions. Unfortunately, the different economic analyses are often not well understood and they rarely assist in a political discussion or in the development of national health strategies.

The cost-effectiveness analysis compares different health interventions by their costs and obtained health effect. It helps to assess which health intervention is worth to be implemented from the economic point of view. The costs are expressed in monetary units, and the health effect in life-years gained. The cost-effectiveness analysis, therefore, followed by sensitivity analysis (which tests the impact of best case and worse case scenarios) becomes a part of the decision-making process. The cost-utility analysis (utility is a cardinal value that represents the strength of an individual's preferences for specific outcomes under condition of uncertainty) is applied when the healthcare area that is likely to provide the greatest benefit has to be identified. The cost-profit or cost-benefit analysis is useful when information is needed to assess which intervention will result in resource savings (that both sides of the equation are in same monetary units).

A clear and very useful explanation of these analyses and their terminology can be found in the series named "What is?" sponsored by an educational grant from Aventis Pharma [www.evidence-based-medicine.co.uk], and, in a more sophisticated version, in [http://www.cche.net/usersguides/main.asp].

The economical analyses, along with survival analysis (Cox model) and many other methods are powerful tools that produce evidence. Although the educational material in the shown sites is only instructive, the references exist that explain the methods, calculations, and limitations, of each approach. Costs in medicine remain an important issue and now are incorporated in any decision analysis and clinical guideline.

QUALITY

The following short list of common definitions is useful for better understanding of quality in health care and medicine:

- Quality – "Degree to which a set of inherent characteristics fulfills requirements" (ISO 9000, 2000, 3.1.1)
- Quality assurance – "Part of quality management focused on providing confidence that quality requirements will be fulfilled" (ISO 9000, 2000, 3.2.11). "Quality assurance indicates the quality of process performance" (HS1-A2, 2004).
- Quality control – "Part of quality management focused on fulfilling quality requirements" (ISO 9000, 2000, 3.2.10). "Quality control indicates the quality of procedural performance" (CLSI, HS1-A2, 2004).
- Quality improvement – "Part of quality management focused on increasing the ability to fulfill quality requirements (ISO 9000, 2000, 3.2.12). "Continuous quality improvement indicates how to achieve sustained improvement" (CLSI, HS1-A2, 2004).
- Quality management – "Coordinated activities to direct and control an organization with regard to quality (ISO 9000, 2000, 3.2.8).
- Quality management system – "Management system to direct and control an organization with regard to quality" (ISO 9000, 2000, 3.2.3). "Quality management system will support all operational paths of workflow" (CLSI, HS1-A2, 2004).
- Quality policy – "Overall intentions and direction of an organization related to quality as formally expressed by top management" (ISO 9000, 2000, 3.2.4.)
- Reliability - the consistency with which the same information is obtained by a test or set of tests in the absence of intervening variables (Tudiver, & al, 2008).

Good quality of healthcare service would not be obtained without serious administrative support. A lot of documents of the Clinical and Laboratory Standards Institute (CLSI, former National Committee for Clinical Laboratory Standards, NCCLS), USA, are developed through a considerable consensus process. After worldwide expert discussion, each document is disseminated for global application [www.nccls.org]. Several CLSI documents describe, in detail, how a health organization that wishes to implement a quality management system can succeed. "These specialized documents are designed for any healthcare service manager who wishes to improve the processes involved in creating customer satisfaction by implementing proven standardized quality system concept" /GP22-A2, 2004, p. 7/.

Continuous quality improvement (CLSI, GP22-A2, 2004) is a model focused specifically on the implementation of clinical service quality system management. It represents any healthcare service as working within two forms of infrastructural quality system matrices. The external matrix is created by external guidance from local and governmental administrative-level policies, processes and procedures. The internal matrix is built up from intrinsic quality system managerial-level policies, processes, and procedures. The internal matrix contains the quality system and underlines service operations rather than healthcare operation.

Another document (CLSI, HS1-A2, 2004) represents organizational hierarchy of quality administration in healthcare establishments. Quality control is the starting level. It is considered as an operational process control technique for measuring the effectiveness of the procedural performance that is expected to fulfill requirements for quality and governmental compliance. It needs quality indicators like precision, accuracy and other statistical variables. Quality assurance is the next level that measures the effectiveness of process performance and provides confidence that the quality requirements are fulfilled. Implementation of a quality management system is the crucial level - the practice facilitating systematic process-oriented improvement. All these levels are included in quality cost management that adds the economic activities – "cost of quality". The highest level is the total quality management. It identifies the cost of quality for obtaining total quality management and insures sustainable high quality "by focusing on long-term success through customer satisfaction" (CLSI, HS1-A2, 2004, p. vii).

In the above motion directed "upstairs" five key activities are implemented in a continuous spiral - quality planning, quality teamwork, quality monitoring, quality improvement and quality review (Plan-Do-Check-Act). The results of the last quality review represent the basis of the next cycle towards the next quality level. All necessary activities have a detailed description in the original document (CLSI, HS1-A2, 2004).

The administration of a healthcare establishment, if decided, should surmount step-by-step the hierarchical ladder, from the lowest level of quality to the highest– total quality management – "An organization-wide approach centered on ongoing quality improvement as evidenced by total customer satisfaction and minimal cost of maximized quality" (CLSI, GP22-A2, 2004, p. xii).

Recently, the MARQuIS project (2009) outlined the EU perspectives in five papers. They commented quality improvement strategies for European cross-border healthcare, national quality improvement policies and strategies, applications of quality improvement strategies in European hospitals, the results of the MARQuIS project, and the future direction of quality and safety in hospital care in EU.

However, the lack of staff motivation is able to transform all administrative efforts for high quality in empty formalism and bureaucratic curtain. If medical professionals understand, joint and support the administrative efforts for implementation of quality management system, the team surely will succeed. In fact it is too early to discuss the effectiveness of this systematic approach towards continuous improvement of the healthcare service. More experience should be obtained for a frank assessment of the described administrative approach for obtaining high quality in healthcare.

Quality Indicators

Measurement of the quality is essential for its improvement. The tools intended to measure the quality of healthcare in fact measure the evidence for quality and confirm that a desirable level is obtained.

- Quality indicators are „observations, statistics, or data defined by the organization or service that typify the performance of a given work process and provide evidence that the organization or service is meeting its quality intentions" (AABB, 2003).
- The thresholds are "statistical measure of compliance of the specific indicator for acceptable outcome" (CLSI, HS1-A2, 2004).

Quality indicators are objective measures for analysis of quality achievement in health service. Their implementation is an attainable, realistic goal for assessing compliance and quantifying improvement.

Some quality indicators concern patient preferences and are obtained by patient interviews. These indicators are important for identification of gaps in quality at the population level and can be useful for improvement of health service. These are mainly indicators related to pain, symptom management and access to care. With palliative care and emergency room visits, they are identified as acceptable for assessment of quality.

The structure indicators are, for instance, the patient-to-nurse ratio, the existing strategies to prevent medication errors, the measurements of patient satisfaction. The process indicators give a quick view of the quality of care. When indicators such like the length of stay in the hospital, duration of mechanical ventilation, the proportion of days with all beds occupied, the proportion of glucose measurement higher than 8.0 or lower than 2.2 mmol/L, are applied to an intensive care unit, they can characterize the quality of total activity of the unit (Steel, & al, 2004).

The outcome indicators are the standardized mortality, the incidence of decubitus, the number of unplanned extubations and others. In each case, however, it is important to assess the validity of data used because the quality ranking of the hospitals depends not only on the indicators used, but also on the nature of the data used. By means of the same indicator, hospitals classified as high-quality using routine administrative data have been reclassified as intermediate or low-quality hospitals using the enhanced administrative data (Glance, & al, 2008). The authors emphasize the need to improve the quality of the administrative data if these data are to serve as the information infrastructure for quality reporting.

A recent study (Grunfeld, & al, 2008) assesses stakeholder acceptability of quality indicators of end-of-life care that potentially are measurable from population-based administrative health databases. A multidisciplinary panel of cancer care health professionals, patients with metastatic breast cancer and caregivers for women died of metastatic breast cancer, is used to assess acceptability among the indicators for end-of-life care. The authors conclude that patient preferences, variation in local resources, and benchmarking should be considered when developing quality monitoring systems. Those quality indicators that stakeholders perceive as measuring quality care will be most useful.

The acceptance of quality indicators in EU is a subject of another study (Legido-Quigley, & al, 2008). It is noticed that a few EU countries have adopted quality indicators, possibly because some contradictions in EU healthcare policy. Health care is a responsibility of the member states, but the free movement of healthcare customers is regulated by the European law. Some initiatives on quality are coming from national governments but others are from health professionals and providers; some solutions are offered by EU laws but others are entirely nationally based. The following convincing example is shown as evidence for the large variations in the perception of the meaningfulness of quality indicators: in Denmark, the quality of care provided by hospitals for six common diseases (lung cancer, schizophrenia, heart failure, hip fracture, stroke, and surgery for acute gastrointestinal bleeding) is measured for hospital assessment; in UK the performance of general practitioners is assessed with the quality and outcomes framework of about 140 measures developed through evidence and professional consensus. Another very important side of the problem deserves attention: "Quality indicator systems have been criticised for focusing on what is easily measured rather than what is important, and for being used in ways that encourage opportunistic behaviour, either by manipulating data or changing behaviour to achieve targets while compromising care". (Legido-Quigley & al 2008).

The best currently available evidence for quality of any medical care might be the evaluation of patient outcomes. The general criteria for conducting studies on patient outcomes are described in a CLSI document (CLSI HS6-A, 2004) and deserve more attention. The document is focused on the planning, conducting and reporting patient outcomes research. It provides a brief review on research methodology of primary patient outcome studies such as observational studies (surveys or cross-sectional studies, case-control studies and cohort studies) and interventional studies (randomized controlled trials and nonrandomized studies). It outlines the role of systematic overviews, meta-analyses, decision analyses, cost-effectiveness analyses and simulations along with a limited reference to some published methodological sources.

A good example of the rules implementation on an outcome study is the PATH project (Veillard, & al 2005). It is currently implemented as a pilot project in eight EU countries in order to refine its framework before its further expansion. The project describes the outcomes achieved, specifically the definition of the concept and the identification of key dimensions of hospital performance. It also designs the architecture directed to enhance evidence-based management and quality improvement through performance assessment, selection of the core and tailored set of performance indicators with detailed operational definitions. It identifies the trade-offs between indicators and elaborates on the descriptive sheets for each indicator in order to support the hospitals in interpreting their results, designing a balanced dashboard, and developing strategies for implementation of the PATH framework. The future implementation of this project could be of significant interest for grading of hospitals by quality and effectiveness.

Patient Safety

The high quality and reliability in health care are inaccessible without suitable activity to insure patient safety. Recently the General Secretariat of the Council of the EU sent a recommendation on patient safety, prevention and control of healthcare associated infections to the Working Party on Public Health [Interinstitutional file 2009/0003 (CNS) 6947/09, 27 February, 2009]. The document offers the important definitions concerning patient safety:

- Adverse event – "incident which results in harm to a patient";
- Harm – "impairment of structure or function of the body and/or any deleterious effect which arises from that";
- Healthcare associated infections – "diseases or pathologies (illness, inflammation) related to the presence of an infectious agent or its products as a result of exposure to healthcare facilities or healthcare procedures";
- Patient safety – "freedom for a patient from unnecessary harm or potential harm associated with healthcare".

The draft document notices an estimation showing that between 8% and 12% of patients in EU Member States admitted to hospitals suffer from adverse events whilst receiving healthcare. That is why the document is focused on the expected action and national policies directed towards improving public health, preventing human illnesses and diseases, and obviating sources of danger to human health: "Community action in the field of public health shall fully respect the responsibilities of the Member States for the organisation and delivery of health services and medical care" the document says. The aim is "to achieve result-oriented behaviour and organizational change, by defining responsibilities at all levels, organizing support facilities and local technical resources and setting up evaluation procedures" [Interinstitutional file 2009/0003 (CNS) 6947/09, 27 February, 2009].

It is also emphasized that the realization of these recommendations needs dissemination of the document content to healthcare organisations, professional bodies, and educational institutions along with improvement of the patient information. The document suggests that each institutional level should follow the recommended approaches. This would ensure that the key elements are put into everyday practice and the patient safety is receiving proper attention.

EVIDENCE

During the last decades several powerful methods for the distinction of evidence from claims in medicine were effectively disseminated.

Evidence can be measured and assessed. For example, the accuracy of the diagnostic tests can be measured by their diagnostic sensitivity (the probability of a positive result amongst target persons) and diagnostic specificity (the probability of a negative result amongst control persons); the post-test probability of disease can be calculated by Bayesian approach from pre-test probability and the new information from the diagnostic test; the ratio of the probability that a given test result is met in a target (ill) person to the probability that the same result is met in a control (healthy) person, is given by the likelihood ratio (LR); the various kinds of effects (risks) for treated and control populations (groups) could be evaluated by the odds ratio; the treatment effect – by the number needed to treat (NNT), that is the inverse of the absolute risk reduction and is translated as "how many patients should be treated to prevent an event". There are many others. Most of these useful methods can be found in the book-series Clinical Evidence [www.clinicalevidence.com], Wikipedia and others Internet or published resources related to clinical epidemiology.

There are other methods that have become more sophisticated. For example, summarizing the results of a number of randomized trials and other independent studies can be done by the statistical technique called meta-analysis. It is used mainly to assess the clinical effectiveness of healthcare interventions as well as to estimate precisely the treatment effect. Meta-analysis is usually applied in systematic reviews, but as any method has some limitations. The outcome of a meta-analysis will be influenced by the inclusion or exclusion of certain trials, and by the degree of adherence to the rigorous standards for the eligibility criteria explicitness and appropriateness that should characterize a meta-analysis (Fried, & al, 2008).

Another example for gathering evidence is the assessment of the future effect of a medical action by decision analysis. It includes building a decision tree, obtaining probabilities and utilities for each outcome, evaluating the outcomes, and performing a sensitivity analysis to compare alternative health strategies (Detsky, & al. 1997, [www.cche.net/usersguides/main.asp], [www.evidence-based-medicine.co.uk] and others).

How to obtain evidence for healthcare costs through clinical economic analysis and measurement of the healthcare quality by quality indicators was already discussed. However, any calculations have limitations and need valid primary data.

EVIDENCE BASED MEDICINE

Evidence-based medicine (EBM) is the conscientious, explicit and judicious use of the best current evidence in making decisions about the care of individual patients (Sackett, & al 2000). In this context "best" means that the quality of the evidence can be measured, and "current" means that the best evidence today might not be the best tomorrow.

EBM instructs clinicians how to access, evaluate, and interpret the medical publications. The clinician can find the relevant answer of the patient problem by performing critical appraisal of the information resources,. After the decision is taken and best health service applied to the patient, the clinical performance can be evaluated and continually monitored. The goal of this process is to improve patient care by more effective and efficient use of clinical information, including diagnostic and prognostic markers, and to ensure effective and safe treatment in compliance with individual patient preferences.

EBM also offers an approach to teaching the practice of medicine. Centre for Health Evidence maintains (on behalf of the Evidence-Based Medicine Working Group) the full text of the series "Evidence-Based Medicine: A New Approach to

Teaching the Practice of Medicine" [http://www.cche.net/usersguides/main.asp]. The series was originally published in the Journal of the American Medical Association (JAMA) between 1992 and 2000 years and was last updated on August 15, 2007. The educational materials have been enhanced and re-introduced in a new interactive website [http://www.usersguides.org]. Access to the site is available by subscription through JAMA. In the „Users' Guides to EBM", the interested medical professional can find a step-by-step explanation how to use electronic information resources, how to select publications that are likely to provide valid results about therapy and prevention, diagnostic tests (including Bayesian approach and likelihood ratios), harm and prognosis, how to use a clinical decision analysis, clinical practice guidelines and recommendations, and many other basic principles of EBM.

A study assessing the efficiency of EBM teaching shows the growing popularity of EBM education, practice teaching and evaluation of learning methods, but also indicates the lack of data on the application of the obtained EBM skills in the clinical practice. It is noticed also that users' perception for the main barriers to EBM practice is the finding of contradictory results in the literature, the insufficient knowledge of English language, the limited access to PCs, and the lack of time and institutional support (Gardois, & al, 2004).

The Objective Structured Clinical Examination (OSCE) measures the family medicine resident lifelong learning skills in evidence-based medicine as an important part of the evaluation of physician skills. The authors describe an innovative assessment tool for evaluating the skills of EBM. It was found that the competencies are overlapped with well known major skills such as translation of uncertainty for an answerable question, systematic retrieval of best evidence available, critical appraisal of evidence for validity, clinical relevance and applicability, and application of results in practice. These skills are tested in a simulated OSCE. The results show that the development of standardized tools for assessing EBM skills is an essential part of the evaluation of physician skills. They also emphasize the importance of the physician's understanding of the different levels of evidence (Tudiver, & al 2008)

An interesting article describes the development and implementation of an evidence-based practice model named CETEP (Clinical Excellence Through Evidence-Based Practice). The model provides the framework for a process that can be easily adapted for use as a tool to document the critical appraisal process. It is focused on nurse's activities that lead to evidence-based practice changes and can be adapted for use in any healthcare organization. CETER emphasizes the process evaluating the applicability of the evidence for the clinical practice. It is shown that using research to incorporate essential components into clinical practice needs serious consideration before changing practice at the bedside. The article encourages nurses to conduct research and use evidence that will have meaning for their practice. It is expected that addressing practice problems or evaluating changes in practice with this model will be empowering. Translation of research to practice is more complex than simply writing a policy or procedure based on a research study and expecting the staff to comply. Successful integration of research into practice requires critical appraisal of study methods and results, and most importantly, consideration of the applicability of the evidence to the particular clinical setting (Collins, & al, 2008).

Table 1 gives a list of sites that are useful for any reader interested in the principles and application of EBM.

EBM practice starts by converting the need for clinical information into answerable questions. The answers are researched through e-information and library resources. If the Internet is accessible, a lot of library resources become available. A simple enumeration includes MEDLINE, Cochrane Databases of Systematic Reviews and Clinical Trials, DARE, ACP Journal Club, InfoR-

Table 1. Some websites, with information related to EBM

http://www.ahrq.gov/clinic	http://www.acponline.org/journals/acpjc/jcmenu.htm
http://www.jr2.ox.ac.uk/bandolier/	http://www.ceres.uwcm.ac.uk/frameset.cfm?section=trip
http://cebm.jr2.ox.ac.uk/	http://www.ebponline.nehttp://agatha.york.ac.uk/darehp.htm
http://www.clinicalevidence.com	http://www.york.ac.uk/inst/crd/ehcb.htm
http://www.cochrane.org/	http://www.evidence-basedmedicine.com
http://www.infopoems.com	http://medicine.ucsf.edu/resources/guidelines
http://www.ICSI.org	http://www.ahrq.gov/clinic/uspstfix.htm
http://www.guidelines.gov	http://www.york.ac.uk/inst/crd/

etriever, InfoPoems, UpToDate, DynaMed and others. The readings found are critically appraised for validity, clinical relevance, and applicability of the evidence. The application of the obtained results in practice and monitoring the effects are focused on the patient.

When researching the evidence one should keep in mind the difference between POEM (Patient-Oriented Evidence that Matters) and DOE (Disease-Oriented Evidence). POEM deals with outcomes of importance to patients, such as changes in morbidity, mortality, or quality of life. DOE deals with surrogate end points, such as changes in laboratory values or other measures of response (Slawson & Shaughnessy, 2000).

The preferable readings in researching the evidence are the high quality systematic reviews that can be found mainly in The Cochrane Database of Systematic Review, The Cochrane Controlled Trails Register, The Cochrane Review Methodology Database [www.york.ac.uk/inst/crd/welcome.htm], [www.cebm.jr2.ox.ac.uk], [www.hiru.macmaster/ca/cochrane/default.htm], [www.ich.ucl.ac.uk/srtu] and other sites.

The systematic reviews are an important source of evidence because their authors take care for finding all relevant studies on the question, assessing each study, synthesizing the findings in an unbiased way, very often after performing a meta-analysis. Expert critical appraisal about the validity and clinical applicability of systematic reviews can be found in the Database of Abstracts of Reviews of Effects (DARE), at the Website of the Centre for Review and Dissemination, University of York [www.york.ac.uk/inst/crd/welcome.htm], the sites shown in Table 1, as well as in [www.mrw.interscience.wiley.com/cochrane/cochrane_cldare_articles_fs.html].

The next preferable readings as sources of evidence are randomized controlled trials (RCT) – the most appropriate research design for studying the effectiveness of a specific intervention or treatment. There is considerable information about how to plan, perform, and report a RCT as STARD checklist of items to include in diagnostic accuracy study (Bossuyt, & al, 2003), and in a randomized trial (Altman, & al, 2001). All other study designs, especially already mentioned outcomes studies (CLSI HS6-A, 2004) can also produce high quality evidence.

The findings of systematic reviews, RCT and other studies provide the evidence for the development of clinical guidelines based on the principles of evidence-based medicine. The clinical guidelines are destined to bridge the gap between research and practice, to base the clinical decisions on a research evidence, and to make this evidence available globally. The clinical guidelines are systematically developed statements designed to help practitioners and patients to decide on appropriate healthcare regarding specific clinical conditions and/or circumstances. Guidelines development, legal implications, implementations, and evaluation, are described in „What is?" series [www.evidence-based-medicine.co.uk], in [www.healthcentre.org.uk/hc/library/guidelines.htm], [www.nice.org.uk], and some others sites.

Table 2. Evidence hierarchy scheme [http//www.guideline.gov] from the guideline of Diabetes mellitus (with small modifications)

LEC*	Study Design or Information Type	Comments
1.	RCT** Multicenter trials Large meta-analyses With quality rating	Well-conducted and controlled trials at 1 or more medical centers Data derived from a substantial number of trials with adequate power; substantial number of subjects and outcome data Consistent pattern of findings in the population for which the recommendation is made – generalizable results Compelling nonexperimental, clinically obvious evidence (e.g., use of insulin in diabetic ketoacidosis); "all or none" evidence
2.	RCT Prospective cohort studies Meta-analyses of cohort studies Case-control studies	Limited number of trials, small number of subjects Well-conducted studies Inconsistent findings or results not representative for the target population
3	Methodologically flawed RCT Nonrandomized controlled trials Observational studies Case series or case reports	Trials with 1 or more major or 3 or more minor methodological flaws Uncontrolled or poorly controlled trials Retrospective or observational data Conflicting data with a weight of evidence unable to support a final recommendation
4	Expert consensus Expert opinion based on experience Theory-driven conclusions, Unproven claims, Experience-based information	Inadequate data for inclusion in level-of-evidence categories 1, 2, or 3; data necessitates an expert panel's synthesis of the literature and a consensus. *Level-of-Evidence Category, **Randomized Controlled Trials.

The guideline development follows the principles of EBM. It starts with a clear definition of key questions about patients involved, alternative strategies, clinical outcomes, and methodological quality of the available evidence. A systematic review of each question should be available, and the evidence in the guideline should be arranged by their levels of power - from randomized controlled clinical trials and basic clinical research to well-conducted observational studies focused on patient-important outcomes and inferences. Nonsystematic clinical studies and expert opinion also are acceptable.

A concise, continuously updated, and easy-to-use collection of clinical guidelines for primary care, combined with the best available evidence, is offered by [http://ebmg.wiley.com]. The collection covers a wide range of medical conditions with their diagnostics and treatments. The high-quality evidence is graded from A (that means "strong evidence exists and further research is unlikely to change the conclusion") to D (that means "weak evidence and the estimate of effect is uncertain"). All reviews cited in the site are coming from The Cochrane Database of Systematic Reviews.

It is likely that a complete source of clinical guidelines is the National Guideline Clearinghouse, United States [http//www.guideline.gov/index.asp]. As recommended by EBM (Sackett, & al, 2000), each guideline contains a description of the methods used to collect and select the evidence and the rating scheme for the strength of this evidence. Such a rating scheme, used in the diabetes mellitus guideline (revised 2007), is given in Table 2 as an example [http//www.guideline.gov].

According to the principles of EBM, guidelines for clinical practice are also subject of critical appraisal and continuous improvement. For example, the recommendations made in the diabetes mellitus guideline (edition 2000) were found to be in agreement when concerning the general management and clinical care of type 2 diabetes, but some important differences in treatment details were noticed. The influence of professional bodies such as the American Diabetes Association was seen as an important factor in explaining the international consensus. It was also noticed that the globalisation of recommended management of diabetes is not a simple consequence of the globalisation of research evidence and deserves more attention (Burgers, & al, 2002).

Sometimes, the principles of EBM might escape the authors of clinical guidelines. The core question of the guideline may not be clearly defined, the outcomes of interest may not be explicit, the systematic reviews may be missing, the quality of the primary studies may contain different kinds of bias or patient values and preferences might be neglected. As a result, the quality of the guidelines may be compromised.

On the other side, data from clinical trials are often focused on specific patient populations and conditions. As a result, patient safety and trial efficiency are maximized, but may not reflect the majority of patients in clinical practice. The information obtained from such an artificial environment to clinical practice can be problematic if transferred directly to the clinical practice

Nevertheless the usefulness of the clinical guidelines was appreciated from medical professionals soon after their dissemination. The existing considerable variations in resources, needs and traditions, stimulated many countries to establish their own processes for development or adaptation of clinical guidelines.

In 2001, the Council of Europe developed a set of recommendations for producing clinical guidelines and for assessing their quality. The international collaboration created the European research project PL96-3669 (AGREE, Appraisal of Guidelines, Research and Evaluation in Europe). The efforts of researchers from Health Care Evaluation Unit at St George's Hospital Medical School in London, Guidelines International Network (an international network for guidelines developing organisations), policy makers, and others have contributed substantially for creating an international collaboration for implementation of the project. The project ultimate goal is to improve the quality and effectiveness of clinical practice guidelines by the introduction of an appraisal instrument, development of standard recommendations for guideline developers, programmes, content analysis, reporting, and appraisal of individual recommendations. The development programme concerns guidelines on asthma, diabetes and breast cancer. All of the guidelines are based on the principals of EBM and are presented in [www.agreecollaboration.org/instrument/] and [http://www.agreecollaboration.org].

In connection with the AGREE, several studies show that guidelines on the same topic may differ, possibly due to different medical practice, insufficient evidence, different interpretations of evidence, unsystematic guideline development methods, influence of professional bodies, cultural factors such as differing expectations of apparent risks and benefits, socio-economic factors, cultural attitudes to health or characteristics of health care systems resources, and patterns of disease (Cluzeau, & al, 2003; Burgers, & al, 2003; Berti, & al, 2003). In such countries, a guideline developed on the basis of the best current evidence and prepared for global dissemination, might appear irrelevant (Fried, & al, 2008).

Several sessions of AHRQ (an USA Federal Agency for Healthcare Research and Quality) are also directed towards assessment of the guideline implementation. The AHRQ website [www.ahrq.gov] contains high quality information for Clinical practice guidelines, Evidence-based practice, Funding opportunity, Quality assessment, Health IT Home, and others. The critical role of guideline implementation is explored. The common conclusions are that access to knowledge must be close to the point of decision and that the importance of guideline implementation into practice depends on using recommendations at the right time for the right patient. The same information may be delivered in different manners and may lead to different results (Slutsky, 2008).

Obviously, the opportunity to obtain the relevant information on time at the point of decision-making might influence critically the patient outcomes. On the other side, national evidence-based guidelines are missing in some countries and optimal evidence is often not available for many clinical decisions.

Another study considers an important and sometimes contradictory aspect of evidence-based medical practice – rational prescribing. It is shown that many factors other than evidence drive clinical decision-making. Amongst them are patient preferences, social circumstances, disease-drug and drug-drug interactions, clinical experience, competing demands from more urgent clinical conditions, marketing or promotional activity, and system-level drug policies. For example, despite the availability of trials and strong evidence for the positive effect of pravastatin and simvastatine, the new statines with less evident effects are often prescribed. It is likely that the lack of time and training for evidence evaluation allows some well-intentioned clinicians to be influenced by promotional information at the time of pharmaceutical product launch (Mamdani, & al, 2008).

The possible interference of industry in clinical trials is well summarized in an expert article. It is shown that the priorities of the pharmaceutical industry, in terms of disease targets and the entities that are chosen to test might not reflect the needs of patients or the community. "The goals of industry can, therefore, become the hidden agenda behind the generation of much of the evidence that is used to construct guidelines. The profusion of clinical trials in lucrative diagnostic categories is testament to this phenomenon" (Fried, & al, 2008).

Whatever a guideline is, the clinician has to translate the available evidence to the management of an individual patient. However, the patient conditions are complex and often presented with chronic or co-morbid complications for which a suitable guideline may not exist. The real patient can be very different from the population included in clinical trials and the real clinician is, in fact, practicing an "opinion-based medicine" (Hampton, 2002).

The evidence-based medicine has made a substantial impact on medical research and practice of medicine through the clinical guidelines. However, the need of regular recalls of EBM concepts and skills becomes necessary for the critical appraisal, validity, and applicability of the guidelines. Only evidence-based recommendations may consider the balance between benefits, risks and burdens, and weigh these considerations using patient and societal, rather than expert, values.

With the aim to avoid discrepancies some organizations use different systems to grade evidence and recommendations. As a result, the current proliferation and duplication of guidelines is wasteful (Townend, 2007). A revision of the current practice for development and dissemination of guidelines seems to be adequate for better understanding and easier application. It is proposed that a uniform grading system (GRADE) achieve widespread endorsement. Then, specialty groups can produce a central repository of evidence that is regularly updated with the available systematic reviews. "From this central resource, regional guidelines could be developed, taking into account local resources and expertise and the values and preferences important in that population" (Guyatt, & al, 2006; Fried, & al, 2008),(www.gradeworkinggroup.org/publications/index.htm; http://www.gradeworkinggroup.org/intro.htm.

The first step in this direction is already completed. The National Guidelines Clearing House, USA, already developed syntheses of guidelines covering similar topics [http://www.ngc.org/compare/synthesis.aspx] (accessed 17 October 2007). BMJ as well requests that authors should preferably use the GRADE system for grading evidence when submitting a clinical guidelines article to the journal [www.bmj.com].

With GRADE the patients and clinicians have the opportunity to weigh up the benefits and downsides of alternative strategies when making healthcare management decisions. Much more about the balance and uncertainty between benefits and risks, decisions about an effective therapy, resource and cost can be learned by UpToDate (an electronic resource widely used in North America), [www.uptodate.com]. "When dealing with resource allocation issues, guideline panels face challenges of limited expertise, paucity of rigorous and unbiased cost-effectiveness analyses, and wide variability of costs across jurisdictions or health-care systems. Ignoring the issue of resource use (costs) is however becoming less and less tenable for guideline panels" (Guyatt, & al, 2006).

CONCLUSION

The e-medical resources are useful and probably will continue to improve. With some crucial governmental support the delivery of healthcare services to patients in rural, lonely, or distant regions with shortages of medical staff will be facilitated. The e-medicine undoubtedly can reduce the cost of on-site communication between patients, doctors, and insurance agencies. In many cases, however, the information about the quality of the supporting evidence of the e-health service will remain limited.

The e-sources will continue to provide excellent specific information for health professionals who have recognized the need to learn and understand how to discover, assess, and use the best current evidence in decision-making about the individual patient care. The principles of EBM deserve to become a way of thinking for governmental clerks, in particular when decisions for population health strategies are made, and for politicians when promises are disseminated.

The invasion of the market principles into the realm of medicine is a reality and the customer satisfaction tends to become a priority. However, common sense and governmental regulations are needed to avoid the transformation of the quality medical care into hedonistic "satisfaction-based medicine". The results from outcome studies and assessments based on quality indicators seem to be a more realistic foundation for measuring the quality of healthcare for both the patients and the societies.

ACKNOWLEDGMENT

Special thanks to Dr. Geroge Daskalov, St Francis Hospital - Hartford CT, USA for help and support.

REFERENCES

Altman, D. G., Schltz, K. F., Mohler, D., & al. (2001). The revised CONSORT statement for reporting randomized trials: Explanation and elaboration. *Annals of Internal Medicine,* 134, 663-694. See also [http://www.annals.org/cgi/content/abstract/134/8/663] and associated Web site [www.consort-statement.org].

AABB. (2003). *American Association of Blood Banks, Standards for Blood Banks and Transfusion Services* (22nd ed). Bethesda, MD. Retrieved from www.aabb.org

Burgers, J. S., Bailey, J. V., & Klazinga, N. S., & al. (2002). Inside Guidelines: Comparative analysis of recommendations and evidence in diabetes guidelines from 13 countries. *Diabetes Care, 25,* 1933–1939. doi:10.2337/diacare.25.11.1933

Burgers, J. S., Cluzeau, F. A., & Hanna, S. E., & al, & the AGREE Collaboration. (2003). Characteristics of high quality guidelines: evaluation of 86 clinical guidelines developed in ten European countries and Canada. *International Journal of Technology Assessment in Health Care, 19*(1), 148–157.

Bossuyt, P. M., Reitsma, J. B., & Bruns, D. E., & al. (2003). Towards complete and accurate reporting of studies of diagnostic accuracy. *Clinical Chemistry*, *49*, 1–6. doi:10.1373/49.1.1

CLSI publication GP22-A2. (2004). *Continuous Quality Improvement: Integrating Five Key Quality System Components; Approved Guideline* (2nd ed.). Wayne, Pennsylvania, USA: CLSI.

CLSI publication HS1-A2. (2004). *Quality Management System Model for Health Care; Approved Guideline* (2nd ed.). Wayne, Pennsylvania, USA: CLSI.

CLSI publication HS6-A. (2004). *Studies to Evaluate Patients Outcomes; Approved Guideline*. Wayne, Pennsylvania, USA: CLSI.

Cluzeau, F. A., Burgers, J. S., & Brouwers, M., & al. (2003). Development and validation of an international appraisal instrument for assessing the quality of clinical practice guidelines: the AGREE project. *Quality & Safety in Health Care*, *12*(1), 18–23. doi:10.1136/qhc.12.1.18

Collins, P. M., Golembeski, S. M., Selgas, M., & al. (2007). Clinical Excellence Through Evidence-Based Practice - A Model to Guide Practice Changes. *Topics in Advanced Practice Nursing eJournal*. *7*(4), Medscape, Posted 01/25/2008. Retrieved from [http://www.medscape.com/viewarticle].

Detsky, A. S., Naglie, G., & Krahn, M. D., & al. (1997). Primer on Medical Decision Analysis. *Medical Decision Making*, *17*, 123–233. doi:10.1177/0272989X9701700201

Fried, M., Quigley, E. M., Hunt, R. H., & al. (2008). Is an Evidence-Based Approach to Creating Guidelines Always the Right one? *National Clinical Practice in Gastroenterology and Hepatology*, *5*(2), 60-61. Nature Publishing Group. Posted 03/10/2008.

Gardois, P., Grillo, G., Lingua C., & al. (2004). Assessing the efficacy of EBM teaching in a clinical setting Santander 9 EAHIL Conference, September 24, 2004.

Glance, L. G., Osler, T. M., Mukamel, D. B., & Dick, A. W. (2008). Impact of the present-on-admission indicators on hospital quality measurement experiance with the Agency for Healthcare Research and Quality. (AHRQ) Inpatient Quality Indicators. *Medical Care*, *46*(2), 112–119. doi:10.1097/MLR.0b013e318158aed6

Grunfeld, E., Urquhart, R., Mykhalovskiy, E., & al. (2008). Toward population-based indicators of quality end-of-life care: testing stakeholder agreement. *Cancer, 112*(10), 2301-8. (PreMedline Identifier: 18219238).

Guyatt, G., Gutterman, D., Baumann, M. H., & al (2006). Grading Strength of Recommendations and Quality of Evidence in Clinical Guidelines Report from an American College of Chest Physicians. *Task Force Chest*, 129, 174-181. Retrieved March 16, 2009 from [http://www.chestjournal.org/content/129/1/174.full.pdf+html]

Guyatt, G. H., Oxman, A. D., Vist, G. E., & al. (2008). Rating quality of evidence and strength of recommendations GRADE: an emerging consensus on rating quality of evidence and strength of recommendations. *British Medical Journal*, 336, 924-926 (26 April), for the GRADE Working Group doi: 10.1136/bmj.39489.470347.AD. Retrieved from [http://www.gradeworkinggroup.org/intro.htm]

Hampton, J. R. (2002). Evidence-based medicine, opinion-based medicine, and real-world medicine. *Perspectives in Biology and Medicine*, *45*, 549–568. doi:10.1353/pbm.2002.0070

ISO 9000. (2000). Quality management systems - Fundamentals and vocabulary. Geneva: International Organization for Standardization.

Itagaki, M. W., Berlin, R. B., Bruce, R., & Schatz, B. R. (2002). The Rise and Fall of E-Health: Lessons From the First Generation of Internet Healthcare. *Medscape General Medicine 4*(2). Retrieved August, 6, 2009 from [http://www.medscape.com/viewarticle/431144] .

Kolbasuk, M., & McGree, N. (2009). Retrieved June 17, 2009, from http://www.docmemory.com/page/news/shownews.asp?num=11826

Legido-Ouigley, H., McKee, M., & Walshe, K., & al. (2008). How can quality of healthcare be safeguarded across the European Union? [Retrieved from]. *British Medical Journal, 336*, 920–923. doi:10.1136/bmj.39538.584190.47

LeRouge, C., Hevner, A., Collins, R., & al. (2004). Telemedicine Encounter Quality: Comparing Patient and Provider Perspectives of a Socio-Technical System. *Proc. 37th Hawaii International Conference on System Sciences*. Retrieved March 25, 2009 from [http://www2.computer.org/portal/web/csdl/doi?doc=abs/proceedings/hicss/2004/2056/06/205660149a.abs.htm]

Mamdani, M., Ching, A., Golden, B., & al. (2008). Challenges to Evidence-Based Prescribing in Clinical Practice. Annals of Pharmacotherapy, 42(5), 704-707. Harvey Whitney Books Company. Posted 07/15/2008. Retrieved from [http://www.medscape.com/viewarticle/576145].

MARQuIS research project. Qual Saf Health Care, 18, i1-i74. (2009) *National Guideline Clearinghouse (NGC)*, Guideline Syntheses (accessed 17 October 2007). Retrieved from [http://www.ngc.org/compare/synthesis.aspx].

Sackett, D. L., Straus, S. E., Richardson, W. S., Rosenberg, W., & Haynes, R. B. (2000). Evidence-*Based Madicine. Now to Practice and Teach EBM.* Second Edition, Churcill Livingstone, Edinburg, London, New York & al., as well as in [http://www.library.utoronto.ca/medicine/ebm/].

Slawson, D. C., & Shaughnessy, A. F. (2000). Becoming an information master: using POEMs to change practice with confidence. Patient-oriented evidence that matters. [Retrieved from]. *The Journal of Family Practice, 49*, 63–67.

Slutsky, J. (2008). Session Current Care - G-I-N abstracts. Retrieved March, 27, 2009 from [http://www.g-i-n.net/download/files/G_I_N_newsletter_May_2008.pdf]

Steel, N., Melzer, D., & Shekelle, P. G., & al. (2004). Developing quality indicators for older adults: transfer from the USA to the UK is feasible. *Quality & Safety in Health Care, 13*(4), 260–264. doi:10.1136/qshc.2004.010280

Townend, J. N. (2007). Guidelines on guidelines. *Lancet, 370*, 740. doi:10.1016/S0140-6736(07)61376-2

Tudiver, F., Rose, D., Banks, B., & Pfortmiller, D. (2004). Reliability and Validity Testing of an Evidence-Based Medicine OSCE Station. *Society of Teachers in Family Medicine meeting*, Toronto, May 14, 2004. Date Submitted: May 22, 2008. Retrieved March 22, 2009 from http://www.stfm.org/fmhub/fm2009/February/Fred89.pdf

UEMS. 2007.19 – Bratislava Declaration on eMedicine. (2009, February 25). Retrieved June 17, 2009,from http://admin.uems.net/uploadedfiles/893.pdf.

Veillard, J., Champagne, F., & Klazinga, N., & al. (2005). A performance assessment framework for hospitals: the WHO regional office for Europe PATH Project. *International Journal for Quality in Health Care, 17*(6), 487–496. doi:10.1093/intqhc/mzi072

Chapter 10
Safety and Security in Professional and Non-Professional E-Health and Their Impact on the Quality of Health Care

Suzana Parente
Portuguese Association for Quality in Health Care, Portugal

Rui Loureiro
Portuguese Association for Quality in Health Care, Portugal

ABSTRACT

E-health involves professionals and non-professionals and raises safety and security issues that affect the quality of health care. Therefore, the chapter provides some basic ideas on e-health safety and security, focusing on the healthcare provider perspective. To clarify some of the controversies and some of the problems in the use of data, arising from the use of e-health without taking into consideration the safety and security issues, we present one novel unpublished case and six cases from the Food and Drug Administration (FDA), Multi-Media Consumer Information, (FDA) Patient Safety News. Topics highlight fraud, impersonation of health care professionals, misuse of data and information, and backups.

INTRODUCTION

E-health is prevalent. It covers everything from patient to professional identification, prescribing, clinical data, accounting to management of medical devices, pharmaceuticals and safety and security of healthcare facilities (e.g. fire, intrusion, flooding). Moreover, the Internet is a key component in every facet of today's life, including even older users (the fastest growing group of Internet users). As a result, it has an impact on the implementation of IT in healthcare, especially regarding the non-professional users of e-health. Furthermore, the development of the Internet from the web 1.0 to 2.0 to the semantic web will undoubtedly play a vital role in the application and misuse of e-health (Goodenough, 2009).

DOI: 10.4018/978-1-61692-843-8.ch010

Social networks like today's Facebook, Twitter, blogs and chat rooms, should also be analyzed for their impact especially in the non-professional e-health sector.

Overall, there are two types of clients in e-health, which include the professional user, healthcare professionals of all specialties, and the non-professional user, who acts as a supplier of data and end user. Consequently, we might distinguish two dimensions e-health, which affect the health care options of a growing number of individuals in modern societies.

1. Professional e-health, which encompasses the use of IT by healthcare professionals and patients.
2. Non-professional e-health, which includes Internet data on diseases, procedures, medical devices, and pharmaceuticals.

On the other hand, ensuring the privacy and confidentiality is an indispensable component of health information systems (Doupi et al., 2005) while safety and security, the most salient issues when quality in e-health is concerned, are not the task of IT specialists. It is also the responsibility of healthcare organizations and healthcare providers (Katsikas et al., 2008).

The evolution from an organization-centered to a process-related and to a person-centered health system involves many aspects of security, safety, privacy, ethics, and quality (Blobel, 2007). Therefore, while discussing about health information systems, we need to implement new technologies in order to face challenges arising from both legal and technological background (Blobel, 2007; Pharow, P. & Blobel. 2009). The lessons learned in the last years clearly show that e-health is more than just a straightforward change from paper records to electronic records. It calls for a paradigm shift and the use of new technologies and procedures (Hildebrand et al., 2006). As a result, interoperability, security and confidentiality are vital for the acceptance of the new approaches, the quality improvement, and the safety of patient's care (Hammond, 2008; Engel et al., 2006). Safety is the cornerstone of quality and an integral consideration in all aspects of care delivery (IOM, 2001).

On clinical grounds, the growing availability of solutions, which monitor remote health-related data, using wireless networks technologies (e.g. ECG, blood pressure monitoring, lab tests) reinforces the e-health importance. Events like the severe acute respiratory syndrome (SARS) and the swine flu pandemic provide excellent case studies of the overall impact of IT on health care. However, reliable information (public or/and professional) coexists with rumors, misleading information, counterfeit medicines, counterfeit medical devices and diagnostic tests.

Finally, it is worthwhile mentioning that IT safety and security involve professionals and non-professionals, and deal with issues like (Adibi, et al., 2008; De Meyer et al., 2008; Savastano et al., 2008):

- hardware security
- password protection of received/sent files
- encryption of communication data
- encryption of stored data (e.g. files, e-mails, data files, image files, audio files)
- e-signatures
- safety copies of stored data(backups)
- software validation
- software license hardware accesses
- software accesses
- redundant processing

However, the chapter will outline the basics of e-health safety and security emphasizing on the provider perspective.

BACKGROUND

E-health is a new word and concept, which arises at the end of the 20th century (Eysenbach, 2001;

Oh et al., 2005). Later, it was introduced in many aspects of human life (e.g. e commerce, e government). However, when we browse the Internet, using the Google search engine, for e-health written in any of the traditional ways (ehealth OR e-health OR "e health") we see millions of entries. If we also check for (ehealth OR e-health OR "e health") AND (safety OR security), (ehealth OR e-health OR "e health") AND security, (ehealth OR e-health OR "e health") AND safety, excluding "patient safety", (ehealth OR e-health OR "e health") AND (safety OR security), excluding "patient safety", we obtain similar results. Finally, safety and security issues seem to affect patient safety in many aspects (e.g. electronic prescriptions, patient identification and logistics).

From a qualitative approach, most of studies on e-health safety and security deal primarily with hardware and software issues or the use of IT in health care for patient safety (e.g. wrong surgery, patient identification, drug mix-ups). On the other hand, we observe small-scale projects at a departmental level with no actual data exchange but the Internet empowers citizens, providing information on medicines, medical devices and procedures (Bauer, 2002).

Overall, it is about time to create a security system, not only on the hardware, software, communication and access, but most importantly on the safety and security of data acquired though professional and non-professional e-health. This seems to be the new frontier for e-health safety and security. As a result, we should consider using techniques and methodologies like risk management and the cost of quality and non-quality (Figure 1), balancing gains, risks and investment in e-health. This should be founded on a framework of value (e.g. ratio between Quality and Resources) as e-health promises enormous benefits through improving efficiency (e.g. reduced manual data information base, faster, convenient, and convenient access to data, long-distance consultation, scheduling and consultation management).

Safety and Security in Health Care

E-health falls short in reliability, and the flow of information, at the national and cross border level

Figure 1. Costs of quality and non-quality (adapted from Schiffauerova, A. and Thomson, V, 2006)

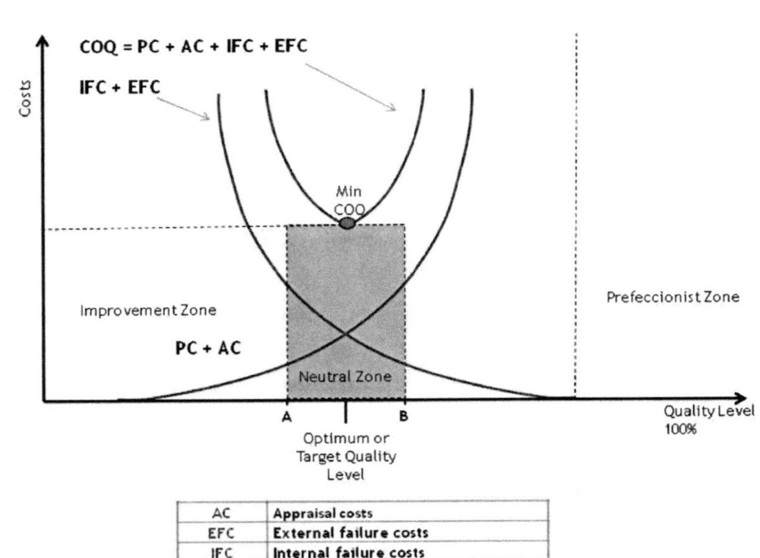

AC	Appraisal costs
EFC	External failure costs
IFC	Internal failure costs
COQ	"Costs of Quality"
PC	Prevention costs

(Hildebrand et al., 2006). The lack of sufficient software knowledge creates risks of inadequate access to data, lack of policies on data use and data collection, unsafe or missing history of backups, inadequate funding for efficient data collection and not helpful software. As a rule, with few exceptions, data are not available on a national basis.

Therefore, in order to clarify some problems and controversies in the use of data arising from the use of e-health, we present one novel unpublished case and six cases extracting information from the Food and Drug Administration (FDA), Multi-Media Consumer Information, (FDA) Patient Safety News.

CASE STUDIES

Case Study 1: Medical Records

A clinical database, regarding intensive care unit (ICU) patients in a surgical and trauma unit was set up in a Portuguese central hospital. The condition of a patient at arrival, including co-existing pathologies, clinical improvement and results at discharge, all invasive procedures, and the therapeutic interventions were recorded. Finally, APACHE and SAPS II scores were also recorded for each patient.

This database started experimentally, but it steadily became the only source of clinical data regarding ICU patients. The database was loaded on a personal computer (PC), which was available to doctors and residents, as well. It was located in the heart of the ICU. Nurses did not work on it since they had access to other computers, located at different areas of the ICU. The computer allowed access to Internet and Intranet in order to view radiology and lab tests results.

One morning, when starting their shift, doctors noticed that they could not retrieve any information from the computer.

Why?

During the night shift, one of the nurses used the computer and accidentally erased the database.

Most of the data could be retrieved from a resident's backup. However, three- month data were lost forever.

It is worthwhile mentioning that there was no formal training of the healthcare professionals before using the system. Moreover, there was not a single person handling the computer, and a backup system.

Case Study 2: Drug Name Confusion: Salagen and Selegiline (FDA show 48#9)

'A pharmacist reported that the similar spelling of the two drug names led him to enter 'selegiline' into the computer instead of 'Salagen'. The error was recognized only after the patient complained that the medication was not helping his dry mouth, and this caused the pharmacist to check the patient's profile' (Food & Drug Administration, 2006).

Case Study 3: Mix-Ups between Insulin U-100 and U-500 (FDA show 79#1)

'depending on the screen size, the prescriber may see only the first few words of the product listing, so the drug concentration may not be visible' (Food & Drug Administration, 2008).

Case Study 4: FDA/ISMP Campaign to Eliminate Dangerous Abbreviations (FDA show 53#8)

'That includes written medication orders, computer-generated labels, pharmacy entry screens, and commercial medication labeling, packaging, and advertising' (Food & Drug Administration, 2006).

work with software vendors to make changes in computer programs for order entry, labeling and medication printouts (Food & Drug Administration, 2006).

Case Study 5: Recalls and Safety Alerts (FDA show 26#2)

'counterfeit contraceptive patches that contain no active ingredient. They have been sold by an overseas internet site. The counterfeit patches were promoted by this web site as Ortho Evra transdermal patches, which are FDA approved, and made by Ortho-McNeil Pharmaceutical, Inc' (Food & Drug Administration, 2004).

'patients about the potential dangers of buying medical products on line' (Food & Drug Administration, 2004).

'They should look for sites that bear the seal "Verified Internet Pharmacy Practice Sites. That shows the site is operating according to the standards of the National Association of Boards of Pharmacy (NABP)' (Food & Drug Administration, 2004).

Case Study 6: FDA Clears Computer-Connected Glucose Meters (FDA show 7#2)

'FDA recently cleared for marketing two glucose test meters for use in conjunction with hand-held computers' (Food & Drug Administration, 2002).

'Of course, it's important that patients know how to operate a PDA before they use this system (Food & Drug Administration, 2002).

Overall, as we can easily deduce from the case studies, patient treatment is not without risk for patients, health professionals and organizations. Moreover, the prevailing approach to medication delivery safety issues is the solution at the point of failure using computerized physician order entry systems (Friedman et al., 2009). As a result, there is a lack of a systemic, holistic approach to addressing medication delivery issues (Cafazzo et al., 2009). However, fragmented solutions do not address the problem especially when the misleading 'looks alike, sound alike' brand names and different concentrations of active ingredients are presented to health professionals.

SOLUTIONS AND RECOMMENDATIONS

A strategy to safer health care outcomes should include:

- a 'positive list' of safe and secure e-health data sources
- e-literacy on both the professional and non-professional level
- risk assessment of all health technology including the use of the data obtained, stored or processed through IT technology
- knowledge of the benefits and limitations of IT applied to health care by professional and non-professional health uses
- user-friendly approach to information technology both at professional and non-professional level, including senior citizens
- continual development and testing of hardware and software, which relates to the safety and security
- empowerment of the health care professionals at all dimensions of the health care provision, including safety and security issues
- establishment of a safety culture in e-health
- evaluation of the ever-growing mass production of affordable diagnostic tools (e.g., blood pressure monitors)
- research on the need and impact of the growing demand for integrating different tools, systems, standards, terminologies, language, cultures

Figure 2. E-health interfaces

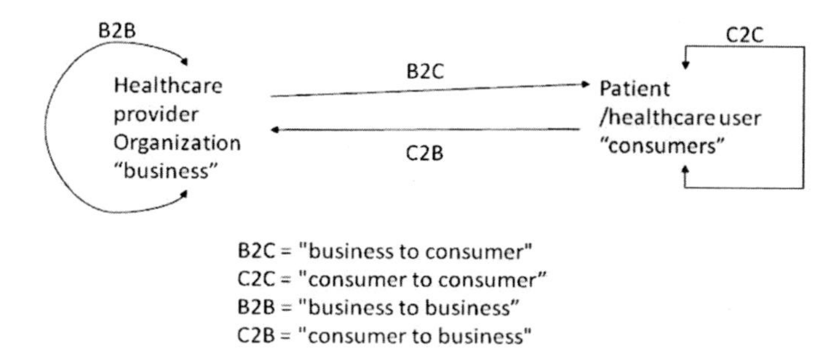

FUTURE RESEARCH DIRECTIONS

Today, safety and security in e-health are primarily focused on hardware, software, communications and access to the data. However, this approach leaves behind safety and security issues, which result from data in both the professional and the non-professional areas of e-health. Moreover, it does not evaluate the effect of the emerging Semantic Web (Burger et al., 2009). As a result, the information technology industry, the health care industry, regulatory bodies, policy makers, health care professionals, and patients experience a 'new' challenge, which is associated with focusing on health outcomes. Therefore, they have to assess the complex relationships deriving from their interactions, which are depicted in Figure 2. In the figure B2C (business to consumer) shows the capability of consumers to interact with their systems on and off line. B2B (business to business) shows the improved possibilities for institution-to-institution transmissions of data. Finally, C2C (consumer to consumer) shows the new possibilities for peer-to-peer communication of consumers.

CONCLUSION

Safety and security are pivotal issues, when quality in e-health is concerned, while a sound system is certainly secure and efficient. Therefore, the close cooperation of healthcare professionals and IT specialists is a pressing issue.

REFERENCES

Adibi, S., & Agnew, G. B. (2008). On the diversity of eHealth security systems and mechanisms. *Conference Proceedings; ... Annual International Conference of the IEEE Engineering in Medicine and Biology Society. IEEE Engineering in Medicine and Biology Society. Conference*, 1478–1481.

Bauer, K. A. (2002). Using the Internet to empower patients and to develop partnerships with clinicians. *World Hospitals and Health Services*, *38*(2), 2–10.

Blobel, B. (2007). Comparing approaches for advanced e-health security infrastructures. *International Journal of Medical Informatics*, *76*(5-6), 454–459. doi:10.1016/j.ijmedinf.2006.09.012

Burger, A., Romano, P., Paschke, A., & Splendiani, A. (2009). Semantic Web Applications and Tools for Life Sciences, 2008-preface. *BMC Bioinformatics*, *10*(Suppl 10), S1. doi:10.1186/1471-2105-10-S10-S1

Cafazzo, J. A., Trbovich, P. L., Cassano-Piche, A., Chagpar, A., Rossos, P. G., Vicente, K. J., & Easty, A. C. (2009). Human factors perspectives on a systemic approach to ensuring a safer medication delivery process. *Healthcare Quarterly (Toronto, Ont.)*, 70–74.

De, Meyer F., & De, Moor G., & Reed-Fourquet, L. (2008). Privacy Protection through pseudonymisation in eHealth. *Studies in Health Technology and Informatics*, *141*, 111–118.

Doupi, P., Ruotsalainen, P., & Pohjonen, H. (2005). Implementing interoperable secure health information systems. *Studies in Health Technology and Informatics*, *115*, 187–214.

Engel, K., Blobel, B., & Pharow, P. (2006). Standards for enabling health informatics interoperability. *Studies in Health Technology and Informatics*, *124*, 145–150.

Eysenbach, G. (2001). What is e-health? *Journal of Medical Internet Research*, *3*(2), e20. doi:10.2196/jmir.3.2.e20

Food & Drug Administration. (2002). *FDA Clears Computer-Connected Glucose Meters*. Retrieved July 31, 2009 from http://www.accessdata.fda.gov/scripts/cdrh/cfdocs/psn/transcript.cfm?show=7#2

Food & Drug Administration. (2004). *Warning on Counterfeit Contraceptive Patches*. Retrieved July 31, 2009 from http://www.accessdata.fda.gov/scripts/cdrh/cfdocs/psn/transcript.cfm?show=26#2

Food & Drug Administration. (2005). *How to Evaluate Health Information on the Internet*, Retrieved July 31, 2009 from http://www.fda.gov/Drugs/EmergencyPreparedness/BioterrorismandDrugPreparedness/ucm134620.htm

Food & Drug Administration. (2006). *Drug Name Confusion: Salagen and Selegiline*. Retrieved July 31, 2009 from http://www.accessdata.fda.gov/scripts/cdrh/cfdocs/psn/transcript.cfm?show=48#9

Food & Drug Administration. (2006). *FDA/ISMP Campaign to Eliminate Dangerous Abbreviations*. Retrieved July 31, 2009 from http://www.accessdata.fda.gov/scripts/cdrh/cfdocs/psn/transcript.cfm?show=53#8

Food & Drug Administration. (2008). *Mixups between Insulin U-100 and U-500*. Retrieved July 31, 2009 from http://www.accessdata.fda.gov/scripts/cdrh/cfdocs/psn/transcript.cfm?show=79#1

Friedman, M. A., Schueth, A., & Bell, D. S. (2009). Interoperable electronic prescribing in the United States: a progress report. *Health Affairs (Project Hope)*, *28*(2), 393–403. doi:10.1377/hlthaff.28.2.393

Goodenough, S. (2009). Semantic interoperability, e-health and Australian statistics. *Health Information Management Journal*, *38*(2), 41–45.

Hammond, W. E. (2008). eHealth interoperability. *Studies in Health Technology and Informatics*, *134*, 245–253.

Hildebrand, C., Pharow, P., Engelbrecht, R., Blobel, B., Savastano, M., & Hovsto, A. (2006). BioHealth--the need for security and identity management standards in eHealth. *Studies in Health Technology and Informatics*, *121*, 327–336.

Institute of Medicine. (2001). *Crossing the Quality Chasm: A new health system for the 21st century*. Washington, DC: National Academy Press.

Katsikas, S., Lopez, J., & Pernul, G. (2008). The challenge for security and privacy services in distributed health settings. *Studies in Health Technology and Informatics*, *134*, 113–125.

Oh, H., Rizo, C., Enkin, M., & Jadad, A. (2005). What is eHealth?: a systematic review of published definitions. *World Hospitals and Health Services*, *41*(1), 32–40.

Pharow, P., & Blobel, B. (2008). Mobile health requires mobile security: challenges, solutions, and standardization. *Studies in Health Technology and Informatics*, *136*, 697–702.

Savastano, M., Hovsto, A., Pharow, P., & Blobel, B. (2008). Security, safety, and related technology - the triangle of eHealth service provision. *Studies in Health Technology and Informatics*, *136*, 709–714.

Schiffauerova, A., & Thomson, V. (2006). A review of research on cost of quality models and best practices. *International Journal of Quality & Reliability Management*, *23*(6), 647–669. doi:10.1108/02656710610672470

Chapter 11
Measuring Safety of Care

Solvejg Kristensen
European Society for Quality in Healthcare, Denmark

Jan Mainz
European Society for Quality in Healthcare, Denmark

Paul D. Bartels
European Society for Quality in Healthcare, Denmark

ABSTRACT

Patient safety initiatives have been launched in a number of countries, mostly focusing on problem identification, learning and improvement. However, so far there has been little focus on monitoring outcomes and surveillance of development of patient safety at the organizational and system level. As a consequence, we still do not know the extent of adverse incidents or patient safety problems, just as we do not know whether the measures introduced have in fact led to improvement. The perspectives of implementing use of e.g. indicators, audits and questionnaires for systematic risk management is, that it will be possible to continuously estimate the prevalence and incidence of patient safety quality problems. The lesson learned in quality improvement is that it will pay back in terms of improvement in patient safety. For this purpose validated methods are needed.

INTRODUCTION

In the1990s, a number of prevalence studies measuring adverse incidents were carried out in the USA and Australia. The studies gave a snapshot of the prevalence of adverse incidents, which was estimated to be 4% and 17% respectively. Since then, prevalence studies have been carried out in a number of European countries as well, generally finding prevalence rates around 10% (de Vries et al., 2008). The differences in findings reflect differences in the methodological approach used in the studies. This type of study can provide a snapshot of safety of care, typically based on knowledge from review of patients' charts - a highly laborious task, which is generally only performed once. Continuous, systematic monitoring of the frequency and nature of safety of care incidents is hardly ever performed.

Patient safety initiatives have been launched in a number of countries, mostly focusing on problem identification, learning and improve-

DOI: 10.4018/978-1-61692-843-8.ch011

ment. However, so far there has been little focus on monitoring outcomes and surveillance of development of patient safety at the organizational and system level. As a consequence, we still do not know the extent of adverse incidents or patient safety problems, just as we do not know whether the measures introduced have in fact led to improvement.

Measuring patient safety focuses on making visible the potential and the actual risks of harm to patients respectively. Various methods are available to measure specific aspects of patient safety locally. The methods are well-known from quality assurance management and usually relate to auditing, questionnaire surveys, and in recent years also indicator monitoring.

Already in 2004 the Committee of Ministers and The Council of Europe made a number of recommendations regarding patient safety (Council of Europe, 2004). One recommendation was to develop reliable and valid indicators of safety of care; this recommendation was enhanced in a new recommendation in 2009, stating (Council of Europe, 2009):

- "to develop a set of reliable and comparable indicators, to identify safety problems, to evaluate the effectiveness of interventions aimed at improving safety and to facilitate mutual learning between Member States; account should be taken of the work done at national level and of international activities such as the Organization for Economic Co-operation and Development (OECD) healthcare quality indicators project and the Community Health Indicators project;
- to gather and share comparable data and information on patient safety outcomes in terms of type and number to facilitate mutual learning and inform priority setting, with a view to helping Member States to share relevant indicators with the public in the future".

It has been documented that measuring performance and outcomes can improve the quality of care (Mainz et al., 2004). Such measuring has supported accountability and transparency, helped to make judgments and set priorities, enabling comparison over time, between providers and of effectiveness of interventions (Mainz, 2004; Mainz & Bartels, 2006). Accordingly, specific measures for systematic surveillance, risk management, monitoring and development of safety of care and patient safety activities are needed (Council of Europe, 2004).

The purpose of this chapter is to give an overview of some aspects of measuring patient safety, and the strengths and weaknesses of the measuring methods applied.

BACKGROUND

The patient safety approach rests on the assumption that many and complex weaknesses at the organizational as well as at the clinical level together may cause an adverse incident, and that they constitute a complicated cause-effect relationship that may shed some light on why incidents occur.

Recently, a general concept has been proposed. It illustrates the complexity of measuring patient safety by including a good deal more points of measuring than usually found in quality assurance, see Figure 1. The concept is based partly on Donabedian's concept of measuring structure, process and outcome, partly on Reason's theory of latent and active errors leading to potential or actual risks of harm to patients. A patient may be harmed by active errors caused by errors arising when an intended plan is performed, or by lack of action. Latent errors are characteristics of or events in the system or organization that increase the risk of active errors. Examples of latent errors at system level include decisions made regarding technology, training and education, communication, work environment and work procedures (Leape & Berwick, 2005).

Figure 1. Points of measuring for patient safety indicated as grey boxes (Brown et al., 2008)

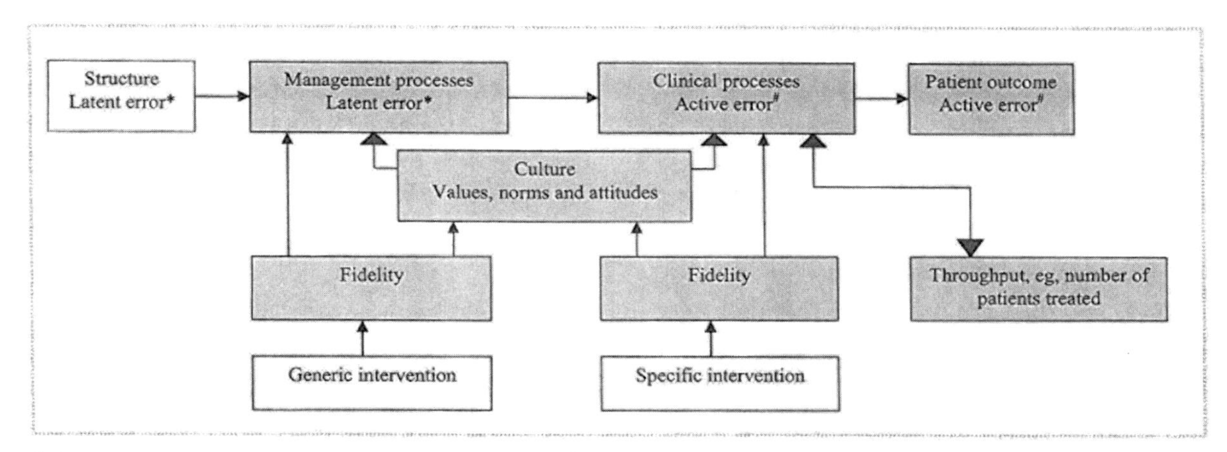

* Latent error: A latent error is a characteristic of or an event in the system or organisation that increases the risk of active failures.

Active error: An active error can harm the patient either through errors arising when an intended plan is performed, or by lack of action.

Measuring can be performed close to the cause in the structure and in the process to examine risk, or close to the effect – outcome – to examine harm to the patient. It is also possible to measure based on intermediary targets such as culture or volume of production (Brown et al., 2008). Ideally, several points of measuring should be used to examine patient safety in a particular area.

MEASURING METHODS USED TO SURVEY SAFETY OF CARE

The Trigger Tool Method

The method was developed at the Institute for Healthcare Improvement in the USA, and it is a tool to identify and monitor the frequency of harm to patients. The method takes its starting point in a review of random samples of patients' medical records in a particular ward. The incidence of patient harm in the sample is determined on the basis of pre-defined information in the records, so-called "triggers", known to occur in connection with patient harm. An example of a trigger could be *Readmission within 30 days*. If readmission is identified, it is evaluated whether it was caused by treatment-related harm to the patient.

The data is presented as patient harm per 1,000 patient days, 100 discharges and the period measured respectively. Actually, the Trigger Tool Method (TTM) rests on a highly structured explicit audit of medical records, and it presupposes that the patient mix is constant during the time of observation. That is why the method is not well-suited for benchmarking purposes; its main strength lies in monitoring outcome of interventions. Studies have described the method as robust and well-suited for that purpose (Griffin & Classen, 2008).

Measuring Patient Safety Culture

Results from a patient safety culture survey describes how managers and staff experience various dimensions of patient safety, e.g. attitude to reporting, communication, learning from incidents and support from management (Madsen & Østergaard, 2004). The method is suitable for identifying problems and as a basis for dialogue and strategic planning at all levels in an organization. It is not a suitable tool to classify the level of patient safety, or for benchmarking purposes.

There is a number of questionnaires available for measuring patient safety culture; they vary in scope, target groups, content as well as documented validity. Some of the frequently used and thoroughly tested questionnaires include the Hospital Survey on Patient Safety Culture from the Agency for Healthcare Research and Quality (AHRQ) and the Safety Attitude Questionnaire from The University of Texas Center of Excellence for Patient Safety Research and Practice. Questionnaire outcomes can be presented as indicators.

Another widely used tool for problem identification and development of patient safety culture is the Manchester Patient Safety Framework from the University of Manchester. It is a tool to help organizations and healthcare teams assess their progress in developing a mature safety culture through workshops.

Although patient safety culture must be regarded as important and fundamental to the quality of processes and outcomes, there is still scant evidence of covariance between culture and other types of measuring patient safety, such as e.g. incidence of medication errors.

Measuring Mortality Rates

The ultimate patient harm is death. The Hospital Standardised Mortality Rate (HSMR) is a method to calculate mortality at hospital level, taking into account differences in patient population mix. HSMR states the number of deaths as a percent of the expected number of deaths (country-wide average). It is possible to follow changes in mortality over time at hospital level, but the method does not allow comparison across hospitals.

HSMR has been used as an outcome measure in connection with broad interventions, e.g. the Institute for Healthcare Improvement (IHI) campaign "100k lives Campaign".

The method depends on a vast number of factors, including mortality outside the hospital, proportion of emergency treatment, number of transfers, patient population, co-morbidity, lifestyle factors etc. The indicator has not been validated to any significant extent, and primarily for case-based methods (Koster et al., 2008). Whether it is possible to demonstrate a real cause-effect relationship between intervention and changes in HSMR remains unclear and, therefore, the value of the HSMR is still disputed (Shojania & Forster, 2008).

Sets of Patient Safety Indicators

Whereas the methods mentioned above are new and specific to the measurement of safety of care, the Patient Safety Indicators (PSI) are clinical quality indicators, but interpreted within the frame of reference of patient safety (Kristensen et al., 2007). They are used e.g. to measure specific problems of patient safety such as infections, falls, screening for suicide risk or risk of complications in well-defined procedures. Sets of PSI are composed to include as many potential organizational and clinical problems as possible to cover as many aspects of safety of care as possible in an area. The methodological requirements and epidemiological principles for development and application of PSI, including data collection, statistical analysis and presentation of results are the same as for quality indicators (Mainz, 2003b; Mainz, 2003a).

Using PSI enables comparison across units, which explains why PSI has attracted considerable interest from international organizations like the EU and OECD.

The OECD's patient safety indicators are based on administrative data and made up at a national level. EU supported the project Safety Improvements for Patients In Europe (SimPatIE) 2005 – 2007. Part of the aim was to develop a set of PSIs (Kristensen et al., 2007). The indicator set from SimPatIE is related to the OECD's, and it is based partly on administrative data, partly on clinical data. The SimPatIE set includes measurement of culture and mortality, as well as theme- or diagnosis-specific problems, e.g. infections or delivery-related complications (Kristensen et al., 2007).

In their 2004 recommendation the Committee of Ministers and The Council of Europe mention development and validation of patient safety indicators as a specific area to be considered for inclusion in research programmes (Council of Europe, 2004). Since then, some work has been done, but more is still needed.

FUTURE RESEARCH DIRECTIONS

Over the last five years, work has been in progress in a number of countries and a good deal of initiatives has been launched to improve patient safety. There is certainly no lack of interest in patient safety: adverse incidents are being analyzed, retrospective and prospective problem-identifying measures taken etc. Having good intentions and willingness to improve is not enough! The true extent of the problems remains unknown, just as we have no way of knowing whether the measures taken so far have, in fact, led to improvement.

In its white paper 'Together for Health: A Strategic Approach for the EU 2008-2013' of 23 October 2007, the Commission identifies patient safety as an area for action (Commission of the European Communities, 2007).

To support the Member States in their local work towards developing safety of care, the Commission has co-financed various action and research projects, e.g. SIMPatIE and the European Network for Patient Safety (EUNetPaS). The SIMPatIE project aimed to use Europe-wide networks of organizations, experts, professionals and other stakeholders in order to establish a common European set of vocabulary, indicators and internal and external instruments for improving safety in healthcare. EUNetPaS builds on results from previous projects, experiences and recommendations, and the project aims to establish an umbrella network of all 27 EU Member States and EU stakeholders to encourage and enhance collaboration in the field of patient safety. EUNetPaS focuses on developing and recommending operational tools for problem identification, analysis, problem solving and effect monitoring within the four key topic area: Culture of Patient Safety, Education and Training in Patient Safety, Reporting and Learning Systems and Medication Safety. The Office for Quality Indicator under the European Society for Quality in Healthcare is a partner in the project and involved in development, evaluation and recommendations on feasible and well-tested instruments to enhance Patient Safety Culture, through the use of indicators and patient safety culture questionnaires and process tools.

CONCLUSION

Measuring patient safety is a new field, and a field in need of much more research-based documentation. However, it seems obvious already at this stage that the complexity of the area calls for a broad approach using on a number of different measuring dimensions. There is no single, ideal method for measuring safety of care.

REFERENCES

Brown, C., Hofer, T., Johal, A., Thomson, R., Nicholl, J., & Franklin, B. D. (2008). An epistemology of patient safety research: a framework for study design and interpretation. Part 3. End points and measurement. *Quality & Safety in Health Care*, *17*, 170–177. doi:10.1136/qshc.2007.023655

Commission of the European Communities. (2007). *White Paper 'Together for Health: A Strategic Approach for the EU 2008-2013*. Retrieved November 2009 from http://ec.europa.eu/health/ph_overview/Documents/strategy_wp_en.pdf.

Council of Europe. (2004). *Recommendation Rec (2006)7 of the Committee of Ministers to member states on management of patient safety and prevention of adverse events in health care.* Retrieved November 2009 from https://wcd.coe.int/ViewDoc.jsp?id=1005439&BackColorInternet=9999CC&BackColorIntranet=FFBB55&BackColorLogged=FFAC75.

Council of Europe. (2009). *COUNCIL RECOMMENDATION of 9 June 2009 on patient safety, including the prevention and control of healthcare associated infections (2009/C 151/01).* Retrieved November 2009 from http://eur-lex.europa.eu/LexUriServ/LexUriServ.do?uri=OJ:C:2009:151:0001:0006:EN:PDF.

de Vries, E. N., Ramrattan, M. A., Smorenburg, S. M., Gouma, D. J., & Boermeester, M. A. (2008). The incidence and nature of in-hospital adverse events: a systematic review. *Quality & Safety in Health Care, 17*, 216–223. doi:10.1136/qshc.2007.023622

Griffin, F. A., & Classen, D. C. (2008). Detection of adverse events in surgical patients using the Trigger Tool approach. *Quality & Safety in Health Care, 17*, 253–258. doi:10.1136/qshc.2007.025080

Koster, M., Jurgensen, U., Spetz, C. L., & Rutberg, H. (2008). ["Standardized hospital mortality" as health quality indicator. An English method has been tested in Swedish patient registries]. *Lakartidningen, 105*, 1391–1397.

Kristensen, S., Mainz, J., & Bartels, P. (2007). *Patient Safety. Establishing a set of Patient Safety Indicators* Aarhus: Sun-Tryk Aarhus University. Retrieved November 2009 from http://www.simpatie.org/Main/pf1175587453/wp1175588035/wp1176820943

Leape, L. L., & Berwick, D. M. (2005). Five years after To Err Is Human: what have we learned? *Journal of the American Medical Association, 293*, 2384–2390. doi:10.1001/jama.293.19.2384

Madsen, M. D., & Østergaard, D. (2004). *Udvikling af metode og værktøj til at måle sikkerhedskultur på sygehusafdelinger. Afrapportering af projekt om sikkerhedskultur og patientsikkerhed i Københavns Amt.* Retrieved November 2009 from http://www.risoe.dk/rispubl/SYS/syspdf/ris-r-1491.pdf.

Mainz, J. (2003a). Defining and classifying clinical indicators for quality improvement. *International Journal for Quality in Health Care, 15*, 523–530. doi:10.1093/intqhc/mzg081

Mainz, J. (2003b). Developing evidence-based clinical indicators: a state of the art methods primer. *International Journal for Quality in Health Care, 15*(Suppl 1), i5–i11. doi:10.1093/intqhc/mzg084

Mainz, J. (2004). Quality Indicators: Essential for Quality Improvement. *International Journal for Quality in Health Care, 16*, 1–2. doi:10.1093/intqhc/mzh036

Mainz, J., & Bartels, P. D. (2006). Nationwide quality improvement--how are we doing and what can we do? *International Journal for Quality in Health Care, 18*, 79–80. doi:10.1093/intqhc/mzi099

Mainz, J., Krog, B. R., Bjornshave, B., & Bartels, P. (2004). Nationwide continuous quality improvement using clinical indicators: the Danish National Indicator Project. *International Journal for Quality in Health Care, 16*(Suppl 1), i45–i50. doi:10.1093/intqhc/mzh031

Shojania, K. G., & Forster, A. J. (2008). Hospital mortality: when failure is not a good measure of success. *Canadian Medical Association Journal, 179*, 153–157. doi:10.1503/cmaj.080010

Chapter 12
An Information Technology Architecture for Drug Effectiveness Reporting and Post-Marketing Surveillance

Amar Gupta
University of Arizona, USA

Raymond Woosley
Critical Path Institute, USA

Igor Crk
University of Arizona, USA

Surendra Sarnikar
Dakota State University, USA

ABSTRACT

Adverse drug events impose a large cost on the society in terms of lives and healthcare costs. In this chapter, the authors propose an information technology architecture for enabling the monitoring of adverse drug events in an outpatient setting as a part of the post marketing surveillance program. The proposed system architecture enables the development of a web based drug effectiveness reporting and monitoring system that builds on previous studies demonstrating the feasibility of a system in which community pharmacists identify and report adverse drug events. The authors define the key technical requirements of such a monitoring and reporting system, identify the critical factors that influence the successful implementation and use of the system, and propose information technology solutions that satisfy these requirements.

DOI: 10.4018/978-1-61692-843-8.ch012

INTRODUCTION

Adverse drug reactions have been estimated to result in more than 2.1 million injuries and 100,000 deaths each year in the US alone (Lazarou, Pomeranz & Corey, 1998). The annual economic cost of adverse drug events is estimated to be more than $75 billion (Johnson & Bootman, 1995). Mitigating the impact of adverse drug events requires the implementation of a comprehensive mechanism for monitoring and detecting adverse drug events. Such a mechanism can save lives and reduce healthcare costs.

Reliable detection of adverse drug events is a difficult problem. Although some adverse drug reactions are detected during early clinical trials, serious adverse drug effects can still go undetected during this phase due to the practical limitations associated with the size and duration of the clinical trials. Recent examples of such cases include Rofecoxib and Cerivastatin (Fontanarosa, Rennie & DeAngelis, 2004). The FDA monitors for adverse drug events in the post-marketing phase through the MedWatch program (www.fda.gov/MedWatch/report.htm). The MedWatch program, which is mainly a voluntary reporting program, suffers from several limitations, the most critical of which are the under-reporting of adverse events and the lack of a denominator reflecting the magnitude of exposure.

In a 1996 article titled "The Clinical Impact of Adverse Event Reporting" the FDA estimated that only 1% of serious adverse drug events are reported to the MedWatch program (Food and Drug Administration [FDA], 1996, p.5). An alternative mechanism for detection of adverse drug events is the use of longitudinal medical records. However, the availability of data from such records has been limited. In addition, the extraction of meaningful conclusions from such data is difficult due to data integrity, heterogeneity, and missing data problems.

Several information-technology based solutions have been suggested to help monitor and reduce the adverse drug event problem. Most of the proposed solutions and studies conducted have been limited to inpatients in a hospital setting. Although a major part of drug dispensing and medications takes place in an outpatient setting, there is limited literature concerning the detection of adverse drug events in an outpatient setting. In this paper, our focus is on methods for the detection of adverse drug events in an outpatient setting and in the post marketing phase using a web-based reporting system. Specifically, our focus is developing the IT architecture for enabling a large-scale data collection mechanism to support the detection and quantification of previously unrecognized side effects and drug interactions for drugs, especially those newly introduced into the market. We propose an IT architecture for enabling a web-based reporting and surveillance solution called the Drug Effectiveness Reporting and Monitoring System (DERMS). The DERMS system is based on a community pharmacy based safety network and proposes the participation of community pharmacies for the collection of clinical response and adverse drug event information from patients. We describe the information technology architecture that forms the supporting infrastructure for the surveillance system and discuss the requirements and factors necessary for a successful implementation of the proposed system.

This paper is structured as follows. In Section 2, we describe the proposed post marketing effectiveness and safety surveillance program and discuss the limitations of the system in its current form. In Section 3, we review previous literature discussing technological solutions to the adverse event detection problem. We briefly describe the Drug Effectiveness Reporting and Monitoring System and propose the enabling IT architecture in Section 4 and discuss the success factors for its implementation in Section 5. We discuss the limitations of the proposed system in Section 6 and make concluding observations in Section 7.

Post-Marketing Surveillance

An effective surveillance process that follows the introduction of a new drug into the market requires the efficient flow of information among the different affected entities including patients, drug companies, the FDA, and healthcare professionals such as doctors, nurses and pharmacists. This should include information on drug usage, patient exposure, interactions, adverse effects, and treatment outcomes. At present, the primary mechanism for disseminating information from the drug companies and FDA is through sales representatives, visiting lecture series, press releases, information services, pharmacy databases that enable the timely dissemination of information relevant to drug interactions, and the official labeling information (package insert).

While the FDA and drug companies are able to use broadcast mechanisms and information services exist for disseminating information to physicians, pharmacists and patients, there are currently no widely implemented mechanism for the reverse flow of information on adverse events and medication and treatment outcomes from patients and healthcare practitioners to the FDA on an on-going basis. This channel is weak and relies heavily on the MedWatch system and other similarly limited mechanisms.

Currently, post-approval monitoring by the FDA is mainly achieved through the Medwatch system, a post-marketing surveillance program. The MedWatch system relies on voluntary submission of reports by patients and healthcare providers. In this program, patients and healthcare providers can submit an adverse event report via several mechanisms including an online report form, fax, phone, and mail. The Medwatch reports, along with adverse event information reported by pharmaceutical companies, are stored in the Adverse Event Reporting System (AERS) database. The database is publicly available for download by clinical reviewers and researchers on a quarterly basis for analyzing drug interactions and monitoring drug safety. (Center for Drug Evaluation and Research [CDER], 2005).

Figure 1. Information flows in the post approval phase

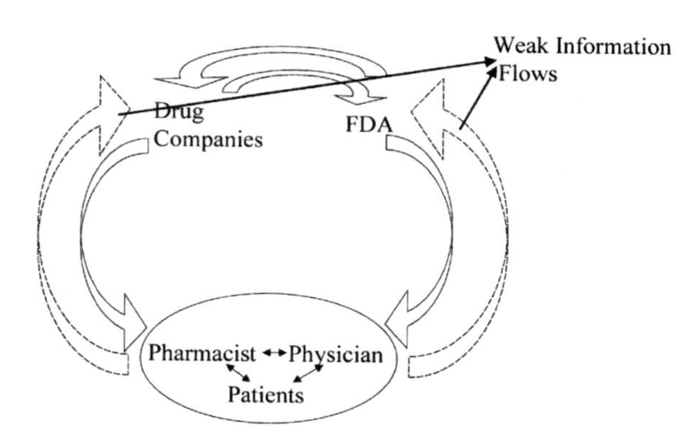

While the MedWatch program has been successful at identifying critical side effects that exhibit in the early stages after drug marketing, it suffers from several major limitations that prevent the faster detection of the adverse drug effects. For example, although 19 drugs were withdrawn from the market between 1997 and 2007 based on MedWatch data, it took an average of 6.6 years post introduction of the drugs into the market to identify their adverse effects and remove these drugs from the market. In addition, the system is far less effective at identifying adverse effects that result from prolonged administration of drugs (Brewer & Colditz, 1999; US Department of Health and Human Services, 1999).

The limitations of the MedWatch system include the poor quality of submitted reports, duplicate reporting of events, under-reporting of adverse events, and the absence of a common denominator, i.e. baseline information, required to make meaningful conclusions from the data (Fontanarosa et al., 2004). In addition, the detection of adverse effects resulting from prolonged use of drugs requires the collection of longitudinal medical records, which are not readily available to the MedWatch system. Longitudinal medical records are necessary for the detection of adverse effects that manifest late in the chronic administration of a drug, such as in the case of Vioxx where the increased risk of heart attacks and strokes on prolonged use was not detected by the MedWatch system but rather through controlled clinical studies.

The MedWatch system is also deficient in providing background information, such as the number of patients being administered a particular medication. Background information, such as the number of events per number of patients exposed, is essential for the scientific evaluation of adverse event data. Other factors contributing to the noise and biased nature of MedWatch data include increases in adverse event reports in response to media publicity and "dear healthcare professional" letters. Given the various limitations of current adverse event reporting mechanisms, there is a need for a comprehensive adverse event data collection mechanism that can result in data of better quality and serve as an early alert system for newly introduced drugs.

PREVIOUS WORK

Several studies have been conducted analyzing the use of Information Technology (IT) in managing Adverse Drug Events (ADE). Literature in this area focuses on the detection of adverse events using computer-based mechanisms and the prevention of ADE using IT tools. Computerization and the use of information technology tools for automating healthcare workflow have resulted in significant improvements in healthcare delivery and in the prevention of adverse drug events (Bates et al., 1999; Bates et al., 2001; Evans et al., 1992). Computerization and healthcare information technology systems such as computerized order entry and clinical decision support systems have led to significant reductions of medical errors and improvements in the quality of care (Bates et al., 2001).

Surveillance mechanisms for the detection of adverse drug events can be classified as outpatient based monitoring mechanisms and inpatient based monitoring mechanisms. Bates et al., (2003) examined the effectiveness of various information technology tools in detecting adverse events in inpatient and outpatient settings. They determined that information technology tools that analyze administrative data recorded using ICD9 codes are of limited value in identifying adverse drug events, while rule based detection mechanisms that rely on laboratory test results and occurrences of antidote use are able to detect a significantly larger portion of the adverse events. Another finding of the study is the need for natural language processing tools to process free text data for the detection of adverse events. A significant portion of the patient related information such as visit notes, admission notes, progress notes, consultation notes, and nursing notes are stored in the form of free text. Although rule-based mechanisms are able to identify a significant portion of the adverse events, they still under-perform chart review based methods for adverse event detection. This is primarily due to the inability of rule-based mechanisms to identify symptom changes, which are mostly recorded in free text form (Classen et al., 1991).

In outpatient care, free text processing tools greatly outperform rule-based mechanisms that rely on ICD-9 codes for the detection of adverse events. Honigman et al., (2001) reported that code-based mechanism can detect only about 3% of the adverse events when applied to outpatient data, while free text processing mechanism were able to identify 91% of the adverse events. Anderson et al., (2002) present results from a simulation study designed to analyze the effect of information technology in reducing adverse events. Their primary focus was on the use of information technology tools in reducing prescription errors through the automation of the prescription workflow using electronic means as well as the prevention of adverse events by verifying prescriptions against a database of known drug interactions. A detailed review of various methodologies for the detection of adverse events is given in Murff et al. (2003).

Although several systems have been developed for the detection of adverse drug events given various patient data, the reporting and collection of adverse drug event information itself has not been extensively investigated. Moreover, most of the proposed systems are limited to inpatient settings and single organizations. There is relatively limited literature analyzing the use of information technology for large scale adverse event reporting in an outpatient setting. A study by Tejal et al., (2000) reports the incidence of adverse drug events in outpatient care to be common and that most such events are not documented in the medical records. A majority of the events are preventable and proper monitoring for symptoms, response, and adequate communication between outpatients and providers can prevent most adverse drug events (Tejal et al., 2003).

A series of studies have been conducted over the past few decades to evaluate alternative mechanisms for collecting and reporting adverse drug events in an outpatient setting. Fisher et al., (1987) conducted a study analyzing the effectiveness of post-marketing surveillance using outpatient adverse drug event reports. They concluded that outpatient based post-marketing surveillance programs that rely on patient-initiated reports can complement existing physician based surveillance systems. Fisher and Bryant (1990) observed that patients can correctly differentiate adverse drug events from other adverse clinical events under certain conditions. They observed that the discrimination between adverse drug events from other adverse clinical events was better when the reporting was initiated by a staff member and the reporting was spontaneous as opposed to an interviewer-mediated systematic enquiry. Data from patient drug attributions has been observed to be consistent with alternative monitoring methods such as physician assessments and epidemiological data, and can also be used to improve the discriminatory power of such methods (Fisher et al., 1994). In addition to the Fisher et al. studies, a recent study by Cohen et al., (2005) analyzed the effect of pharmacist intervention in a community pharmacy setting. The study showed a considerable reduction in adverse events by conducting an audit of discharged patients and a subsequent 9-month follow-up.

A community pharmacist based outpatient post marketing surveillance system potentially has several uses, including early detection of adverse drug reactions, discovery of new therapeutic benefits of the newly introduced drugs (Fisher & Bryant, 1992) and comparison between alternative medications (Fisher et al., 1993, Fisher et al., 1995). However, the previous studies were limited to short time periods and did not explore the use of emerging information technologies to leverage the surveillance and monitoring mechanism.

Critical Path Institute (C-Path, 2005) has proposed a community pharmacy based surveillance model that is characterized by the following aspects: (1) the data collection is performed in an outpatient setting and involves community pharmacies, which are visited by patients more frequently than hospitals. (2) The community pharmacy based model focuses on pharmacists and pharmacy technicians to collect large-scale data on adverse events and drug effectiveness. (3) The model is designed to collect baseline information and information on background rates to help conduct rigorous data analysis.

In this paper, we propose a web-based information system, i.e. the Drug Effectiveness Reporting and Monitoring System (DERMS). The DERMS system was one of the models developed for the Critical Path Institute. Although it is currently not a part of the CPSN, the DERMS system can be adapted to serve as a general pharmacy based patient safety system.

DRUG EFFECTIVENESS REPORTING AND MONITORING SYSTEM

In this section, we give a brief overview of the Drug Effectiveness Reporting and Monitoring

System described previously in (Gupta el al., 2007), describe the key processes of the DERMS system and propose a system architecture for supporting the key processes to be implemented in the DERMS system.

Overview

The key requirements of the DERMS system are derived from the community-pharmacy based model for post-marketing surveillance proposed by the Critical Path Institute. The community pharmacy based model includes a large-scale data collection mechanism that involves pharmacists and pharmacy technicians to identify and collect adverse event information. After medical evaluation, pharmacists and pharmacy technicians usually constitute the first point of contact with patients as outpatients. Hence, they can potentially collect and maintain evolving historical information on the patient's medication history. Such history would include comprehensive information on the various types of medications taken by the patient, along with the corresponding duration of use for each medication. Such records can serve as an alternative source of information for evaluating the long-term effects of clinical medicines. The perceived direct and indirect benefits of such as system include the following: (1) the creation of longitudinal medical records by integrating patient medication history with baseline and periodically collected follow-up information on the patient's medical condition, and (2) Faster detection of adverse events using a systematic monitoring procedure implemented at the point of medication dispensing and (3) assessment of comparative effectiveness.

Key Processes

The drug effectiveness reporting and monitoring system is characterized by three key processes that include the data collection process, surveillance and monitoring process and surveillance administration process. We describe each of these processes in detail below.

Surveillance Administration Process. The surveillance administration process basically captures the key tasks of the agency responsible for administering the surveillance mechanisms and the infrastructure. The surveillance administration process involves the identification of newly introduced drugs that need to be monitored. It also includes the identification of appropriate data items that need to be captured and the design and development of questionnaires for eliciting and capturing adverse event information. The questionnaires developed in this process are used in the data collection process which we describe next.

Data Collection Process. The data collection process is illustrated in Figure 2. The process is initiated when a patient visits a pharmacy to fill a prescription. If the prescribed drug has been selected by a surveillance administrator for surveillance, the pharmacist proceeds to collect further information about the patient with the patients consent. For patients who are not already in the system, a basic patient information questionnaire is used to collect information on patient demographics.

A baseline information questionnaire is administered at the start of a medication to collect basic information about the patient's health status before beginning the new medication. At the time of each refill, a follow-up questionnaire is administered to the patient to record the patient's health status and query for any adverse drug effects. In the case of severe adverse drug effects a MedWatch report is filed by the Pharmacist. Each of the questionnaires administered to the patient was designed during the surveillance administration process.

The questionnaires vary based on the type of the drug being monitored. In order to design these questionnaires, the research team studied previous examples and the work of others. This included the examination of post-marketing surveillance programs of the FDA, as well as of allied research and

Figure 2. Data collection process

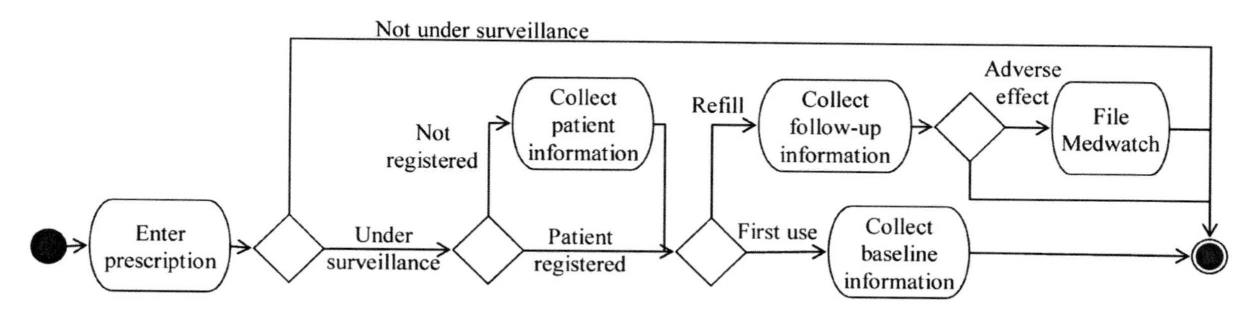

monitoring endeavors. Further, the research team studied questionnaires designed by researchers of the Arizona Center for Education and Research on Therapeutics (AzCERT). Based on different needs, five types of forms were delineated. These were: the basic patient information form; the baseline information questionnaire; the routine follow-up questionnaire; the special follow-up questionnaire; and the adverse event reporting form. The special follow-up questionnaire is used for medications that are known to have potential harmful side effects usually occurring after a certain period has elapsed. A screenshot of the data collection process within the DERMS system is shown in Figure 3.

Surveillance and Monitoring Process. While the data collection process is executed by the Pharmacist, the surveillance and monitoring process is primarily executed by research and quality improvement organizations. An overview of the process is given in Figure 4. In this process, the data collected during the data collection process is analyzed by researchers to identify possible drug interactions and signals suggesting serious side effects.

Following the analysis, three possible actions are supported by the DERMS system. In the case of suspect data points or outliers, a researcher can contact the concerned pharmacy for follow-up information. In the case of confirmed adverse effects, a report can be sent to the FDA's office of drug safety (ODS). If the researcher requires the collection of additional information through follow-up questionnaires, the surveillance administration can be contacted for modifications or the design of specialized follow-up questionnaires to be administered during the surveillance process. A screenshot from the surveillance process within the DERMS system is shown in Figure 5.

Figure 3. Data collection forms

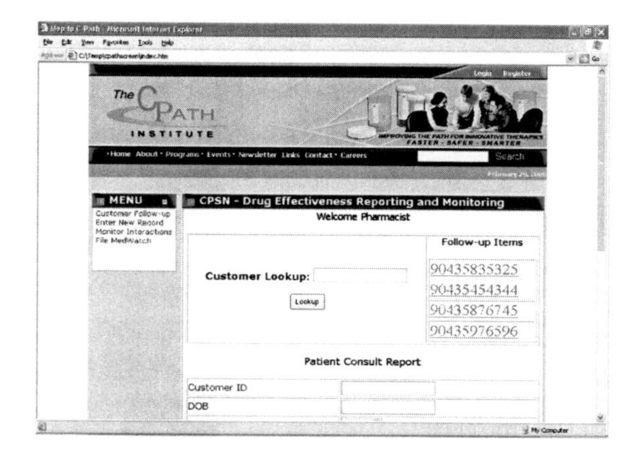

System Architecture

In order to support the above mentioned key processes, we propose a three-layer system architecture as illustrated in Figure 6. It consists of a core infrastructure layer, an application layer and an interface layer. The core IT infrastructure supporting the drug effectiveness reporting and monitoring system consists of a centralized relational database and file system for storing the surveillance data and associated documents. The core infrastructure also includes an application

Figure 4. Surveillance process

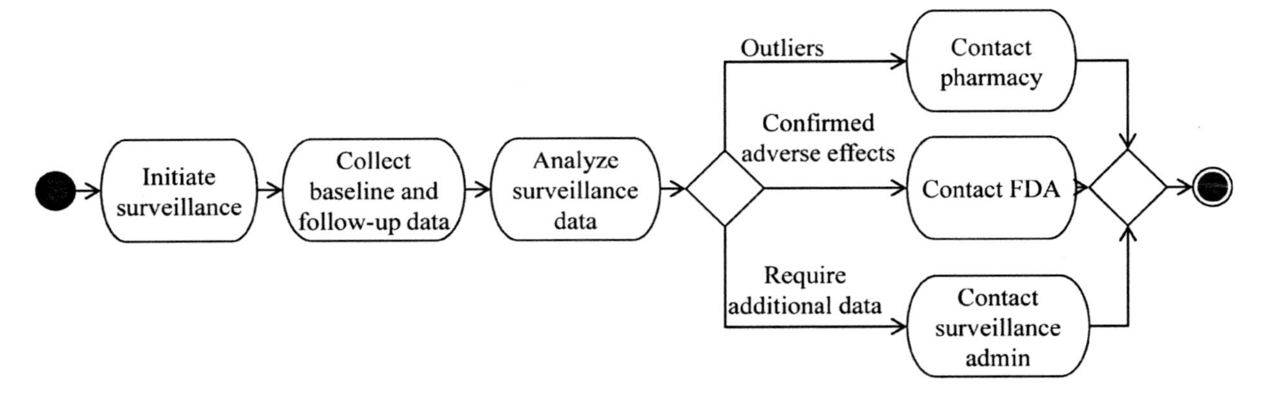

server, a workflow engine and a statistics and data-mining module that help execute the business logic implemented in the DERMS modules. Three application modules corresponding to the key processes supported by the DERMS system are included in the application layer. They implement the business logic and processes that support the data collection, administration and surveillance and monitoring mechanisms.

The interface layer consists of a HTML interface accessible through a web browser, a web service interface, and an email interface. The HTML interface is the primary web-based interface used by the pharmacists to execute the data collection process. The web service interface can be used to interface with pharmacy information systems to directly retrieve data from pharmacy systems. The web service interface can also be by researchers to interface with statistical and analysis software. The email interface is used for communication between various entities involved in the data collection, administration and surveillance and monitoring processes.

Critical Success Factors

The proposed large-scale post-marketing surveillance system involves the participation of multiple stakeholders and is influenced by several factors that determine its adoption and successful implementation. We reviewed literature in the area of event reporting systems (Barach & Small, 2000),

Figure 5. Surveillance visualization screenshot

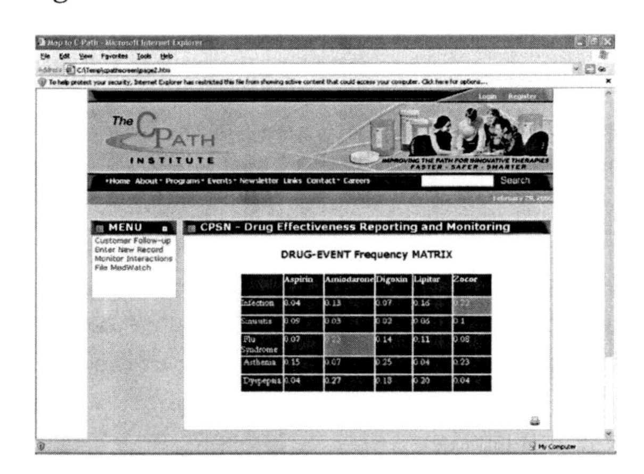

Figure 6. System architecture

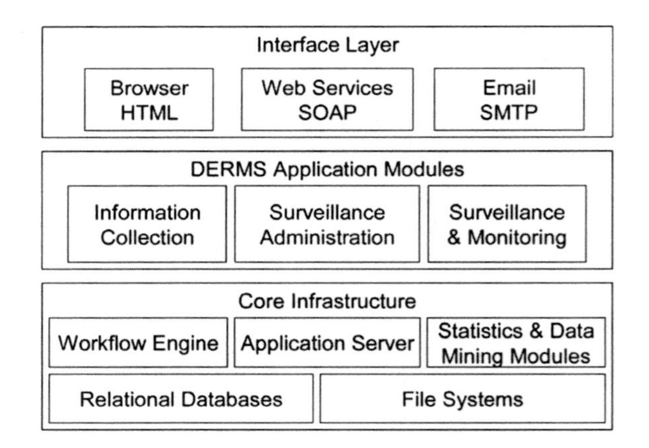

post-marketing surveillance methods (Fisher et al., 1987), pharmaco-epidemiological studies involving the participation of community pharmacists (Farris et al., 2002; Oh et al., 2002; Schommer et al., 2002; Weinberger 2002) and information technology adoption (Menachemi et al., 2004) to determine the key factors that influence the successful implementation of such a system.

Barach and Small (2000) draw lessons from an analysis of various non-medical critical event reporting systems and prescribe a set of guidelines for the design of medical event reporting systems. They identify six different factors as being critical to the successful adoption and high quality of a medical event reporting system: "immunity (as far as practical); confidentiality or data de-identification (making data untraceable to care-givers, patients, institutions, time); independent outsourcing of report collection and analysis by peer experts; rapid meaningful feedback to reporters and all interested parties; ease of reporting; and sustained leadership support." We analyze each of these factors and identify the critical elements of the community pharmacy based surveillance model to derive the technological requirements of the DERMS model.

Immunity: A key barrier to adoption of an incident reporting system is the fear of reprisal or a lack of trust for an individual and fear of litigation for organizations. As such, immunity to the greatest extent possible is important for successful adoption of an incident reporting system. In the context of the community pharmacy-based adverse event reporting system, this translates into immunity for pharmacists and the community pharmacy participating in the reporting program. From a technical requirements point of view, enabling immunity requires the use of mechanisms that provide confidentiality to users, anonymity to the pharmacists and pharmacies, and mechanisms that prevent the traceability of patients by unauthorized users.

Confidentiality: Confidentiality of data is an important element for a successful reporting system. For healthcare applications, confidentiality implies protecting the privacy rights of the patients by de-identifying patient data. However, de-identification of data sometimes leads to duplication of records. Therefore, data management mechanisms that enable de-duplication of records and the identification of unique individual records while preserving patient privacy need to be developed. Access control mechanisms and data encryption technologies need to be provided in order to ensure the security of data and prevent unauthorized use of the data.

Evaluation: Barach and Small (2000) report that independent collection of reports and analysis by peer evaluation is an important factor influencing the quality of an incident reporting system. In the community pharmacy based approach, this is achieved by outsourcing the data evaluation to regional quality improvement organizations, data collection to community pharmacies, and monitoring and overview to an independent administrative entity. Providing the above features would require a scalable and flexible mechanism that would enable multiple diverse entities to seamlessly exchange data by integrating heterogeneous applications and data sources and at the same time provide privacy, data security, and prevent unauthorized access. Recent developments in information technology such as workflow system, web services, service oriented architecture (SOA) and grid computing can provide a successful implementation to support the independent collection and evaluation features of the community pharmacy based system.

Feedback: Feedback to incident reporters and all participating stakeholders is necessary for successful adoption and implementation of an incident reporting system. The reporting and data analysis modules, along with workflow and communication tools can be used to provide meaningful feedback to the interested participating users.

Reporting: Two major factors need to be considered when designing the data collection process: the ease of reporting the data and the quality of the data being collected. Previous studies

(Bates et al., 2003) have shown that typical hospital incident reports and ICD-9 based reporting mechanisms are inadequate for detecting adverse drug events. Reporting mechanisms need to be customized for each drug and drug combinations to collect relevant symptomatic information. While the data fields determine the quality of the data being collected, the design of the report affects the adoption of the reporting system. Complexity and amount of time spent reporting is a major barrier to large scale adoption of a reporting system. The reporting system needs to be designed such that it leverages the users familiarity with other computer based systems, minimizes the amount of data to be manually entered and the overall reporting time.

Leadership: Continued leadership is necessary to maintain and manage an incident reporting system and to effectively respond to changing needs. Monitoring and communication capability are key to enabling effective leadership. In the DERMS system, an administrative module is provided to initiate and monitor the surveillance process. Graphical tools, integrated email, and messaging mechanisms can be used to provide this functionality.

Workload Minimization: A key barrier to adoption of the system is the addition to workload because of increased reporting responsibilities. Time and motion studies indicate that pharmacist spend around 6-7% of their time in computer entry activities (Murray et al., 1998). A study by Oh, et al., (2002) estimates that pharmacists need to spend an additional 3 minutes of time for patient consultation and adverse drug effect monitoring. As long as the additional computer order entry time is minimal, resistance to adoption should be minimal.

The introduction of additional workload is a key problem especially in locations with shortages in pharmacist. However, the following mechanisms can be considered to alleviate the problem. First, the additional workload can be distributed between a pharmacists and a pharmacy technician such that the computer entry activities are handled by a pharmacy technician while the activities related to the elicitation and identification of adverse events are delegated to a pharmacist. Second, depending on resource constraints, the surveillance mechanism can be limited to patients who are prescribe certain newly introduced drugs thereby lowering the additional workload.

Incentives: Previous studies have indicated that the provision of financial incentives has had a positive effect on patient counseling activities of pharmacist resulting into reduced adverse events (Farris et al., 2002). As such, financial incentives can serve an additional factor in promoting the adoption of a community pharmacy based system. In addition to financial incentives, job satisfaction, is a key driver in increased pharmacist involvement in patient counseling and drug therapy reviews. A study by Schommer (2002) concludes that pharmacists prefer to spend more time on patient consultation and drug use management instead of medication dispensing and business management.

Factors Influencing Pharmacy Participation

The successful adoption and continued use of the proposed system by community pharmacies and pharmacists is dependent on several factors. In order to promote the successful adoption of the new surveillance system, the features of the system also need to be aligned with the interests of the community pharmacy and the professional interests of the pharmacists. Based on previous studies on IT adoption, we hypothesize that while organizational buy-in is necessary for initial adoption of a new system, its continued use is dependent on the perceived usefulness of the system and its alignment towards the skill and professional interests of the pharmacists.

Several operational factors also need to be considered for the successful implementation of the proposed surveillance system. For example, a paper describing randomized control trials con-

Table 1. Critical success factors

Success Factor	Implementation	Possible IT Solutions
Immunity	Anonymity of reporters, participants	Data Encryption and de-identification. Access control.
Independent Reporting and Evaluation	Involvement of Community Pharmacies, Quality Improvement Organizations and administrative entity.	Workflow systems, Mediators and Web Services for heterogeneous data and application integration. Access control and relational views.
Confidentiality	Patient Privacy, Data de-identification	Data element identification and Probabilistic de-duplication algorithms.
Feedback	Summary reports and information	Reporting modules and data validation and verification algorithms
Ease of Reporting	Minimal reporting time, Capture of key and minimal data elements	Assistive technologies and intuitive user interfaces.
Leadership	Surveillance Administration, Dashboards, Real-time monitoring of key metrics, problem detection and communication capability.	Communication modules, Monitoring and reporting modules.
Workload Minimization	Financial Incentives, Workload distribution between Pharmacists and Pharmacy Technicians	Integration with pharmacy systems to minimize computer entry.

ducted to evaluate the effectiveness of pharmaceutical care programs in Indianapolis (Weinberger, 2002) highlights several operational difficulties that occur in programs involving community pharmacies. The study, initiated at a major pharmacy chain, analyzed new pharmaceutical care programs aimed at giving the pharmacists a greater role in providing the patients with better healthcare. The data were initially transmitted from the pharmacy chain to the Indianapolis Network for Patient Care (INPC) for purposes of consolidation and analysis. As this experimental study progressed, the pharmacy chain was acquired by a larger national pharmacy chain. Apart from the problems caused by differences in computer systems of the two organizations, there were problems created by major differences in their management policies. For example, the parent pharmacy required the patients to give their categorical affirmative response before patient data could be utilized in any manner. In order to address this new requirement, a decision was made to offer a sum of $60 as incentive to patients who were willing to let their data to be used for purposes of this experimental study. With this incentive, 21% of the patients responded to the offer, with approx 70% of them agreeing to let the data be used, and the balance 30% declining the offer. In order to increase the response rate, the pharmacy personnel initiated follow-up efforts. Finally, 20%of the persons originally contacted agreed to accept the offer of $60 in lieu of data be utilized for the experimental study.

The above experience emphasizes four critical success factors for achieving progress in this area. First, senior management must accept the need for such studies and be prepared to explicitly support the endeavor through its entire life-cycle; without such close involvement, the effort will fail. Second, pharmacists should view this function as an integral part of their job of dispensing drugs and interacting with patients on issues related to drugs; in order to make this scenario feasible, financial incentives may need to be provided to pharmacists. Third, the policies of major pharmacy chains vary significantly from each other; discussions need to occur among them in order to generate consensus on this critical issue that impacts human lives. Fourth, new mechanisms need to be developed to share relevant chains across otherwise competing entities in a manner that meets applicable guidelines for information, security, and safety, while simultaneously ensuring that the risks to human lives is minimized.

LIMITATIONS

At the beginning of this paper, we had identified some of the weaknesses of the current MedWatch system. The concept demonstration prototype described in this paper mitigates some of the problems, but several of them still remain and need further research and attention. The areas requiring further attention are discussed in the following paragraphs.

First, the automated assimilation of the information from diverse information systems, each characterized by its own design and significantly different from others, will require use of advanced concepts from the realm of integration of heterogeneous information systems. Similarly, state-of-the-art ideas related to data mining and knowledge discovery will need to be employed. The scalability of the concept demonstration prototype needs to be examined in detail in order to evaluate the potential feasibility of utilizing the proposed approach over an extended geographic area.

Second, the prototype system tracks drugs that are provided to customers over-the-counter at retail outlets of major pharmaceutical chains. If this concept is extended to smaller chains and individual shops, it will need to deal with a still greater variety of legacy hardware and software. The problem is further complicated by the fact that patients now acquire drugs by mail, both from outlets in the US and abroad, using web-based and telephone-based mechanisms to place the concerned purchase orders for drugs. No effective mechanism currently exists for tracking the purchase of such drugs.

Third, our approach lacks the ability to track samples of drugs that have been provided by the prescribing physician to the patient. Such dispensing of drugs by physicians may need to be monitored, especially for drugs that have only recently been introduced. The same web-based interface could be used to enter the requisite information by personnel in the physician's office. Also, some pharmaceutical companies now provide magnetic cards that can be redeemed at pharmacies for samples of drugs. If this new concept is used for all samples, the limitations of monitoring drug samples will be overcome.

Fourth, our proposed system relies heavily on pharmacists for their expertise and good will in talking with to patients, eliciting the requisite information from them, and reporting it using the web-based interface.

Fifth, patients may currently obtain drugs from multiple pharmacy outlets that belong to different chains. Without a common identifier, it is difficult to track that the medicines were indeed purchased for use by the same patient. The most obvious identifier would be the social security number in the US. However, current regulations and concerns for patient privacy prevent such usage. New options need to be explored.

CONCLUSION

In this paper, we propose an IT architecture that forms the enabling infrastructure for a new post-marketing surveillance tool for newly introduced drugs called the Drug Effectiveness Reporting and Monitoring System. We briefly define the key characteristics of the DERMS system and propose a system architecture for supporting the key processes implemented in the DERMS system. We then analyze the critical success factors for the DERMS-based post marketing surveillance mechanism and identify supporting IT solutions.

Future work in this area involves further investigation of the critical success factors and development of instruments to validate the hypothesized critical success factors. In addition, large-scale implementation of such as system requires further investigation of the privacy and security issues related to data collection, storage and sharing processes. Recent developments in this area include the FDA's new Sentinel Initiative (http://www.fda.gov/Safety/FDAsSentinelInitiative/), which includes a comprehensive approach to gather data from diverse healthcare data holders to evaluate medical safety issues. We intend to explore extensions to the DERMS system that can enable it to inter-operate with the Sentinel System.

REFERENCES

Anderson, J. G., Jay, S. J., Anderson, M., & Hunt, T. J. (2002). Evaluating the capability of information technology to prevent adverse drug events: a computer simulation approach. *Journal of the American Medical Informatics Association, 9*, 479–490. doi:10.1197/jamia.M1099

Barach, P., & Small, S. (2000). Reporting and preventing medical mishaps: lessons from non-medical near miss reporting systems. *British Medical Journal, 320*, 759–763. doi:10.1136/bmj.320.7237.759

Bates, D. W., Cohen, M., Leape, L. L., Overhage, J. M., Shabot, M. M., & Sheridan, T. (2001). Reducing the frequency of errors in medicine using information technology. *Journal of the American Medical Informatics Association, 8*, 299–308.

Bates, D. W., Evans, R. S., Murff, H., Stetson, P. D., Pizziferri, L., & Hripcsak, G. (2003). Detecting adverse events using information technology. *Journal of the American Medical Informatics Association, 10*, 115–128. doi:10.1197/jamia.M1074

Brewer, T., & Colditz, G. A. (1999). Postmarketing surveillance and adverse drug reactions: current perspectives and future needs. *Journal of the American Medical Association, 281*, 824–829. doi:10.1001/jama.281.9.824

C., & Bates, DW. (2000). Incidence and preventability of adverse drug events in nursing homes. *American Journal of Medicine*, 109, 87-94.

Center for Drug Evaluation and Research. (2005). Adverse event reporting system. Retrieved from http://www.fda.gov/cder/aers/default.htm

Classen, D. C., Pestotnik, S. L., Evans, R. S., & Burke, J. P. (1991). Computerized surveillance of adverse drug events in hospital patients. *Journal of the American Medical Association, 266*, 2847–2851. doi:10.1001/jama.266.20.2847

Cohen, M. M., Kimmel, N. L., Benage, M. K., Cox, M. J., Sanders, N., Spence, D., & Chen, J. (2005). Medication safety program reduces adverse drug events in a community hospital. *Quality & Safety in Health Care, 14*, 169–174. doi:10.1136/qshc.2004.010942

Evans, R. S., Pestotnik, S. L., Classen, D. C., Bass, S. B., & Burke, J. P. (1992). Prevention of adverse drug events through computerized surveillance. *Proceedings- The Annual Symposium on Computer Applications in Medical Care.* 437-41.

Farris, K. B., Kumbera, P., Halterman, T., & Fang, G. (2002). Outcomes-based pharmacist reimbursement: reimbursing pharmacists for cognitive services. *Journal of Managed Care Pharmacy, 5*(8), 383–393.

Fisher, S., & Bryant, S. G. (1990). Postmarketing surveillance: accuracy of patient drug attribution judgments. *Clinical Pharmacology and Therapeutics, 48*, 102–107.

Fisher, S., & Bryant, S. G. (1992). Postmarketing surveillance of adverse drug reactions: patient self-monitoring. *The Journal of the American Board of Family Practice*, *5*, 17–25.

Fisher, S., Bryant, S. G., & Kent, T. A. (1993). Postmarketing surveillance by patient self-monitoring: trazodone versus fluoxetine. *Journal of Clinical Psychopharmacology*, *13*, 235–242. doi:10.1097/00004714-199308000-00002

Fisher, S., Bryant, S. G., Kent, T. A., & Davis, J. E. (1994). Patient drug attributions and postmarketing surveillance. *Pharmacotherapy*, *14*, 202–209.

Fisher, S., Bryant, S. G., Solovitz, B. L., & Kluge, R. M. (1987). Patient-initiated postmarketing surveillance: a validation study. *Journal of Clinical Pharmacology*, *27*, 843–854.

Fisher, S., Kent, T. A., & Bryant, S. G. (1995). Postmarketing surveillance by patient self-monitoring: preliminary data for sertraline versus fluoxetine. *The Journal of Clinical Psychiatry*, *56*, 288–296.

Fontanarosa, P., Rennie, D., & DeAngelis, C. (2004). Postmarketing surveillance — Lack of vigilance, lack of trust. *Journal of the American Medical Association*, *292*(21). doi:10.1001/jama.292.21.2647

Food and Drug Administration. (1996). The clinical impact of adverse event reporting. Retrieved from http://www.fda.gov/downloads/Safety/MedWatch/UCM168505.pdf

Gandhi, T. K., Burstin, H. R., Cook, E. F., Puopolo, A. L., Haas, J. S., Brennan, T. A., & Bates, D. W. (2000). Drug complications in outpatients. *Journal of General Internal Medicine*, *15*(3), 207–208. doi:10.1046/j.1525-1497.2000.04199.x

Gandhi, T. K., Weingart, S. N., Borus, J., Seger, A. C., Peterson, J., & Burdick, E. (2003). Adverse drug events in ambulatory care. *The New England Journal of Medicine*, *348*(16), 1556–1564. doi:10.1056/NEJMsa020703

Gurwitz, J. H., Field, T. S., Avorn, J., McCormick, D., Jain, S., Eckler, M., Benser, M., Edmondson, A.

Honigman, B., Lee, J., Rothschild, J., Light, P., Pulling, R. M., Yu, T., & Bates, D. W. (2001). Using computerized data to identify adverse drug events in outpatients. *Journal of the American Medical Informatics Association*, *8*, 254–266.

Johnson, J. A., & Bootman, J. L. (1995). Drug-related morbidity and mortality. A cost-of-illness model. *Archives of Internal Medicine*, *155*(18), 1949–1956. doi:10.1001/archinte.155.18.1949

Lazarou, J., Pomeranz, B., & Corey, P. (1998). Incidence of adverse drug reactions in hospitalized patients. *Journal of the American Medical Association*, *279*, 1200–1205. doi:10.1001/jama.279.15.1200

Menachemi, N., Burke, D., & Brooks, R. G. (2004). Adoption factors associated with patient safety-related information technology. *Journal for Healthcare Quality*, *26*(6), 39–44.

Murff, H. J., Patel, V. L., Hripcsak, G., & Bates, D. W. (2003). Detecting adverse events for patient safety research: a review of current methodologies. *Journal of Biomedical Informatics*, *36*(1-2), 131–143. doi:10.1016/j.jbi.2003.08.003

Murray, M. D., Loos, B., Tu, W., Eckert, G. J., Zhou, X. H., & Tierney, W. M. (1998). Effects of computer-based prescribing on pharmacist work patterns. *Journal of the American Medical Informatics Association*, *5*(6), 585–586.

Oh, Y., McCombs, J. S., Cheng, R. A., & Johnson, K. A. (2002). Pharmacist time required for counseling in an outpatient pharmacy. *American Journal of Health-System Pharmacy*, *59*(23), 2346–2355.

Schommer, J. C., Pedersen, C. A., Doucette, W. R., Gaither, C. A., & Mott, D. A. (2002). Community pharmacists' work activities in the United States during 2000. *Journal of the American Pharmacists Association*, *42*(3), 399–406. doi:10.1331/108658002763316815

US Department of Health and Human Services. (1999). Managing the Risk from Medical Product Use, Creating a Risk Management Framework. Retrieved from http://www.fda.gov/downloads/Safety/SafetyofSpecificProducts/UCM180520.pdf

Weinberger, M., Murray, M. D., Marrero, D. G., Brewer, N., Lykens, M., & Harris, L. E. (2002). Issues in conducting randomized controlled trials of health services research interventions in nonacademic practice settings: the case of retail pharmacies. *Health Services Research*, *37*(4), 1067–1077. doi:10.1034/j.1600-0560.2002.66.x

Chapter 13
Exploring Linkages between Quality, E-Health and Healthcare Education

Christopher L. Pate
St. Philip's College, USA

Joyce E. Turner-Ferrier
St. Philip's College, USA

ABSTRACT

This chapter explores the concept of e-health as it relates to healthcare delivery, healthcare quality and education. Although the concept of e-health is emerging and lacks clear definition, a body of literature in healthcare policy and organization has focused on many of themes and ideas that are relevant to the study of e-health. This chapter introduces several frameworks and concepts that are essential for an inquiry into the relationships between e-health and quality-related outcomes in healthcare and educational settings. This chapter addresses these relationships by discussing and defining the concept of e-health, discussing central linkages between e-health and quality-related healthcare outcomes, and highlighting key themes between health education, technology and quality.

INTRODUCTION

Changes in healthcare delivery have become so widespread and frequent that the idea of change in healthcare has become one of anticipation and expectation rather than interruption and surprise. Consumers, providers, organizations and societies have seen changes in the definitions of vital concepts related to healthcare delivery, like health and quality, which have in turn altered the methods by which healthcare organizations and communities align and create the structures and processes necessary to provide healthcare services to supported populations. In addition to changing definitions, the healthcare sector remains influenced by changing expectations and interests of the numerous and diverse set of stakeholders found within the healthcare sector.

The concept of e-health is one of the more recent concepts to emerge in the healthcare sector and, like many other aspects of healthcare delivery, is a concept that clearly embodies a combination of ideas and theoretical approaches. Eysenbach defines the concept as:

DOI: 10.4018/978-1-61692-843-8.ch013

...an emerging field in the intersection of medical informatics, public health and business, referring to health services and information delivered or enhanced through the Internet and related technologies. In a broader sense, the term characterizes not only a technical development, but also a state-of-mind, a way of thinking, an attitude, and a commitment for networked, global thinking, to improve health care locally, regionally, and worldwide by using information and communication technology (2001).

Harrison and Lee (2006) provide a similar definition with a leaning towards the structural aspects of e-health applications. Harrison and Lee refer to e-health as:

...an all encompassing term for the combined use of electronic information and communication technology in the health sector...this term refers to the that technology used for clinical, education, research, and administrative purposes, both at the local site and across wide geographic regions (p. 283).

Although the literature provides no definitional consensus on the concept, a great deal can be learned about the implications of e-health through an existing literature that has focused on innovations, information technology, quality, and healthcare education. These subjects can guide our understanding of the growth and importance of this concept as it relates to the larger goals of healthcare, particularly the goal of improving and understanding healthcare quality. In considering e-health a recent innovation, we also turn to theoretical frameworks related to systems, quality and diffusion of innovations. The use of specific theoretical frameworks provide meaningful ways to understand the complexity and potential of e-health as a significant tool in improving healthcare and as a powerful enabler to improving education in healthcare, which ultimately will have an impact on healthcare outcomes.

After completing this chapter, readers should be to:

1. Provide a definition of the concept of e-health and the relationship between e-health and the larger healthcare system
2. Evaluate potential relationships between e-health, healthcare, education, and quality.
3. Discuss the concept of quality and how the concept relates to e-health initiatives
4. Describe the linkages between e-health, technology and healthcare education

BACKGROUND

The fact remains that the healthcare industry remains in a state of flux. Communities, nations, political leaders, system beneficiaries, healthcare providers and other important stakeholders continue to influence and alter the way that healthcare operates. Not only do these stakeholders influence how healthcare systems are planned, but they also influence the way that healthcare is and will be delivered. Perhaps most importantly, these stakeholders help establish the larger strategic goals, which in turn drive the development of objectives as well as the means by which these goals are achieved. Innovations, like e-health, can provide the procedural and technological means to further health system goals.

Innovations in healthcare are naturally designed to improve one or more aspects of healthcare delivery.

The characteristics frequently discussed include the costs of care, access to healthcare services, and quality of care. Certainly, the variety of normative positions held by leaders and other stakeholders of healthcare systems may also drive innovations. For example, viewing equity as the foremost priority of healthcare systems may call for innovations that identify and potentially alleviate health disparities that are strictly the result of way that healthcare is delivered. Holding efficiency as priority may call for innovations that improve the productive capacity of healthcare organizations without adversely affecting the quality of care. In the latter case, technological innovations—like those associated with the concept of e-health—can potentially improve production at lower costs at a fixed level of quality. On the other hand, technological innovations may also improve quality while incurring higher costs.

Understanding the linkages between e-health and quality is complicated in part because no definitional consensus exists for either of these terms. The lack of common meaning can present challenges from both practical and academic perspectives. Academically, the lack of common meaning can serve as a motivating force and call for meaningful dialogue to create knowledge. From a pragmatic point of view, different conceptualizations held by different stakeholders can also lead to meaningful dialogue with the aim of arriving at definitional resolution. On the other hand, the lack of consensus can create inter and intra-organizational dysfunctions as organizations cling to and attempt to leverage their own positions for self-gain. Establishing a common language may serve as a powerful platform that enables e-health to more effectively enable organizations and communities to reach broadly established goals, like quality improvement.

What is also clear about healthcare is that the interdependent and complex nature of healthcare delivery calls for structured ways to analyze the strategic goals, processes, technologies, outcomes, and other features of the healthcare system. Systems theory is often used a theoretical framework that serves as a starting point for analysis (Austin & Boxerman, 1998; Ginter, Swayne, & Duncan, 1998). This particular framework plainly underscores the complexities of healthcare, but also provides a simple and powerful way of evaluating key relationships. As Ginter, Swayne, and Duncan suggest, use of systems theory allows managers and leaders to focus on the most relevant aspects of a particular challenge while retaining sight of the larger context in which the issue or challenge presents itself.

In its essence, systems theory provides an elementary way of viewing the relationship between inputs and outputs. In its most basic form, system inputs are converted to and drive outputs, which in turn provide a feedback mechanism to the level and quantity of inputs needed. In an open system design, the entire system is monitored and influenced by an external environment, which may alter the nature of the system (see Austin & Boxerman, 1998; Ginter, Swayne, & Duncan, 1998). Austin and Boxerman's use of the cybernetic system framework is a natural extension of the systems model and provides a way in which to examine the concept of e-health as it relates to the attributes of the healthcare system, education, and quality.

The cybernetic system has several features of interest to e-health, quality and education. First, the model provides us with a simple framework that allows us to envision the linkages between providers, support staff, supporting technology, patients and outcomes. Second, the model allows us explicitly recognize the fact that the relationships between the drivers are not strictly sequen-

Figure 1. General cybernetic system framework (adapted from Austin, C.J., & Boxerman, S.B. (1998). Information systems for health services administration (5th ed.). Chicago, IL: Health Administration Press.

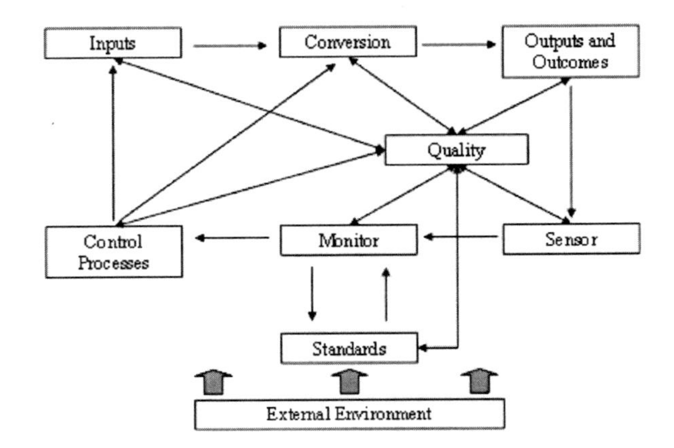

tial. Feedback and adjustments given outcomes are necessary to improve the system. Third, the model exemplifies the fact that relationships in healthcare settings are inherently interdependent and complex. Last, the model specifically includes the concept of quality, which is an essential component of organizational performance that must be considered in any evaluation of outcomes, whether the context is in healthcare or in healthcare education.

What is most striking in the analysis of the relationships between quality, healthcare and education is the numerous similarities between the institutions of healthcare and education (Johnson, 1993). Education is one of the most critical aspects of healthcare delivery, whether the education comes in the form of interaction between the patient and provider, between the patient and healthcare organization, or between the healthcare organization and the larger community. Education can reduce information asymmetries and provide patients with essential information with the potential to alter behavior and ultimately improve healthcare outcomes and quality of life. But education of healthcare providers and professionals is also important in improving quality, and the quality of education is a key factor in creating a competent, professional healthcare workforce.

QUALITY AND E-HEALTH

The concept of quality is one that elicits many perceptions and ideas; however, the volume of research and literature on this topic has failed to reach an operational consensus on its meaning. On the one hand, the concept of quality is driven and framed at a localized level. For the healthcare organization that supports a community, the idea of quality can be driven by the needs and wants of the supported community. Local information-related needs have also been consistent with organizational structures in healthcare settings (Wong, Legnini, & Whitmore, 2000) and adoption of technologies (Fitzgerald, Ferlie, & Hawkins, 2003), each of which in turn have the potential to improve quality.

To address quality or other needs from a local level, providers and healthcare organization may develop specific strategies, interventions, goals, and objectives that reflect the quality-related considerations of the supported community. In educational settings, the same type of analogy exists: To the extent that the educational institution responds to the perceived needs of the community and links these needs to quality efforts, the educational institution may derive and understand the concept through a localized process. Improving the quality of healthcare through health information technology and related innovations will naturally depend upon the extent to which technologies are adopted, and adoption of innovations will be framed by decision making and social forces at local levels (Fitzgerald, Ferlie, & Hawkins, 2003; Frank, Zhao, & Borman, 2004).

Donabedian's (2005) well-known structure-process-outcome (SPO) framework (See Table 1) provides a meaningful way of viewing the concept of quality and can provide a way in which healthcare organizations can engage in critical discussions about the specific roles that e-health applications can play in improving healthcare delivery. Structural measures of quality are those that are considered "input measures of an organization's capacity to permit or promote effective work" (Flood, Zinn, Shortell, & Scott, 2000, p. 365), and e-health technologies and supporting equipment clearly fall under this quality domain. Because of

Table 1. Quality domains and indicators

Quality domain	Indicators
Structure	Resource availability, resource quality, management systems, policies
Process	Extent to which healthcare delivery complies with process standards
Outcome	Healthcare outcomes typically based on group results

Note. Source Varkey, Reller, & Resar (2007)

interdependencies between the quality domains under the SPO model (Flood, Zinn, Shortell, & Scott) and because of the focus and importance of processes and outcomes in healthcare, the value of e-health applications may ultimately hinge upon the ability to make substantial improvements in these two dimensions.

Although the SPO model provides a powerful framework for analysis in healthcare settings, educational settings have not specifically embraced the SPO as a framework, perhaps because of the framework's focus on clinical and healthcare specific concepts. However, distinctions between inputs, processes, and outcomes are noted categorizations in education (Dolmans, Wolfhagen, & Scherpbier, 2003). Another conceptualization in educational settings is through the classifications proposed by American Society for Quality, which identifies quality domains in terms of accountability, curricular alignment, assessment and student satisfaction (Brown & Marshall, 2008).

E-Health in Healthcare Settings

One of the most significant benefits of e-health and related information technology applications is the capacity of these products and services to improve outcomes and quality in healthcare settings. The Institute of Medicine (IOM; 2001) identified several ways that information technology can yield such benefits. These include enhanced or increased capability of healthcare providers and organizations to improve:

- Safety
- Effectiveness
- Patient-centeredness of care
- Timeliness of care
- Efficiency
- Equity in healthcare provision (pp. 164 - 165)

Information technology applications can be found in both the administrative and clinical sides of healthcare systems. Within administrative divisions, specific applications have been developed and used in to support logistical functions, facilities management and planning, human resources management, and patient administration (Malec, 1998). Clinical applications include computer-based patient records, electronic order entry, automated results reporting, clinical services support systems, and other related applications (Austin & Boxerman, 1998).

Between the two administrative and clinical domains, the growth of applications has reportedly been strongest in the administrative areas. Wong, Legnini and Whitmore (2000) indicate that incentives facing healthcare administration and management naturally led to the adoption of electronic information systems to support administrative goals. Bates (2002) notes that "payment issues, rather than clinical needs, have driven most investment in IT in healthcare" (p. 1). Under a constrained financial environment, close examination of revenues, costs, productivity, and reimbursement rates can provide healthcare managers with the ability to calculate and project a number of financial indicators for the particular system or facility. Operational objectives, such as cost minimization, profit maximization, cannot be achieved unless the organization has a system to capture revenue and cost data. Godin (1997) suggests that although administrative health technologies are often cost-control focused, clinical information systems also impart the sense of control from a "big brother" viewpoint (p. 878), which certainly ties into privacy and confidentiality concerns from a policy perspective.

From a clinical perspective, electronic applications have the primary function of providing information to clinicians (Wong, Legnini, & Whitmore, 2000) and from a clinical decision-making lens, the technologies "present(s) the dawning of a new age of quality initiatives" (Carruthers & Jeacocke, 2000, p. 159). With an objective of assisting healthcare professionals in decision-making at the provider-patient encounter level, e-health applications are closely aligned with the concept of expert systems. The programs found within these types of systems promote "intelligent problem-solving behavior within a narrow area of expertise" (Grabinger, Jonassen, & Wilson, 1992, p. 366). From a healthcare perspective, an expert system would supply the provider with clinical feedback regarding potential treatment options, related clinical findings, recommended pharmaceutical support for a given diagnosis, and potential. Ultimately, clinical decision systems have the potential to improve "quality of care by reducing human errors or minimizing the effect of those that do occur" (Wong, Legnini, & Whitmore, 2000, p. 244).

In a systematic review of the relationship between health information technology and quality, Chaudhry et al. (2006) found two key themes about this relationship. First, health information technology has been shown to improve adherence with clinical guidelines. Supporting adherence is based upon the associated decision-making processes and functions are inherently built into adherence (Chaudhry et al., p. E-14). Second, technologies have also increased the ability of organizations to improve quality of care by increasing monitoring of through "large scale screening and aggregation of data" (p. E-16).

Bodie and Dutta (2008) remark that the "markers of literacy and markers of healthcare quality are closely related (and) provides ground for theoretical development and pragmatic attention" (p. 177). Bodie and Dutta (2008) explain that organizations must consider the need to increase health literacy. Health literacy as defined by the World Health Organization (WHO) refers to the "cognitive and social skills which determine the motivation and ability of individuals to gain access to, understand and use information in ways which promote and maintain good health" (Nutbeam, 1998, p. 10). The most readily cited definition of health literacy is offered in the Healthy People 2010 report as "the capacity to obtain, interpret, and understand basic health information and services and the competence to use such information and services to improve health" (US Department of Health and Human Services, 2000, p. 181).

Bodie and Dutta (2008) also assert that disparities in healthcare provision are reflected in e-health settings as in traditional settings due to the existence of the same deficiencies in access, socioeconomics, and education for underserved populations. Successful marketing requires organizations to devise mechanisms to improve marketing information to include levels that would make using e-health more attractive and understandable to the underserved, which would increase their market share of consumers.

Bodie and Dutta's (2008) integrative model of e-health use (See Figure 2) is a suggested model for increasing health literacy, which is consistent with the numerous interdependencies in healthcare as well as the systems model that introduces this chapter.

Bodie and Dutta (2008) states that e-health literacy is important because it functions as both an influencer of motivation and user ability in healthcare consumption. Hemming and Langille (2006) assert,

The conceptual framework shows the complex and interactive relationships between: determinants of health (education, early child development, aging, personal capacity, living/working conditions, gender, and culture); actions to promote health (communication, capacity development, community development, organizational development, and policy); literacy (general, health, and other); and the indirect and direct effects of literacy. These all impact a person's overall health.

Educational Linkages

Education plays a central role in healthcare, and e-health applications can play a critical role in improving healthcare outcomes because of the ability of these applications to improve the education component of healthcare delivery.

Figure 2. An integrative model of e-health use (adapted from Bodie & Dutta, 2008, p. 189)

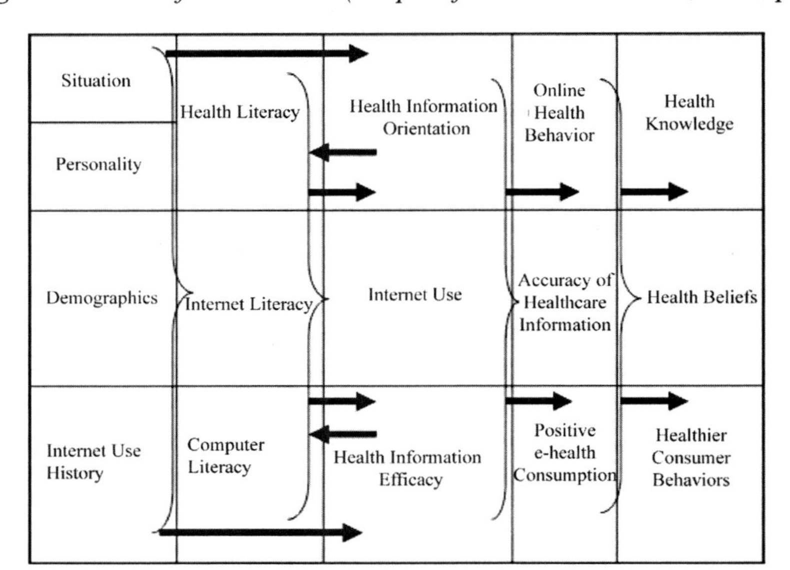

From a patient care perspective, education is a critical component of nearly all aspects of the patient-provider encounter. Education is a necessary, but not sufficient aspect of, preparing providers, administrators, and support staff for success in the healthcare industry. Perhaps pre-entry education should be considered as the minimal requirement for entry into the healthcare system—a great deal of what is required for success in healthcare environments will be learned once entry to the healthcare system is gained. On-the-job education continues throughout a career in healthcare. Healthcare professionals require ongoing education to meet licensure and credentialing requirements and similarly, healthcare organizations must show evidence of education and development for organization and facility-level accreditation. Most relevant to our discussion of e-health and education is the fact that changes in the structures and processes associated with healthcare delivery require education to allow providers and staff to adapt to and implement interventions.

Another key way to think broadly about e-health and educational linkages relates to the ways in which e-health applications and technologies can be introduced into educational settings. On the one hand, the technologies, applications, concepts and ideas can be represented in programs of instruction and curricula for prospective and current providers and technicians. On the other hand, these topics could be introduced in such a way as to educate students on the mechanics of the applications—that is, the focus would move from simple instruction to modeling and application. The focus here would entail hands-on learning. Visualizing the classroom and the technologically advanced forms of classroom delivery as two broad categories leads to the development of a simple model to further examine relationships between e-health and education. The classification scheme depicted in Figure 3 summarizes this method of classification.

In a summary of the findings of several commissions focused on healthcare education, Stephenson et al. (2002, p. 38) states "that improvements will come when health care providers work more effectively in teams and when they have the competencies to practice in increasingly accountable and technological environments." One of the ways to develop these skills is to provide instruction and training in educational environments that

Figure 3. A four quadrant model of e-health and methods of delivery

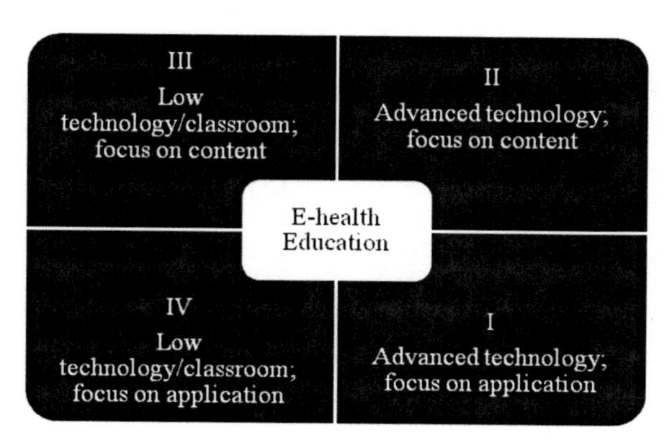

would align with the concept of advanced technology with a focus on application (Quadrant I in Figure 3). A variety of technological applications have the potential for improving education in healthcare. In a meta-analysis focusing on distance education in allied health programs, Williams (2006) provided a summary classification of the educational methods used in distance education. These broad classifications underscore the diverse types of technological applications available to healthcare institutions, higher education, and other organizations interested in healthcare education.

For healthcare providers that are far-removed from physical institutions that provide healthcare training, the same types of technology that can serve to improve patient care can also improve access to healthcare training resources. Improved access to these resources is being facilitated by delivery through video-teleconferencing, audio-teleconferencing, email, the Internet (Sheppard & Mackintosh, 1998), synchronous social networking technologies (McLeod & Barbara, 2005). Sheppard and Mackintosh (as cited in McLeod and Barbara, 2005) note that "technology offers the opportunity to 'maximize interactivity' and overcome the barriers of time, cost and distance to rural and remote health professionals" (p. 276). Interestingly and not surprisingly, the very mechanisms used to deliver preparatory education for healthcare professionals is also found to have ongoing relevance as for use post a formalized plan of education. For example, McLeod and Barbara (2005) noted that students provided with chat functions to support fieldwork training for occupational therapy and speech pathology programs reported a stronger connection with instructors and peer support from other students. Students in McLeod and Barbara's indicated a desire to use the same technology in practice settings (p. 280).

Use of the PDSA framework is a robust method of developing interventions to improve quality in healthcare settings and "the most commonly used approach for rapid cycle improvement in health care" (Varkey, Reller, & Resar, p. 736). Components or activities associated with the PDSA framework are also noted features of quality improvement efforts in educational settings. Dolmans, Wolfhagen, and Scherpbier (2003) remark that

Table 2. Classification of distance education activities

Classification	Activities and Methods
Interaction	Focus on methods of communication, including email, audio and video conferencing, synchronous social networking (e.g., chat, instant messaging)
Introspection	Instructional activities involving simulations, lab exercises, group projects, demonstrations and reflective writings
Innovation	Activities focusing on two or more learning styles (e.g., visual, auditory, tactile)
Integration	Includes activities such as role playing, case studies and other skill-building techniques
Information	Activities such as tests or comprehension checks to determine whether and the extent to which knowledge or skills were transferred

Note. Olcott, 1999, as cited in Williams, 2006, pp. 129 - 130

conducting measurements, making judgments, and developing priorities for improvements are essential steps to improve quality in education. Price (2005) also notes that the PDSA method has direct linkages with the development and implementation of healthcare-related education.

Smothers, Greene, Ellaway, and Detmer (2008) observe that "the continuum of healthcare education is fragmented, consisting of disconnected organizations with various goals ranging from education to assessment and regulation" (p. 151). The systems approach to healthcare delivery has also been recognized as a critical way to structure educational interventions for healthcare education. For example, the Accreditation Council on Graduate Medical Education (ACGME) and the American Board of Medical Specialties (ABMS) have aligned critical competencies around a systems approach (Price, 2005). The competencies identified as systems-related components by the ACGME and ABMS include the following:

- Understanding how care practices affect other professionals, the organization, and the larger society
- Understanding how differences in delivery systems influence costs and allocation of resources
- The provision of quality, cost-effective care
- Advocating for patient care quality
- Partnering with managers in the assessment, coordination, and improvement of performance (Price, 2005, p. 260)

The ACGME and ABMS consider the use of technology as one feature of the competency based framework described above (Price, 2005). Another framework with close ties to Donabedian's SPO framework is the quality and outcomes framework (QOF), which has been used as a framework in the evaluation of medical training practice in the UK (Swanwick, Ahluwalia, Rennison, & Talbot, 2007). Although this particular framework at this point does not specifically evaluate the physical resources associated with training, the framework does focus on the information-related aspects of clinical care that are inherent in many e-health applications.

The inclusion of information technology as a relevant competency with a broad framework in healthcare education is not unusual, but, like the problem with the lack of consensus with quality in healthcare settings, the pursuit of quality in healthcare education is influenced to a large extent by the view of quality taken by interested stakeholders. Accrediting bodies of technical programs, like the US Committee on Accreditation for Respiratory Care (CoARC), the US Commission on Accreditation of Allied Health Education (CAAHEP), the US Accreditation Council for Occupational Therapy Education (ACOTE), and others have developed their own set of standards to evaluate the quality of health science programs. Although focus on programmatic outcomes is a critical component of quality evaluation, the extent to which students in the health professions are competent to practice in the field is certainly an overriding consideration.

Use of simulation technology, which would fall into Quadrant I in Figure 3, also has natural linkage with e-health. For instance, students in the field of health information technology have access to a wide range of technologies that are physical, electronic, or virtual simulations of the technologies used in healthcare settings. Use of these technologies in educational settings provides students with the opportunity to engage in learning and skills-building activities in an environment that prepares for actual use of the technologies in healthcare settings. One of the key benefits to use of such technologies is the fact that providers and technicians are learning in environments that pose no risk to patient care. However, the use of high-technology applications in simulation is not well-developed in educational settings. Wachter (2004) suggests that the extent to which use of these applications is developed may depend upon the degree to which the utilizations of these technologies (simulation) results in changes in practice.

DIFFUSION, INTEGRATION AND BARRIERS

Whether in healthcare settings or in settings designed to provide education to healthcare providers, the potential of e-health to serve as a strategic enabler will not be realized if the technologies and processes associated with e-health are not adopted by the respective systems. Achieving improvements in quality-related outcomes can only occur if the applications, technologies, and systems are diffused. From a sociological perspective, the process of diffusion contains the following elements:

1. Acceptance
2. Time for adoption
3. Item identification
4. Adopting entities
5. Specific communication channels
6. Social structure
7. System of values (Katz, Levin, & Hamilton, 1963).

Knowledge of diffusion frameworks can assist in identifying methods and considerations associated with the integration of e-health applications in healthcare settings. These frameworks can also be helpful for understanding the diffusion of knowledge from a healthcare education perspective. Rogers' theoretical framework of diffusion has been frequently cited as a means of understanding innovations in healthcare (Fitzgerald, Ferlie, & Hawkins, 2003; Godin, 1997; Smothers, Greene, Ellaway, & Detmer, 2008) and educational settings (Frank, Zhao, & Borman, 2004). As defined by Rogers (Rogers, 1995 as cited in Frank, Zhao & Borman, 2004), the concept of diffusion refers to "the process by which an innovation is communicated through certain channels over time among members of a social system" (p. 150).

Integration

E-health integration into healthcare systems requires careful consideration and planning. Sternberg (2002) asserts there are seven steps to success with e-health assimilation into a healthcare delivery system. These include (a) strategy development, (b) creation of usable content, (c) thinking about design, (d) selection of the right technology, (e) proper implementation, (f) increase in marketing and (g) integration. However, prior to initiating the Sternberg's proposed steps, the organization must develop a clear vision for what the technology is going to be used for in the organization's future plan and how the effects of the technology will be measured. Strategic development must consider e-health as a multipurpose tool that will assist the organization to achieve the overall future plan to enhance and sustain the organization as it competes for consumers in the online market.

Generally speaking, the change process includes development, implementation, and an ongoing continuous quality improvement/evaluation process. Change requires developing a plan for inclusion of workers through appropriate training and employee investment. Organizational leadership must invest the time and energy into e-health education for employees and consumers. Kee and Newcomer (2008) outline organizational responsibility in successful change processing as four critical elements, diagnosing change risk and organizational capacity, strategizing and making the case for change, implementing and sustaining change, and reinforcing change by creating a change-centric, learning organization.

Given that e-health represents a fundamental change in the ways in which healthcare is delivered, organization design can inform aspects of the change process. Education is a critical step in the organization design process. The organization design process is one that "provides a systematic, conceptual, and process framework that allows a company to effect a paradigm shift" (Jewell & Jewell, 1992, p. 222). The critical steps for effecting change include:

1. Establishment of direction and commitment
2. Assessment
3. Planning
4. Education
5. Development of changes
6. Implementation of changes
7. Ensuring continuous change (p.222).

The first step in the change process is perhaps the most critical and relevant to a larger goal of system-wide adoption of e-health. The goal of e-health adoption in healthcare organizations, or for that matter the adoption of innovative methods for the instruction of e-health, requires sponsorship, commitment, and top-down support in order to reach the established goal. Jewell and Jewell (1992) specifically link the first step in the process to elements of the organization's strategy (e.g., mission, vision, philosophy) and emphasize that leadership and management have an essential and crucial role in ensuring that the planned change can be adopted as envisioned. Change management principles are just as important in the development and implementation of educational interventions for healthcare. Students of in the fields of allied health and nursing are expected to have the ability to adapt to change, whether change is measured in terms of resources, professional role, or knowledge development in the field of study (Huebler, 1994 & Selker, 1995, as cited in Harris, Adamson, & Hunt, 1998).

Creation of technological standards has been cited as one of the critical steps toward integration (Institute of Medicine, 2001). Clearly, the ability of healthcare organizations to share data will depend upon the ability of the organizations to use common data elements and systems that can efficiently transmit data between and within organizations. Mearian (2009, p. 14) identified use of "evidence-based order systems" as another important way of standardizing patient treatment. Interestingly, the standardization has similar analogues in terms of healthcare education. Smothers, Greene, Ellaway and Detmer (2008) note that "through standards implementation, educators can collaborate across institutions, address the growing need for greater access to a shared knowledge base, better track learning outcomes, and integrate education into practice" (p. 150). Like the need for interoperability in healthcare, interoperability in healthcare education is also paramount in order to improve or achieve educational outcomes.

The impact of social influence must also be considered in any effort to adopt and implement new technologies. Frank, Zhao and Borman's (2004) research on the influence of social capital and diffusion of innovations in education settings underscores the importance of social aspects of change. Using a multiple regression to analyze the influence of social and institutional factors on computer use, this research found that access to technical expertise as well as perceived social pressures were significant predictors of use. Although perceptions of the potential of technology are critical in implementation of innovations (Frank, Zhao & Borman), it is interesting to note that social interaction helps frame localized understanding of studies related to the effectiveness of innovations (Fitzgerald, Ferlie, & Hawkins, 2003).

From a quality perspective, it is critical that a sustained effort is in place to ensure that the a desired level of quality is achieved from the intervention or innovation. Dolmans, Wolfhagen, & Scherpbier (2003) state that the success of quality assurance depends upon the extent to which evaluation is systematic, carried out in a structured manner, and integrated into the organization's regular patterns of work.

Barriers

In spite of the idea that e-health applications have the potential to yield substantial benefits to in healthcare delivery, a number of barriers impede the growth and adoption of these applications. Four key barriers are tied to incentives, costs, organizational structures, and policies.

The presence and types of incentives facing an organization play a tremendous role in the decision-making process and choices made by organizations. One of the key barriers to development and implementation of e-health applications is the lack of "legal and financial incentives" (Diamond & Shirky, 2008, p. w384). Although incentives have led to the development and implementation of administrative systems, the lack of incentives has created a lag in development and implementation of clinical systems. The linkage between reimbursement policies also has the potential create a disincentive for development. Bates (2002) notes:

Perhaps the most difficult and problematic barrier to adoption of quality-related IT is that incentives for adopting such changes are lacking under the current reimbursement system...under fee-for-service reimbursement, there is no financial incentive for hospitals to reduce adverse event rates...under prospective or capitated reimbursement, justifying investment in technology that will result in longer-term benefit may be hard for capital-strapped organizations (p. 6).

In a summary of key activities and issues related to health information technology, the State Health Watch (2008) reports that funding is the most critical barrier to widespread adoption. Healthcare organizations and providers may simply lack the capital necessary to develop, purchase or implement costly e-health applications (Institute of Medicine, 2001). Although funding can refer to the direct costs associated with the purchase of technologies, other cost considerations include those associated the training and education of personnel to use these technologies and systems as well as the development of systems that meet prescribed technology standards (Anderson, 2007). The development of e-health applications that are compatible with currently used software and operating systems requires recognition that older systems, which have become widely institutionalized, must be replaced or upgraded. The costs associated with the replacement or upgrade can be substantial. Referring to what are known as legacy systems, the Institute of Medicine (2001) states that "there is no easy way to shift from such systems to state-of-the-art information systems based on an open client-server architecture, personal computer networks, and more flexible, nonproprietary protocols" (p. 174). Underscoring the costs associated with development of systems at localized levels, the costs of development at larger levels are substantial. Mearian (2009) reports estimates of $75 to $100 billion for implementation in the United States.

As previously noted, information technology has found support and incentives for growth in administrative aspects of healthcare (versus the lack of and competing incentives in clinical services), and a similar finding has occurred in educational settings. Privateer (1999) notes that "many colleges and universities have used information technology tools to improve existing administrative procedures but have not given equal effort to re-engineering the academic side of the house" (p. 64). Second, Privateer suggests that the use of academic technologies to improve outcomes in education is constrained because of the view that these technologies are viewed from a cost-benefit perspective, with little about the benefits that can be provided. For healthcare organizations facing constrained budgets and unproven evidence regarding the relationship between costs and quality, the decision to adopt can be easily framed in a cost-benefit perspective. Lacking evidence of quality and effectiveness, the allocation of scarce resources to costly technologies would be difficult to justify.

Whereas the current structuring of the healthcare system has created a lack of incentives to advance safety (Wachter, 2004), the incentives facing the individual stakeholders also influence the manner in which e-health solutions are adopted. Brandenburg and Binder (1992) note that "while use of such technology offers tremendous promise for improving human performance, it also threatens and disrupts traditional power structures and decision processes...implementation of emerging technology usually requires a change process that is extremely sensitive to all the stakeholders" (p. 666). Sensitivity to all stakeholders requires a recognition that healthcare organizations not only support diverse communities, but—also as a collective body—consists of a diverse and heterogenous grouping of organizations, firms, associations, individual providers, and other entities. From an interorganizational perspective, healthcare organizations differ on a number of important ways that would prevent adoption and implementation of e-health applications that could be broadly used to improve quality of care. Obviously these differences include those related to the information technology infrastructure, but also include other drivers of adoption such as resources, core strategies, leadership capabilities, and workforce characteristics. The Institute of Medicine (2001) notes that not only do workers vary in terms of knowledge and experience, but also in terms of "receptivity to learning or acquiring new skills" (p. 175). The same types of barriers presented by organizational heterogeneity in healthcare settings is also present in healthcare education. Smothers, Greene, Ellaway and Detmer (2008) observe that "the continuum of healthcare education is fragmented, consisting of disconnected organizations with various goals ranging from education to assessment and regulation" (p. 151). Frank, Zhao and Borman's (2004) study of the influence of social capital on diffusion of innovations in schools observed interorganizational heteterogeneity from a slightly different perspective. This research noted that "schools differed in the populations they served, their configurations, their architecture, their leadership, their institutional histories, and their relationships to their districts" (p. 158). This same type of interorganizational variation is also typical for discussions about healthcare organizations.

According to Anderson (2007), regulation of e-health data is now on the forefront of issues tackled by the healthcare industry, yet policy-related aspects of e-health adoption present considerable barriers to widespread adoption of e-health applications (Institute of Medicine, 2001; State Health Watch, 2008). The IOM reports that lack of policies relating to "privacy, security, and confidentiality" (p. 171) represents a significant barrier for adoption and implementation of health information technology. The development of effective policies, specifically those related to privacy, security, and standards, are essential to facilitate adoption and implementation of health information technology: Barriers exist when the policies are either non-existent, when the policies are not adopted, or when these are not enforced.

The potential benefits of e-health technologies and application can motivate providers and consumers into a hurried pace to find solutions to removing barriers. Overcoming these barriers for providers will require interventions through subsidies and performance incentives by payers and government; certification and standardization of vendor applications that permit clinical data exchange; removal of legal barriers through standardization and accreditation guidelines; and greater security of medical data to convince practitioners and patients of the value of electronic medical records (Anderson 2007, p. 5). The business or economic aspect generating revenues for providers provide incentives for research for more efficient and nondiscriminatory delivery of healthcare across all cultural, social, political, and economic barriers. Consumers need access and education to overcome the barriers to e-health accessibility. Educational programs sponsored by providers and government agencies must be initiated and maintained for underserved communities to bring consumers in these areas current with technological advances.

CONCLUSION

The concept of electronic healthcare delivery is a rapidly changing method of providing healthcare for the masses using Internet services. Establishment of direction and commitment to e-health is imperative and unavoidable for the health care community. The direction has been set by the more than 110 million consumers of e-health on the Internet today (Stahl & Spatz, 2003) and healthcare providers who have embraced the efficiency, consumer competency and speed that technology has brought to healthcare practice. Healthcare systems are rapidly developing new and innovative infrastructures to support electronic health delivery and consumption while carefully marrying e-health concepts to the traditional hardcopy methods of health services delivery. Vital to the development of e-health infrastructure is an implicit understanding of the relationships between e-health, quality, and the roles that education plays in the complex relationship between health outcomes and its complex set of inputs.

As the healthcare industry moves rapidly toward adopting e-health, overcoming barriers to e-health will necessary in order to achieve large-scale adoption of e-health applications. Efficient, accessible e-health service delivery is a common goal shared by healthcare organizations and consumers alike. This goal cannot be achieved without education for both providers and consumers. Healthcare professionals are increasingly recognizing the benefits of e-health for healthcare organizations, systems, and consumers in the financial and educational arenas. E-health holds unlimited possibilities waiting to unfold as new technologies are developed and instituted in the healthcare industry and as both providers and consumers are better educated to methods of access and use.

Ultimately the success of e-health—and educational efforts related to e-health--will depend upon the extent to which healthcare and academic outcomes are achieved and sustained.

REFERENCES

Anderson, J.G. (2007). Social, ethical, and legal barriers to e-health. *International Journal of Medical Information, 76* (5, 6), 480 – 483.

Austin, C. J., & Boxerman, S. B. (1998). *Information systems for health services administration* (5th ed.). Chicago, IL: Health Administration Press.

Bates, D. W. (2002). The quality case for information technology in healthcare. *Medical Informatics and Decision Making, 2*(7), Retrieved May 2, 2009, from http://www.pubmedcentral.nih.gov/articlerender.fcgi?artid=137695

Bernstein, M., McCreless, T., & Côté, M. (2007, Winter). 2007). Five constants of information technology adoption in healthcare. [from Academic Search Complete database]. *Hospital Topics, 85*(1), 17–25. Retrieved May 3, 2009. doi:10.3200/HTPS.85.1.17-26

Bodie, G.D., & Dutta, M. J. (2008). Understanding health literacy for strategic health marketing; eHealth disparities, and the digital divide. *Health Marketing Quarterly, 25*(1/2), p175-203, 29p. Retrieved August 23, 2009 from Academic Search complete.

Brandenburg, D. C., & Binder, C. (1992). Emerging trends in human performance interventions . In Stolovitch, H. D., & Keeps, E. J. (Eds.), *Handbook of human performance technology: A comprehensive guide for analyzing and solving performance problems in organizations*. San Francisco, CA: Jossey-Bass Publishers.

Brown, J. F., & Marshall, B. L. (2008). Continuous quality improvement: An effective strategy of program outcomes in a higher education setting. *Nursing Education Perspectives*, *29*(4), 205–211.

Campbell, G.S., Sherry, D., Sternberg, D J. (2002). A hospital Web site that works. *Marketing Health Services, 22*(2), 40-2. Retrieved February 26, 2009, from ABI/INFORM Global database. (Document ID: 121772167).

Carruthers, A., & Jeacocke, D. (2000). Adjusting the balance in health-care quality. *Journal of Quality in Clinical Practice, 20*(4), 158-160. http://tiger.spc.alamo.edu:2052

Chaudhry, B., Jerome, W., Shinyi, W., Maglione, M., Mojica, W., & Roth, E. (2006). Systematic Review: Impact of Health Information Technology on Quality, Efficiency, and Costs of Medical Care. *Annals of Internal Medicine*, *144*(10), E12–W18. http://search.ebscohost.com.

Croft, D., & Peterson, M. (2002). An Evaluation of the Quality and Contents of Asthma Education on the World Wide Web. *CHEST, 121*(4), 1301. http://tiger.spc.alamo.edu:2052

Damberg, C., Ridgely, M., Shaw, R., Meili, R., Sorbero, M., Bradley, L., et al. (2009, April 15). Adopting Information Technology to Drive Improvements in Patient Safety: Lessons from the Agency for Healthcare Research and Quality Health Information Technology Grantees. *Health Services Research, 44*(2p2), 684-700. Retrieved September 30, 2009, doi:10.1111/j.1475-6773.2008.00928.x

Diamond, C., & Shirky, C. (2008). Health Information Technology: A Few Years Of Magical Thinking? *Health Affairs*, *27*(5), w383–w390. http://search.ebscohost.com, doi:10.1377/hlthaff.27.5.w383. doi:10.1377/hlthaff.27.5.w383

Dolmans, D.H.J.M., Wolfhagen, H.A.P., & Scherpbier, A.J.J.A (2003, July). From Quality Assurance to Total Quality Management: How Can Quality Assurance Result in Continuous Improvement in Health Professions Education?. *Education for Health: Change in Learning & Practice (Taylor & Francis Ltd), 16*(2), 210. Retrieved September 28, 2009, from Health Source: Nursing/Academic Edition database.

Donabedian, A. (2005, December). Evaluating the Quality of Medical Care. *The Milbank Quarterly*, *83*(4), 691–729. Retrieved August 30, 2009. .doi:10.1111/j.1468-0009.2005.00397.x

Ellaway, R., & Masters, K. (2008). AMEE Guide 32: e-Learning in medical education Part 1: Learning, teaching and assessment. *Medical Teacher*, *30*(5), 455–473. http://tiger.spc.alamo.edu:2052, doi:10.1080/01421590802108331. doi:10.1080/01421590802108331

Eysenbach, G. (2001). What is e-health? *Journal of Medical Internet Research*, 3(2). Retrieved March 4, 2009 from http://www.jmir.org/2001/2/e20/

Fitzgerald, L., Ferlie, E., & Hawkins, C. (2003). Innovation in healthcare: How does credible evidence influence professionals? *Health & Social Care in the Community*, *11*(3), 219–228. doi:10.1046/j.1365-2524.2003.00426.x

Flood, A. B., Zinn, J. S., Shortell, S. M., & Scott, W. R. (2000). Organizational performance: Managing for success . In Shortell, S. M., & Kaluzny, A. D. (Eds.), *Health care management: Organization design and behavior* (4th ed., pp. 356–389). Albany, NY: Delmar.

Ginter, P. M., Swayne, L. E., & Duncan, W. J. (1998). *Strategic management of health care organizations* (3rd ed.). Malden, MA: Blackwell Publishers, Inc.

Godin, B. (1997). The rhetoric of a health technology: The microprocessor patient card. *Social Studies of Science*, *27*(6), 865–902. doi:10.1177/030631297027006002

Grabinder, R. S., Jonassen, D., & Wilson, B. G. (1992). The use of expert systems . In Stolovitch, H. D., & Keeps, E. J. (Eds.), *Handbook of human performance technology: A comprehensive guide for analyzing and solving performance problems in organizations*. San Francisco, CA: Jossey-Bass Publishers.

Harris, L., Adamson, B., & Hunt, A. (1998). Assessing quality in higher education: Criteria for evaluating programmes for allied health. *Assessment & Evaluation in Higher Education, 23*(3), 273. http://tiger.spc.alamo.edu:2052

Harrison, J., & Lee, A. (2006, November). The role of e-health in the changing health care environment. [from Academic Search Complete database.]. *Nursing Economics*, *24*(6), 283–289. Retrieved May 2, 2009.

Institute of Medicine. (2001). *Crossing the quality chasm: A new health system for the 21st century*. Washington, DC: National Academies Press.

James, B. (2005, January 2). E-health: Steps on the road to interoperability. *Health Affairs*, *24*, 26–30. Retrieved March 4, 2009. doi:.doi:10.1377/hlthaff.W5.26

Jewell, S. F., & Jewell, D. O. (1992). Organization design . In Stolovitch, H. D., & Keeps, E. J. (Eds.), *Handbook of human performance technology: A comprehensive guide for analyzing and solving performance problems in organizations*. San Francisco, CA: Jossey-Bass Publishers.

Johnson, J. W. (1995). Health care and higher education: A chilling parallel. *EDUCOM Review*, *28*(5), 42–45.

Katz, E., Levin, M. L., & Hamilton, H. (1963). Traditions of research on the diffusion of innovations. *American Sociological Review*, *28*(2), 237–252. doi:10.2307/2090611

Kee, J. E., & Newcomer, K. E. (2008). Why do change efforts fail? [from ABI/INFORM Global database.]. *Public Management*, *37*(3), 5–12. Retrieved December 18, 2008.

Maheu, M. M., Whitten, P., Allen, A. (2001). *E-Health, Telehealth, and Telemedicine: A Guide to Start-up and Success: Jossey-Bass Health Series*. San Francisco. Retrieved June 15, 2009 from Academic Search complete.

Malec, B. T. (1998). Administrative applications . In Austin, C. J., & Boxerman, S. B. (Eds.), *S.B. (1998). Information systems for health services administration* (5th ed.). Chicago, IL: Health Administration Press.

Mearian, L. (2009). Cost of Obama E-health Plan Could Reach $100B. *Computerworld, 43*(5), 12-14. http://tiger.spc.alamo.edu:2052

Muramoto, M., Campbell, J., & Salazar, Z. (2003). Provider Training and Education in Disease Management: Current and Innovative Technology. *Disease Management & Health Outcomes*, McLeod, S., & Barbara, A. (2005). Online technology in rural health: Supporting students to overcome the tyranny of distance. *Australian Journal of Rural Health, 13*(5), 276-281. http://tiger.spc.alamo.edu:2052

Price, D. (2005, May). Continuing medical education, quality improvement, and organizational change: implications of recent theories for twenty-first-century CME. *Medical Teacher*, *27*(3), 259–268. doi:10.1080/01421590500046270

Privateer, P. M. (1999). Academic technology and the future of higher education: Strategic paths taken and not taken. *The Journal of Higher Education*, *70*(1), 60–79. doi:10.2307/2649118

Sheppard, L., & Mackintosh, S. (1998). Technology in education: What is appropriate for rural and remote allied health professionals? *The Australian Journal of Rural Health*, *6*(4), 189–193. doi:10.1111/j.1440-1584.1998.tb00311.x

Smothers, V., Greene, P., Ellaway, R., & Detmer, D. (2008, March). Sharing innovation: the case for technology standards in health professions education. *Medical Teacher*, *30*(2), 150–154. doi:10.1080/01421590701874082

Stahl, L., & Spatz, M. (2003, January). Quality Assurance in eHealth for Consumers. [from Health Source: Nursing/Academic Edition database.]. *Journal of Consumer Health on the Internet*, *7*(1), 33. Retrieved September 27, 2009. doi:10.1300/J381v07n01_03

Stephenson, K., Peloquin, S., Richmond, S., Hinman, M., & Christiansen, C. (2002). Changing Educational Paradigms to Prepare Allied Health Professionals for the 21st Century. *Education for Health: Change in Learning & Practice (Taylor & Francis Ltd)*, *15*(1), 37-49.

Sternberg, D. J. (2002). Seven steps to e-health success. [from ABI/INFORM Global.]. *Marketing Health Services*, *22*(2), 44–47. Retrieved August 23, 2009.

Survey of states finds boom in e-health strategies. (2008, July). *State Health Watch*. Retrieved March 4, 2009, from Academic Search Complete database.

Swanwick, T., Ahluwalia, S., Rennison, T., & Talbot, T. (2007). The Quality and Outcomes Framework (QOF) and the assessment of training practices as learning organisations. *Education for Primary Care*, *18*(2), 173–179.

Varkey, P., Reller, K., & Resar, R. (2007, June). Basics of Quality Improvement in Health Care. [from Academic Search Complete database.]. *Mayo Clinic Proceedings*, *82*(6), 735–739. Retrieved September 30, 2009. doi:10.4065/82.6.735

Wachter, R. (2004). The End Of The Beginning: Patient Safety Five Years After 'To Err Is Human'. *Health Affairs*, 23534–23545.

Williams, S. (2006). The Effectiveness of Distance Education in Allied Health Science Programs: A Meta-Analysis of Outcomes. *American Journal of Distance Education*, *20*(3), 127–141. doi:10.1207/s15389286ajde2003_2

Wong, H. J., Legnini, M. W., & Whitmore, H. H. (2000). The diffusion of decision support systems in healthcare: Are we there yet? *Journal of Healthcare Management*, *45*(4), 240–253.

Chapter 14
Gastrointestinal Motility Online Educational Endeavor

Shiu-chung Au
Tufts Medical Center, USA

Amar Gupta
University of Arizona, USA

ABSTRACT

Medical information has been traditionally maintained in books, journals, and specialty periodicals. Now, a growing number of people, including patients and caregivers, turn to a variety of sources on the Internet, most of which are run by commercial entities, to retrieve healthcare-related information. The next area of growth will be sites that focus on specific fields of medicine, featuring high quality data culled from scholarly publications, operated by eminent domain specialists. One such site is being developed for the field of Gastrointestinal Motility; it further augments the innovations of existing healthcare information sites with the intention of serving the diverse needs of lay people, medical students, and experts in the field. The site, called Gastrointestinal Motility Online, leverages the strengths of online textbooks, which have a high degree of organization, in conjunction with the strengths of online journal collections, which are more comprehensive and focused, to produce a knowledge base that can be easily updated, but still provides authoritative and high quality information to users. In addition to implementing existing Web technologies such as Wiki- and Amazon-style commenting options, Gastrointestinal Motility Online uses automatic methods to assemble information from various heterogeneous data sources to create a coherent, cogent, and current knowledge base serving a diverse base of users.

INTRODUCTION

For the last several decades, Harrison's Principles of Internal Medicine, published by McGraw Hill, has served as a major source of information in the field of Gastrointestinal Motility. This book and its online presentation have been, and continue to be, used by many medical colleges to train the next generation of medical doctors; practitioners in this field also frequently refer to them.

Traditionally, papers and articles in specialty medical journals supplemented the material in

DOI: 10.4018/978-1-61692-843-8.ch014

textbooks like Harrison. The latter book would itself be updated periodically to reflect the state of the art in medicine and the various specialties, providing a consensus opinion of the standard of care.

The advent of computers and Internet has given rise to online sources of information such as UpToDate (http://www.uptodate.com/) and WebMD (http://www.webmd.com/). While gaining tremendous following and being updated frequently, these sources of online information relate to the medical field as a whole and not to particular specialties. Furthermore, the information on these sites is generally maintained by personnel of the respective organizations, not by specialists in specific disciplines of medical science. These organizations are usually set up as commercial entities, rather than non-profit ones.

The progressive transformation of information has seen many journals that were previously in paper format opting to use new electronic technologies; most of them now come out both in paper and electronic formats. Searchable electronic archives, such as PubMed (http://www.pubmedcentral.nih.gov/), now place a plethora of information into the hands of researchers and physicians. However, such searches are very time consuming and often produce irrelevant or poorly supported articles. Sites like Harrison's Online (http://www.accessmedicine.com/) serve as information directories that can be searched, hoping to place most suitable information on a medical topic in a user's hand. Students have gradually come to expect information in quick and readily available forms without having to bother about inter-library loans or even hardcopy versions at all.

The goal of the endeavor described in this article was to adapt emerging technologies to improve methods of teaching gastrointestinal material to students and to serve as a more effective source of relevant and accurate information for medical practitioners and specialists.

Evidence-Based Medicine

A study from the School of Information Management and Systems at UC Berkeley estimates that, in 2003, the World Wide Web contained about 170 terabytes of information on its surface alone, equivalent to seventeen times the size of the information in the Library of Congress (Lyman & Varian, 2003). With this increasingly information-rich society, the most precious ability for students and learners is no longer to find the information, but to discern the most relevant pieces of information and to integrate them into practice. The American Library Association describes "information literacy" as the ability of individuals to "recognize when information is needed and have the ability to locate, evaluate, and use effectively the needed information" (American Library Association, 1989).

The medical domain version of information literacy is evidence-based medicine.

Evidence-based medicine (EBM) is the integration of best research evidence with clinical expertise and patient values (Guyatt et al., 1992). The Centre For Evidence-Based Medicine in Toronto, Canada, states that the origins of evidence-based medicine date back to post-revolution Paris (CEBM, 2007), but that the current growth is most closely attributed to the work of a group lead by Gordon Guyatt at McMaster University in Canada in 1992. EBM publications, reflecting interest in this field, have grown from a lone publication in 1992 to thousands in 2007.

Studies have become increasingly critical of the value of textbook sources (Antman et al., 1992). Didactic continuing medical information may be ineffective at changing physician performance (Davis et al., 1997), and clinical journals may lack practical application (Haynes, 1993). In addition, physicians are faced with an increasing burden on their time, forced to diagnose patient findings within a matter of minutes (Sackett & Straus, 1998), and can only afford to set aside half an hour or less per week for general medical reading (Sackett, 1997). The staggering mass of information being discovered is also daunting: 500,000 articles are added to the commonly used Medline medical journal database every year, and "if a physician read 2 articles each day, every day for a year, (s)he would still find herself or himself 648 years behind" (Lindberg, 2003). As research increases the quantity of information available, medical practitioners are compelled to find efficient methods to educate themselves.

The Centre for Evidence Based Medicine has cited several examples of strategic, educational, and technical improvements in medicine that have enabled the current explosion in interest in this field. These include the emergence of new strategies for evaluating information; the creation of systematic reviews; the growing emphasis on continuing medical education and lifetime learning; and the advent of online journals, meta analysis of multiple studies, and ready access to such resources through electronic archives. Rapid dissemination of accurate and comprehensive compilations of research results enables medical practitioners to make informed decisions that are supported by the latest research results, and not by outdated trials.

In light of the increasing number of medical journals, and especially specialties, the sheer quantity of information threatens to overwhelm medical practitioners. The concept of information mastery has been coined to describe the set of skills that physicians must nurture in approaching, analyzing and incorporating or rejecting new information. The issues mentioned above are not limited to the medical arena alone: Former Vice-President Al Gore described the state of information management as "resembling the worst aspects of our agricultural policy, which left grain rotting in thousands of storage files while people were starving" (Gore, 1992).

The Center for Information Mastery at the University of Virginia asserts that the usefulness of medical information is dependent upon its relevance, validity, and the work required to obtain it, as specified in Equation 1 (Slawson et al., 2007).

$$\text{Usefulness of Medical Information} = \frac{(\text{Relevance})(\text{Validity})}{\text{Work}}$$

Equation 1: Usefulness (Slawson et al., 2007)

Further, the increasing quantity of research being performed by commercial enterprises, as well as other organizations with potential conflicts of interest, requires information be filtered for validity before incorporation into medical canon. Finally, increased effort involved in accessing the relevant pieces of information reduces the accessibility of such information. In addition, healthcare organizations are siloed, gaining the advantage of sub-optimizing local departments, possibly at the cost of the whole (Senge, 1980); this complicates the problem further.

Information Retrieval and Decision-Making

As Stephen Hawking observes in *The Universe in a Nutshell*, the rate of growth of new knowledge is exponential. While 9,000 articles were published annually in 1900 and around 90,000 in 1950, there were 900,000 scientific articles published per annum in 2000 (Hawking, 2001). The explosive growth of information is challenging both the information repositories designed to hold it, and the ability of users to access relevant information.

At the time of this writing, Wikipedia serves as the de-facto standard for online general encyclopedias, and is among the top ten most-visited Web sites (Alexa Internet, 2007a). Its open-source, volunteer-without-accountability approach led to initial concerns about information validity, but these concerns have been largely addressed. Nature magazine studied Wikipedia and Encyclopedia Brittanica and found that the two of them were largely similar in accuracy (Giles, 2005). The growth of Wikipedia's information base further enhances the quality and breadth of coverage, and supports the possible future use of Wikipedia or Wiki-style architecture as an academically respectable source of reference.

In contrast to the indexed and contributed semi-structured format of Wikipedia, Google relies on search-keyword phrases. The usefulness of Internet-crawling indexers, like Google, is based upon the ability to retrieve and capture information from many sites, and to retrieve relevant pages on query. Google's initial strength and rise to stardom was achieved through its superior PageRank algorithm, which still remains a carefully guarded trade secret; this algorithm provides an uncannily relevant list of matches to any user query, ranging from commonplace query phrases to obscure esoteric trivia and even misspellings.

In a small supermarket today, shoppers are bombarded with a selection of 285 varieties of cookies and 95 varieties of chips, leading the consumer to a state of decision overload (Schwartz, 2004). There is a growing need to restructure data to meet the informational and management requirements of an organization or group of people (Carlson, 2003).

Medical Information Repositories

For the medical arena, PubMed is the most widely used information database in the world, accounting for 1.3 million daily queries by 220,000 unique users (Lindberg, 2003). It is a free access search engine, provided by the U.S. National Library of Medicine as the main access point to the Medline database, a cataloged repository of medical literature classified using the descriptors known as Medical Subject Headings (MeSH). A broad range of search features are offered, including combined searches, exclusions, classification by type of article (original research versus review) and related articles. Another feature of the Medline database, known as MedlinePLUS, provides generalized information on health topics, and is aimed at the public or at practitioners outside their specialty domain. At the current time, PubMed serves as the gold standard in comprehensive medical information, despite its dated interface.

HighWire Press, a Stanford-originated endeavor, distributes thousands of journals, and provides its own search engine. In a recent study, the relevance of articles retrieved from HighWire was found to be greater than that of PubMed, but with the disadvantage of a slower retrieval Speed (Vanhecke et al., 2006).

In order to make a comparative evaluation between different approaches, it is appropriate to characterize the information recall ability using three parameters: precision, recall, and fall-out.

Precision (Equation 2) can be defined as the proportion of all retrieved documents that are relevant.

$$\text{precision} = \frac{|\{\text{relevant documents}\} \cap \{\text{retrieved documents}\}|}{|\{\text{retrieved documents}\}|}$$

Equation 2: Precision (Wikipedia, 2007)

Recall (Equation 3) captures the concept of complete retrieval of all relevant documents.

$$\text{recall} = \frac{|\{\text{relevant documents}\} \cap \{\text{retrieved documents}\}|}{|\{\text{relevant documents}\}|}$$

Equation 3: Recall (Wikipedia, 2007)

Fall-out (Equation 4) is a measure of the number of documents that are retrieved but are unrelated to the issue being searched.

$$\text{fall-out} = \frac{|\{\text{non-relevant documents}\} \cap \{\text{retrieved documents}\}|}{|\{\text{non-relevant documents}\}|}$$

Equation 4: Fall-out (Wikipedia, 2007)

Medical research, while generally emphasizing maximal precision and minimal fall-out, occasionally requires increased recall, in the case of obscure diseases, or unusual side effects of medications. Medline serves as a canonical list for such purposes, but at the cost of significantly lower precision.

Medical practitioners using Google for their searches will often find themselves frustrated at the large quantity of articles on obscure and irrelevant topics. A researcher searching for a pharmacologic treatment of a syndrome will turn up with thousands of articles dealing with various sub-types, biochemical-signaling processes involved, and even support groups, before finding a therapeutic treatment. Due to the nature of the search engine and the storage methods, there are concerns about Google's or any search engine's ability to maintain a collection of such information. Carlson (2003) showed that due to the relatively small collection of documents indexed by an average search engine, a significant amount of relevant information would not be returned even in the presence of a perfectly formulated search phrase.

In order to accommodate domain-specific areas, Google has introduced the concept of "Refine Your Search" (http://www.google.com/coop). Without altering its main core search methodology, Google allows users to more quickly locate the type of information desired (i.e., treatment or symptoms). These refinement tools, provided by vendors and other private individuals or agencies that are deemed authoritative, subsequently label Web sites with appropriate descriptor tags. The potential conflict of interest created by these corporate associations is a matter of concern, due to omissions or maliciousness of the labeling.

The range of challenges and issues that characterize the medical domain include:

- The presence of an extensive array of synonyms for various drugs and diseases that require semantic knowledge to be encoded into the search engine in order to link concepts that are not lexically related
- The naming of disease subtypes (often after a major contributor or discoverer), requires that hierarchies be constructed to allow users looking for the subclasses of disease to find information on the main umbrella disease, and vice versa.
- The growth in the understanding of generalized syndromes results in a corresponding need reclassification based on new etiologies of disease, thereby suggesting a dynamic organizational structure for the online medical information systems.

In view of the growing difficulty in locating desired pieces of information, individuals performing research are in increasing danger of information overload. As such, the next generation of medical information access tools must aim to improve the ability to retrieve the right chunks of information quickly, with zero or minimal extraneous information; this concept is termed as increasing the signal to noise ratio in the field of electrical engineering.

VISION AND GOALS FOR GASTROINTESTINAL MOTILITY ONLINE

Gastrointestinal (GI) Motility Online is an example of a medical information system that seeks to provide access to high quality medical information online related to a particular medical specialty, by centralizing the information and presenting relevant information that is customized to the user's information requirements.

The field of Gastrointestinal Motility is complex and interdisciplinary, involving a variety of experts. The possible user base includes laypersons, patients, medical students, biomedical scientists, physiologists, pathologists, pharmacologists, biomedical students, researchers, pharmaceutical staff, house staff, specialty fellows, internists, surgeons, and gastroenterologists. Each role requires a different approach to depth, scholastic relevance, and clinical direction in terms of information presentation. For example, students are interested in innovative research or review papers; researchers would like to know the most recent developments, and practitioners might be more interested in using the information for differential diagnosis purposes. GI Motility aims to serve as a collaboration of medical professionals, approaching diseases and patients from different angles.

In a library, a user interacts with the data in books very differently from the way that she or he interacts with data in an online presentation. The user expects the book to be focused and to address the topic in a linear fashion. Online, the same user navigates quickly, using hyperlinks, to explore secondary topics. In fact, the user *expects* a different presentation and a different style of information; as a result, the nature of the interactions will differ even with the same content. One of the aims of Gastrointestinal Motility Online is to address these different styles and to present the desired subset of information in the manner that the user might expect. For example, a user might be interested in viewing articles from the perspective of case-based, symptom-based, or test result-based diagnosis in order to apply the information to a particular problem at hand. In essence, the vision of Gastrointestinal Motility Online is to present information as framed by the interaction with the particular user at the particular point in time.

The first step in the vision of Gastrointestinal Motility Online was to collect the information in a manner that will be consistent with the goal to acquire the reputation for the highest quality of knowledge. The information base is assembled entirely from material provided by internationally acknowledged experts. All chapters including synopses, articles, and reviews are written by reputed authorities. The pool of information is envisaged to be shared between different types of users and for different purposes. The design of the system emphasizes a one-stop information approach that enables the users to derive information at various depths. This applies to onsite information, as well as to information at offsite locations.

Details of Effort: A two-phase approach is being utilized for the creation of the information system: the first involves full leveraging of commercial technology as it exists today, and the second involves further research on aspects that can be incorporated in future versions of our system. In the absence of a better term, the term gastrointestinal knowledge repository is used for the final system, as well as for the initial concept-demonstration prototype system.

For the first phase, the acquisition of knowledge proceeded with the establishment of titles and themes for chapters, as determined through discussions involving the concerned authors and the editors for this project (Dr. Goyal and Dr. Shaker). The creation of the gastrointestinal motility knowledge repository began with calls to key gastrointestinal experts inviting them to submit a chapter, in electronic form, for inclusion in this knowledge repository. The inputs from the contributing authors were reviewed by these two editors and by others, on an anonymous peer review basis. Under the aegis of an unrestricted grant from Novartis Corporation, the two editors worked closely with the staff of Nature Publishing Group on a number of tasks that ultimately led to the creation of the following Web site: http://gimotilityonline.com.

The creation of the site involved an automated conversion process to adapt MS-Word and rich text documents into a Web presentable format, with special emphasis placed on images, tables, and video. The majority of the investment for development lay in formatting and typesetting; the design itself was of less concern as it followed existing Web branding and style guidelines of Nature Publishing Group. Rights for images needed to be obtained; images, tables and video needed to be edited to fit a standard look and feel. After receiving author contributions, the project required approximately 18-24 months to complete, with 9-12 months required for the editorial process itself. The current site consists of 1,000 HTML pages, 1,000 images, 500 Powerpoint presentations and 40 videos. Articles are cross-linked by topics, and the current volume is equivalent of about 700 pages of text. This volume is increasing as this endeavor continues to progress.

Site Purpose

The ostensible purpose of the site is to disseminate information on the specialty of gastrointestinal medicine, primarily to gastrointestinal medical practitioners and to other interested parties. The ambition for the site is for it to become the central hub of information on this specialty, aggregating information from many sources, authors, and journals into one central location with the objective of becoming a de facto standard for online gastrointestinal information.

A secondary role is the development of a community of gastrointestinal specialists and other interested parties, who can form an online collaborative, expand upon the information repository, and facilitate peer communications and discussions. In addition, the site aims to explore and to expand the concept of online information repositories, especially the optimal integration of current generation of electronic journals and online textbooks.

Site Audience

The primary site audience is the set of gastrointestinal specialists, associated medical staff, and staff under training. Members of this primary user base would initially visit the site because of a recommendation from a colleague or because another site (search or advertisement) directed the user to it. Occasional patients are expected, but are unlikely to become the primary users of this site.

Initially, the core attractions for users to this site are the quality and depth of information coupled with the ease of access and the low cost; these same factors will also help to retain the user base. Since most physicians and healthcare specialists spend relatively little time online (six hours per week on average), the signal to noise ratio of the site and the ease of locating a desired piece of information (through the information architecture) must be both very high to impress the user base (Fridman, 2000). The primary user of the site is unlikely to demand high interactivity; instead, the interest will be on locating and extracting the information as quickly as possible. As such, the site must be efficiently organized, streamlined, and equipped with powerful search and index functions.

After drawing a user initially, repeat visitors would use the site to browse new topics of interest, as well as to entrust the editorial staff to select articles that represent innovative research in the relevant field. An interacting community base would evolve over time and eventually cause a change in the workflow. Specialists would then visit the site to explore the comments from their colleagues on the topics expressed and to leave their own authoritative inputs on different articles, eventually contributing entire articles as much as a good electronic journal aspires to do today.

While being relatively low in terms of being technically savvy, a typical user of Gastrointestinal Motility is likely to be very comfortable with using the Internet for retrieval of scholarly information through PubMed, online textbooks, and ready references such as UpToDate. A sleek, uncluttered design is likely to be the most attractive, even though it may not support applications involving high load times, such as Flash or embedded videos. Users are comfortable reading large articles online, but they also expect printable versions to be available, on an as-needed basis.

The user base, while highly intelligent, is relatively small in numeric terms, and is characterized by a small presence on the Web. The process of attracting a critical mass to build and to maintain a user community is a high priority task; this involves contacting a high percentage of all members of this specialist community.

Site Content

Gastrointestinal Motility Online is a site that provides information on both medical practice and the fundamentals of the gastrointestinal tract. The information must provide both breadth and depth on the topic, and should ultimately serve as an encyclopedia of the domain-specific knowledge.

Information Architecture: As in a library, information must be properly accessible in order to have value. The architecture of the information is partly determined by the methods that the users will use to query the evolving knowledge base. In a library, the name of the author and the title of the book are important. In a journal, the age of the article or the issue in which it was published may be essential. In Gastrointestinal Motility Online, the most likely user scenarios involve searching for information by anatomical section or syndrome. The timing is also important; recent material is favored over older material. Since relevance of the article is also important, the name of the journal and the name of the author are also used prominently in searches.

Furthermore, classification schemes or hierarchies to group-related topics are essential to narrow the branching process used by the search technique. The determination of related information is a complex topic. In order to address the latter issue, medical organizations are creating medical ontologies, such as unified medical language system (UMLS), to quantify and to impose structure on conceptual relationships. With this classification, the selection criteria can be hierarchically built up or finely specified to obtain desired results. A lengthier discussion of this topic appears later in this article.

Look and Feel: The look and feel of the site needs to convey the sense of scholarly authority, but with a sleek technological approach. Medical personnel have high standards concerning the accuracy of articles, and a professional presentation aids in supporting this perception. A site that is gaudy or shows too many bells and whistles, or involves a long load time, reflects poorly on the content, as do garish colors or lack of color.

Images and video must be consistent and should be available to download as needed for reference and for closer examination. The level of interactivity available should be low, as most gastrointestinal specialists have small online presence. Natural language queries, such as those used with AskJeeves (http://www.ask.com/), are unnecessary, as long as the search and browse features are precise and efficient. Pages may be presented as either textbook or journal articles, based on the preference of the user.

Extracting Content, Metadata, and Cross Referencing: One of the most powerful functions of the Internet is the ability for Web users to span several related articles quickly because of cross-referenced links. A user interested in the preparation of a particular chicken recipe can quickly reference how to sauté and with what form of pan, moving quickly to sources to buy the appropriate cast-iron skillet or wok to benefits and comparisons of different brands and retailers. A Wiki of only gastrointestinal specialists, with limited control from an editor, would be appropriate for the collection and dissemination of information; Gastrointestinal Motility Online is striving towards that goal.

A particularly useful feature in Gastrointestinal Motility Online, not available in online journals, is its cross-referencing tool. Articles that are closely related or broach a topic in greater depth can be quickly accessed by a cross reference within the Gastrointestinal Motility Online domain. These links are established by content extraction tools that create metadata and relate that data between different documents. Footnotes are available at the bottom and allow for a broader topical search; however, the inline linking of articles is particularly appealing for tracking particular items or syndromes of interest.

Search Capabilities

Search features are incorporated in Gastrointestinal Motility Online, but are considered secondary to the organization of the information. A dynamic keyword search for anatomical sections of the gastrointestinal tract is less likely to reveal useful information on general function than a manual perusal of the literature through the prepared subject browse option. The efficient organization of the information, based on the anticipated needs and access patterns of users, is an essential feature for building a knowledge repository. By acknowledging that specialists would be more likely to query by anatomy or syndrome, one needs mechanisms for structured order, as compared to mechanisms that order by article size, author name, or recent usage. An additional feature, incorporated within the community-building module, is a user rating system that allows users to rank the importance of articles so that users browsing information can be directed to the most useful and informative articles.

One difficulty with searches is the likelihood that a particular phrase will appear in nearly all documents unless the search is very specific. In cases where the gastrointestinal tract is analyzed as an interactive system, the phrases for anatomical locations may occur multiple times as reference points, but the central theme of the article may not be easy to determine by word frequency. As a result, a number of semantic tools, described later in this article, are used to analyze articles and to classify them appropriately.

Experts of the Nature Publishing Group (NPG), who possess prior experience in online information presentation, based on the online version of Nature magazine, helped to develop the initial vision of the online knowledge repository. The base site is hosted by Nature Publishing Group. While the site was being developed, commercial tools were available to handle both the production of electronic journals and static textbook efforts like AccessMedicine/Harrison's Online (http://www.accessmedicine.com/) and WebMD. However, the gastrointestinal knowledge repository falls somewhere in between these two cases; accordingly, few over-the-shelf tools and algorithms were available for immediate use. As such, a significant fraction of the interface and architecture had to be innovated and refined, through experimentation.

Many of the existing tools for creating electronic journals are geared towards collation of articles, graphics, and layout work. These tools reduce the time needed by the authors and editors for the processes of uploading, formatting, and editing. In the development of Gastrointestinal Motility Online, the use of a software suite facilitated handling of images and consistency of look and feel. One area where tools are lacking is the ability to organize information into a coherent topical fashion, as in a textbook. Searching on a keyword is especially difficult on a physician specialty site, where the dialect is limited and the concepts are reused multiple times. As such, editorial staff must impose additional control to prevent the site from becoming a write-only knowledge repository.

Collections of electronic journals, such as Ovid (http://www.ovid.com/site/index.jsp), have been primarily targeted for libraries and research centers. The primary purpose of Ovid is to serve as a warehouse of information, albeit uncategorized. Gastrointestinal Motility Online's current state differs from that of Ovid in terms of the presentation of the material: the former system is specifically formatted to provide an online view as well as a hardcopy output. The long-term goal of Gastrointestinal Motility Online is to collect a comprehensive knowledge on subjects (as Ovid does), as well as to add more intelligent search tools or information utilities. While Ovid does not organize information except into broad categories, Gastrointestinal Motility Online refines classifications, provides responses to search queries that are more accurate, and supports tools that use the knowledge in compelling ways, such as for differential diagnosis.

The advantages of sites built in a textbook style, such as AccessMedicine, is the hierarchical organization and ready access to information. The evolution of online textbooks has generated significant activity on the sites, as teaching tools. Gastrointestinal Motility Online uses over 40 illustrative videos, which are not typical of a journal, but fit the online textbook paradigm. Online textbooks are excellent repositories of information, except that updating the sites to incorporate new information is generally cumbersome because of the level of interactivity involved.

At a broader technological level, eBooks represent a technology that has been adapted to deliver information electronically. Medical eBooks can be argued to be a natural outgrowth of the eBook movement to electronic media: volume and space requirements are reduced, key phrase searching can be performed, and portability is enhanced. Nevertheless, few medical texts are adapted as eBooks.

Although eBooks have grown in popularity, they have not grown as rapidly as projected by consultants; this could be because of the following reasons:

1. Most readers see no need to replace print books.
2. Due to the limited screen size, limited battery life, and navigation interface issues with eBooks, many people still find paper books easier to handle.
3. Digital rights management causes compatibility and portability problems when attempting to move the eBook from desktop to PDA or laptop.
4. Current pricing of eBooks does not account for the reduced value relative to paper books. When readers finish reading a paper book, they can give it to a friend or sell it to a used bookstore; neither is possible with most eBooks.

-(Crawford, 2006)

Additionally, delivery of information may not be simply online, but online and to a mobile user using a PDA or other portable device. The constraints involved in transmitting and displaying information on a limited display panel create a new set of challenges. In most markets other than healthcare, the primary applications for PDAs are for scheduling and contact management (as a busy executive might use in lieu of a pen-and-paper daily planner), or as a portable browser or e-mail client (as in the case of technologists and engineers). In such cases, the application of the PDA works within the bounds of the limited display and the modern constraint of minimal bandwidth, often serving as a surrogate cell phone of sorts.

However, in medicine, the PDA is often stretched beyond its limits. The current trend is the delivery of detailed information pages into a portable format, downloadable to PDA. Since medical practitioners can no longer maintain a complete mental catalog of all drugs and particularly obscure clinical symptoms or diseases, PDAs assist physicians in their duties without requiring a quick trip to a computer terminal or a large paper binder archive. Harrisons and UpToDate have both moved rapidly in this area, and the list of available drug databases is already large. PDAs fill the role of drug lookup very well, as well as serve as a primer for obscure diseases. The difficulty lies with more graphically intense data that may not display properly, or may need to be downloaded on the fly. In such cases, medical information systems are pushing the technological limits of PDAs.

PDA sales as a whole, however, are in decline, except as a niche application. Analysts such as IDC and Gartner have predicted downtrend trend in sales of PDA. Dell has withdrawn its PDA line from production (Mechaca, 2007). In the long term, the PDA may carefully constrain its niche to feature more of the portable planner features and less multimedia and display power, rendering it less useful to medical practitioners. Until the advent of revolutionary new display technologies,

Table 1. The Online Endeavor "Gastrointestinal Motility Online" is a hybrid, adopting the best qualities of online textbooks, such as Harrison's Online, and journal collections, such as PubMed. Organized, Well Edited, Frequently Updated and Comprehensive Information are self-explanatory. Search features specifically refer to the ability to search for a keyword or phrase. Differential diagnosis refers to the ability to integrate clinical patient presentations and create a list of possible problem diagnoses.

	Online Textbook	Journal Collections	Hybrid – GI Motility Online
Organized	X		X
Well Edited	X		X
Frequently Updated		X	X
Comprehensive Information		X	X
Search Features	X	X	X
Differential Diagnosis			X

such as holographic displays or direct-to-eye projection technologies, the ability for PDAs to contribute to medical reference appears to be technologically limited.

As shown in Table 1, Gastrointestinal Motility Online is a hybrid that lies between the two models of electronic journals and online textbooks, exclusively focused on providing authoritative information in an organized fashion within a specific domain. Using this system, a gastrointestinal researcher can find the most recent journal articles because of the frequent updates, and a gastrointestinal clinician can easily locate a detailed diagram of the lower esophageal sphincter. In addition, topical information can be cross-linked between papers—a typical feature of textbooks and very pertinent for teaching and presentations.

CONCEPTS AND INNOVATIONS

The exploration of the technological space between electronic journals and online textbooks is a relatively new idea. All new ideas face challenges in terms of deployment and adoption. Consider the fax number. As the number of fax machines increases, the value of the fax increases—this illustrates the fact that networks attain greater value with larger number of users. The difficulty faced by Gastrointestinal Motility Online and other specialty interest sites is in terms of initial growth and development of specific communities of interest. These sites must be aesthetically attractive, informative, efficient, and up-to-date.

The case of Gastrointestinal Motility Online illustrates one form of evolution of online journals and textbooks into an active online scientific community. Site loyalty is achieved and maintained by the reputation of the authors and contributors. Gastrointestinal Motility Online needs only to achieve a critical user mass before gaining the benefits of Web sites like e-Bay (http://www.ebay.com/) or Amazon (http://www.amazon.com/) in terms of de facto authority and brand recognition. For sites, which are less commercially oriented, the loyalty of the user base is perhaps even more heavily emphasized. Two notable sites, which have grown rapidly without such a strong commercial bias, are Wikipedia and Imdb.

Wikipedia has been both maligned and praised for its loyal community and efforts to create a free encyclopedia that is accurate and up to date without any commercial affiliations. Wikipedia began in 2000 as a complementary project for Nupedia, in which articles were written by experts and reviewed by a formal process (Wikipedia, 2007). In 2001, Larry Sanger proposed on the Nupedia mailing list to create a wiki as a "feeder" project for Nupedia (Sanger, 2001); this spawned rapid growth. By 2001, Wikipedia contained approximately 20,000 articles and 18 language editions and, as of 2007, English Wikipedia contains over 1.7 million articles, making it the largest encyclopedia ever assembled. The site relies on the goodwill of its members to write, update and contest articles, and has thus far proven that the Internet community as a whole is willing to contribute towards the database, albeit haphazardly (recent events are more likely to be covered in detail, while significant historical figures languish). Given the size and relatively stable growth of the project, the prospect of a peer-reviewed and written information repository might not be so cynically doomed.

The International Movie Database (IMDB), a site in the top 20 (Alexa Internet, 2007b) U.S. Web sites visited, is the largest Internet compilation of movie information (approximately 900,000 titles and 2.3 million names) (IMDB, 2007). IMDB draws a significant portion of its information from the participation of its user base. Beyond subjective reviews, users are also asked to supply cast and crew lists, production details, and actor biographies. IMDB grew from two lists that started as independent projects in early 1989 by participants in the Usenet newsgroup rec.arts.movies. Each list was maintained by a single person, recording items e-mailed by newsgroup readers, and posting updated versions of his list from time to time. The lists were eventually combined, and by late 1990, the lists included almost 10,000 movies and television series. As the contributions continued to grow rapidly, the IMDB formed as an independent company in 1995 and was later purchased by Amazon Inc. (Wikipedia, 2007b).

The approach of the IMDB system closely resembles the envisioned system for GI Motility Online, with the user population submitting proposed changes, followed by an editorial process. Database content is generally provided and updated by a vast collection of volunteer contributors. There are only 17 members of the IMDB who are dedicated to monitoring received data, although 70% of IMDB's staff serve as editors (IMDB, 2007), reviewing changes, verifying the information before posting the changes, and policing the forums.

Peer review is considered to be one of the most even-handed and least biased methods of scrutinizing articles for publication. The development of a community, as well as the ability for members of that community to voice their opinions about professional papers is pivotal to the dissemination of accurate information. The model of Amazon or eBay is to allow users to comment, and thereby to signify reliability and approval. Gastrointestinal Motility Online allows users to provide feedback, both critical and supportive, in order to enhance the relevance of articles.

According to Harris Interactive poll, only one-fourth of physicians use the Internet to communicate with their patients (Computing in the Physician's Practice, 2000). In the same poll, although 89% of physicians use the Internet in their practice in search of information, they spend only six hours per week to browse medical developments. Accordingly, Gastrointestinal Motility Online has been configured to serve as an encyclopedic source, as well as a high-value news feed. AccessMedicine uses a Podcast update model, with 10-minute broadcasts generated daily for use in family practice. Gastrointestinal Motility Online caters to a smaller specialty group with correspondingly less frequent pace of developments, and is therefore less time sensitive.

Automation

Automated content generation or extraction from other publications is not feasible, due to the stringent need to maintain relevance and quality. Thus, deployment of a pure peer-reviewed wiki-style community is precluded by the need to maintain quality. If membership of the wiki is restricted to those users whose credentials are accepted, or if changes must be approved at an editorial level, then a wiki would facilitate the rapid exchange of information as well. In the second part of the endeavor, the goal is to enable machine-assisted updating of the material in the gastrointestinal knowledge repository. Currently, all updates must be initiated manually. The pressure to update, but to update accurately applies to many situations: addition of new material, editing of existing material, and deletion of parts of existing material as new study results become available. Initial thoughts and test results are documented in Sharma (2005).

As the site evolves, the need to keep the site relevant to a particular group of specialist physicians may conflict with the preferences of another significant category of users: the researchers. Gastrointestinal Motility Online intends to use user-based customized layout, as presented by Sarnikar et al. (2005). The filtering of details from the main knowledge repository is not intended to block or hide information, but to provide a more relevant source. Classification and weighting are accomplished by a rules-based system that can assess whether an article is clinical or basic science-related. Login will also provide both the ability to contribute and comment on articles, and to obtain a specialized view depending on the type of user. The application of user-based site layouts is not innovative, but is important to the domain of medical informatics because physicians attach such a high priority on relevance.

Given the large number of articles published weekly and the difficulty in ascertaining relevance and quality, a number of automated tools will be used to optimize the updating process. Sarnikar et al. (2005) present one technique that will assist in filtering journal results, and maintaining and updating the site. Their method selects articles ranked by relevance using a combination of both rule-based and content-based methods, using the following principles:

1. Profiles are modeled in the form of rules.
2. The purpose of the rule-based profile is to identify a sub-set of documents of interest to a user.
3. Each role has a set of predefined rules associated with it.
4. Rules specify knowledge sources to access (e.g., nursing journals for Nurses).
5. Rules can specify knowledge depth and knowledge breadth.
6. Rules can specify semantic types of primary importance to roles.

Profiles are used in the gastrointestinal motility context to separate information into categories: for example, new clinical findings versus basic science. Articles may be assigned a category and a relevance weight, given categorization rules based on Unified Medical Language System (UMLS) synonym lists and the categories *sign or symptom, diagnostic procedure, therapeutic or preventive procedure and disease or syndrome semantic types*. In addition to a text search in the abstract, Sarnikar and Gupta (2007) also assign weights to the type of journal. These tools can select and filter relevant articles for presentation as an RSS XML news feed to editors or automatically assemble relevant articles for use by the editors or Web site administrators. While these tools will aid the editor, there is yet no replacement for the role of humans in decisively selecting and classifying information.

Ontologies and semantic networks are prerequisites to the development and classification of information repositories. Ontologies serve many purposes (Kumar, 2005) including:

- Reuse and share domain knowledge
- Establishing classification schemes and structure
- Making assumptions explicit

They further enable analysis of information and complement the stricter terminology that is used in straightforward text searches. Examples of ontologies in use today include the National Library of Medicine's Medical Subject Heading (MeSH), disease specific terminologies such as

National Cancer Institute's PDQ vocabulary, drug terminologies such as the National Drug Data File, and medical sociality vocabularies such as the Classification of Nursing Diagnoses and the Current Dental Terminology. In Gastrointestinal Motility Online, the ontological hierarchy will be used to distinguish between sections of the gastrointestinal tract, from the stomach and esophagus to the large intestine and colon (Kumar, 2005).

A key enabler for development of automatic information processing is the set of ontologies presented in the UMLS semantic network that rely upon the concepts built in the UMLS concept hierarchy. Hierarchical and clustered ontologies allow software to construct knowledge trees, conglomerating relevant knowledge. An overview of the UMLS is available at The Unified Medical Language System: What is it and how to use it? (http://www.nlm.nih.gov/research/umls/presentations/2004-medinfo_tut.pdf).

UMLS is an aggregate of over 134 source vocabularies, including the classifications from such lists as ICD-10 and DSM: IIIR-IV. It represents a hierarchy of medical phrases that can be used to classify most medical articles and textbook entries. For example, using UMLS, the following phrases are grouped similarly: *Deglutition Disorders, Difficultyin swallowing, Difficulty in swallowing (context-dependent category), Dysphagia NOS, Dysphagia NOS (context-dependent category), Can't get food down, Cannot get food down, Difficulty swallowing, Difficulty swallowing (finding), Dysphagia, Dysphagia (Disorder), Swallowing difficult, Swallowing Disorders* (Aronson, 2001).

The system described in Sharma (2005) uses techniques of Natural Language Processing (NLP) to construct a semantic understanding surpasses text searching. Using the Automated Integration of Text Documents in the Medical Domain (ATIMED) system, the content and order of phrases are related lexically using a concept called Word-Net. Word-Net operates on the verbs, subjects and objects of the sentences, comparing sets and subsets of subject-verb-objects collections in order to determine topic relatedness.

Word-Net further uses a lexical dictionary to determine similarity in all verb pairs and then subject-verb-action pairs. Sharma (2005) uses the following two sentences as examples: *Dysphagia is a disease and defined as a sensation of sticking or obstruction of the passage of food. Dysphagia is related to obstruction of passage of food.* Since both sentences contain similar objects and subjects, and use the verb "is", the sentences is deemed similar. However, within the current mechanism, the phrase, "*Dysphagia relates to obstruction of passage of food*" would result in a poorly scored correlation or low match because the action verb is not similar (Sharma, 2005).

Finally, the same technique allows the creation of new documents by collating sentences and paragraphs from various documents. An initial method of grouping sentences uses the quantity of concepts expressed. This method is further refined by evaluating the sentences based on the following criteria: *similar-subjects, similar-objects, similar-subjects-objects,* and *similar-objects-subjects.* Based on the structure of English grammar, these techniques have been reliably shown to collate relevant data into a readable format.

A diagram of the method is shown in Figure 1.

A sample output, based on the use of this technique, is provided below:

REGURGITATION is defined as the spontaneous appearance of gastric or esophageal contents in the back of the throat or in the mouth. In distal esophageal obstruction and stasis, as in achalasia or the presence of a large diverticulum, the regurgitated material consists of tasteless mucoid fluid or undigested food (Sharma, 2005).

The context interchange of heterogeneous sources of information being collated for different classes of users leverages tools from an additional branch of information technology. One level of development is the creation of maps between

Figure 1. Integration of semantic understanding to generate new information (Adapted from Sharma, 2005)

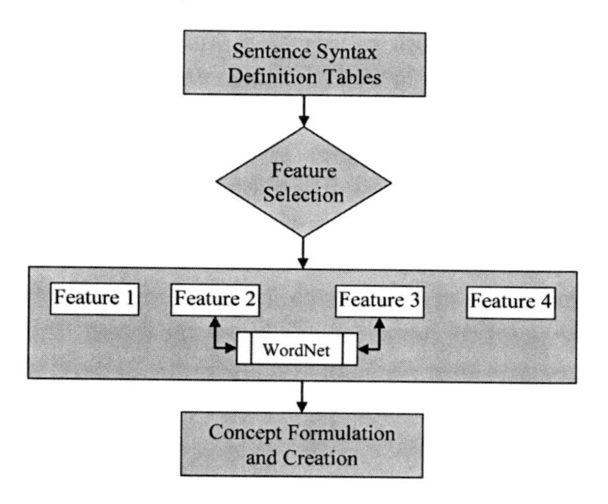

inputs and outputs, in much the same way that a dictionary might map between languages. The conversion of *n* sources to *m* outputs can grow to be an exponentially difficult problem; this can be addressed with the use of intelligent heuristics and protocols to selectively prune the data. Difficulties become particularly apparent with changes in any client schema that cause a cascade of changes in the mappings (Sarnikar, 2005). Using an independently developed predefined mediating schema would restrict the amount of information that could be exchanged. Apart from relational schema, a client schema could also be specified as a hierarchical schema or as an XML-based message (Sarnikar & Gupta, 2007). In the context of Gastrointestinal Motility Online, the specific source contexts are innovative journal papers, reviews, and textbook articles. The output contexts are specialist clinicians, researchers, students, and other health professionals. Developing a schema to accurately represent journal abstracts and determine the relevance of those abstracts is another method of exchanging contexts. Innovation in this domain will allow Gastrointestinal Motility Online to maintain updated, consistent-quality references without requiring an editor to read every journal article published immediately.

LESSONS LEARNED

The GI Motility Online site benefited from a mature development environment for Web-based information retrieval.

Interface: In the case of GI Motility Online, the user base is a readily identifiable group, trained in a similar fashion, with specific needs and expectations of organization and formatting. The following two aspects influenced the design process:

- Pagination is a critical issue for online didactic materials. As people do not like the interface to online books (Crawford, 2006), the development of the site must reflect the reading style and needs of its users. In the case of GI Motility Online, there are currently no page delimiters; this is encouraging users to print the material to be used as a reference. A solution of delivering a formatted print-ready PDF could be applied, but the cost begins to climb with the number of different formats and delivery options supported.
- Tables must be handled intelligently. Tables are used in many medical publications to rapidly and clearly present information. The trend in the mid-1990s for netiquette was to inline the tables with the text, but this can create awkward gaps or poor formatting choices. GI Motility Online chooses the path of Harrison's Online, in linking to the tables outside the main document to preserve readability.

Based on their respective training, many physicians expect a particular language and layout of medical information. The highest-value information for each physician may vary based on specialty, and user-customization of graphical widgets. Since GI Motility Online aims to support a broad base of users with many different roles and information needs, reusable widgets, of the type available in customizable Web-portals, may potentially solve these varying needs.

Workflow: As stated previously, over nine months was required for simply editing the site information, moving documents back and forth between editors, experts and developers. The method involved several inefficient technologies, such as mailing CDs and sending large files through mail servers. The advantage of such hands on interaction and communication is the result: the authors of the site are particularly pleased by the polished appearance of the delivered product.

Electronic collaboration between different sites was difficult due to the nature of document formats, which does not produce a consistent print layout on different computers, and layout formats, which do not allow easy markup or revision to the document.

The use of a standardized input format and efficient conversion of the RTF-formatted documents into Web viewable formats was crucial to the development of the Web site. Though conversion of documents is a minimally complex task, the production of a site that allows conversation on the fly to support concurrent editing and proofing between multiple users is a challenge. Online publishing companies, such as Atypon, offer suites of software to facilitate publishing workflow, allowing multiple authors to upload articles, multiple editors to revise articles, and art editors to manage graphics, in an organized fashion.

Meta-Information: The World Wide Web provides a tremendous asset in connecting related articles seamlessly. In determining related pages, an active agent, a human, machine or some combination thereof, must isolate the crucial elements of a page and capture that as meta-information, preferably categorized. Organized meta-information allows automated tools to develop connections and links to potentially relevant information.

Extracting crucial elements of a page is best handled by encouraging authors to define keywords, as with scientific articles. Although many automated agents have historically been unsuccessful in information extraction, the medical domain provides some assistance with standardized ontologies, which allow agents to categorize information in a framework, reducing some identification errors.

Maintenance: Many articles in mainstream sites, such as ESPN.com, offer the opportunity for users to comment and leave feedback. This increases user participation and value to the site, but raises additional issues that need to be addressed such as:

- Profanity or other inappropriate comments must be censored
- Sites are more open to attack and security leaks due to their increased functionality
- Bandwidth usage increases, and may debilitate the site

In addition, a version control framework must be established for sites that allow updates, in order to rollback unwanted changes. Furthermore, hardware resources must be allocated to store site changes.

CURRENT USAGE AND FUTURE DIRECTIONS

Anecdotal evidence provided by the lead creator of GI Motility Online, Dr. Raj Goyal, highlights that the representatives of Nature Publishing Group describe the site as being popular, and that site visits to GI Motility Online are increasing. Due to the delicate nature of conversation with his peers in gastroenterology, Dr. Goyal cannot be certain, but he states that initial impressions are unanimously positive and enthusiastic. Dr. Goyal notes that the majority of the traffic to GI Motility Online currently arrives from Google, and indeed, Google's first returned site in response to "GI Motility" is GI Motility Online (Google, 2007). GI Motility Online does not currently permit any advertising; if this policy is revised, the usage patterns may change. Further, the numbers for site visits are expected to increase if the site were to be more supported by Nature Publishing Group.

The stakeholders are satisfied with the quality of the product, and are ambitiously pursuing an extension of the product to broaden coverage to other parts of the GI tract.

Dr. Goyal has received inquiries to publish the material in a hardcopy format. Custom-built books or full-page colored slides offer additional utility to medical educators, specialists, nurses, and students, and may also offer a revenue stream. These custom-built printable books are a logical extension of the current "print what you want" photo fulfillment services that are popular on photo sharing sites or album hosting services. Given that Harrison's Principles of Internal Medicine contains over 2,000 colored pages in book form, there may be a future for customized books in medicine.

Retrieval: New algorithms for search and ranking are not merely lexically-based, but also combine closely related concepts and relationships between ideas. This facilitates the creation of a richer search language that can account for relationships, such as causation, consequence, association, treatment, or opposite. For example, hypothermia is directly opposite hyperthermia, and may be caused by thalamic alterations. Such basic chains of relationships could be easily captured, if the language and storage of meta-information about articles could contain the necessary underlying details.

Presentation: Using Tufte's principles (Tufte, 2001), the real estate of a screen needs to be more efficiently used. Currently, most search-engine results do not often give the sense of the relevance of the article, of the correct sections, or the tone of the article. The information density of the return pages is low, causing users to scroll through potentially hundreds of articles to find relevant information. Graphical interfaces are likely to be a solution, as the ability of the Internet to handle higher bandwidth applications grows. In medical research in particular, an interface, which allows users to quickly see search results of the primary concept and even related concepts, may dramatically affect usability.

Online Sharing: Bulletin board systems, which flourished during pre-Internet days, have re-emerged on the Internet as forums, and are a popular source of information. Corporations with significant Internet presence, and especially gaming companies like Nintendo (http://forums.nintendo.com/nintendo/), have begun adding and using these forums as a method of improving public relations and offering support.

Intranet and Internet file sharing systems have also flourished, as bandwidth rates increase. The rise of Youtube is one phenomenon, but the comfort of using the Internet to disseminate multimedia (such as GI endoscope video) appears to be more solidified. These high bandwidth applications have grown in acceptance, and despite the threat of viruses in downloaded files, file-sharing traffic is increasing daily.

Megaupload and Rapidshare, two prominent file sharing services, are now ranked #18 and #27 in the reliable Alexa ranking (Alexa Internet, 2007b) of most visited Internet sites in the U.S. However, these services are predominantly used by non-commercial entities. Commercial enterprises may be hesitant due to slow adoption, security issues, bandwidth maximums, or unprofessional presentation. Such file sharing sites will certainly cater in the future to commercial entities, perhaps by providing specially developed sites, or providing branded services. The future of the Internet, and especially the ability to deliver high bandwidth, will increasingly rely upon specialized sites with high-capacity and high-bandwidth connections close to Internet backbones.

Collaboration: Collaboration in the domain of GI motility will drive improvements in language tools, with many GI specialists throughout the world, who may need to collaborate via the Internet or phone services. Currently, Altavista and Google offer Web-based text translation, but more intelligence or domain-specific knowledge may be required. One common example in GI translation is translating the world "oral" to mean "verbal", when in fact, the correct reference is to the mouth cavity. Overall, however, text translation between languages is generally adequate for initial communication.

Oral translation is a high value direction to pursue, but at the same time, is a very difficult task. Psycholinguistics research is still unraveling the complexities of language parsing, and the ability of current artificial intelligence to understand language is severely limited. Nevertheless, translators in this area will prove essential and highly desirable for the next generation of online collaborators.

Similarly, one of the holy grails of artificial intelligence development is the creation of an artificial system capable of interpreting human language. Within specialized domains with limited vocabularies, artificial readers become more feasible, but the medical domain is particularly difficult, due to its large specialized vocabulary. Development in this area would provide rewards for medical researchers, allowing the creation of agents, which would allow researchers to process more information by selecting and even summarizing articles.

Organizationally, scientific research in domains such as medicine would benefit tremendously from the creation of a centralized authority to monitor, synthesize and rate research. The current system of research funding in America places research at the whim of special-interest private funding and sometimes misdirected public funding in overly popular or extremely esoteric areas. Regulating and directing research might also help avoid repeating inconclusive research, which does not get published (and thus may be repeated).

CONCLUSION

Gastrointestinal Motility Online is an evolving knowledge base related to Gastrointestinal Motility disorders. The current phase of the endeavor focuses on the collection and organization of knowledge from many different sources. Knowledge-mining tools are being developed to utilize this information as it becomes available to add fast, relevant access and other utilities to the information repository.

The continuous change in standards of care and knowledge due to rapid discoveries in the basic and clinical sciences prompts for a system that is more flexible than a textbook, while demanding thoroughness and accuracy. Knowledge mining tools and other advanced technologies to aid in the conversion and integration of articles and research into the mainstream science are being integrated into Gastrointestinal Motility Online, and look to impact the breadth and speed of knowledge-base upgrades. Gastrointestinal Motility Online serves to balance the needs of its user base while embracing the academic rigor in a novel application of technology to the science of medicine.

ACKNOWLEDGMENT

The authors would like to thank Dr. Raj Goyal for his invaluable input and contribution to GI Motility Online and this article. The authors also thank Richard Martin for his helpful comments and proofreading of the text.

REFERENCES

Alexa Internet. (2007a). *Three-month traffic statistics for wikipedia.org.* Retrieved from http://www.alexa.com/data/details/main?q=&url=wikipedia.org

Alexa Internet. (2007b). *Top Sites United States.* Retrieved from http://www.alexa.com/site/ds/top_sites?cc=US&ts_mode=country&lang=none

American Library Association. (1989). *Presidential Committee on Information Literacy - Final Report.* Retrieved from http://www.ala.org/ala/acrl/acrlpubs/whitepapers/presidential.htm

Antman, E., Lau, J., Kupelnick, B., Mosteller, F., & Chalmers, T. (1992). A comparison of results of meta-analyses of randomized control trials and recommendations of clinical experts. *Journal of the American Medical Association, 268*, 240–248. doi:10.1001/jama.268.2.240

Aronson, A. (2001). Effective mapping of biomedical text to the UMLS Metathesaurus: The MetaMap program. In *Proceedings of the 2001 AMIA Symposium* (pp. 17-21).

Carlson, C. (2003). Information overload, retrieval strategies and Internet user empowerment . In Haddon, L. (Ed.), *The Good, the Bad and the Irrelevant (COST 269)* (*Vol. 1*, pp. 169–173). Helsinki, Finland.

CEBM. (2007). *Why the sudden interest in EBM?* Retrieved from http://www.cebm.utoronto.ca/intro/interest.htm

Computing in the Physician's Practice. (2000). Retrieved from http://www.harrisinteractive.com/harris_poll/index.asp?PID=58

Crawford, W. (2006). *Why aren't ebooks more successful?* Retrieved from http://www.econtentmag.com/Articles/ArticleReader.aspx?ArticleID=18144

Davis, D., Thomson, M., Oxman, A., & Haynes, R. (1997). Changing physician performance: A systematic review of the effect of continuing medical education strategies. *Journal of the American Medical Association, 274*, 700–705. doi:10.1001/jama.274.9.700

Evidence-Based Medicine Working Group. (1992). Evidence-Based Medicine Working Group: Evidence-based medicine. A new approach to teaching the practice of medicine. *Journal of the American Medical Association, 268*, 2420–2425. doi:10.1001/jama.268.17.2420

Fridman, S. (2000). *Doctors lag when it comes to computer use - Industry trend or event.* Retrieved from http://www.findarticles.com/p/articles/mi_m0HDN/is_2000_March_28/ai_60907019

Giles, J. (2005). *Internet encyclopedias go head to head.* Retrieved from http://www.nature.com/news/2005/051212/full/438900a.html

Google. (2007). *Search returned "GI Motility."* Retrieved from http://www.google.com/search?hl=en&q=GI+Motility

Gore, A. (1992). Infrastructure for the global village. *Scientific American, 265*, 150–153.

Hawking, S. (2001). *The universe in a nutshell.* New York: Bantam Books.

Haynes, R. (1993). Where's the meat in clinical journals? [Editorial]. *ACP Journal Club, 119*, A22–A23.

IMDB. (2007). *How/where do you get your information? How accurate/reliable is it?* Retrieved from http://imdb.com/help/show_leaf?infosource

Kasper, D., Fauci, A., Longo, D., Braunwald, E., Hauser, S., & Jameson, J. (2005). *Harrison's principles of internal medicine* (16th ed.). New York: McGraw-Hill.

Kumar, A. (2005). *Ontology-driven access to biomedical information (ODABI)*. Undergraduate Thesis, University of Arizona.

Lindberg, D. (2003). *NIH: Moving research from the bench to the bedside*. Presentation to the Subcommittee on Health.

Lyman, P., & Varian, H. (2003). *How much information?* Retrieved from http://www2.sims.berkeley.edu/research/projects/how-much-info-2003/index.htm

Mechaca, L. (2007). *Goodbye, Axim*. Message posted to http://direct2dell.com/one2one/archive/2007/04/11/11397.aspx

Sackett, D. (1997). Using evidence-based medicine to help physicians keep up-to-date. *The Journal for the Serials Community*, *9*, 178–181. doi:10.1629/09178

Sackett, D., & Straus, S. (1998). Finding and applying evidence during clinical rounds: The evidence cart. *Journal of the American Medical Association*, *280*, 1336–1338. doi:10.1001/jama.280.15.1336

Sanger, L. (2001). *Let's make a wiki*. Message posted to http://web.archive.org/web/20030414014355/http://www.nupedia.com/pipermail/nupedia-l/2001-January/000676.html

Sarnikar, S., & Gupta, A. (2007). *A context-specific mediating schema approach for information exchange between heterogeneous hospital systems*. Forthcoming in International Journal of Healthcare Technology and Management.

Sarnikar, S., Zhao, J., & Gupta, A. (2005). Medical information filtering using content-based and rule-based profiles. In *Proceedings of the AIS Americas Conference on Information Systems (AMCIS 2005)*, Omaha, NE.

Schwartz, B. (2004). *The paradox of choice*. New York: HarperCollins Publishers.

Senge, P. (1994). *The fifth discipline: The art and practice of the learning organization*. New York: Doubleday/Currency.

Sharma, R. (2005). *Automatic integration of text documents in the medical domain*. Undergraduate Thesis, University of Arizona.

Slawson, D., Hauck, F., Strayer, S., & Rollins, L. (2007). *What is information master?* Retrieved from http://www.healthsystem.virginia.edu/internet/familymed/docs/info_mastery.cfm#Information

Tufte, E. (2001). *The visual display of quantitative information*. Cheshire, CT: Graphics Press.

Vanhecke, T., Barnes, M., Zimmerman, J., & Shoichet, S. (2006). *PubMed vs. HighWire Press: A head-to-head comparison of two medical literature search engines*. Computers in Biology and Medicine.

Wikipedia. (2007a). *Information retrieval*. Retrieved from http://en.wikipedia.org/wiki/Information_retrieval.

Wikipedia. (2007b). *Wikipedia*. Retrieved from http://en.wikipedia.org/wiki/Wikipedia.

Chapter 15
An Evaluation of E-Learning in Healthcare

George Athanasiou
University of Patras, Greece

Nikos Maris
Technical University of Crete, Greece

Ioannis Apostolakis
National School of Public Health, Greece

ABSTRACT

As new technologies enable a radical transformation of the learning process, new learning approaches and techniques appear, and the need for quality assurance of all learning assets emerges. Although, the existing e-learning standards have managed to cover most of the different aspects of the e-learning process, the shift to new paradigms such as collaborative and community learning sets the need for new standards. The main goal of e-learning standards is to enable and ensure interoperability and re-usability of solutions, systems, objects and processes. E-learning is an extremely useful tool for the healthcare community since it allows professionals, researchers, companies and individuals to improve their skills and expand their knowledge. However, it has faced several difficulties mainly due to the heterogeneity of educational needs. The different user groups have different requirements from e-learning, different availability and resources and consequently different quality standards. In this chapter, the authors emphasize on the quality assurance, and the community aspect of e-learning.

INTRODUCTION

E-learning can be used by medical educators to improve the efficiency and effectiveness of educational interventions in the face of social, scientific, and pedagogical challenges. It has gained popularity in the past decade; however, its use is highly variable among medical schools and appears to be more common in basic science courses than in clinical clerkships (Moberg & Whitcomb, 1999; Ward et al., 2001). The effectiveness of e-learning, especially in medicine, has been demonstrated primarily by studies concerning higher education, government, corporate, and military environments (Gibbons & Fairweather, 2000; Bernard et al., 2004). However, these

DOI: 10.4018/978-1-61692-843-8.ch015

studies have limitations, especially because of the variability in their scientific design (Bernard et al., 2004; Letterie, 2003). Often they have failed to define the content quality, technological characteristics, and type of specific e-learning intervention being analyzed. In addition, most of them have included several different instructional methodologies, which complicated the analysis of educational outcome (Piemme, 1988). Most of these studies compared e-learning with traditional instructor-led approaches (Johnson et al., 2004; Bernard et al., 2004).

Yet three aspects of e-learning have been consistently explored: product utility, cost-effectiveness, and learner satisfaction. Utility refers to the usefulness of the method of e-learning. Several studies outside of health care have revealed that most often e-learning is at least as good as, if not better than, traditional instructor-led methods such as lectures in contributing to demonstrated learning (Wentling et al., 2000). Several studies from the pre-Internet era, including two meta- analyses are cited (Gibbons & Fairweather, 2000) that compared the utility of computer-based instruction to traditional teaching methods. The studies used a variety of designs in both training and academic environments, with inconsistent results for various outcomes. Yet learners' knowledge, measured by pre-post test scores, was shown to improve. Moreover, learners using computer-based instruction learned more efficiently and demonstrated better retention.

Recent reviews of the e-learning (specifically Web-based learning) literature in diverse medical education contexts reveal similar findings. Chumley-Jones et al.(2002) reviewed 76 studies, published in the medical, nursing, and dental literature, on the utility of Web based learning. According to the authors, one-third of the studies evaluated knowledge gains, most using multiple-choice written tests, although standardized patients were used in one study. In terms of learners' achievements in knowledge, Web-based learning was equivalent to traditional methods. Of the two studies evaluating learning efficiency, only one demonstrated evidence for more efficient learning via Web-based instruction (Chumley-Jones et al., 2002).

A substantial body of evidence in the non-medical literature has shown, on the basis of sophisticated cost analysis, that e-learning can result in significant cost savings, sometimes as much as 50%, compared with traditional instructor-led learning (Gibbons & Fairweather, 2000). Savings are related to reduced instructor training time, travel costs, and labor costs, reduced institutional infrastructure, and the possibility of expanding programs with new educational technologies (Gibbons & Fairweather, 2000). Only one study in the medical literature evaluated the cost-effectiveness of e-learning as compared with text-based learning. The authors found that the printing and distribution of educational materials is less costly than creating and disseminating e-learning content (Chumley-Jones et al., 2002; Reddy & Wladawsky-Berger, 2001).

Finally, several studies concerning both medical and nonmedical students revealed high satisfaction from e-learning and increased satisfaction in comparison to traditional learning. The ease of use and access, navigation, interactivity, and user-friendliness are some additional benefits for learners (Gibbons & Fairweather, 2000; Chumley-Jones et al., 2002). However, in most cases e-learning was perceived as a supplement to traditional instructor-led training, thus stating the need for a blended-learning strategy (Gibbons & Fairweather, 2000; Chumley-Jones et al., 2002; Walker et al., 2003).

The chapter provides a set of e-learning standards, a reference framework for the description of quality approaches and an introduction on how the e-learning process can be founded on pedagogical standards. The novelty of our approach lies in the fact that it combines the merits of evaluation, self-support and collaboration for improving the quality in learning and makes it an applicable solution for the highly volatile healthcare community. The multi-layered structure, allows healthcare learning communities to state their needs and capabilities and make full exploitation of each other during the evaluation of the learning process, content and outcomes.

BACKGROUND

From Traditional to Collaborative Learning

It is undeniable that improving the quality, flexibility and delivery rate of healthcare services is of great benefit to society. In opposition to the Industrial Society, where goods are transported for one peer to another, in the Information Society the primary good is information, which is retrieved, collected, processed and redistributed. In order to find, analyze and deliver the appropriate information we should combine the effective use of Information and Communication Technologies (ICT) with the use of appropriate knowledge.

The formation of knowledge is achieved by education, i.e. the effort to provide information, which aims at learning. In the traditional learning process, the individual is passive receiver (Negroponte, 1996) of the scientific knowledge, which is transformed firstly into course knowledge (syllabus) and secondly into instructed knowledge for the student, by the teacher (Figure 1). The "transformation" of knowledge emphasizes the need of a teacher, who is responsible (Komis, 2006) to evaluate, to process and to disseminate the knowledge. As a consequence, the teacher needs evaluation models and standards for assessing the quality of the teaching process.

However, some learning psycho-pedagogical models (e.g. the sociocultural theory) have suggested that learning occurs from the continuous interaction of the individual with his socially, culturally and historically defined environment. The collaborative activities are the main contributors in the process of constructing the knowledge, according to the Activity Theory (Vygotsky, 1934), When collaborative learning is employed there is no such transformation of knowledge and consequently the evaluation and quality assessment models are insufficient.

Community based, and e-learning models are very helpful in cases where learning could not be reachable by a person. This exclusion from traditional learning can be due to several reasons; in the case of healthcare professionals, for example, the individual needs for education and learning updates differ from one field of expertise to another, whereas in the case of public awareness for healthcare issues, citizens may not be able to move to the educational centers, may not have enough time to spend for education or even may not access education due to disabilities. Flexible learning models that combine e-learning solutions with virtual community structures have already been proposed (Apostolakis et al., 2008) as alternatives to traditional learning, that allow learners to decide what to learn, how and in what

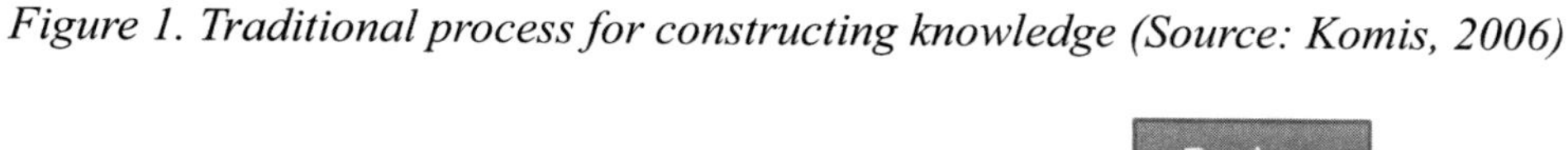

Figure 1. Traditional process for constructing knowledge (Source: Komis, 2006)

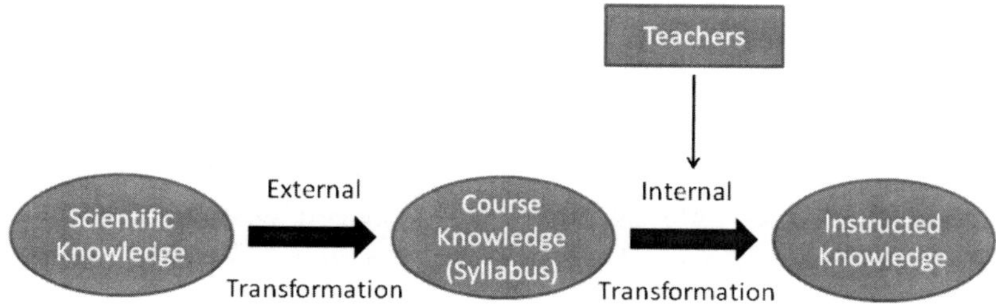

Figure 2. Learning categories

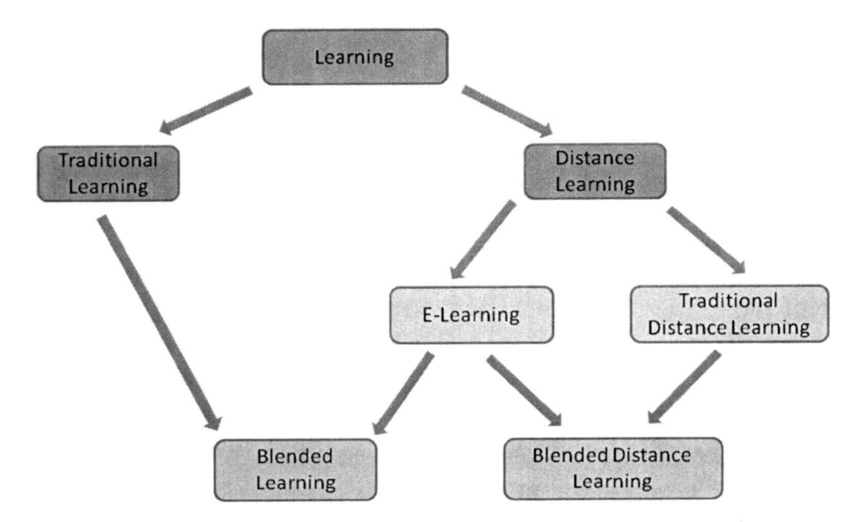

tempo and help them cover the growing need for healthcare education and public awareness whilst supporting the aforementioned requirements. The evolution in mobile devices gave to learning a ubiquitous sense and made it accessible to even more people.

Community based learning is not restricted in a single category of learning, although it spans the distant learning part of the tree in (Figure 2), it can also employ traditional learning methods. All forms of tele-learning, either synchronous (which takes place in real time) or asynchronous are employed by communities and mixed (blended) learning comes in assistance when it is necessary. The difference in the community approach is that it allows the community members to choose one or even more solutions in parallel in order to achieve the best possible result.

E-Learning and Quality Standards

E-learning quality – and educational quality in a wider context – is a diverse concept. It is not an absolute and well defined concept but rather depends on the situation in which it is employed. No country has reached a social, political or academic consensus on what educational quality is. Different methods are used to assure quality, ranging from market-oriented instruments, government-driven consumer protection mechanisms and accreditation concepts to institutional strategies and different instruments. Approaches can have an explicit intentional character or can be rather implicit – when quality development is left to individuals' professional competences.

The definition of quality always takes place as a normative act, referring to a particular context. Consequently, situations and interests always influence its definition. In the sector of social and educational services quality becomes a negotiable issue between various propounded academic theories and subjective, political and social interests (Ehlers & Pawlowski, 2006).

To critically analyze quality, it is helpful to identify the basic points of the debate. We can distinguish between three fundamentally different aspects in the discussion (Ehlers, 2003a; Ehlers, 2003b):

- different interpretations of quality
- different stakeholders with different perspectives on quality
- different forms of quality (input-, process-, output-quality)

Figure 3. The three aspects of debate (Source: Ehlers, 2003a)

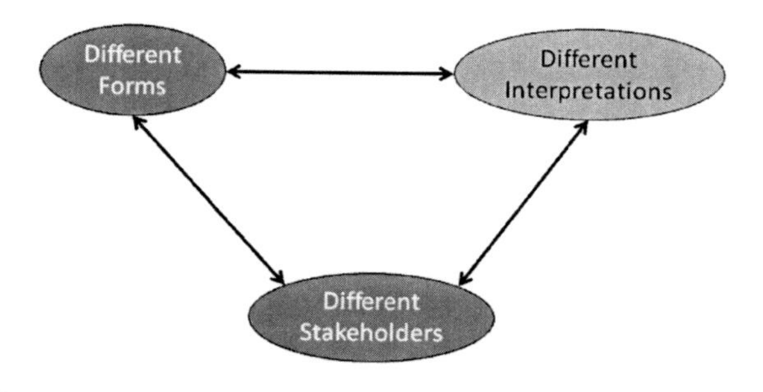

Together these three aspects provide a general framework of reference for the described debate (Figure 3).

One dimension is the different interpretation of the meaning of quality. Numerous definitions from various fields are available. For example, economics adopt the product based definition, which views quality as a physical characteristic of an object. The quality of a piece of jewelry then depends on its gold fraction and the quality of a whisky on the duration of its storage. There is also a user-based approach which relates to individual customer preferences. Under this interpretation, optimal fulfillment of demand signifies the best in quality: An often borrowed book, therefore, attains a higher quality than a seldom borrowed volume. We also have the production-based approach which sets standards, compliance with which equals quality. Here, the main focus is on functionality. All books which do not fall apart then have the same quality (Ehlers & Pawlowski, 2006; Pawlowski, 2006).

In education, we can currently identify several meanings of quality (Harvey & Green, 2000):

- quality as an exception, describing the surpassing of standards, quality as perfection, describing the state of flawlessness, quality as functionality, referring to the degree of utility,
- quality as an adequate return, measured by the price-performance or cost-benefit ratio,
- quality as transformation, describing the above mentioned co-producer relationship between the learner and the learning environment and referring to the learners' progress in terms of a learning process.

However, there are not only different interpretations of quality but also different perspectives for each different stakeholder: the enterprise that trains its employees, the tutors supervising an e-learning-program, the human resource managers who establish a framework for continuing education in their sector, and the learners. Each of these players generally has divergent interests and differing quality requirements and interpretations. It is, therefore, important to regard quality not as a static element but as a negotiation process between different stakeholders involved in the social process (Ehlers & Pawlowski, 2006; Pawlowski, 2006).

Last but not least, quality can also refer to different educational processes or levels. We can cite the different levels of the famous quality triad by (Donabedian, 1980):

- e-learning prerequisites (input or structure quality): availability or capability of the technological infrastructure, qualification of tutors,
- the learning process (process quality): the interaction of learners, learning formats, corporate learning culture, the learning content and desired training goals,
- the result (output/ outcome quality): the increase in learners' professional competence.

Defining quality is not an easy task and definitely cannot be solved by a standard quality assurance process. Quality criteria should be carefully defined from the begging, but they should be constantly revised and adopted in the future, in order to appraise e-learning-services and formats. A key factor for e-learning, therefore, will be a concise quality orientation which spans all processes and puts learners first. Learners' (professional) development is at stake – regardless of formal or informal environments (Ehlers & Pawlowski, 2006).

In conclusion, quality in e-learning brings together the fields of education, technology and economy. Multiple e-learning standards are needed due to the diversity of quality requirements in the healthcare domain (ex.: in the education of healthcare professionals).

E-Learning and Virtual Learning Communities (VLCs) in the Healthcare Domain

Virtual learning communities (VLCs) combine the flexibility of distance education with the modern psycho-pedagogical learning model, namely collaborative learning (Figure 4). They employ ICT in order to create knowledge and spread it to the community through collaboration. Their main objectives comprise: delivery of education, question resolution and exchange of views and beliefs. The importance of each objective varies depending on the specific needs of each learning community in terms of professional, social and educational development. Traditionally, the members of a VLC have an identity and follow specific ethics. In the case of healthcare VLCs, they comprise of professionals, researchers, companies, patients and care givers, who try to improve their knowledge, answer everyday medical issues and require consultation. Although, identification of each individual member is a requirement for validating the quality of consultation, the protection of individual's sensitive information is also of greater importance. This results in a trade-off between virtual and real personality for the different community members. According to their role in the community, members of a VLC should reveal (e.g. doctors) or conceal (e.g. patients) parts of their identities, as explained in the following subsection.

Figure 4. Virtual learning community (Source: Apostolakis et al., 2008)

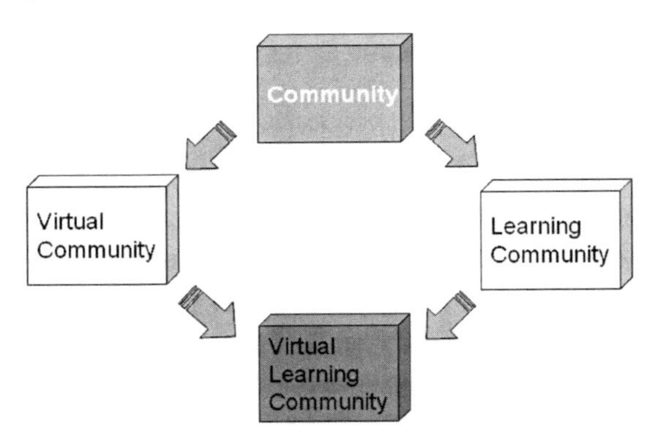

Although healthcare VLCs do not differ significantly from other communities, they still have several differences in the way they evaluate the educational assets and processes. In a VLC personal experiences, applied expertise and advises are the main assets of the community. The exchange and dissemination of good practices and knowledge is the main learning process, which broadens the circle of interest of the community and contributes to the community knowledge. A VLC develops freely and maintains the undiminished interest of its members.

In the case of a VLC for healthcare, the source of knowledge is of greater importance. The validity of information, the credibility of knowledge contributors and the freshness of knowledge are the three most important factors that help a VLC for healthcare to thrive. In order to increase control on the quality of the aforementioned assets, specific roles are defined in the community. The rights and obligations are subject to each member's role within the VLC. Depending on the level of accessibility to the community services the following roles can be defined for a VLC:

- **Administrator**
    - Has full access to the functions and configuration of the VLC, while is responsible for its smooth operation.

- **Tutor**
    - Organizes the learning process, collects and reorganizes the knowledge assets.
- **Moderator**
    - Manages the communication among the community members, corrects or deletes incorrect information and pinpoints the rules to the members.
- **Trainee**
    - Initiator: Often has the initiative to start a debate (conversation) and define the framework in which it will be conducted.
    - Facilitator: Offers solutions to problems and ensures that the conversations are not of topic.
    - Complicator: Highlights the weaknesses and shortcomings of the current debate and proposes alternative approaches.
    - Closer: Makes the final conclusions and closes the debate
    - Passive User: Monitors the discussion and operates passively
- **Visitor**
    - Navigates in the virtual environment without showing an identity.

In the case of a healthcare VLC, several extra roles are defined in order to guarantee the quality of content and processes and evaluate the results of each learning process.

As stated (Papadopoulou et al., 2007), virtual learning communities are emerging every day in many health related domains. They are divided in 4 groups based on the objectives of their members. Virtual health care delivery teams, in which health care providers of different disciplines (such as physicians, nurses, social workers, physical therapists, etc.) create a team to combine their knowledge and expertise in order to provide a comprehensive plan of care (Demiris, 2006). As an example, virtual medical teams for the continuous treatment of home care patients are developed (Pitsillides et al., 2004). The second type of health care communities is the virtual research teams, where health care researchers and professionals meet using new ICT technologies in order to communicate and exchange information. As an example we can refer to The Virtual Radiopharmacy (VirRAD) (ViRAD, 2007) developed in the framework of an eLearning program. Afterwards there is the virtual disease management, which aims at enhancing the care plan and the provider-patient relationship while emphasizing prevention of deterioration and complications using evidence –based practice guidelines. As an example we can refer to the home asthma telemonitoring (HAT) system (Finkelstein et al., 2001). Finally, there are support groups (Eysenbach et al., 2004), where people with interests gather "virtually" to share experiences, ask questions, or provide emotional support and self help. As of April 2004, Yahoo Groups listed at least 25.000 electronic support groups in health and wellness sections.

EVALUATION OF E-LEARNING

Several methodologies have been proposed in the past for the evaluation of e-Learning activities. However, none of them focused on virtual learning communities. Moreover, most of the existing methodologies are mainly guidelines for the evaluation process or the criteria composition and do not provide specific evaluation criteria.

Indicatively, some evaluation models are reported below:

- Embedding Learning Technologies Institutionally (ELTI) (Deepwell, 2007)
- MIT90 (Morton & Michael, 1991)
- Methodology of the Observatory on Borderless Higher Education (OBHE, 2008)
- Pick&Mix (Bacsich, 2005)

- E-Learning Maturity Model (eMM) (Marshall & Mitchell, 2007)

As far as the evaluation of e-health is concerned, several models have been proposed in the past, such as the model for the certification of the health related websites, which was introduced in Bakavos & Apostolakis (2007). That model concerned certification of e-health services provided over a network of health participants and mainly aimed to improve protection of citizen.

Finally, influenced by the e-Learning Maturity Model, Athanasiou et al (2008) have proposed some evaluation criteria for the evaluation of VLCs, which mainly focus on the effectiveness of learning process. Those criteria dealt with: (a) detailed description of the knowledge domain, (b) improvement of interaction between members, (c) emphasis on the pedagogical approach of the learning process and (d) self-evaluation of the VLC.

Standards have been around in education and training for decades. They are used by institutions and governments to ensure that learning is predictable, fair, consistent, and economic and achieves at least a minimum level of quality acceptable to society. These are laudable goals for any organization; however in the world of education, standards are sometimes interpreted by the teaching staff as an attempt to limit their creativity, freedom and ability. After all, we cannot treat the education of children in a school the same way we treat the production of cars in a factory (Holmes, 2006).

The debate on standards has become even more fraught with the introduction of ICT, which has added a technological dimension to learning. So it is best for us to separate right from the beginning the discussion on educational standards from the one on technical standards. Discussion on the former, as already mentioned, has been continuing for decades and is becoming even more difficult as we aim to compare and contrast the different educational policies at a European level. However, it remains a fundamental question associated with education and training, and in this context e-learning and the use of ICT is just a side issue. With the latter (technical standards), the situation is quite different. There is an appreciation that if the technology is to work and to become transparent in the learning process, then we must have international standards.

The European Commission has been supporting Europe's involvement in the development of global technical standards for e-learning for many years. Through the Information Society Technologies (IST) Programme, for example, with the ARIADNE project. Through the e-learning Initiative and the EQO project (EQO, 2004; Holmes, 2006). Most importantly, through support for the CEN's working group on learning technologies.

Standards for Quality and for e-learning have been discussed in the last decade: On the one hand, cost-reduction, secure investments, and new market potentials are expected. On the other hand, there is the fear of limitations for innovative solutions. Standards are often misunderstood, especially in the education community. They are perceived as restricting flexibility or creativity or huge additional effort. However, new generations of quality standards provide only a basic framework and help organizations to develop quality systems according to their particular requirements. In the same way, learning technology standards provide descriptive specifications to develop interoperable solutions. A variety of standards has been developed and adopted for different contexts and have improved the flexibility and effectiveness of e-learning. The following figure (Figure 5) shows a classification for standards in the field of learning, education, and training (Ehlers & Pawlowski, 2006; Pawlowski, 2006).

Existing Models for Content Quality, the IMS Learning Design and the DIN Didactical Object Model

Only a few interoperability standards try to capture the learning scenario within a framework, which enables instructional designers to propose

Figure 5. Standards' classification (Source: Pawlowski, 2006)

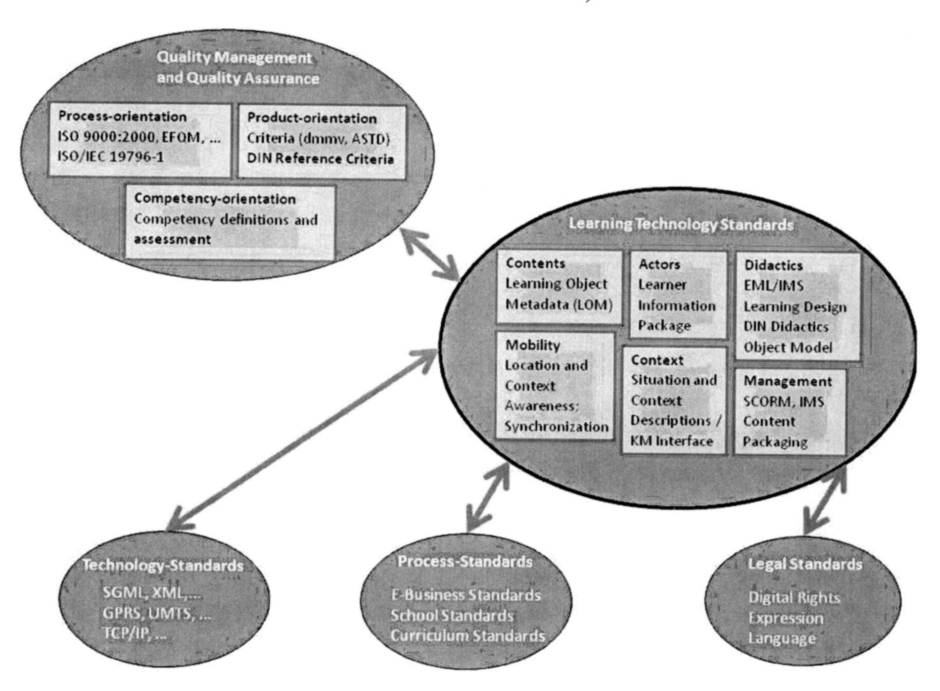

a comprehensive plan of such a learning flow as a teaching-learning-process. The term "Educational Interoperability Standards" is used for those standards (various specifications). Sometimes they are referred to as "Educational Modeling Languages" – in short EML (Klebl, 2006; Ehlers & Pawlowski, 2006).

A learning scenario is a social setting dedicated to learning, education or training. It is a process of interaction between people in a specific learning situation using resources for learning within a designed environment. People in the role of learners perform activities directed towards learning objectives using resources for learning. Learners may work on their own or in a group of learners. They may be supported by teaching staff.

The core concepts of IMS-LD and DIN-DOM (DIN, 2005) starting from objectives and scope of both specifications are presented in this section. The specifications themselves consist of documents which describe context, conceptual model, information model as well as examples and description of best-practice. For further reading, some summarizing articles can be recommended. The "Designer's Guide" gives an excellent introduction to IMS Learning Design (Koper et al., 2003). An overview can also be found at (Olivier & Tattersall, 2005). For both specifications, the information model itself is provided as a binding in XML. This binding (in both cases implemented as XML-schema) can be used to create plans for units of study which are compatible to the particular specification. Both documents and XML-schema files are available on the web.

Objectives and Scope of IMS Learning Design

The specification IMS Learning Design starts with a very comprehensive objective:

The objective of the Learning Design Specification is to provide a containment framework of elements that can describe any design of a teaching-learning process in a formal way (Koper et al., 2003).

Given this rather extensive objective for the specification of IMS Learning Design, eight more specific goals come from this broad objective (Klebl, 2006):

- "Completeness"
- "Pedagogical Flexibility": explains the notion of support for a wide variety of approaches to learning.
- "Personalization": emphasizes adaptability within learning scenarios for the individual learner.
- "Formalization", "Reproducibility", "Interoperability", "Compatibility" and "Reusability": denote essential organizational and technical requirements for reuse, exchange and trade of plans for learning scenarios.

Objectives and Scope of DIN Didactical Object Model

The main objective of DIN Didactical Object Model is to support exchange, comparability and transparency of instructional concepts, learning scenarios and teaching-learning methods in different areas (DIN, 2005). In order to achieve this, elements of a learning scenario have to be described within unifying and understandable categories for different actors in both the instructional design process and the learning scenario itself. Two aspects of the intended use are differentiated (DIN, 2005):

- Instructional designers as well as teaching persons may use the DIN-DOM for designing, operating and evaluating learning scenarios.
- Teaching persons as well as persons responsible for educational and training matters may use the clear description conformance to the DIN-DOM for decisions of use and choice according to educational intentions and situational needs.

As stated above, the specification DIN-DOM relates explicitly to IMS Learning Design. Therefore, objectives and goals of IMS Learning Design are not repeated. Instead, the relations to instructional design processes and decisions are accentuated (Klebl, 2006; Ravitch, 1995).

Interoperability Standards and Quality

There is an indirect relation between Educational Interoperability Standards and Educational Quality. Some aspects of this indirect relationship can be stated as follows (Klebl, 2006):

- **Integrated learning scenarios:** An Educational Interoperability Standard provides a differentiated and comprehensive framework for designing and operating integrated learning scenarios. Learner activities, interaction within a group of learners and different supporting roles of teaching staff like tutoring, coaching and informing are taken into account within the description of a learning scenario. Following the premise that the named aspects enhance learning, as the contemporary discussion on learner-centered approaches like situated learning and social-constructivist learning suggest, one can hardly deny that Educational Interoperability Standards contribute to the quality in computer supported learning scenarios.
- **Broader range of methods for teaching and learning:** An Educational Interoperability Standard enables the integration of one or more instructional designs in a learning scenario, e.g. problem-oriented-learning, collaborative learning, project method. Within a pedagogi-

cal meta-model, a formal description of a teaching-learning-process is largely open to different approaches towards teaching and learning. Hence, an increase in the variety of methods for teaching and learning can be expected. This leads to a variety of methods for the learner, in elaborated cases up to the adaptive selection of learning methods according to individual learning preferences.

- **Learner's competence in learning:** If learning methods in a learning unit are described as an outcome of instruction design, it can be useful to represent the learning methods to the learner in the graphical user interface. A learner, informed about the process of teaching and learning, will probably acquire knowledge about his or her own learning process. This knowledge can be thought of as meta-cognition which leads to the development of learning skills.
- **Free market economy for educational services and products:** Since Educational Interoperability Standards promote the transparency for teaching-learning processes within the instructional design process, they support the comparison of services and products in an educational market. In an idealized free market, the possibility to compare educational services and products will lead to innovation and quality.
- **Quality management:** An Educational Interoperability Standard serves as a standardized instrument within instructional design processes to document educational concepts, pedagogical models and lesson plans. Hence, an Educational Interoperability Standard is an indispensable device for quality management. Instructional design processes are managed according to reference processes in order to continuously create high quality outcomes.
- **Best practice sharing:** The ability to describe a formalized and standardized learning scenario allows reuse and sharing of successful approaches to teaching and training. Regardless whether reuse, exchange and sharing is done cooperatively, e.g. between colleagues in an educational institution or commercially, e.g. from educational content providers to educational institutions, approved concepts or separate learning scenarios can spread more easily (Liber, 2002).

The Quality Standard for E-Learning ISO/IEC 19796-1

The Quality Standard ISO/IEC 19796-1 is the basic framework, which has been employed for quality development and for the description of quality approaches (Pawlowski, 2006). It comprises several Quality Management and Quality Assurance Standards for e-learning and defines how they can be employed in organizations. Although, many organizations have adapted general standards like ISO 9000:2000 or the EFMQ Excellence Model, the ISO/IEC 19796-1 standard has gained attention since it provides a "reference framework for the description of quality approaches" (RFDQ) (ISO/IEC, 2005). It indicates the aspects that should be covered and assists organizations to find the most appropriate solutions for each aspect. It can be thus used as an instrument to develop the quality in the field of e-learning.

The ISO/IEC 19796-1 standard consists of three parts:

- A description scheme for quality approaches
- A process model as a reference classification
- Reference Criteria for evaluation

It assumes that each organization defines its "Quality profile" first, which comprises of objectives, methods, relations, people to be involved etc. and consequently adapts this profile to the running needs and requirements. Since it does not provide specific requirements or rules – given that it is a framework – its role is to guide actors through the process of quality development in the field of e-learning (Pawlowski, 2006).

Consequently, it requires the definition of the "Description Model" a scheme that describes quality approaches (guidelines, design guides, requirements etc), and documents all quality concepts in a transparent way. Based on the CEN/ISSS CWA 14644 (CEN/ISSS, 2003; CEN/ISSS, 2005), the "Description Model" serves as a base for building a harmonized scheme for describing quality approaches.

Then it demands the definition of the "Process Model", which includes the relevant processes within the life-cycle of information and communication systems for learning, education, and training. The model is divided in seven parts, which map the different steps of developing learning scenarios (ISO/IEC, 2005; Pawlowski, 2006).

Finally, ISO/IEC 19796-1 enlists several reference criteria (media, data security, law and ethics, learning psychology related etc.) for the assurance of quality of learning products in a comprehensive criteria catalogue.

Pedagogical Evaluation of Learning Content

A realistic example of evaluating the learning content, assuring quality, is the Peer Evaluation of the Learning Object Pedagogical Quality in the Virtual Polytechnic (Leppisaari & Vainio, 2007). According to that study, 50 production teams, comprising 450 teachers from the Finnish Virtual Polytechnic designed several learning objects for different subject areas and different learning scenarios. The learning content produced by each team were peer evaluated by other teams on a regular basis, via face-to-face meetings between team coordinators and representatives, thus strengthening the role of collegial evaluation in the content evaluation process (Leppisari & Vainio, 2007).

The peer evaluation pairs came from the same educational field, which included social sciences, business and administration, business information management and information technology, culture, social services, health and sports. The evaluation was performed on the overall work of the team in the e-Production and Moodle environments. The electronic evaluation form was mainly focused on the pedagogical quality assessment of the designed learning objects and courses.

The complete evaluation framework, studied in Leppisaari and Vainio (2007) apart from the quality of content, aimed to assess its reusability in different contexts (Holmes & Gardner, 2006). As a result, learning objects were designed using basic 'learning material segments', which can be used in different learning processes and at different stages of the learning process. They were relatively atomic and separate entities, thus facilitating reusability. Compared to traditional online material, the use of learning objects offered greater possibilities to tutors and to the educational applications they employed.

Different quality assessment models, quality criteria and assessment tools, for example, MERLOT (www.merlot.org), a peer-review process model, and LORI, Learning Object Review Instrument (Haughey & Muirhead, 2005; Nesbit et al., 2002), have been constructed to evaluate the quality of learning objects. In the peer evaluation model introduced in Leppisaari & Vainio (2007), authors employed pedagogical quality evaluation criteria especially designed for the polytechnic content production context. The pedagogical quality in this context mainly targeted to the applicability of the material for teaching and learning and the support of the professional expert development process. The evaluation process tested whether the structure of learning objects facilitates the construction of a meaningful learning process and meets the polytechnic education quality standards. In these terms, reviewers asked for authentic, objective oriented and support construction of knowledge (Leppisaari et al., 2006a, Leppisaari & Vainio, 2006b).

The aim of most related educational content evaluation frameworks is to investigate how learning objects promote a learner's learning process, in terms of authenticity, intentionality and knowledge construction. This can be achieved by testing whether the content and activities: (a) push the learner in learning situations, (b) support the learner's conscious and objective-oriented knowledge construction, (c) support construction of knowledge. These three factors are further discussed in the following.

- **Authenticity**

The main requirement for authentic learning is an environment that offers learners the opportunity to deploy work practices, methods, cognitive processes and authentic sources and materials in real-life situations (Oliver et al., 2006; Bennett et al., 2002). Meaningful learning can be promoted through educational activities that require the combination of acquired knowledge and skills in unexpected problems.

- **Intentionality**

Intentionality refers to the direct linking of the learning content, activities to the students' goals, and personal objectives. Careful examination and prioritization of goals is necessary to build an intentional learning. On the other hand, the flexibility of content and activities, will allow tutors to develop customizable solutions to each individual needs. Although, the learner's behavior is guided by his/her own intentions and not by any external agent, a flexible content structure will allow adaptation to everyday needs and realistic problems that the learner considers important to solve (Jonassen et al., 1999; Tirri & Nevgi, 2000; Ally, 2004).

- **Knowledge Construction**

According to constructivists, learning is a process of knowledge construction in which the learner has an active role and learning is based on his/her cognitive activity. An individual builds new knowledge on the basis of previous knowledge, based on his/her own initiative and actions, in interaction with the surrounding environment (Tirri & Nevgi, 2000; Ally, 2004; Hakkarainen et al., 2004).

The peer evaluation model and the flexibility provided by learning objects form an ideal base for the evaluation of learning in the virtual learning environment.

Pedagogical Evaluation of the Learning Process

The evaluation of the learning process was correctly proposed, by going from the quality of e-Learning to eQuality of learning (Ravet, 2007). This work, instead of using traditional methods to evaluate the new status, aimed to advance the reflection on how technologies can contribute to the improvement of quality of learning. Its broad scope encompassed all processes linked to learning: formal and informal, face to face and at a distance, initial and continuous, individual and organizational learning and suggested how technologies can be employed to support these processes using different levels, which range from pedagogy to administration and infrastructures.

The work of Ravet, raised several questions that need to be answered when evaluating the processes of a virtual learning community. First, we should check whether industrial models of quality can be applied to the knowledge economy or we would rather reinvent new ones. Then we should reposition the role of technologies in quality processes, from simple companions of the process to radical reformers and distinguish between domains where new technologies are being assimilated by old quality systems and others for quality systems are accommodated (transformed) to exploit the full potential of new technologies. In this direction we should study whether innovative social practices can be applied in the evaluation process. Moreover, we should clarify the similarities and differences between learning technologies and training technologies and form quality assessment respectively. Finally, we should think of the consequences in moving from the quality of learning, to quality as learning.

To open this discussion and invite the reflections of learning and quality practitioners, the European Foundation for Quality in E-Learning has decided to publish a Green Paper on eQuality (Ravet, 2007), which proposed to shift the focus from the quality of eLearning to eQuality as learning, i.e. reflect on how digital technologies could provide support for improving all forms of learning – instruction and training, face to face, at a distance, or mixed, formal and informal, personal and organizational – making the quality process itself a personal and organizational experience. Taking this one step further, we suggest an evaluation model which capitalizes on the structure of the educational community and can be ideally applied in VLCs.

Quality Assessment in Self Supportive Healthcare Communities

In this subsection, we provide a brief description of a virtual community for healthcare as a basis for our suggestion for a community-based evaluation model, which can be applied on the VLC. In a community for healthcare three distinct roles are assumed: (a) Care providers, the professional members of the community, i.e. doctors and nurses, who advice, treat and support the community members as part of their work, (b) Care givers, the friends or family of the member who voluntarily participate in order to receive guidance or provide support to other members and (c) Care consumers or "receivers", the patients. They need medical help and ask for it either directly or indirectly. Several categories of patients need special and continuous care, especially patients with uncured diseases, who are in need of psychological support all the time. It is also important for patients to discuss their issues with other patients and receive useful advices and support.

The above structure contains huge potential which can be exploited in favor of the community members (Varlamis & Apostolakis, 2007). The main notion behind communities is that they enforce collaboration of individuals and behind self supportive communities, is that expert members (i.e. researchers and scientists) are able to disseminate their findings and guide industry and practitioners in favor of patients. Volunteers can exchange information and useful hints concerning patient caring and support while patients or members with disabilities can disseminate their practical knowledge and provide psychological support to other patients.

The heart of a healthcare VLCs is a Web-based portal where members can access the full range of knowledge resources, maintain member-to-member networking groups, share professional practice solutions, and conduct association business. A virtual community builds over a web-based portal, and allows distant and continuous membership (Leimeister et al., 2004). In such communities, members demand better support in terms of quality, quantity and efficiency. On the other side, the intrinsic need of patients to help co-patients, of doctors to help their colleagues and of associations to work in common can help the community to be self-supported and do not seek for external assistance. In order to improve the quality of content and processes, the VLC should maintain the history of all the actions in the community. This information is very useful for doctors and researchers, who have direct access to their patients profile and history of discussions, but also to the evaluators of the educational outcome.

Quality Improvement Using the Supportive Structures

The outcome of the e-learning process is of critical importance in the healthcare domain. In order to enhance and maintain its quality, the e-learning process has to be described in a way that is standard and comparable with other e-learning processes. As different roles mean different goals, we view them as different communities. Some roles participate in a community but not in the entire community, thus simplifying the description of the whole e-learning process.

Each community does not necessarily follow a collaborative e-learning process or an e-learning process at all (e.g. blended learning). Similarly, it can have a quality assessment plan or not. In contrast to what mentioned above, several communities are not necessarily self-supportive, but they have the ability to evaluate the learning process of another community (Ravet, 2007).

The idea of combining evaluation results from other communities in order to achieve improved overall quality and reliability through supportive structures lies in the fact of analyzing an e-learning process by separating it into two or more layers. On the first layer, there are several communities and each one of them has a different responsibility (role). These communities are the subjects of the evaluation process, and are going to be evaluated by other communities (evaluation community partners) in the upper layer (see Figure 6). The upper layer is concerned (only) with the coordination, cooperation and support between these communities. The sum of all the aforementioned layers could form a bigger community, in which the sub-communities have their specific role. The above proposed point of view is presented analytically in the figure below (Figure 6):

As shown in the above figure, there may be more than one layer, which not only work autonomously, but interoperate with each other in order to achieve certain goals. The bottom layer includes the sub-communities, which are needed for the description of the whole (big) community. In the middle layer several sub-communities collaborate on performing the evaluation of the learning content and/or of the learning process. Their functionality, in a high level of abstraction, is similar to the evaluation process that used peer evaluators, as suggested in Leppisaari and Vainio (2007). Finally, the top layer comprises sub-communities which are responsible for the co-operation, co-ordination and support of all underlying sub-communities. The gain from this multi-tiered structure is that the whole community achieves self-evaluation and self-support, along with complete collaboration and interoperability.

There are many benefits of such a learning process. First of all, combining the benefits of collaborative learning a better learning outcome is achieved. Secondly, by self-evaluation, the learning content and processes become better and better. As a result, their quality improves, focusing on better pedagogical approaches, which ensures the reliability of the whole learning process. Furthermore, the layer which is responsible for co-operation and support offers smooth interoperability and collaboration, which enhances the above benefits.

FUTURE RESEARCH DIRECTIONS

The chapter provides a set of e-learning standards, a reference framework for the description of quality approaches, and explains how an e-learning process can be implemented based on pedagogical standards. The novelty is the combination of benefits of evaluation for improving quality, self-support and collaboration in learning and the full exploitation of them by the separation of the whole learning process in layers.

However, further research should be done on the implementation of layers in big communities in order to find and correct potential drawbacks in practice. Additionally, as e-Learning does not

Figure 6. Proposed point of view for improving quality

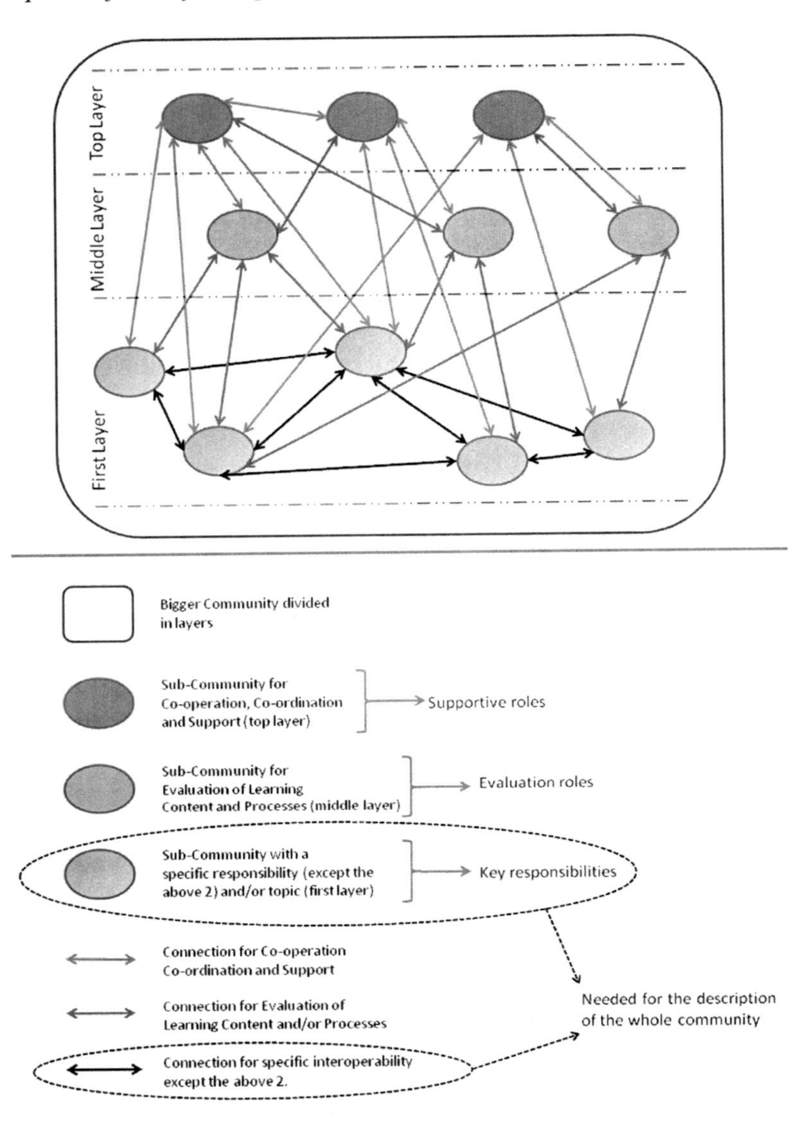

seem to entirely replace traditional learning, in the near future, the idea of Blended Learning will prevail in Learning Procedures and VLCs (Blended-VLCs). Therefore, the above mentioned layer-based approach for Blended-VLCs requires more research.

CONCLUSION

The outcome of the e-learning process is of critical importance to the health-care domain. In order to enhance and maintain its quality, the e-learning process has to be described in a way that is standard and comparable with other e-learning processes. As different groups of community members (roles) have different goals, each subgroup can be seen as different communities. Some roles participate in a community but not in the whole community, thus simplifying the description of the whole e-learning process. Each community does not necessarily follow a collaborative e-learning process or an e-learning process at all. The most common paradigm is blended learning. Additionally, each community is not necessarily self-supportive but one specific community may evaluate the learning process of another specific community, following the peer evaluation model. The idea of combining content evaluation for quality, process evaluation for quality and self-support helps on achieving improved overall quality and reliability. The supportive structures, allow focusing on better pedagogical standards.

Changes in health-care delivery and advances in medicine require the continuous training of all participants. The complexity and breadth of medical education content, together with the scarcity of experts, make the adoption of e-learning a realistic proposition. Part of the quality of a health-care system is the quality of the adopted e-learning process.

REFERENCES

Ally, M. (2004). Foundations of Educational Theory for Online Learning. In Anderson T. & Elloumi F. (Eds.), *Theory and Practice of Online Learning.* Athabasca University. Retrieved January 30, 2009 from http://cde.athabascau.ca/online_book/.

Apostolakis, I., Varlamis, I., & Papadopoulou, A. (2008). *Virtual learning communities*. Athens: Papazisis Publishers.

Athanasiou, G. S., Maris, N. I., & Apostolakis, I. A. (2008). Evaluation of Virtual Learing Communities for Supporting e-Learing in Health Care Domain. In *Proceedings of 6th ICICTH* (pp 287-293), Samos, Greece.

Bacsich, P. (2005). *Benchmarks for e-learning in UK HE - adaptation of existing good practice.* Presented at the e-Learning workshop of the Association for Learning Technology Conference. Retrieved September 10, 2009 from http://www.matic-media.co.uk/pubsandpres-2005.htm.

Bakavos, I., & Apostolakis, I. (2007). *Model of the certification procedure for internet health related websites*. In Proceedings of 5th ICICTH (pp 164-169), Samos, Greece.

Bennett, S., Harper, B., & Hedberg, J. (2002). Designing real life cases to support authentic design activities. *Australian Journal of Educational Technology*, *18*(1), 1–12.

Bernard, R., Abrami, P. L., Lou, Y., & Borokhovski, E. (2004). How does distance education compare with classroom instruction? A meta-analysis of the empirical literature. *Review of Educational Research*, *74*, 379–439. doi:10.3102/00346543074003379

CEN/ISSS. (2003). *Workshop Learning Technologies. Quality Assurance Standards*. Brussels: CEN.

CEN/ISSS. (2005). *Learning Technologies Workshop, Project Team "Accessibility properties for Learning Resources"*. Retrieved January 25, 2009 from http://www2.ni.din.de/sixcms/detail.php?id=5984.

Chumley-Jones, H. S., Dobbie, A., & Alford, C. L. (2002). Web-based learning: sound educational method or hype? A review of the evaluation literature. *Academic Medicine*, *77*(10suppl), S86–S93. doi:10.1097/00001888-200210001-00028

Deepwell, F. (2007). Embedding Quality in e-Learning Implementation through Evaluation. *Journal of Educational Technology & Society*, *10*(2), 34–43.

Demiris, G. (2006). The diffusion of virtual communities in health care: Concept and challenges. *Patient Education and Counseling*, *62*(2), 178–188. doi:10.1016/j.pec.2005.10.003

DIN. (2005). Deutsches Institut für Normung e.V. (ed.). *e-Learning. Qualitätssicherung und Qualitätsmanagement im e-Learning*. Berlin: Beuth.

Donabedian, A. (1982). *Explorations in Quality Assessment and Monitoring*. Chicago: Health Administration Press.

Ehlers, U. D. (2003a). Quality in E-Learning – The Learner as a key quality assurance category. *Vocational Training European Journal, 2003/II*.

Ehlers, U. D. (2003b). *Qualität beim E-Learning*. Retrieved January 15, 2009 from http://www.lernqualitaet.de/qualität ehlers.pdf (15/1/2009).

Ehlers, U. D., & Pawlowski, J. M. (2006). Quality in European e-learning: An introduction . In Ehlers, U.-D., & Pawlowski, J. M. (Eds.), *Handbook on Quality and Standardization in E-Learning* (pp. 1–8). New York: Springer-Verlag. doi:10.1007/3-540-32788-6_1

EQO. (2004). French-European workshop. *Comparing Quality models adequacy to the needs of clients in e-learning*. Retrieved January 15, 2009 from http://www.eqo.info/?fuseaction=news.extraspecial_062004

Contribution to the implementation of relevant Quality approaches in the European Higher Education Retrieved January 15, 2009 from http://www.enpc.fr/fr/formations/ecole_virt/nte/rencontresGEVP/index.htm

Eysenbach, G., Powell, J., Englesakis, M., Rizo, C., & Stern, A. (2004). Health related virtual communities and electronic support group: systematic review of the effects of online peer to peer interactions. *British Medical Journal*, *328*, 1166–1172. doi:10.1136/bmj.328.7449.1166

Finkelstein, J., O'Connor, G., & Friedmann, R. H. (2001). Development and Implementation of the home asthma telemonitoring (HAT) system to facilitate asthma self-care. *Studies in Health Technology and Informatics*, *84*, 810–814.

Gibbons, A., & Fairweather, P. (2000). Computer-based instruction. In Tobias, S., Fletcher, J. (Eds), *Training & Retraining: A Handbook for Business, Industry, Government, and the Military* (pp 410-422). New York: Macmillan.

Hakkarainen, K., Palonen, T., Paavola, S., & Lehtinen, E. (2004). *Communities of Networked Expertise*. Amsterdam: Elsevier.

Harvey, L., & Green, D. (2000). Qualität definieren. Fünf unterschiedliche Ansätze. *Zeitschrift fur Padagogik*, *41*, 17–39.

Haughey, M., & Muirhead, B. (2005). The pedagogical and multimedia designs of learning objects for schools. *Australasian Journal of Educational Technology*, *21*(4), 470–490.

Holmes, B. (2006). Quality in a Europe of diverse systems and shared goals . In Ehlers, U. D., & Pawlowski, J. M. (Eds.), *Handbook on Quality and Standardization in E-Learning* (pp. 15–28). New York: Springer-Verlag. doi:10.1007/3-540-32788-6_2

Holmes, B., & Gardner, J. (2006). *E-Learning. Concepts and practice*. London: Sage Publications.

ISO/IEC. (2005). *Technical report about proposed standards concerning Participant Information data models*. Retrieved from http://jtc1sc36.org/doc/36N0965.pdf

Johnson, C. E., Hurtubise, L. C., & Castrop, J. (2004). Learning management systems: technology to measure the medical knowledge competency of the ACGME. *Medical Education*, *38*, 599–608. doi:10.1111/j.1365-2929.2004.01792.x

Jonassen, D. H., Peck, K., & Wilson, B. G. (1999). *Learning with Technology: A Constructivist Perspective*. Merril: Prentice-Hall.

Klebl, M. (2006). Educational interoperability standards: IMS learning design and DIN didactical object model . In Ehlers, U.-D., & Pawlowski, J. M. (Eds.), *Handbook on Quality and Standardization in e-Learning* (pp. 225–250). New York: Springer-Verlag. doi:10.1007/3-540-32788-6_16

Komis, V. (2006). *Introduction to education of information technology*. Athens: Kleidarithmos Publishers.

Koper, R., Olivier, B., & Anderson, T. (2003). *IMS Learning Design Information Model*. Retrieved January 25, 2009 from http://www.imsglobal.org/learningdesign/ldv1p0/imsld_infov1p0.html.

Leimeister, J. M., Daum, M., & Krcmar, H. (2004). Towards mobile communities for cancer patients: the case of krebsgemeinschaft.de. [IJWBC]. *International Journal of Web Based Communities*, *1*, 1–9.

Leppisaari, I., Silander, P., & Vainio, L. (2006a). Autenttisuus ammattikorkeakoulun virtuaaliopetuksen haasteena. In M. Ylikarjula (Ed.) *Ihmettelya ja oppimista tutkimuksen aarella*: Opettaja oman tyonsa tutkijana –symposiumin III artikkelit (pp. 17-36). Keski-Pohjanmaan ammattikorkeakoulun julkaisuja.

Leppisaari, I., & Vainio, L. (2006b). *Online mentoring - to Developing Teachers' Online Pedagogy Expertise in Content Producing Teams*. In C.M. Crawford (Ed.), *Proceedings 17th International Conference of Society for Information Technology and Teacher Education* (pp. 2314-2321), Orlando, Florida.

Leppisaari, I., & Vainio, L. (2007). Teachers as Peer Evaluators of Learning Object Pedagogical Quality in the Virtual Polytechnic. In *Proceedings of Educause Australasia*, Melbourne, Australia. Retrieved January 10, 2009 from http://www.caudit.edu.au/educauseaustralasia07/papers/Teachers%20as%20Peer%20Evaluators%20of%20Learning.pdf.

Letterie, G. S. (2003). Medical education as a science: the quality of evidence for computer-assisted instruction. *American Journal of Obstetrics and Gynecology*, *188*, 849–853. doi:10.1067/mob.2003.168

Liber, O. (2002). The revolutionary possibilities of eLearning standards . In Bachmann, G., Haefeli, O., & Kindt, M. (Eds.), *Die Virtuelle Hochschule in der Konsolidierungsphase* (pp. 197–208). Münster, New York, München, Berlin: Waxmann.

Marshall, S. J., & Mitchell, G. (2007). *Benchmarking International E-learning Capability with the E-Learning Maturity Model*. In Proceedings of EDUCAUSE Australasia, Melbourne, Australia. Retrieved January 10, 2009 from http://www.caudit.edu.au/educauseaustralasia07/authors_papers/Marshall-103.pdf.

Moberg, T. F., & Whitcomb, M. E. (1999). Educational technology to facilitate medical students' learning: background paper 2 of the medical school objectives project. *Academic Medicine*, *74*, 1146–1150. doi:10.1097/00001888-199910000-00020

Morton, S., & Michael, S. (1991). *The Corporation of the 1990s: Information Technology and Organizational Transformation*. New York: Oxford University Press.

Negroponte, N. (1996). *Being digital*. New York: Random House.

Nesbit, J., Belfer, K., & Vargo, J. (2002). A Convergent Participation Model for Evaluation of Learning Objects. *Canadian Journal of Learning and Technology 28(3)*. Retrieved January 20, 2009 from http://www.cjlt.ca/index.php/cjlt/issue/view/11

OBHE (Observatory on Borderless Higher Education). (2008), Retrieved January 20, 2009 from http://www.obhe.ac.uk.

Oliver, R., Herrington, J., & Reeves, T. C. (2006). Creating authentic learning environments through blended learning approaches . In Bonk, J., & Graham, C. R. (Eds.), *The handbook of blended learning* (pp. 502–515). San Francisco: Pleiffer.

Olivier, B., & Tattersall, C. (2005). The Learning Design Specification . In Koper, R., & Tattersall, C. (Eds.), *Learning Design. A Handbook on Modeling and Delivering Networked Education and Training* (pp. 21–40). Berlin, Heidelberg, New York: Springer.

Papadopoulou, A., Varlamis, I., & Apostolakis, I. (2007). Models and Practices for the development of e-learning communities in healthcare. In proceedings of the 5th ICICTH (pp. 170–174). Greece: Samos.

Pawlowski, J. M. (2006). Adopting quality standards for education and e-learning. In U.-D. Ehlers & J. M. Pawlowski (Eds.), Handbook on Quality and Standardization in E-Learning (pp. 65–77). New York: Springer-Verlag. doi:10.1007/3-540-32788-6_5doi:10.1007/3-540-32788-6_5

Piemme, T. E. (1988). Computer-assisted learning and evaluation in medicine. Journal of the American Medical Association, 260, 367–372. PubMed doi:10.1001/jama.260.3.367doi:10.1001/jama.260.3.367

Pitsillides, A., Pitsillides, B., Samaras, G., Dikaikos, M., Christodoulou, E., Andreou, P., & Georgiadis, D. (2004). DITIS: A collaborative virtual medical team for home healthcare of cancer patients . In Istepanian, R., Laxminarayan, S., & Pattichis, C. (Eds.), *M-Health: emerging mobile health systems*. New York: Kluwer Academic/Plenum.

Ravet, S. (2007). *From quality of eLearning to eQuality of learning*. Retrieved September 22, 2009 from http://www.qualityfoundation.org/index.php?m1=2&m2=28&page_id=34.

Ravitch, D. (1995). *National standards in American education: A citizen's guide*. Washington: Brookings Institution Press.

Reddy, R., & Wladawsky-Berger, I. (co-chairs) (2001). *Transforming Health Care through Information Technology*. Arlington, VA: National Coordination Office for Information Technology Research & Development.

Rifkin, J. (2004). *The European Dream: How Europe's Vision of the Future is Quietly Eclipsing the American Dream*. Cambridge: Polity Press.

Tirri, K., & Nevgi, A. (2000). *In search of a Good Virtual Teacher*. Annual European Conference on Educational Research, Edinburgh, United Kingdom. Retrieved from http://www.eric.ed.gov/ERICDocs/data/ericdocs2sql/content_storage_01/0000019b/80/16/b6/9f.pdf

Varlamis, I., & Apostolakis, I. (2007). *Self supportive web communities in the service of patients*. In Proceecings of IADIS International Conference on Web Based Communities (pp 133-140). Salamanca, Spain.

VirRAD - The Virtual Radiopharmacy - a Mindful Learning Environment (2007). Retrieved from http://community.virrad.eu.org/.

Vygotsky, L. (1934). *Thought and language*. MIT Press.

Walker, R., Dieter, M., Panko, W., & Valenta, A. (2003). What it will take to create new Internet initiatives in health care. *Journal of Medical Systems*, *27*, 95–103. doi:10.1023/A:1021065330652

Ward, J. P., Gordon, J., Field, M. J., & Lehmann, H. P. (2001). Communication and information technology in medical education. *Lancet*, *357*, 792–796. doi:10.1016/S0140-6736(00)04173-8

Wentling, T., Waight, C., Gallaher, J., La Fleur, J., Wang, C., & Kanfer, A. (2000). *E-Learning: A Review of Literature.* University of Illinois National Center for Supercomputer Applications, Urbana- Champaign, IL Retrieved January 30, 2009 from http://learning.ncsa.uiuc.edu/papers/elearnlit.pdf.

Chapter 16
E-Health Communities for Learning Healthy Habits:
How to Consider Quality and Usability

Åsa Smedberg
Stockholm University, Sweden

ABSTRACT

There are e-health communities of many different kinds available on the Internet today. Some e-health communities are for people who need to change their established bad, or unhealthy, habits such as the ones for people suffering from overweight or smoking. To develop and maintain a healthier life-style is not an easy task to succeed with, it involves being able to change everyday situations. E-health communities can assist in this process through continuous interactions between community members. However, whether these e-health communities actively support learning depends on the ways they help community members reflect upon their habits, underlying reasons and motivational factors. In this chapter, the author presents a framework for how to evaluate these e-health communities from a learning perspective. The framework covers different types of conversation topics, ways to respond and community knowledge.

INTRODUCTION

E-health communities of different kinds are used on a daily basis by many people. The communities have different purposes depending on the type of subject they address. E-health communities for people with unhealthy behaviors, such as people suffering from overweight and obesity and people who find it hard to quit smoking, these communities need to be evaluated from a learning perspective. Both the conversations for learning purposes and the content of the advice and recommendations need to be evaluated. The main mission of this chapter is therefore to discuss learning aspects of e-health communities, and to lay out recommendations regarding what to measure in terms of conversational acts and content of posted issues. The ideas behind the presented framework have been empirically tested on e-health communities in Sweden and other European countries. The chapter includes references to results from these studies.

DOI: 10.4018/978-1-61692-843-8.ch016

BACKGROUND

The Internet has become much used by people who like to meet others who share similar interests. Web-based communities of different kinds have therefore become popular arenas. The definition of a traditional community is a place for groups and individuals to meet with others who share the same interests to cooperate and satisfy each other's needs. The web-based community becomes then a community that uses the Internet to mediate interaction between the groups and individuals who participate in the community. The web-based community should be able to support a sense of togetherness among the community members (Preece, 2000). Web-based communities can also be regarded as virtually social networks useful for empathetic support, information sharing and problem solving (Andrews, 2002).

One type of web-based communities is the one used by people who like to discuss health-related issues. This group of users has grown rapidly in number and constitutes a large and increasing group on the Internet today (Fox & Fallows, 2003). This growing interest for health-related issues on the Internet has led to patients as well as citizens getting more and more empowered (Fox, Ward & O'Rourke, 2005; Korp, 2006). The Internet and the more available health information and conversations on health issues have also brought empowerment to minority and marginalized groups in the society, such as elderly people (Loader, Hardey & Keeble, 2008) and black women in the United States (Mehra, Merkel & Bishop, 2004). The e-health communities are used on a daily basis by people with different physical and mental conditions. Among these e-health communities, there are also those for people who suffer from established bad, or unhealthy, habits, such as smoking or bad eating behavior, for example (Smedberg, 2004, 2008a). Through these e-health community systems, people are able to share experiences, learn together and give advice on how to cope with different health conditions. The communities let both strong and weak tie relations be developed (Haythornthwaite, 2006).

The great importance of these online systems is also mirrored in the development of national portals for health services. There are NHS Direct Online and Net Doctor sites, for example. Through these sites, the public can access health information sources and medical-trained people, and also patients and citizens with similar concerns who can share personal perspectives. The aim is to offer appropriate and even proactive health management for the general public (Milicevic, Gareis & Korte, 2005).

Studies have shown how patients who interact online with other patients benefit from this (Walther, Pingree, Hawkins & Buller, 2005). For example, chronically ill patients manage to cope with stressful life situations better when communicating online with other patients in so called self-help groups (Josefsson, 2007). The patients can then act both as consumers and producers of medical information. Different coping activities on the Internet include seeking information about illnesses, treatments, medicine, etc., and also looking for social support and advice from others. As a consequence, the patients can more easily find strength in their position to challenge the medical expertise.

However, there are studies that indicate differences in the way people act in e-health communities of different kinds, with different types of health issues being discussed. In a one-month long comparative study of two Usenet newsgroups on health issues, one addressing a mental disorder and one a life-threatening physical illness were compared (Burnett & Buerkle, 2004). The results showed that the conversations on the physical illness were almost without exception filled with compassion and support, while the conversations concerning the mental condition often were filled with flames and reflecting interpersonal conflicts. This relation between settings and effects on social life is studied in Social Informatics (Kling, 2000; Kling, 2001). The technology can be used in many ways and lead to many different social outcomes. It is not obvious or predetermined in what ways the technical system will affect the participants. Another discipline is the Community Informatics that deals with issues about the usage and effects of computer-mediated communities in particular (Bishop, Bruce & Jones, 2006; Loader & Keeble, 2004, e.g.). A characteristic of Community Informatics is that it emphasizes community building and social interactions enabled by the technology rather than the mediating technology itself, and the relationships between media and community development are the focus of the studies (Loader & Keeble, 2004).

LEARNING THROUGH E-HEALTH COMMUNITIES

Through e-health communities, interacting people can share and develop knowledge and understanding, practices and experiences together. However, learning together with others demands for attention and sensibility to one another. People who want to learn together must pay attention to one another's needs, and they have to ask for problem specific and personal information, for example. This is crucial for the community participants, in order for them to adjust advice and personal narratives to help each other (McDermott, 2000). The participants are able to look for concerns, ask questions and present ideas and counter-ideas when needed, by using language effectively. Examples of speech acts important in a conversation include requests, negotiations to clarify needs and concerns, promises, acts to meet concerns and acceptances (Austin, 1962; Medina-Mora, Winograd, Flores & Flores, 1992; Winograd & Flores, 1987).

Also having opposing ideas is useful for learning and for the evolvement of a community (Baker, Quignard, Lund & van Amelsvoort, 2002). There must be a combination between the competence of the community and experience of the world, i.e., between the standards of the community and the personal and diverse experiences from the outside of the community (Wenger, 2004). Learning takes place through the tension between competence of the community and our experiences. Consequently, to argue and to let different views be represented in conversations have therefore shown to be important for a balanced and supportive online group (Soller, 2001). In this context, to have opposing ideas is something useful for the learning situation of a community (Baker, Quignard, Lund & van Amelsvoort, 2002; Wenger, 2004). Also, strong tie relations need to be combined with weak tie relations (Haythornthwaite, 2007). Characteristics of strong ties are frequent communication, access to similar information, shared values and approaches, social and emotional support together with openness and self-disclosure. Weak ties, on the other hand, are characterized by less frequent communication between strangers or not so close friends or colleagues. Even though strong tie relations are important to enhance knowledge among the participants, also weak ties are needed in order to let the community experience new inputs in terms of different ideas and approaches.

When considering the effectiveness of communities in general, three different dimensions can be seen (Wenger, 2004). One is learning energy that includes identification of knowledge gaps and also definition of shared visions, the second one is social capital that includes events that aim to weave the community together and enhance the development of trust, and the third one is self-awareness of community participants as well as of the community as a whole, something that is developed through accumulated experiences and a reflective mode. When learning a new and healthy practice is concerned, the second dimension, social capital, can also play another role for the community. By having face-to-face meetings, such as work out exercises, cooking activities, and the like, these bonding activities can also play a role for developing practical skills in real life.

Learning Healthy Habits

Trying to learn new things and also trying to help others in their learning processes can be a challenge. This has been pointed out by many pedagogues and researchers. However, an even more delicate task to succeed in is to help each other reflect upon and change behavior such as a bad, or unhealthy, habit. Even though factual knowledge is needed, it is not enough if we cannot find a way to handle specific situations of our everyday life. Over the years, the difficulties regarding how to succeed in changing established bad habits have been discussed among medical professionals and in medical sciences. The question of how to get rid of bad eating habits and how to develop a healthier way of living in order to lose weight is one such difficulty. In fact, bad eating habits, too little exercising, and overweight and obesity as a consequence, has become a serious problem to many people (Timperio & Crawford, 2004). It is a problematic situation since unhealthy life-styles can lead to critical health conditions for the ones concerned. Therefore, changing the established bad habits is important in order to reduce the risks of getting severe illnesses later. Heart conditions, diabetes, asthma and lung conditions are examples of health implications of unhealthy life-styles. Preventive health care is therefore essential to stop people from becoming patients of the health care system. Different systematic approaches have been used, such as treatment programs for overweight and obese people. Unfortunately, it has turned out to be difficult to succeed with changing behaviors on a long-term basis; most of the ones with weight problems who have gone through treatment programs regain weight after finishing the program (Byrne, Cooper & Fairburn, 2004). There are different factors that inhibit successful weight loss, for example, a negative mood caused by dissatisfaction with the achieved weight, a tendency to judge self-worth in terms of weight and shape and an effort to reduce negative moods by eating without being hungry (Byrne, Cooper & Fairburn, 2004). Unhealthy eating behavior caused by negative moods is typical for eating disorders; while underweight people tend to eat less to cope with negative emotions, overweight people eat more (Geliebter & Aversa, 2003).

Accordingly, long-term impact is difficult to succeed with through traditional programs. The habits need to be challenged on an everyday basis and also positive emotions are important for the success. For people wanting to lose weight and to stick to a healthy life-style, ongoing social support is therefore one factor of importance (Baughman, Logue, Sutton, Capers, Jarjoura & Smucker, 2003). The discrepancy between the *theory of action* and *theory-in-use* is a general problem for behavioral changes (Argyris, 1994; Argyris, 2005). The theories-in-use are those mental models that are practically being used by individuals in everyday life situations, while the theory of action relates to the beliefs and understanding of practices that people talk about as their own. Especially in stressful situations, the discrepancy between these models becomes evident.

If we want to develop a new life-style, such as learning to eat healthier, exercise or stop smoking, we need to question the way we live today. When trying to learn a new behavior with help from others, we have to question each other's behavior and understanding of problems (Argyris, 1994; Senge, 2004). This is important in order to trigger critical thinking, and reflect upon the underlying models, the assumptions and values, that affect our behavior. This is sometimes called double-loop learning (Argyris, 1994, Argyris, 2005). To explain, criticize, share and motivate are all necessary parts of learning new behaviors together with others (Soller & Lesgold, 2000), and interpersonal relations should not prevent the participants from expressing different views and positions (Baker, Quignard, Lund & van Amelsvoort, 2002; Wenger, 2004). When practicing the models, we engage in single-loop learning. This means that we try to work on our ability to perform, and develop our practical skills, within our mental understanding and beliefs. Both single-loop and double-loop learning are needed if we want to succeed in more profound types of changes, such as changing life-style.

The use of the Internet for learning purposes can help the one who wants to learn, the e-learner, to exercise more control over his or her learning situation (Haythornthwaite, 2006). When individuals become familiar with the new cyber life, they get used to the freedom of choosing what, when and from whom they learn. It is in this context that the national health portals and the web-based communities for health purposes can play an important role. Figure 1 illustrates the domain of e-health communities for learning in order to develop healthy established habits.

Figure 1. Continuous learning through e-health communities to achieve sustainable healthy habits

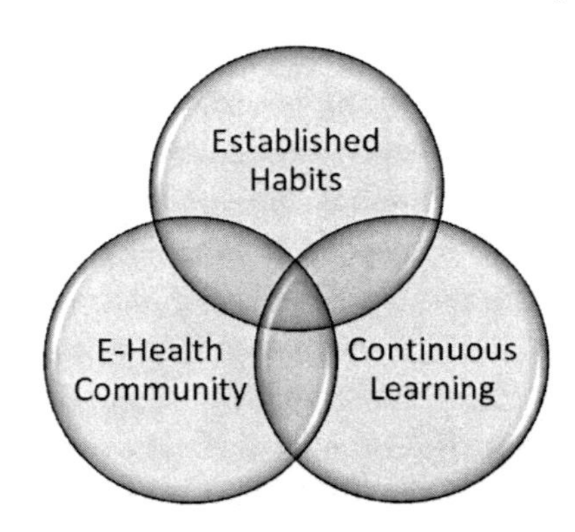

FRAMEWORK FOR EVALUATING E-HEALTH COMMUNITIES

The idea of having people with common concerns coming together online to discuss health issues and exchange knowledge and experiences is appealing and, in general, a good thing. However, the question is whether the online conversations can be regarded as helpful to the community members who are about to learn a new and healthier behavior. E-health communities for people who want to change unhealthy habits into healthier ones need to be evaluated from a learning perspective. Examples of e-health communities of this kind are those targeting people with overweight or obesity and people who find it hard to quit smoking. Both the conversations for learning purposes and the content of the advice and recommendations need to be evaluated. What will be presented in the following sections are therefore recommendations regarding what to measure in terms of communicative acts and content of postings.

The framework presented uses ideas of discourse analysis. Discourse analyses focus on the use of language as a social function, and it is based on the idea that all linguistic material is action oriented (Preece, 2000). It addresses the question "what is the function of this text?". In the e-health community context, the discourse analyses include studies of *how the community members make requests and respond to each other*, and to what degree they agree, counteract, etc. To understand the basic foundation of online communication for sharing experience and information, we need to consider the role of the participants and the way they ask questions and respond to questions from others. Patterns of conversations are mapped. Since having different opinions expressed in an e-health community is important for learning among the individuals, responses of this kind are to be detected. Through classification of conversational acts, the different types can be identified.

Besides the patterns of conversational acts, also the accumulated community knowledge needs to be addressed. Firstly, systematic analyses need to be made of the different topics, or conversation issues, raised in the e-health community. The reason for these analyses is to find out about *what is discussed*, and in what ways the issues relate to learning. Secondly, *the content of responses* (advice, information, etc.) is to be studied and compared to what is known as expert knowledge in the specific field. There are other online systems that the community contents can be evaluated against, in a more or less automatic manner. We will present how the contents of the answers given by medical experts in an 'Ask the Doctor' system can be used for this purpose.

The ideas behind the presented framework have been empirically tested on e-health communities present in Sweden and other European countries (Smedberg, 2007a-b; Smedberg, 2008a-b). In the following sections, references to results from these studies will be presented.

Evaluating Community Dialogues from a Learning Perspective

Communication is an important tool when we want to learn together with others. Different mental models can then be put against each other; we can compare values, opinions and experiences, and we can negotiate the meanings, for example. We can also use the fact that new possibilities can be revealed through the interactions we have with other people. There is no predefined amount of possibilities, but they are created when people meet, either face-to-face or online. By listening and asking questions, we can better understand why people approach life and situations in the way they do. We can also get others to reflect upon past experiences with questions and comments, and thereby help them become observers of their own behaviors and assumptions. When doing this, we can eventually stop patterns of bad or unhealthy behaviors from being repeated in the future. Consequently, in order to achieve effective online interaction in collaborative groups, the participants need to have conversational skills. In fact, studies have shown that the differences between a supportive and non-supportive student group refer to the ways the group members engage in conversations (Soller, 2001). Characteristics of importance for a supportive group were shown to be related to conversational activities: the number of questions posted by the participants, questions met by answers from the others, and also conversations arguing about understanding more than acknowledging the statements from the others.

In the following section parts, we will present different types of conversation topics and response acts in e-health communities, and reflect on their relevance for learning new habits.

Different Types of Conversation Topics

Through empirical studies of e-health community conversations on established bad habits, different types of conversation topics have been detected (e.g., Smedberg, 2008b). The two main types of topics are requests of personal character and the more neutral requests. The personal questions address specific problems and concerns of the one who asks the others for help, while the neutral postings ask for factual knowledge, about a certain diet or medicine, for example. Regarding the questions on personal matters, three sub categories were observed: questions on setbacks, obstacles and incentives. The sub categories on personal matters could have been defined in other ways; however, the three categories were chosen since they could be said to represent areas of importance for learning a new behavior. Setbacks, obstacles and incentives are categories that most evidently correspond to the ideas of double-loop learning that is highly important for learning a new behavior. These conversation topics aim to reflect upon repeated patterns of breakdowns, foreseen problems (feedforward) and motivational factors, i.e., reflections on different things that the community members face when they try to practice new habits. Besides having requests as start-ups for conversations, there are also conversations that start with a statement.

The following are short explanations of each detected type of topic together with some examples from e-health conversations (see Table 1). The examples have been collected from empirical studies of e-health communities on overweight and smoking conducted over the past years.

Table 1. Community topics, explanations and examples

Community Topic	Explanation	Examples from Conversations on Established Bad Habits
Fact queries	Requests for factual knowledge	Requests for side-effects of medicines, how often one should exercise and eat, how to detect signs of addiction, about unexpected physical changes when giving up smoking or losing weight, whether it is common to gain weight after quitting smoking, about skin problems when quitting smoking
Setbacks	Personal experiences of recurrent breakdowns, problems and mistakes	Problems related to changing life-style, not managing to lose weight, to regain weight despite great efforts, unable to develop exercising habits or to stop smoking
Obstacles	Seen or foreseen difficulties to overcome	How to eat slowly, difficulties to exercise due to physical disabilities, holidays and gatherings with friends and family that the participants saw could be problematic for keeping new eating habits
Incentives	Induce action or motivate effort due to fear of punishment/ negative effects or expectation of reward	Motivational factors, value systems, those things that are of importance for the members' struggle to stop smoking or reduce weight, requests to challenge the other members to achieve a certain weight loss, requests concerning whether they want to change behavior for their own sake or for the approval of someone else
Statements	Statements of facts or personal opinions	Successful diets and personal experiences of periods of non-smoking habits, recommendations regarding literature and TV programs, welcoming phrases and cheerful words, expressions of appreciation of having found community support

Different Types of Responses

Also important to consider are the ways that the community members carry on the conversations. Through empirical studies, different ways in which community members respond to postings from others have been identified (e.g., Smedberg, 2008a). The responses are given to start-up requests and statements and also to thoughts and advice from responding community members (responses to responses). There is one type of response where the community members agree with the sender and express their sympathy with the thoughts, ideas and troubles presented. These responses offer confirmation of problems and ideas and also sympathy with the others. Among the responses characterized by sympathy, you can also find the ones expressing gratitude to the others. These responses explicitly show appreciation for received advice, recommendations and the like. A second type of response combines expressions of sympathy with the sharing of experiences and advice. Furthermore, there are examples of responses where the community members question the ideas or problem formulated by the first sender. This third type of response reflects critically upon the situation described, and opposing ideas are often introduced. Finally, a fourth type of response comes from community members who much more explicitly reject the first sender's ideas and his or her understanding of the situation. In these responses the "right" ways of thinking or doing, according to the senders of the responses, are often presented. Regarding learning new and healthier habits, responses that can help the sender to reflect upon his or her situation and current habits are most valuable. In general, the reflections and counter ideas can therefore be regarded as helpful in the learning process.

In order to illustrate different response acts, we here present an example of an online conversation held by people in an overweight community on the Swedish Net Doctor site. The following is a translated transcript of the conversation.

Request: Is there someone out there who has the same problem with food? I am always hungry; when I eat it only takes about half an hour before I am hungry again! It is like I have a hole in my stomach! I have tried all different sorts of diets, Atkins, low carbohydrate diet, nothing works!

Response1: It can be that you are subjected to the so-called Rebound effect:

- Intake of fast carbohydrates such as rice, potato, pasta
- The blood system uses these extra fast
- The body is tricked to release insulin in order to quickly lower the level of blood sugar
- The level of blood sugar is lowered quickly
- The body receives signals about the blood sugar level and turns on the signals of hunger.

This is a negative circle. It is even that your breakfast affects the level of insulin until lunch. What to do then? Start the day by having dark bread, porridge or soured milk without sugar. Perhaps a fruit like grape. Have lunch and dinner with slow carbohydrates such as a whole meal pasta, unpolished rice, beans, etc. These allow slow secretion of insulin, something that lets you feel full longer. Important is also that ALL meals NEED to include protein, even breakfast. Ham sandwich, egg, or the like. Don't forget the fat which also gives a lower level of insulin. Try to eat some fat with every meal, a teaspoonful of oil on the salad or half an avocado or a mackerel sandwich. This also helps to keep insulin under control and enhance weight reduction. [...]

Response2: You don't suffer from gastric catarrh or something like that? I have stomach problems, and I feel hungry all the time. I have gastric catarrh and take medicine, so now my problems with having a sense of hole in my stomach have disappeared. Go and see a doctor, you may also have a sort of stomach problem, and there are cures for that. Try it and see! /Trinan

Response3: It was as if I had written it myself:-o It usually takes half an hour after I have eaten before I feel hungry again...don't know why, but it has started to get better anyway.

Response4: I have the same problem but I try to decide beforehand at what times I will eat and what I will have to eat, between these I allow myself to be hungry. It is not easy, but you get used to it.

Response5 (response to response4): I am always hungry too, it is really tough, I try to hold on. Good luck!

In the conversation above, the sender of the request described a situation characterized as a setback. The sender experienced a more or less constant feeling of hunger despite different diets tried. The replies from the other community members differed slightly in character. Two of them offered sympathy and confirmation of the expressed problem (responses 3 and 5), further two offered advice (responses 1 and 4), and one (response 2) offered a counter-idea and how to interpret the situation in a different way. The community member with the counter-idea suggested that the experience described could be a symptom of something else, and advised therefore the sender of the request to have a second thought regarding problem definition.

Evaluating Community Knowledge

As discussed so far, there are different ways that people with a certain interest use the e-health community to support, share experiences and to help each other develop healthier habits. Experiences that guide the community members' advice, and recommendations that the members have found on the Internet or elsewhere, can of course be more or less useful and more or less true to scientific results. Giving wrong or less useful responses can be misleading and contra productive. To evaluate the community members' ability to present relevant factual knowledge and recommendations can somehow be a delicate task. One way to go is

Table 2. Comparison of e-health community on overweight and ask the expert system (Based on Smedberg, 2007b, p. 315)

Type	Ask the Expert System Vs. E-Health Community	E-Health Community Vs. Ask the Expert System
Replicated questions largely with the same advice given	50%	14%
Replicated questions with different advice given	3%	10%
Replicated questions without answer	1%	-
Not replicated, but complementary information given	27%	16%
Not replicated, and with no relation	19%	60%

to compare the content of community responses with the responses given by medical experts.

A web-based system for questions and answers between the public and medical experts is the 'Ask the Expert' or 'Ask the Doctor' system. This type of system enables people to get in contact with medical experts to get factual knowledge and medical advice (Bromme, Jucks & Wagner, 2005). It is also used for information-seeking purposes and browsed for questions and answers already posted in the system. In health care, the experts can be physicians, psychologists and dieticians, for example. Studies have shown that Ask the Expert services in the health care sector can be of much value to seekers of health information who need to gain new knowledge and guidance (Marine, Embi, McCuistion, Haag & Guard, 2005). The system offers even a new type of continuous relationships between patients and medical experts (Marco, Barba, Losa, de la Serna, Sainz, Lantigua, et al., 2006). This kind of health system is therefore also interesting to consider when dealing with online learning for people with established bad habits.

In order to investigate the relations between the two types of systems, the e-health community and the Ask the Expert system, studies were made in the field of overweight issues (Smedberg, 2007a-b). Starting point of one of the studies was the usage of an e-health community on overweight on the Swedish Net Doctor site, and the Ask the Expert system on the same site. The first 50 conversations from the targeted open and non-moderated e-health community were collected, starting from January 2006. The conversational issues in the community were compared to the questions and answers (Q&As) available in the archive of Ask the Expert system. In the Ask the Expert system, all words were searchable. Corresponding Q&As were systematically searched for by using keywords and keyword phrases. Only questions being answered by an expert were published on the site and thereby part of this study. To compare results, another study started with the Ask the Expert system targeting overweight issues and looked for differences and similarities in the corresponding e-health community. The results showed that common questions about diets, exercises and weight reduction medicine in the Ask the Expert system were met by corresponding questions and also similar answers in the online conversations. In general, the community members showed great insight into different health issues and problems that were found in both systems. The results from the studies can be seen in Table 2.

However, when comparing corresponding answers in the two systems, the way the answers were presented turned out to be different. The medical expert often gave a more detailed description in his or her answer to a question, such as declaring the amount of fat in food and how the body reacts in medical terms, whereas the community contributions combined facts with practical advice and experiences. Some of the Ask the Expert questions with no corresponding ones in the e-health community were concerned with specific medical conditions. In most cases, this difference between the systems seemed quite natural, since medical-trained people best can handle questions that demand for in-depth medical knowledge.

Another way to evaluate community knowledge is to have medical experts examine the community conversations. Similarities and differences between the e-health community knowledge and the medical expertise have been investigated by medical experts through their evaluation of the community members' postings (e.g., Hwang, Farheen, Johnson, Thomas, Barnes & Bernstam, 2007). When postings with advice and recommendations in 18 online communities on weight-loss were studied, the results gave that online communities on overweight involve, to a large extent, advice congruent with medical guidelines and accepted knowledge of the field (Hwang, Farheen, Johnson, Thomas, Barnes & Bernstam, 2007). The results showed that most advice posted on highly-active web-based communities on weight loss is not erroneous or harmful. Through many replies to a question, the chance of having community members correct an erroneous is also more likely to occur.

E-HEALTH COMMUNITY FOR LEARNING PURPOSES: A SUMMARIZED PICTURE

The way the different parts of learning work together is seen below, in Figure 2. Models for healthy habits are mainly developed through the knowledge of health experts and factual knowledge, while the individual models of the e-health community members are created and recreated by practicing different methods, evaluating results, and experiencing breakdowns, obstacles and issues of motivation or incentives. Often, the community member's theory of action is similar to the healthy models of the experts, while the theory-in-use is the one that generates personal stories of difficulties of different kinds. Through community conversations, the members can reflect on personal stories together. Participating in both e-health communities and Ask the Expert systems can also help the community members keep up with scientific knowledge of the field. As the community members engage in different Internet activities, the expertise and their own reflections on practices can be used together. Community knowledge that guides advice and recommendations between the community members can thereby be more congruent with existing knowledge of the health field. Learning in the e-health community setting is therefore to be regarded together with health information sites and systems in which health experts respond to questions.

Figure 2. Learning new habits as an ongoing cogwheel of interrelated parts

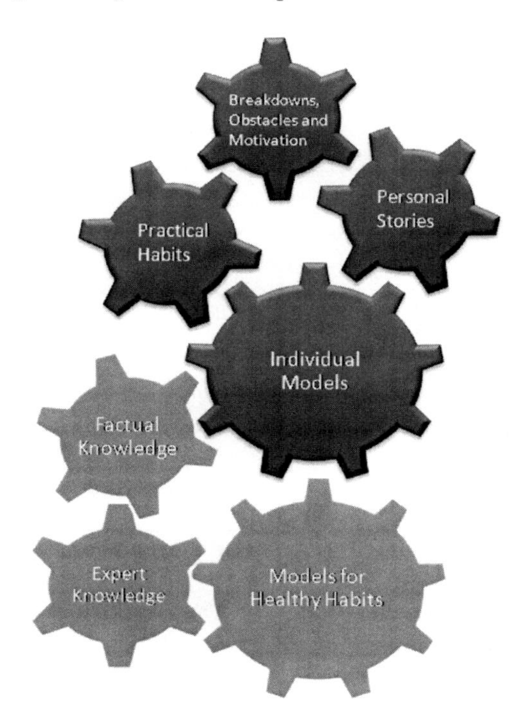

As pointed out in this chapter, learning a new and healthier habit is not an easy task to succeed with. There are several things to consider when

Table 3. Assessing usability of e-health communities for people with established bad habits

Community Element	Community Relevance	Relevance for Learning Healthy Habits
Topic Type		
-Fact queries	Affect the agenda: neutral questions	Sharing of factual knowledge
-Setbacks	Affect the agenda: personal and emotional questions	Reflection on repeated breakdowns
-Obstacles	Affect the agenda: personal and emotional questions	Preparation/mobilization for future actions, to avoid breakdowns: feedforward
-Incentives	Affect the agenda: neutral, personal and emotional questions	Motivation for engaging in healthy habits, underlying reasons for different behaviors
-Statements	Affect the agenda: neutral as well as personal issues	Factual knowledge and general inspiration through success stories
Response Type		
-Empathy	Community bonding	Emotional support, coping with mistakes
-Advice	Engagement in the others	Handling of practical situations
-Opposing ideas	Openness to 'experiences of the world'	Critical reflections on assumptions and current practices
-Rejections	Can be seen as harmful to community bonding	Can create too strong reactions to existing ideas/practices, only relevant in specific learning settings
Responses in number	Engagement, a large number contributes to strong tie relations	Affects the number of suggested solutions, ideas, practices, etc.
Community Knowledge	Affects trust in the community support	Brings accuracy and direction towards existing health guidelines, qualitative advice and recommendations
Experiences of the Community Members	Sharing of problems and solutions to develop community	Reflections on the participants' habits
Strong tie as well as weak tie relations	Contributes to trust as well as community change	Self-disclosure as well as new/deviating ideas
Events outside the community (F2F)	Weave the community together and enhance trust	Support of practical habits and skills in real life situations

designing and evaluating e-health communities for people who want to develop healthy habits together. Community elements that are relevant to consider are presented in Table 3. For each element, its relevance to the community and to learning healthy habits is summarized.

FUTURE RESEARCH DIRECTIONS

The present e-health communities address patients and citizens who like to communicate together on different health issues. The communities are normally non-moderated due to the time-consuming work that a moderator role would require. However, e-health communities could be used in other ways, with new types of technical features and with additional actors as well.

In-depth knowledge of the characteristics of e-health communities, and of the ongoing online conversations, gives designers of community settings a tool to strengthen the learning activities of the community. In the future, we will probably see more complex forms of e-health communities that take advantage of different types of technical features for searching external information and knowledge, and for inviting experts to community discussions, and the like. Future integration between different types of systems, such as e-health communities and Ask the Expert systems, will probably further enhance learning, and provide the users with a more holistic view of a particular health field.

Also, the relations between the online and physical life will become more transparent in the future through the usage of mobile applications. This will develop the e-health communities further. Especially for people with established unhealthy habits, but also for patients who need to learn how to adapt their living to new treatments and medication, being able to get in contact with others more easily will most likely further help people develop sustainable practices in real life situations.

CONCLUSION

In this chapter, we have focused on e-health communities for people with established bad, or unhealthy, habits. We have showed how a combination of online community, communication and learning theories can be applied to the area of e-health communities in order to identify critical community elements. The results also showed the importance of having different types of topics and different ways of responding in balance. Especially topics that are related to reflections on existing practices are important for learning a new life-style. Also, although bonding activities are important in a community, this must be combined with community members expressing opposing ideas. Single- as well as double-loop learning needs to be supported through the e-health community.

A framework for evaluating quality and usability of e-health communities for people with established bad habits needs to consider the conversational skills and engagement of the community members as well as the knowledge of health issues that the members express through advice and recommendations. The framework presented in this chapter addresses this. The categories of topics and responses presented have been applied in empirical studies, and were believed to serve the purpose. However, the categories can certainly be further adjusted, and perhaps divided, in order to map other types of e-health community settings.

REFERENCES

Andrews, D. C. (2002). Audience-specific online community design. *Communications of the ACM*, *45*(4), 64–68. doi:10.1145/505248.505275

Argyris, C. (1994, July-August). Good communication that blocks learning. *Harvard Business Review*, 77–85.

Argyris, C. (2005). Double-loop learning in organizations: A theory of action perspective . In Smith, K. G., & Hitt, M. A. (Eds.), *Great minds in management: The process of theory development* (pp. 261–279). Oxford, UK: Oxford University Press.

Austin, J. L. (1962). *How to do things with words*. Cambridge, MA: Harvard University Press.

Baker, M., Quignard, M., Lund, K., & van Amelsvoort, M. (2002). Designing a computer-supported collaborative learning situation for broadening and deepening understanding of the space of debate. In *Proceedings of the Fifth Conference of the International Society for the Study of Argumentation, 25-28 June 2002* (pp. 55-61). Amsterdam, Netherlands.

Baughman, K., Logue, E., Sutton, K., Capers, C., Jarjoura, D., & Smucker, W. (2003). Biopsychosocial characteristics of overweight and obese primary care patients: do psychosocial and behavior factors mediate sociodemographic effects? *Preventive Medicine*, *37*(2), 129–137. doi:10.1016/S0091-7435(03)00095-1

Bishop, A. P., Bruce, B. C., & Jones, M. C. (2006). Community inquiry and informatics: Collaborative learning through ICT. *The Journal of Community Informatics*, *2*(2), 3–5.

Bromme, R., Jucks, R., & Wagner, T. (2005). How to refer to 'diabetes'? Language in online health advice. *Applied Cognitive Psychology, 19*(5), 569–586. doi:10.1002/acp.1099

Burnett, G., & Buerkle, H. (2004, January). Information exchange in virtual communities: A comparative study. *Journal of Computer-mediated Communication, 9*(2). Retrieved August 19, 2009 from http://jcmc.indiana.edu/vol9/issue2/.

Byrne, S., Cooper, Z., & Fairburn, C. G. (2004). Psychological predictors of weight regain in obesity. *Behaviour Research and Therapy, 42*(11), 1341–1356. doi:10.1016/j.brat.2003.09.004

Fox, N. J., Ward, K. J., & O'Rourke, A. J. (2005). The 'expert patient': Empowerment or medical dominance? The case of weight loss, pharmaceutical drugs and the Internet. *Social Science & Medicine, 60*(6), 1299–1309. doi:10.1016/j.socscimed.2004.07.005

Fox, S. & Fallows, D. (2003, July 16). *Internet health resources*. Pew Internet & American Life Project.

Geliebter, A., & Aversa, A. (2003). Emotional eating in overweight, normal weight, and underweight individuals. *Eating Behaviors, 3*(4), 341–347. doi:10.1016/S1471-0153(02)00100-9

Haythornthwaite, C. (2006). The social informatics of elearning. Paper presented at *Information, Communication & Society (ICS) 10th Anniversary International Symposium, 20-22 September 2006*. Retrieved from the Illinois Digital Environment for Access to Learning and Scholarship (IDEALS) Web site: http://hdl.handle.net/2142/8959.

Haythornthwaite, C. (2007). Social networks and online community . In Joinson, A., McKenna, K., Postmes, T., & Reips, U.-D. (Eds.), *The Oxford handbook of Internet psychology* (pp. 121–137). New York: Oxford University Press.

Hwang, K. O., Farheen, K., Johnson, C. W., Thomas, E. J., Barnes, A. S., & Bernstam, E. V. (2007). Quality of weight loss advice on Internet forums. *The American Journal of Medicine, 120*(7), 604–609. doi:10.1016/j.amjmed.2007.04.017

Josefsson, U. (2007). Coping online – Patients' use of the Internet. Doctoral thesis, 37, Dep. of Applied Information Technology, IT-University of Göteborg, Sweden.

Kling, R. (2000). Learning about information technologies and social change: The contribution of social informatics. *The Information Society, 16*(3), 217–232. doi:10.1080/01972240050133661

Kling, R. (2001). Social informatics. *Encyclopedia of Lis.* Amsterdam: Kluwer Publishing. Retrieved from http://rkcsi.indiana.edu/.

Korp, P. (2006). Health on the internet: Implications for health promotion. *Health Education Research – Theory & Practice, 21*(1), 78-86.

Loader, B. D., Hardey, M., & Keeble, L. (2008). Health informatics for older people: A review of ICT facilitated integrated care for older people. *International Journal of Social Welfare, 17*(1), 46–53.

Loader, B. D., & Keeble, L. (2004). *Challenging the digital divide? – A literature review of community informatics initiatives*. York, England: Joseph Rowntree Foundation.

Marco, J., Barba, R., Losa, J. E., de la Serna, C. M., Sainz, M., & Lantigua, I. F. (2006). Advice from a medical expert through the Internet on queries about AIDS and hepatitis: Analysis of a pilot experiment. *PLoS Medicine, 3*(7), 1041–1047. doi:10.1371/journal.pmed.0030256

Marine, S., Embi, P. J., McCuistion, M., Haag, D., & Guard, J. R. (2005). NetWellness 1995-2005: Ten years of experience and growth as a non-profit consumer health information and Ask-an-Expert service. In *AMIA 2005 Symposium Proceedings, 22-26 October 2005*. Washington DC, USA.

McDermott, R. (2000). Knowing in community: 10 critical success factors in building communities of practice. *IHRIM Journal*, March 2000. Retrieved from http://www.a-i-a.com/capital-intelectual/KnowingInCommunity.pdf

Medina-Mora, R., Winograd, T., Flores, R., & Flores, F. (1992). The Action Workflow Approach to workflow management technology. In *Proceedings from the 1992 ACM Conference on Computer-Supported Cooperative Work*, 281-288. Retrieved from http://portal.acm.org.

Mehra, B., Merkel, C., & Bishop, A. P. (2004). The internet for empowerment of minority and marginalized users. *New Media & Society*, *6*(6), 781–802. doi:10.1177/146144804047513

Milicevic, I., Gareis, K., & Korte, W. B. (2005). Making progress towards user-orientation in online public service provision in Europe . In Cunningham, P., & Cunningham, M. (Eds.), *Innovation and the Knowledge Economy: Issues, Applications, Case Studies*. Amsterdam, The Netherlands: IOS Press.

Preece, J. (2000). *Online communities – Designing usability, supporting sociability*. Chichester, UK: Wiley & Sons, Ltd.

Senge, P. M. (2004). The leader's New Work: Building learning organizations. In K. Starkey, S. Tempest, & A. McKinlay (Eds.), *How Organizations Learn: Managing the search for knowledge* (pp. 462-486), 2nd. London, UK: Thomson Learning.

Smedberg, Å. (2004). Learning through online communities: A study of health-care sites in Europe . In Cunningham, P., & Cunningham, M. (Eds.), *eAdoption and the Knowledge Economy: Issues, Applications, Case Studies* (pp. 1333–1339). Amsterdam, The Netherlands: IOS Press.

Smedberg, Å. (2007a). *How to combine the online community with Ask the expert system in a health care site – A comparison of online health systems usage*. IEEE Computer Society Press.

Smedberg, Å. (2007b). To design holistic health service systems on the Internet. In *Proceedings of World Academy of Science, Engineering and Technology*, November 2007 (pp. 311-317). Retrieved from: http://www.waset.org/journals/waset/v31/v31-56.pdf.

Smedberg, Å. (2008a). Learning conversations for people with established bad habits: A study of four health-communities. *International Journal of Healthcare Technology and Management*, *9*(2), 143–154. doi:10.1504/IJHTM.2008.017369

Smedberg, Å. (2008b). Online health-communities on bad habits for preventive care. In *Proceedings of the 4th Kuala Lumpur International Conference on Biomedical Engineering (Biomed2008), 25-28 June 2008* (pp. 291-294). Kuala Lumpur, Malaysia.

Soller, A. (2001). Supporting social interaction in an intelligent collaborative learning system. *International Journal of Artificial Intelligence in Education*, *12*(1), 40–62.

Soller, A., & Lesgold, A. (2000). Modeling the process of collaborative learning. In *Proceedings of the International Workshop on New Technologies in Collaborative Learning*. Awaji-Yumebutai, Japan. Retrieved from http://www.cscl-research.com/Dr/documents/Soller-Lesgold-NTCL2000.doc.

Timperio, A., & Crawford, D. A. (2004). Public definitions of success in weight management. *Nutrition & Dietetics*, *61*, 215–220.

Walther, J. B., Pingree, S., Hawkins, R. P., & Buller, D. B. (2005). Attributes of interactive online health information systems. *Journal of Medical Internet Research*, *7*(3). doi:10.2196/jmir.7.3.e33

Wenger, E. (2004). Communities of practice and social learning systems . In Starkey, K., Tempest, S., & McKinlay, A. (Eds.), *How organizations learn: Managing the search for knowledge* (2nd ed., pp. 238–258). London: Thomson Learning.

Winograd, T., & Flores, F. (1987). *Understanding computers and cognition: A new foundation for design*. Boston, MA: Addison-Wesley Publishing Company.

ADDITIONAL READING

Andriessen, J., Baker, M. J., & Dan Suthers, D. (2003). Argumentation, computer support, and theeducational context of confronting cognitions . In Andriessen, J., Baker, M. J., & Suthers, D. (Eds.), *Arguing to learn: Confronting cognitions in computer-supported collaborative learning Environments* (pp. 1–25). Dordrecht, The Netherlands: Kluwer Academic Publishers.

Bishop, J. (2005).The role of mediating artefacts in the design of persuasive e-learning systems. *Proceedings of the internet technology & applications 2005 conference*, North East Wales Institute of Higher Education, Wrexham.

Bishop, J. (2007). Increasing participation in online communities: A framework for human–computer interaction. *Computers in Human Behavior*, *23*(4), 1881–1893. doi:10.1016/j.chb.2005.11.004

Boyd, D. M., & Ellison, N. B. (2008). Social network sites: Definition, history, and scholarship. *Journal of Computer-Mediated Communication*, *13*, 210–230. doi:10.1111/j.1083-6101.2007.00393.x

Bradley, G. (2006). *Social and community informatics: Humans on the Net*. London: Routledge.

Dannecker, A., & Lechner, U. (2007). Online and offline integration in virtual communities of patients – An empirical analysis. In Steinfield, Pentland, Ackerman & Contractor (Eds.), *Communities and Technologies 2007: Proceedings of the Third Communities and Technologies Conference*, Michigan State University. London: Springer, 151-170.

De Cindio, F., Gentile, O., Grew, P., & Redolfi, D. (2003). Community networks: Rules of behavior and social structure. *The Information Society*, *19*, 395–406. doi:10.1080/714044686

Figallo, C. (1998). *Hosting web communities*. New York: John Wiley & Sons.

Johnson, G. J., & Ambrose, P. J. (2006). Neo-tribes: The power and potential of online communities in health care. *Communications of the ACM*, *49*(1), 107–113. doi:10.1145/1107458.1107463

Kling, R. (1999). What is social informatics and why does it matter? *D-Lib Magazine*, *5*(1). doi:10.1045/january99-kling

Noar, S. M., & Zimmerman, R. S. (2004). Health behavior theory and cumulative knowledge regarding health behaviors: Are we moving in the right direction? *Health Education Research*, *20*(3), 275–290. doi:10.1093/her/cyg113

Preece, J. (1998). Empathic communities: Reaching out across the Web. *Interaction*, *5*(2), 32–43. doi:10.1145/274430.274435

Preece, J. (1999). Empathic communities: Balancing emotional and factual communication. *Interacting with Computers*, *12*, 63–77. doi:10.1016/S0953-5438(98)00056-3

Preece, J. (2001). Sociability and usability in online communities: Determining and measuring success. *Behaviour & Information Technology*, *20*(5). doi:10.1080/01449290110084683

Preece, J., Nonnecke, B., & Andrews, D. (2004). The top 5 reasons for lurking: Improving community experiences for everyone. *Computers in Human Behavior*, 2.

Smedberg, Å. (2009). The use of an online health community on overweight: A member perspective, *Proceedings of IADIS International Conference Web Based Communities 2009 (WBC 2009), 21-23 June 2009* (pp. 51-58).

Wagner, T. (2005). How to refer to 'diabetes'? Language in online health advice. *Applied Cognitive Psychology*, *19*(5), 569–586. doi:10.1002/acp.1099

Wright, K. B., & Bell, S. B. (2003). Health-related support groups on the Internet: Linking empirical findings to social support and computer-mediated communication theory. *Journal of Health Psychology*, *8*(1), 39–54. doi:10.1177/1359105303008001429

Chapter 17
Standards in Telemedicine

O. Ferrer-Roca
University of La Laguna, Spain

ABSTRACT

For many years, medical teams working on telemedicine have made a strong effort to define the telemedicine Body of Knowledge (BoK), and generate compatible standards that allow delivering telemedicine with adequate medical quality. The authors expect, after the European Commission statement on the Prague 2009 declaration, a new era for telemedicine. The essential barriers, which have already been encountered, include Literacy, Standard connectivity and Quality control. In the present chapter, the authors will address the item of Literacy regarding the type of standards in each of the topics of the Telemedicine Body of Knowledge.

INTRODUCTION

In 1998, we wrote, "the welfare expenses cannot be endlessly increased, whilst an efficient health provision system in the context of the information society, will mark a new trend to configure health care practice in the next century" (Ferrer-Roca & Sosa-Iudicissa, 1998).

In this century and in spite of ICT improvements, the provision of health at distance is not taken as a regular medicine delivery but a "special" service, many times included in the new technology units (UINT= Unit of informatics and new technology) of the hospitals.

DOI: 10.4018/978-1-61692-843-8.ch017

If training and teaching schemes have to cope with society demands of *health quality (HQ)*, *health equity (HE)*, *efficient health delivery (HED)*, and *health security* (HS) medical training should devote a substantial part to e-health and telemedicine.

The main components of the Telemedicine-BoK as we defined in 1998 are listed in Table 1.

The health sector defines *telehealth* as an integrated term including any telematic application for health. It includes therefore any *medical informatics* and *health informatics*. The interna-

Table 1. Body of knowledge of telemedicine

CHAPTER	CONTENTS
1	History of Telemedicine
2	Minimal Technical Requirements
3	Main Telemedicine Applications
4	Basic Technical Knowledge
5	Quality Control and Assessment
6	Use and Indication of Telematic Tools in Telemedicine: Internet
7	Training, including Distance Training, Teleworking and Teleteaching
8	Data Security and Privacy
9	Liability and Legal Aspects
10	Health Economics in Telemedicine
11	Technology Transfer and Social Aspects
12	Emerging Issues

tional consultation carried out by the WHO in 1997, came out with a definition of "health telematics": as a composite term for health related activities, services and systems carried out over a distance by means of information and communications technologies, for the purpose of global health promotion, disease control and health care, as well as education, management and research for health. This also embraces the telematics in health research and health services management, as well as specific applications for "telemedicine" and "tele-education in health". In the Table 2, we include a list of telehealth applications. Under each term, we can include provision or confirmation of diagnosis, surveillance, epidemiology, management, clinical and research information, literature search and retrieval, health and wellness, health and medical educational contents.

BACKGROUND

Redefinitions for 2009

Most terms previously used are outdated and substituted nowadays by the common word of *e-health*, that include an endless list of "*e-*" words such as: e-prescription, e-assistance, e-delivery, e-mail, e-patient etc. In fact, not everyone understands the same using the term of e-health and therefore it is important to define their limits.

For the purpose of the paper we define:

- E-health as *health in Internet*, meaning access to anything related with health with or without quality control.
- E-health system as *e-government in healthcare*, meaning any citizen-health bodies transactions not only administrative but also for collection of results (laboratory, final reports, hospital release, e-prescription….)
- E-healthcare as *telemedicine*, meaning health delivery with the required quality standards and lack of risks for patient and users including confidentiality and security. Items such as knowledge discovery, personalized-health, etc… belong to this and it is under the responsibility of the medical doctors, medical colleges and health authorities to achieve the required quality of healthcare.

The potential scope of telemedicine is therefore enormous and can be summarized in four main aspects presented in Table 3.

ROBOTICS & COMPUTER ASSISTED MEDICINE

i.e. CAS / AEP[8]/ Intelligent devices

If you take into consideration the above scheme, many of the items treated in the field of telemedicine should be taken out. For that reason, it is important to define the limit of competences regarding e-administration for the healthcare items including electronic transactions or citizens' information and advertisement from the

Table 2. Telehealth applications

	CATEGORY	USERS
1	All forms of medicine at distance:	Physicians
	Teleconsultations, telepathology, teleradiology, telepsychiatry,	Health care professionals
	Teledermatology, telecardiology etc. Distant exploratory systems: EC[1], holter etc. Robotic surgery and telesurgery and CAS[2] etc. All forms of telementoring	Health care institutions Medical outsourcing
2	Inter-institutional, patient and clinical records and information systems	Health care institutions
	Electronic health and clinical records and data bases accessible by network	Health care professionals
	Laboratory results access	Health care workers
	Pathology results access	Physician's office
	Patient images access Text-mining and automatic disease classification /metadata annotation. PoC[3] controlling: vital signs and other parameters	Researchers Intensive care units
3	Public Health and Community Health Information networks (CHINS) Multiple-use health information networks	Government Epidemiologists
	Assisted Electronic prescription (AEP)	Public health professionals
	Health GRID for genetics, oncology, etc…	Physicians offices
	Knowledge discovery in patho-pharmacology p-Health	Pharmacies Clinics and CHINS
		Personal health policies
4	Tele-education and multimedia applications for health professionals	University and colleges
	and patients and networked research data bases. Internet services.	Associations
	Knowledge discovery. Data mining.	Researchers
	Patient EHR access and laboratory results access.	Physicians
		Health Care professionals
		Patients
5	Telemonitoring, telecare networks, Alarm systems, GPS[4] location PAN[5] telemetric devices: Diabetes, GI endoscopy, Telephone – SMS triages	Customers Elderly Chronically ill
	Home-care. Emergency networks	Disaster victims Accident victims
	Hospital PoR[6] of medical ambulances	Telenursing
	Telementoring in emergency actions	Call centre users
	Disaster relief and emergencies (POC[7]s teleassistance)	Call centre operators

telemedicine aspects in the hands of the health-care workers doctors or assistant people. Some electronic transactions nevertheless are purely in hands of the doctors such as clinical-records or prescriptions as well as knowledge discovery or personalized treatments based on proteomics or genomics.

In an efficiently networked healthcare system, doctors and nurses should get competencies and qualifications in distant attendance, control and treatment in order not to put in danger their own

Table 3. Scope of the telemedicine

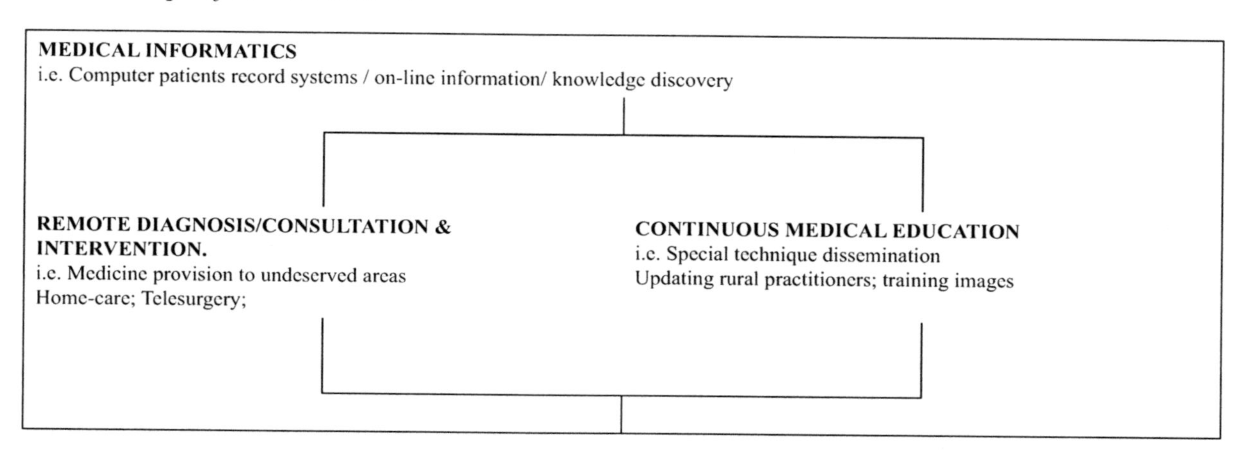

security and the health and security of the patients. Competencies in a topic have always been classified as follows:

1. General competencies to be able to use the tools and know the risks.
2. Specific competencies to be able to indicate applications, test them and change/adapt the tools.
3. Professional competencies to be able to design and implement strategies, software and hardware devoted to telemedicine assistance.

According to this design, all nurses and doctors should have to have general competencies and get during their carrier specific competencies in each of the basic medical knowledge and thereafter the specific competencies linked to their own specialties.

Obviously, professionals in the field of telemedicine should provide this knowledge. Those professionals have to have a role in each of the specialties or departments. As an example close to me, it will not be possible to run a fully automatic pathology department capable of handling and tracking biological specimens for personalized diagnosis and treatment unless a patho-informatics service is in place. This service handle specimen tag and informatics recognition, machine handling for automatic cutting, inclusion, staining and slide preparation; digitize and archive digital slides, together with electronic diagnosis with automatic metadata incorporation for data mining in and out of the Hospital information system (HIS), specimen anonimization and tracking, tissue microarray incorporation and protein and gene detection and archive working a GRID environment with other research groups in personalized treatment.

In fact, to focus on the Body of Knowledge of telemedicine we should take as a reference the publications of the ISI Journal citation Reports Science Edition, which are included in the group of HEALTH CARE SERVICES & SCIENCES where all Telemedicine Journals are included. By contrast, MEDICAL INFORMATICS is lacking of all basic knowledge link to telemedicine with only 20 journals and a limited impact factor. Finally, most technical aspects are better referred in the Journals of ENGINEERING, ELECTRICAL & ELECTRONIC that includes around 229 journals. This again poses the question of when the carrier of Medicine is going to be updated including Information Technologies items directly related with telemedicine.

PRAGUE 2009 DECLARATION

Motivation

The motivation of the promotion of the telemedicine by the EC that ended in the Prague declaration was based on:

- **The Recommendation (COM (2008)3282 final)** of July 2, 2008 on **interoperability**: applied to the clinical record but it is comparable to all aspects of the Telemedicine). It specified that its lack is one of the major obstacles to obtain economic and social advantages of the telemedicine.
- **The Communitarian Politics:** The initiative i2010 of growth and deployment of ICTs. According to the 'Leading markets in Europe', the e-health & telemedicine is one of the most important sectors in the creation and marketing of innovative products and services.

Recommended Policies: The Decalogue

The aspects to be addressed by EU countries according to the EC are a Decalogue:

1. **Infrastructure:** A change and adaptation is required that warrants the levels of quality and security in the provision of health care,
   - With framework conditions, organizational structures and complex application procedures.
   - With national and regional strategies in the field of e-health/telemedicine for cohesion and territorial development.
   - With assignation of resources in e-health/telemedicine, including direct incentives and financial mechanisms of indirect incentives to allow adoption, acquisition or modernization of the systems.
2. **Planning** with five years in advance of the activities directed to guarantee the interoperability. This is the limit market by the CE to guarantee the political coherence that often is a previous requisite to improve investment and innovation.
3. **Re-engineering:** Incorporating users and interested parties (local and regional authorities, healthcare professionals, patients and industry) in interoperability; establishing mechanisms for direction and control, management, public-private association of call for tenders, planning, application, evaluation, training, information and education.

   Due to the fact that interoperability is based, among others, on accomplishing **standard norms,** health care professionals and involved parties should know them.
4. **Technical Compatibility** of the systems, pre-requisite for the interoperability. Therefore the member-states should:
   - Have a memory of the existing infrastructure and technical standards.
   - Include a study of models and standards of structured information.
   - Establish the open standards and forced the standardization bodies in similar direction.
   - Considering the mandate M 403 (Standardization mandate to CEN, CENELEC and ETSI in the ICTs involved in electronic health).
5. **Semantic interoperability** is essential for the quality and security of patients, public health, clinical investigation and health care management. As a consequence, they should:
   - Use international clinic-medical terminologies, nomenclatures and classification of diseases including those related with pharmaco-surveillance and clinical trials.

- Standardized the semantic interoperability using data structures (arquetypes and sheets), and subconjunct of terminology systems and ontologies adapted to user demands;
- Developed a system of sustainable reference concepts (ontology) that take into account the variation of professional languages, juridical terminologies and classical coding systems;
- Have methodologies and tools to easily incorporate the semantic content to daily applications and train the professionals;
- Establish solid systems of evaluations and control.

6. **System certification**: Include the conformance procedures issued by authorities recognized trans-border (of autonomous communities or nations). Those should:
    - Apply existing standards and gain user confidence;
    - Establish nationwide evaluation and certification mechanisms;
    - Demand the industry/enterprise to build self-conformance statements for their products;
    - MD (medical devices) certification requires a CE mark, where software and telecommunications are included. Resolution of call for tenders should take into consideration the certification of quality of the enterprises. Enterprises fulfilling quality requirements should be registered and listed and should have periodical audits.
7. **Personal data protection:** following 95/46/CE and 2002/58/CE directives, should consider the legal safeguard to design and deployment of health care systems.
    - Furthermore, a specific juridical framework to manage healthcare data should be considered.
8. **The Telemedicine legal Framework** should consider:
    - The risk analysis for data management and in-house solutions;
    - The autodetermination as a patient right;
    - The degree of data availability.
    - The level of protection in accessing and manipulating data and trusted ID systems for patients and professionals;
    - Storage of data and samples following legal demands;
    - Audit requirements.
9. **Supervision and evaluation** of the interoperability, security and risk. Demand
    - An observatory to supervise, evaluate, determine the technical and semantical interoperability;
    - Alternatively, an interoperability certificate, issued by the competent authority.
    - To assess applications with a qualitative and quantitative criteria.
    - **Health Technology Assessment (HTA)** should not be limited to cost-benefit, efficiency and clinical value of the Evidence-based Medicine (EBM). Those bodies should also be competent in risk quantification, transaction quality and standardization or norms requirements.
    - Specific services could be built to solve those problems assuring the technical-delivery quality, auditing, and tracking the biological specimens in and out of the biobanks.
10. **Education and sensitization**. The member-states should:
    - Sensitize ICT producers and providers, health care providers, public health institutions, insurance companies and all involved parts;

- Fix the education requirements and knowledge and training of decision bodies in the field of healthcare policies and healthcare professionals;
- Educate and train in the areas of: registry of electronic operations; storage and treatment of clinical information; demand of informed consent of patients and limit of the use of biosamples and data.
- Propose comparable information and training activities to patients.

The ten points could be summarized in three: (1) Use standards to assure quality, interoperability and efficiency. (2) Assure the legal framework in security, data protection and health delivery and (3) Control risk management putting in place the control and certification mechanisms.

The three actions standards are the CORE premise.

STANDARDS IN TELEMEDICINE

The degree of maturity of a technology is linked to the *quantity and quality of researchers together with the number of available standards and protocols and the professional acceptance*. Telemedicine is not yet mature since quality of researchers is still limited as well as the professional acceptance. In spite of the fact that telemedicine has already arrived to an important degree of development because, technically speaking, it is feasible, precise, the sensitivity and specificity is similar to regular medicine provision, the clinical results of its benefits are deploying and cost-benefits are still being collected.

As mentioned, the number of standards is linked to degree of maturity. As we will see in the chapter, most of the standards belong to other technological fields (telecommunications, informatics etc…) and only very few are telemedicine specific such as the Plug and Play IEEE 11073 or ISO/PRF TS 22600 for privilege and access control, etc…

The section of the chapter regarding the body of knowledge, with the exception of the history, provides specific standards that will help on two fundamental items when applied to telemedicine:

- Favoring connectivity and integration of applications
- Assuring quality

In the present section, we will list in the joint table the type of standards recognized in each topic of the body of knowledge, but also can be studied in specific web sites (Medical device standards Portal – USA, 2009; American National Standards Institute – HITSP, 2009).

SEMANTICS

Healthcare applications have stable, granular code sets across several conceptual domains. However, most terminologies used in telemedicine assistance technology are not included, because we develop a specific ontology for telemedicine (Ferrer-Roca et al., 2005) based on the body of knowledge.

Some of the domains and their code sets in Medicine are:

Laboratory Tests and Observation Code Sets:

- Logical Observation Identifiers Names and Codes (LOINC)
- Systematized Nomenclature of Medicine—Clinical Terms (SNOMED-CT)

General Medical Code Sets:

- International Classification of Diseases (ICD-9 and ICD-10)
- MEDCIN point of care terminology
- Medical Subject Headings (MESH)
- Systematized Nomenclature of Medicine—Clinical Terms (SNOMED-CT)

Medication Code Sets (including Medication allergies):

Public

- National Drug Codes (NDC)
- NHS Read Codes
- Health Canada Drug Product Database (DPD)
- US Veterans Administration Drug File (NDF-RT)

Commercial (in alphabetic order)

- First Data Bank National Drug Data File (NDDF)
- Gold Standard (Alchemy)
- Lexi-Comp
- Medi-Span Master Drug Database (MDDB)
- Micromedex DRUGDEX
- Multum Lexicon
- Systematized Nomenclature of Medicine--Clinical Terms (SNOMED-CT)

Units of measure:

Table 4. Standards related with each topic of the BoK of Telemedicine by O.Ferrer-Roca

N	TOPIC	STANDARDS
1	**History of Telemedicine**	Not applied
2	**Minimal Technical Requirements**	
	Ergonomy	ISO9241 **ISO** 9241-410:2008 **ISO** 9241-20. **Ergonomics** of human-system interaction **ISO** 9241 y 13406. Series y1992 **Ergonomic** requirements Monitors **ISO** 10651-2, ISO10651-2. Lung ventilators **ISO** 11064-1, ISO11064-1. **Ergonomic** design of control centers OSHA **ergonomics** requirements - **ISO** 9241, AZSI B11 **ISO** 14155-1 COWs or Computer on wheels Tablet-PC
	ID	PUI[9]; TCI[10]; LOINC[11]
	Audio	MP3; UL 1492; Audio USMLE Step 2; ATSC HDTV standards and supports 8-channel digital audio; G.711; G.723; G.722; G.728; AAC-LD
	Video	MPEG-2 (ISO / IEC 13818-7); MPEG-4 part 3 (ISO / IEC 14496-3) DICOM. ITU H.324 (POTS): video H.263 ; audio G.723; ITU H.320 (ISDN): Audio G.711- G.723; video H.261- H.263; ITU H.323 (LAN): VoIP, Video H261 & H263 H.360 end to end QoS. ITU H610 (ADSL) ITU H241: HD: vídeo AVC / H.264 (MPEG-4 part.10, ISO / IEC 14496-10). ISO IEC 14496 CODING H.120, 768-2000 kbps, small picture H.261, baseline video compression MPEG-1-Video part (ISO/IEC 11172-2) H.262=MPEG2-Video, high rate video MPEG-2- Video part (ISO/IEC 13818-2) H.263, improved lower rates; Same core as original video part of MPEG-4 MPEG-4 Video part (ISO/IEC 14496-2) H.264/AVC Advanced video coding MPEG-4 Part 10 AVC (ISO/IEC 14496-10)
	Compression	JPEG2000

continued on following page

Table 4. continued

N	TOPIC	STANDARDS
	Wireless	Bluetooth; EN 50 371; EN 300 328; EN 301 489-1&17 ZigBee, WIFI: IEEE 802.11 a, b, d, g, h, d; IEEE 802.11 n-MIMO. The ISO 14443 and 15693 standards and EPCglobal's Gen 2 standard, protocols for testing ultra-wideband (UWB) and Wi-Fi RFID devices RFID: ISO/IEC 15693 and ISO/IEC 18000-3 IEEE 1471:2000: Standard Architecture view and view points IEEE 802.11b WIFI and WLAN IEEE 802.15.4 Zig Bee IEEE 802.15.3a UWB Ultrawide band IEEE 802.16 a/e WIMAX
	ICM-Electromagnetic	UN-11 telework & telemeasure (PIRE = 500 mW). UN-30 short-access. UN-85 of RLANs inside (PIRE=200 mW) or outside (PIRE=1W). UN-129 for RFID (PIRE =500mW)
	Telecomm	G.991.1 (G.hdsl) - High bit rate Digital Subscriber Line (HDSL) transmission system on metallic local lines. G.992.1 (G.dmt) - Asymmetrical Digital Subscriber Line (ADSL) Transceivers. G.992.2 (G.lite) - Splitterless Asymmetrical Digital Subscriber Line (ADSL) Transceivers. G.992.3 Asymmetric digital subscriber line transceivers - 2 (ADSL2.dmt) G.992.4 Splitterless asymmetric digital subscriber line transceivers - 2 (ADSL2.lite) G.992.5 – Asymmetric Digital Subscriber Line (ADSL) Transceivers – Extended Bandwidth ADSL2 (ADSL2plus) (Jan '03) G.995.1 - Overview of Digital Subscriber Line (DSL Recommendations). G.991.2 (G.shdsl) - Single pair High bit rate speed Digital Subscriber Line G.993.1 (G.vdsl) - Very high bit-rate Digital Subscriber Line G.994.1, G.996.1 and G.997.1 for tests, management and handshake G.983-x series Optical systems for access networks Broadband PON. Passive Optical Network up to 622 Mbit/s symmetrical / asymmetrical G.984.1 – General Characteristics of Gigabit-capable PONs G.984.2 –Gigabit-capable PONs: Physical media dependent layer specification
	Medical & Health care Robotics	Robot assisted surgery: da Vinci surgical system FDA approved 2000. Robotic Sterostaxis (electrophysiology, biopsy) Catheter Robotics RCMS ISO/TC 184/SC 2/WG 7 ISO 80601-2-XX series DICOM WG 24- Dicom in surgery COWs, computer on Wheel Socially assistive robotics (SAR) Human-Robot Interaction (HRI) *human-machine collaborative systems*
	Health Cards	ISO 7816 & EMV2 2000
	Cryptography	DES[12]: 3DES EDE CBC; Secure Hash Algorithm (SHA); AES SHA-224, SHA-256, SHA-384, SHA-512, SHA-1, RIPEMD-160 QES (Qualified Electronic Signature) DID[13]
	Security	ISO/DIS 17090; ISO/PRF TS 22600; RSA electronic signature system; ISO/TS 17090; UNE/ISO/IEC 15408; UNE/ISO/IEC 17799:2005; ISO/IEC 18014 X.509 ; SSL / HTTPS encryptions; Card-Verifiable-Certificates (CVC)
	Medical Devices	UNE209001: IN2002; CE-label (European Commission Enterprise and Industry European Standards, 2009) ISO 1497n1 ISO 13485

continued on following page

Table 4. continued

N	TOPIC	STANDARDS
	Transport	standard E.800 definitions, QoS[14], NP[15] and QoE[16] SG 12: End to end quality, as perceived by the users. It is fully addressed to Quality, and WP3/12 is dedicated to QoS for IP. SG 13: WP4/13 is dedicated to Network Performance NP SG 2: Mainly on operational aspects of QoS and SLA. New QoS handbook and activities on the impacts of routing on QoS. QSDG: 1 forum meeting each year and QSDG Magazine SG 4: Management of QoS and SLA. SG 9: QoS for cable networks and video assessment. SG 11: QoS signaling. SG15: System-specific requirements for network and transport equipment. SG 16: QoS Mechanisms for H.323-based multimedia systems. Quality of speech and video coders. SG 17: Frame Relay QoS. G.1000 'Communications Quality of Service: A framework and definitions ' G.1010 'End-User multimedia QoS categories ' E.860 'Framework for service level agreement' Y.1541 'IP Performance objective and allocations' Y.1540 ' IP Packet transfer and availability performance parameter" M.3341 ' Requirements for QoS/SLA management over TMN X-interface for IP-based services M.2301 *IP Network Provisioning & Maintenance*
	Medical Informatics	ISO 9126;EN/ISO/IEEE 1073; ISO/IEC 2382-01; ISO/TS; UNE-EN ISO 13606 18303:2002 CHA[17] IHE or Integrated Health Enterprise Sensor Event Platform (Websphere) Open Health
	Text mining	Predictive Model Markup Language (PMML) XML for Analysis and OLE DB for Data Mining SQL/MM Part 6: Data Mining Java Data Mining (JDM) - Java Specification Request 73 (JSR-73) CRoss Industry Standard Process for Data Mining (CRISP-DM) OMG Common Warehouse Metadata (CWM) for Data Mining Web services (SOAP/XML, WSRF, etc) Grid services (OGSA, OGSA/DAI, etc.) Semantic Web Standards (RDF, OWL, etc.) Standards for KDD workflow Standards for process workflow Standards for data transformations Standards for real time data mining Standards for data webs Open Source Efforts: R ; Weka ; GNU Octave
	Data management	XML; HL7; ICD10; MESH;
	Risk management	UNE 71502:2004; ISO/IEC 27004; ISO/IEC 15408; ISO/IEC 27001:2005; ISO/CD TS 25238
	Domotic	X.10; EN 50090-ISO/IEC 14543-3; ZeegBig; Z-wave; EN 13321-1; PLC[18]: Home-plug 1.0; Home-plug 1.0 Turbo; Home-plug AV at 200 Mbps; IMS- Internet Protocol Multimedia Subsystem, Open IPTV Forum; Digital Living Network Alliance (DLNA).
	Web 2.0	GoogleHealth
3	**Telemedicine Applications**	ISO 9126

continued on following page

Table 4. continued

N	TOPIC	STANDARDS
	EHR	ISO13606;EN-TS14796; OpenEHR; EN/ISO/IEEE 1073; prEN 12967 HISA; ENV 12612 Messages for the Exchange of Healthcare Administrative Information EN 13606 EHRcom[19] prEN 13940 CONTsys[20] prEN 14463 ClaML[21] EN 14720 Service request and report messages EN 14822 GPIC[22] EN 1828 Categorial structure for classifications and coding systems of surgical procedures. ISO- TR 18307 Health informatics - Key characteristics for interoperability and compatibility in messaging and communications standards ASTM-CCR[23]; ISO 8601(date/time); NCPDP-script[24] CCHIT [25] **HL-7:** HL7-CDA2-CCD[26] ; HL7-21731-RIM[27]; HL7-AQL[28]; HL7-CTS[29] ; HL7-OMG-HSSP[30]; HL7-CCOW[31]; HL7 CMET[32]; HL7 CMS[33]. E1239 Standard Practice for Description of R-ADT[34] for EHR E1284 Standard Guide for Construction of a Clinical Nomenclature for Support of EHR E1384 Practice for Content and Structure of EHR E1633 Specification for Coded Values Used in EHR E1714 Standard Guide for Properties of a UHID[35] E1715 Standard Practice for An Object-Oriented Model for RADT Functions in EHR E1744 Practice for View of Emergency Medical Care in the EHR E1762 Standard Guide for Electronic Authentication of Health Care Information E1869 Standard Guide for Confidentiality, Privacy, Access, and Data Security Principles for Health Information including EHR E2171 Standard Practice for Rating-Scale Measures Relevant to the Electronic Health Record E2183 Standard Guide for XML-DTD Design, Architecture and Implementation E2184 Standard Specification for Healthcare Document Formats E2211 Standard Specification for Relationship Between a Person (Consumer) and a Supplier of an EHR E2369 CCR Specification for CCR[36] E2473 Practice for the Occupational/ Environmental Health View of EHR EUA[37]
	Laboratory reports	**ELINCS** EHR-Lab Interoperability and Connectivity Standards
	Vital Signs	EN/ISO/IEEE 1073 ENV 13734:2000 Health Informatics – Vital signs information representation EN 1064:2005 Communication protocol for computed assisted ECG
	Virtual Slides	JPEG200; SSVS[38]
	PACS-Picture archiving & communication system	DICOM DICOM SR DICOM Structured Reporting
	HIS-Hospital Information Sys.	EN/ISO/IEEE 1073; ENV13939
	PIS- Pathology Information Sys.	EN/ISO/IEEE 1073; ENV13939 **ISO** TR 18112:2006, **Clinical Laboratory** Testing and in Vitro ISO/IEC 17000 ISO/IEC 17011 ISO/IEC 17025 as an essential standard for accreditation ISO/TC 212, Clinical Laboratory Testing and In Vitro Diagnostic Test Systems

continued on following page

Table 4. continued

N	TOPIC	STANDARDS
	LIS- Laboratory Information Sys	EN/ISO/IEEE 1073; ENV13939; ENV1613; ISO 18812; LIS09-A Standard Guide for Coordination of Clinical Laboratory Services in EHR & networking LoC= Lab on Chip ISO 15189:2003 ISO/IEC 17025 ASTM E1381-02 Standard Specification for Low-Level Protocol to Transfer Messages Between Clinical Laboratory Instruments and Computer Systems ISO/IEC 11179 standard
	MIS, minimal invasive surgery	EN/ISO/IEEE 1073; ENV13939; VITAL
	CAS, computer aided surgery	EN/ISO/IEEE 1073; ENV13939; VITAL
	PoC (point of care)	EN/ISO/IEEE 1073; ENV13939; VITAL HL7- CCOW IEEE 11073-10201 PoC medical device communications - DIM[39] CLSI[40] PoC laboratory control ISO 15197 Quality Assessment SMBG[41] NCCLS National Committee for Clinical Laboratory Standards NIST-CAB[42]= National Institute of Standards and Technology -Consortium on Advanced Biosensors
	PoR (point of reception)	EN/ISO/IEEE 1073; ENV13939; VITAL
	RS, Robotic surgery	EN/ISO/IEEE 1073; ENV13939; VITAL
	pHealth	IEEE2407 o PHI (*Personalized health informatics*) ISO/IEEE11073 (X73-PHD *–personal health devices*)
4	**Basic Technical Knowledge**	
	Plug & Play	EN/ISO/IEEE 1073
	Messaging	HL7; EN/ISO/IEEE 1073;
	Health Cards	ISO 14443-Proximity Health Cards ISO/IEC 7816 Smart Card standard ISO/IEC 7811 Identification Cards **ISO**/IEC 24727 Card Services framework (eEHIC[43]) BSI TR-03105 EMVCo Contactless Level 1 EMVCo Contact Level 1 and Level 2 ISO 17025, ISO 10373 **ISO** 15693 CEN/TS 15480 EU Citizen cards ENV 12018 Health card logic structure ISO/IEC 7816-2 Secure Module Card (SMC)

continued on following page

- Unified Code for Units of Measure (UCUM)

Procedures:

- Current Procedure Terminology (CPT)

Specialty Code Set Examples:

- Current Dental Terminology (CDT)
- Diagnostic and Statistical Manual of Mental Disorders (DMS-IV)

All can be studied in the Unified Medical Language System (UMLS) list of sources. There are over 100 terminology sources, without counting the homegrown terminologies that are still in use in many institutions for various domains.

Table 4. continued

N	TOPIC	STANDARDS
	Tracking systems	RFID ISO18000 RFID standards ISO/IEC 18004:2006; ISO/IEC15961 ISO/IEC 24710 ISO/IEC 24791- Software system infrastructure ISO/IEC 29160- RFID emblem ISO/IEC 24730- Real time location IoT[44] & GS1 standards ISO /IEC 29100 MIIM[45] ISO/IEC 15693 Identification cards -- Contactless integrated circuit cards – Vicinity cards ISO/IEC 14443 Identification cards -- Contactless integrated circuit cards – Proximity cards ISO/IEC 21481 *Information technology -- Telecommunications and information exchange between systems -- Near Field Communication Interface and Protocol -2 (NFCIP-2)* ISO/IEC 18000-3 Mode 3 (EPCglobal HF Gen 2) RFID ETSI ERM TG34 AIM Global CENELEC TC106x * Electromagnetic fields in the human environment CEN TC225 * AIDC technologies EDItEUR EPCglobal™ ; ITU-R ; IATA ; IEEE ; GS1 ISO/IEC JTC1/SC31/WG2 * AIDC – Data Structure ISO/IEC JTC1/SC17/WG8 * Identification cards and related devices - integrated circuit cards without contacts ISO/IEC JTC 1/SC27 ISO TC23/SC19/WG3 * Animal Identification ISO TC104 * Freight containers ISO TC122 * Packaging and JWG * Supply Chain Applications ISO/TC184/SC4 ISO TC204 * Intelligent Transport Systems Universal Postal Union EDItEUR ETSI EN 300 220 - ETSI EN 300 330 - ETSI EN 300 440 - ETSI EN 302 208 - ETSI TR 102 436 - ETSI TS 102 562 - ETSI TR 102 649
	Bar-coding	ISO/IEC 15417 Bar code symbology specification - Code 128 ISO/IEC 15420 Bar code symbology specification - EAN/UPC ISO/IEC 15424 Data carrier identifiers (including symbology identifiers) ISO/IEC 15424 Bar code symbology specification - PDF417 ISO/IEC 16022 Bar code symbology specification - Data Matrix ISO/IEC 16023 Bar code symbology specification - Maxicode ISO/IEC 16388 Bar code symbology specifications - Code 39 ISO/IEC 16390 Bar code symbology specification- Interleaved 2-of-5 ISO/IEC 18004 Bar code symbology QR Code ISO/IEC 24723 EAN.UCC Composite bar code symbolic Specification ISO/IEC 24724 Reduced Space Symbology (RSS) bar code symbology specification ISO/IEC 24728 MicroPDF417 bar code symbology specification ISO/IEC 24778 Aztec Code bar code symbology specification
	Medical Imaging	DICOM JPEG200
	Domotics	ISO/IEEE11073 (X73-PHD–*personal health devices*); X.10; EN 50090-ISO/IEC 14543;

continued on following page

Table 4. continued

N	TOPIC	STANDARDS
	Optical Biopsy	UH-OCT[46]; US[47]; PAM[48]; DOT[49], CE[50]
	Ambient Intelligence	SOUPA (Standard Ontology for Ubiquitous and Pervasive Applications) ISO 9241 H.323; MPEG-7 Near Field Communications (NFC): Bluetooth SIG; IEEE, 802.3 OSGi VME or Virtual mobile environments Standard Self Organizing Map (SOM) EMMA[51]. Agent- related technologies and standards (WSDL, OWL-S, WSMO, UDDI, JXTA, FIPA, LARKS, etc.) Registry types (UDDI, LDAP, ebXML) FIPA[52] set of standards Perceptive particle swarm optimization – PPSO, standard PSO (SPSO)
	Semantics-Terminology	ISO 13606-2-ADL [53]; HL7 CDA[54],SNOMED-CT,LOINC[55], ICDx ISO CD 15225:2000 – Nomenclature – Specification for a nomenclature system for medical devices for the purpose of regulatory data Exchange ISO/DTS 22789:2007, Health informatics – Conceptual framework for patient findings and problems in terminologies ISO 1804 for nursing terminologies, CEN EN 1068 Registration of coding systems CEN EN 12 264 for the definition of a Categorial structure, CEN EN 1828 Categorical structure for surgical procedures, CEN EN 12 611 for clinical laboratory, CEN EN 13 940 for continuity of care CEN EN 15 521 for human anatomy ISO/CD 25720 Genomic sequence variation markup language ISO/NP TS 27527 Health Informatics -- Provider Identification
5	**Quality Control and Assessment**	
		ISO 13485 Compliant Quality Management System ; ISO/TS 16949, Good Manufacturing Practice (GMP) ISO 15189:2003
	HIT or Health Care Information Technology	HITSP-Healthcare Information Technology Standards Panel. CCHIT- Certification Commission for Healthcare Information Technology.
	ISO 9001-medical requirements	21 CFR Part 11 (see risk management).
	ISO 9001-Laboratory requirements	ISO 9001:2000 Quality management systems-Requirements ISO 9000:2005 Quality management systems-Fundamentals and vocabulary ISO 13485:2003. Risk management EN 45001General criteria for the operation of testing laboratories /ISO 25 ISO 15189:2007 Medical laboratories – Particular requirements for quality and competence ISO 15190 standard on clinical laboratory safety ISO 15197 Blood glucosae monitoring systems for self testing ISO/IEC 17025: 2005 General requirements for the competence of testing and calibration laboratories ISO 20776:2007 Laboratory testing & In vitro diagnosis infectious diagnosis ISO/TR 22869:2008 Clinical laboratories ISO 22870:2006 Point-of-care testing (POCT) – Requirements for Quality and competence 21 CFR 58 Good Laboratory Practice for Non-Clinical Lab Studies iPassport Laboratory EQMS[56] 21 CFR Part 606 Good manufacturing for Blood & blood components Committee for Clinical Laboratory Standards (NCCLS) **EQALM** (**E**uropean committee for External **Q**uality **A**ssessment **P**rogrammes in **L**aboratory **M**edicine)

continued on following page

Table 4. continued

N	TOPIC	STANDARDS
	Risk Management	ISO 13485; ISO/IEC 15443 ; UNE71502:2004; ISO/IEC 27004; ISO /CD TS 25238; **21 CFR Part 11.** Based on the FDA's risk-based assessment for regulatory compliance 21 CFR 820 Quality System Regulation 21 CFR 806 Medical Devices; Reports Of Corrections And Removals 21 CFR 803 Medical Device Reporting 21 CFR 808 Exemptions From Federal Preemption Of State And Local Medical Device Requirements 21 CFR 814 Premarket Approval of Medical Devices
	CE Label	ISO/IEC 17025 General requirements for the competence of testing and calibration laboratories ISO/IEC 17021:2006 Conformity assessment -- Requirements for bodies providing audit and certification of management systems
	Benchmarking	JCAHO; PSI; PPE
	AAL, Ambient Assistance living	X.10; Digital Living Network Alliance (DLNA) certification IEC 62481-1 and IEC 62481-2 WPAN, IEEE 802.15.4 is under development
	EBTm[57],	
	Device management	ISO 13485;
	Electro-Magnetic fields & SARS	EN 50371 and EN 62311 ANSI C63.19 ISO/PRF TR 21730- Health informatics -- Use of mobile wireless communication and computing technology in healthcare facilities -- Recommendations for electro-magnetic compatibility (management of unintentional electromagnetic interference) with medical devices
6	**Telematic Tools in Telemedicine: Internet**	
	Data mining Semantic Web	Open Archives Initiative Protocol for Metadata Harvesting (OAI-PMH) and has been ratified as IETF RFC 5013, ANSI/NISO Standard Z39.85-2007, and ISO Standard 15836:2009. ISO 3166 ISO 639
	Metadata registry	ISO/IEC 11179 emphasizes, among other features, the use of non intelligent identifiers (RE: ISO/IEC 11179-5 and 111179-6) for data elements specified for sharing
	Knowledge discovery	
	Web services, GRID technology & Cloud	XML, WSDL, SOAP, SADL, MSDL, ASIDL, OCS[58] OGSI[59] standards
	Distant 3D reconstruction	
	Cloud computing	REST, RSS, ATOM, ATOM-PP
	IoT (internet of things)	The GS1 System of standards includes: GS1 Identification Keys: numbering schemas for products, locations, patients, care-givers, and assets GS1 Bar Codes: several types of bar code, linear and 2-dimensional, for use by GS1 members depending on the application GS1 EPCglobal: supporting the use of radio frequency identification RFID GS1 GDSN: ensuring global data synchronization and accurate product data across supply chain partners GS1 eCom: supporting electronic document interchange technologies
7	**Training, including Distance Training, Teleworking and Teleteaching**	
	Multimedia data sharing	ISO-15938-12:2008 (MPQF), we implicitly refer also to ISO-24800-3 (Part 3 of JPSearch)

continued on following page

Table 4. continued

N	TOPIC	STANDARDS
	Multimedia Querying	ISO-15938-12:2008 (MPQF[60]),
8	**Data Security and Privacy**	
	Public key infrastructure	ISO /DIS 17090 **Security on health informatics** **ISO/CD TS 21298-** Health informatics -- Functional and structural roles ISO/IEC 9594-8 (X.509)- Authentication by means of cryptographically derived credentials (PKI)
	Registry Authorities	ISO 646; ISO/IEC 7812; ISO/IEC 10036 ; **ISO**/IEC 6523- RAI[61] ISO/IEC 11179- Metadata registry for global electronic information interchange; **ISO**/TS 19127 IRDI is an internationally unique Identifier
	Certify authorities	Revocation Lists
	Privilege management	ISO/ PRF TS 22600 Health informatics -- Privilege management and access control
	Digital signature	**Title 21 CFR Part 11 of the FDA**
	Time stamping	ISO/IEC 18014; ISO 8601
	IS- Information Security	ISO/IEC 38500:2008, for the corporate governance of information and communication technology; ISO27000- Vocabulary ISO27001:2005, ISMS[62] - BS7799 in UK. ISO/IEC 27002:2005 (prior ISO/IEC 17799) - IS controls, ISO/IEC 27003-Implementation ISO/IEC 27004- Security indicators ISO/IEC 27005:2008, IS risk assessment, and BS3110-British Risk Management Standard. ISO/IEC 20000:2006 IT service management based on ITILv3, independently certificated. BS25999:2007, British Business Continuity Management Standard; ISO/IEC 24762, IT disaster recovery standard, and BS25777, the British IT Service Management Continuity Standard. CMMI[63] A quality management tool to describe typical organizational behavior at each of five levels of process 'maturity'. ASIS international guidelines ISO/IEC 15443 Information Technology- Security techniques. ISO/IEC-TR 15446:2004 Information Technology- Security techniques- Guide for the production of Protection Profiles and Security Targets ISO/IEC 15408:2005 Information technology- Security techniques- Evaluation criteria for IT security ISO/IEC 18014 Time stamping ISO/IEC 27001:2005 Information Security management systems- Requirements ISO/IEC 27004 Information Security Management measurements
9	**Liability and Legal Aspects**	
	Biological specimen tracking	EPC[64], GS1Healthcare; ISO 18000-2, 18000-3 Mode 2, 18000-4, 18000-6 and 18000-7; ISO 24730-2 and 24730-5 real-time locating system (RTLS) standards; The ISO 14443 and 15693 standards and EPCglobal's Gen 2 standard will also be included, as will protocols for testing ultra-wideband (UWB) and Wi-Fi RFID devices
	LOPD	
	LOAP	
		UI[65], used within the context of the DICOM Standard, are registered values as defined by ISO 9834-3 to ensure global uniqueness
10	**Health Economics in Telemedicine**	

continued on following page

Table 4. continued

N	TOPIC	STANDARDS
	Utility	CUA[66]; CVA[67]
		Quality live: QALY[68]; DALY[69], HALY[70]
		ISO 13485:2003 Quality Management. (ISO 9001:2000 for healthcare)
	Cost-Benefits	CEA[71]; CBA[72]
11	**Technology Transfer and Social Aspects**	
	Technology cycle	PLM Product lifecycle management. PCV Product centric view Business Process Reengineering (BPR)
	ERP[73]	G21: IS auditing guideline. ISAKA auditing standards. COBIT's information criteria Business Process Reengineering (BPR)
	Enterprise 2.0	B2B (business to business). Integration service providers
12	**Emerging Issues**	
	Nanodevices	ISO FDX –B ISO 15693 I ISO 7816 tarjeta proximidad Microchips iso and 21.1 MP chip ISO/IEC 7811 Identification Cards ISO/IEC 17025:2005 ISO 13485 ISO/TS 16949 and ISO/IEC 17025 ISO 14001:2004 ISO IEC 14496 CODING OF AUDIO VISUAL OBJECTS
	Lab on Chip (LoC)	ISO standards: 14443A 14443B, and 15693
	Implantable devices	
	IoT (Internet of Things)	EPC ™ /RFID[74]. Bar coding: **ISO** 15426; **ISO** 15394:2009; **ISO**/IEC 15416 IRDI is an internationally unique Identifier ISO/IEC 11179-6 Metadata of data elements Data Semantics: ISO/IEC 11179 (Metadata Registries) Terminology: ISO 704 (Principles of Terminology) ISO 1087-1 (Vocabulary for terminology work) ISO/TC 37/SC 4 (Language Resources Management) Interoperability: ISO/IEC 19763 (Framework for Metamodel Interoperability) ISO/IEC 20944 (Interoperability and bindings)
	Pervasive computing	PHD, IEEE 11073 family, AAL. ISO/IEEE240-PHI Event Driven Architecture (EDA)
	Cloud computing with VMware	IaaS[75], DaaS[76], PaaS[77],... SLA[78]

Semantic Interoperability

The semantic interoperability is a problem not only in Medical informatics applications but also in the Medical terms itself.

METATHESAURUS is the conceptual backbone in which medical terminology terms are correlated with the same or similar conceptual meanings from different sources.

In the *Metathesaurus maps* the source codes provided by the creators of the different code sets to unique strings (SUIs), normalized lexical terms (LUIs) and distinct concepts (CUIs). This information is located in the first file, the MRCONSO.

(Metathesaurus Relational Concepts and Sources). The second is the MRREL file that contains the relationships between concepts that supports the traversal of a source's ontology.

Pervasive and Mobile Computing

Information technology is moving towards pervasive and mobile computing, not only at home, but at the hospital and at the work place. On this progressive development the *issue of interferences* of wireless signals introduced before is an essential one (see below).

In medicine, personal monitoring scenarios require standardized features and functionalities. Its integration and implementation have been carried out using the Point of Contact standard ISO/IEEE11073 (X73). The result is the Personalized Health Informatics ISO/IEEE240-PHI and the Personal Health Data (PHD) standard the latter based on the 11073 family of standards also called Plug & Play for medical devices. It is applied to small devices with limited resources of processor, memory and power of the short-range wireless technology (see below WSN). Adapt the Domain Information Model and nomenclature of the 11073 to create the new standard that facilitates the remote patient monitoring with a mature technology-service.

However, there is still a lack of development in areas such as standardization of the sensor's communication interface, integration into electronic healthcare record systems or incorporation into ambient-intelligent scenarios.

In ambient intelligence, the Ambient Assisted Living (AAL) is an essential application where, among others, pervasive computing vision plays a role. The most reliable system is a wireless sensor network (WSN) on platforms (i.e. SunSPOT) building a specific services architecture. This architectural model allows the decoupling of applications in components such as ECG's monitor, position system or location awareness etc...

In Domotics the Intelligent Home control (IHC) standard have developed being commercialized in Europe and other countries under Schneider-Electric, or their dependent enterprises (LK in Holland, Alombard in France, Lexel in Holland & UK,...) The so-called "Thinclient", a very small device (minimum software and an operative system) with few electronics is able to open a session capable of administering the devices from the HTPC (Home Theater Personal Computer) server. The Internet Protocol Multimedia Subsystem-IMS based on System Initiation Protocol-SIP-standard, defines how IP networks manage voice calls and data transfer maintaining separated the underlying network services. This could integrate mobile and Wi-Fi.

In virtualization (either VMware or Cloud computing) where the software can simultaneously simulate various operative systems in one hardware simultaneously or use limited-computing portable systems to let the Cloud to take care of it either to distribute the task or to carry out in complex devices or store in huge systems.

Most people cannot distinguish what is a CLOUD-computing and what is a GRID-computing. In a simplistic manner, one thinks of a CLOUD as a virtualization and of a GRID when complex heavy-computing work is required.

GRID computing is ideal when a huge computation power is required in an application. By contrary virtualization is ideal when a numerous simultaneous applications are used most of them consuming a limited computation potential.

In the CLOUD, it is irrelevant whether a Grid or VMware structure is used. You just start the application in the Cloud and allow the Cloud to search the required tools.

The Cloud uses any virtualization architecture: Grid, SaaS (software as a service), PaaS, IaaS (Infrastructure as a Service), DaaS (Database as a Service) etc...all can run in the Cloud simultaneously. The cloud is build with any block consider to be of interest for a task.

GRID: Grid and grid-like technologies—including virtualization, automation, service oriented architecture (SOA) and distributed computing—are all part of the IT infrastructure to enable knowledge-based, global economy. Open Grid Service Infrastructure (OGSI) standards (Dobrev et al., 2002) are based on XML-based Web service protocols for interconnecting resources and defining the way in which elements of a network of computers can interact. In domotics, OGSI is used as a home-gateway but not in the *internal* infrastructure. It has limitations since publish/subscribe protocol does not suit for domotics. In fact, it is possible to provide subscription, but there is no notion of topics, which is a problem since home environment, has very rich ontologies.

Events generated by sensors should be fused, for security reasons, to generate higher-level events (i.e.: if someone is laying down the fall event is trigger if there is also an acceleration event). To fuse sensor data, a rule engine is connected to the WS-Notification interface. The hierarchy of events (event tree) is managed in a separated component. Notice that the event tree is a dynamic structure that can be modified at run time by the event server, but also by clients via appropriate WSDL calls. Client registration to events is stored in an appropriate database in the event server. Registrations to atomic or complex events can be made anytime. Registration may expire or be cancelled. The WS-Notification protocol includes the possibility of having *preconditions* and *selectors* connected with the registration of an event and controlling its generation and delivery. For instance, a client could register to the event of the home user fall, only under the condition that it is night.

Published Standards, Guidelines and Benchmarking

Up to now the latest publications on Telemedicine standards include the so called ATA "Core standards for telemedicine applications", those are the list of standards that we collected in 1998 in the Handbook of Telemedicine and that updated in the new releases in 3 different languages (Spanish, Russian and Greek) as well as in the latest proceedings of the Winter Course of the CATAI of 2007 based on Standards in Telemedicine, 2008 based on Quality control in Medicine. Biobanking and the 2009 proceedings dealing with the role of telemedicine in Superresolution and Optical Biopsy.

It is of paramount importance to realize that from the medical point of view there is no benchmarking in telemedicine, and no accreditation in telemedicine established by the Joint Commission on accreditation of Health Care organizations (JCAHO). That means that we cannot compare the results of medicine with or without telemedicine for the patients because there are no indicators established such us *mortality-index*, *remission-index* or *complication-index* associated to the *risk* or any other parameters that could be used to compare.

Furthermore, there are not PSIs or Patient Security Indicators or even worse, there are no PPEs or Patient Prevention Errors that are closer to the use of *e-health-systems* (i.e.: over dosage or prevention of adverse reactions with AEP or Assisted Electronic prescription…)

Very limited publications deal with well-designed trials that analyze patient benefits of face-to-face consultation versus telemedicine (Ferrer-Roca et al., 2009). This means that the EBM (evidence-based medicine) in telemedicine-EBTM is very limited, maybe with one exception: The clear benefits of the Tele-ictus or Stroke Units based on telemedicine, show for increasing number of patients for whom anticoagulant treatment was indicated, the speed up of diagnosis and treatment.

Healthcare Provider IT Strategies service offers in-depth coverage of the technologies that provide the most clinical value in terms of quality, cost, time, and agility and are transforming precare, point of care (POC), and postcare today.

CE LABEL: A Legal Requirement for Medical Devices in Europe

There are 17 European CE directives that specifically apply to manufacturers with the principal being for the medical devices:

- The Medical Devices Directive (MDD) applies to all general medical devices not covered by the Active Implantable Medical Devices Directive or the In Vitro Diagnostics Directive. 93/42/EEC & the new directive 2007/47/CE that extend the label requirements to software and telecommunications.
- The Active Implantable Medical Devices Directive (AIMDD) 90/385/EEC applies to all active devices and related accessories intended to be permanently implanted in humans.
- The In Vitro Diagnostics Directive (IVDD) 98/79/EC applies to all devices and kits used away from the patient to make a diagnosis of patient medical conditions.

The certification includes:

- Technical documentation/file or design dossier
- Device type examination
- Product quality assurance (based on ISO 13485)
- Production quality assurance (based on ISO 13485)
- Full quality assurance (ISO 13485)
- Batch verification/release

Further details of the CE market label in European Commission Enterprise and Industry European Standards.

The CCHIT® & CCHIT-Certified® labels are U.S. certification bodies that include all e-Health and Telemedicine products integrated inside the HIT (Health Information Technologies) including the Electronic Health Record (EHR). Certification criteria furnish a consensus baseline for these main aspects of an EHR. Certified products must demonstrate to trained, objective jurors all of the capabilities called for by the criteria.

That said, the criteria development and testing process builds on a number of checks and balances to position certification requirements so that they advance the progress of EHR capabilities while being careful not to require IT vendors to do the impossible.

The process for building a continually solid basis for EHRs, especially in the area of interoperability, takes a healthy appreciation for progressively scheduling higher levels of sophistication at the optimum pace and in the most logical sequence. The phased approach and tactical timeline can be found at the 'Introduction to Health IT Certification' (Certification Commission for Healthcare Information Technology, 2009).

Finally, the pharmaceutical industry had started a process of computer validation and management of the information technology in the healthcare and pharmaceutical industry with the following validation calendar, starting in 2009.

- January: Validation Planning (VMP, VP)
- February: Requirements Management and Process Mapping
- March: Specifications (including Migration and System Upgrades)
- April: Risk Management Process
- May: Supplier Evaluation / Audits / Subcontracting / Service Levels / Quality Plan
- June: Software Development (CMMI, ISO, Tools, Source Code Handling etc.)
- July: Software Testing (Development)
- August: Release Management and Hand-Over
- September: IQ: IT Infrastructure (Qualification)
- October: System and Acceptance Testing

- November: Go Live and Validation Reporting (Training)
- December: Support, Repair and IT Management Services
- January 2010: Results and generation of Validation White Paper (Draft for Review)
- March 2010: Validation White Paper (Final)

In Spain, for example, there is a trend for SIS (Sistemas de informacion Sanitaria) certification based on semantic interoperability, which builds on translation parses. This is part of the quality label and certification of the electronic health record systems in Europe (EuroRec, 2009). The standard for the message format was the CEN TC251, ENV 13606 standard, which is now being incorporated into the HL7 standard for clinical record transfer.

The UK experience in achieving a Standard Query Language for Primary Care systems is wider. The vendor must submit its software to an Accreditation process (NHS Connecting for Health, 2009). Part of this accreditation involves the inclusion of a 'HQL' (HEalth Query Language) interpreter. This allows a health community to extract anonymized data in a standard format for clinical audit, commissioning, governance etc. There is a crown copyright implementation of HQL called MIQUEST (Morbidity and Inquiry Export Syntax).

Furthermore, the GS1 UK Healthcare User Group (GS1, 2009) is leading the utilization and development of global standards for the UK healthcare industry, with the primary focus on automatic product identification to improve patient safety, as we will mention in the next paragraph regarding RFID. They are developing, promoting and implementing a global industry response for solutions in preventing medical errors, combating counterfeits and improving supply chain efficiencies throughout the healthcare industry.

RFID & EMI (Electromagnetic Interference)

Interferences are caused by the radio waves of one device, which distort the waves of another. Cells phones, wireless computers and even robots in factories can produce radio waves that interfere with RFID tags. Therefore, it is essential to incorporate new standards that enable interoperability.

RFID has an important role to play in healthcare. Auto-ID systems can help improve infection control and reduce dispensing errors. They can help monitor maintenance activities and locate critical equipment. CoreRFID's healthcare solutions include real time asset location, staff tracking; maintenance management and supplies logistics control systems.

Details of the human interaction can be studied in the CENELEC TC106x Electromagnetic fields in the human environment and the ISO RFID standards can be studied in (ISO RFID Standards, 2009; EPCglobal Inc, 2005; RFID Standards, 2009).

In the UK, as mentioned before, the Global Supply Channel- GS1 group (GS1, 2009) search for automatic identification, traceability, and data synchronization in health care include:

- GS1 Identification Keys: numbering schemas for products, locations, patients, caregivers, and assets
- GS1 Bar Codes: several types of bar code, linear and 2-dimensional, for use by GS1 members depending on the application
- GS1 EPC[79]global: supporting the use of radio frequency identification-RFID
- GS1 GDSN: ensuring global data synchronization and accurate product data across supply chain partners
- GS1 eCom: supporting electronic document interchange technologies

REFERENCES

Aiello, M., & Dustdar, S. (2008). Are our homes ready for services? A domotic infrastructure based on the Web service stack. *Pervasive and Mobile Computing*, *4*(4), 506–525. doi:10.1016/j.pmcj.2008.01.002

American National Standards Institute – HITSP Specifications. Retrieved September 30, 2009 from http://wiki.hitsp.org/docs/

Certification Commission for Health Information Technology. Retrieved September 30, 2009 from http://www.cchit.org/media

Chadwick, P. E. (2007). *Regulations and standards for wireless applications in eHealth*. Paper presented at the 29th Annual International Conference of the IEEE Engineering in Medicine & Biology Society.

Chang, H. H., & Chang, C. S. (2008). An assessment of technology-based service encounters & network security on the e-health care systems of medical centers in Taiwan. *BMC Health Services Research*, *8*, 87. doi:10.1186/1472-6963-8-87

Clarke, M., Bogia, D., Hassing, K., Steubesand, L., Chan, T., & Ayyagari, D. (2007). *Developing a standard for personal health devices based on 11073*. Paper presented at the 29th Annual International Conference of the IEEE Engineering in Medicine & Biology Society. Committee for Healthcare eStandards. Retrieved September 30, 2009 from http://www.chestandards.org/

Crowe, J., Hayes-Gill, B., Sumner, M., Barratt, C., Palethorpe, B., Greenhalgh, C., et al. (2004). *Modular Sensor Architecture for Unobtrusive Routine Clinical Diagnosis*. Paper presented at the Proceedings of the 24th International Conference on Distributed Computing Systems Workshops.

Dobrev, P., Famolari, D., Kurzke, C., Miller, B. A., Dobrev, P., & Famolari, D. (2002). Device and service discovery in home networks with OSGi. *IEEE Communications Magazine*, *40*(8), 86–92. doi:10.1109/MCOM.2002.1024420

Dobrev, P., Famolari, D., Kurzke, C., Miller, B. A., Dobrev, P., & Famolari, D. (2002). Device and service discovery in home networks with OSGi. *IEEE Communications Magazine*, *40*(8), 86–92. doi:10.1109/MCOM.2002.1024420

ENISA. (European Network and Information Security Agency)-Cloud computing Risk Assessment. Retrieved September 30, 2009 from http://www.enisa.europa.eu/act/rm/files/deliverables/cloud-computing-risk-assessment/

EPCglobal Inc. EPC™ Radio-Frequency Identity Protocols Class-1 Generation-2 UHF RFID Protocol for Communications at 860 MHz – 960 MHz, Retrieved March 30, 2005 from http://www.epcglobalinc.org/standards/uhfc1g2/uhfc1g2_1_0_9-standard-20050126.pdf

European Commission Enterprise and Industry European Standards. Retrieved September 30, 2009 from http://ec.europa.eu/enterprise/policies/european-standards/documents/harmonised-standards-legislation/list-references/

EuroRec: European Institute for Health Records. Retrieved September 30, 2009 from http://www.eurorec.org/services/standards/standards.cfm

Ferrer-Roca, O. (2009). Control de calidad y patoinformatica. *Rev Española Patologia*, *42*(2), 85–95. doi:10.1016/S1699-8855(09)70161-8

Ferrer-Roca, O., Figueredo, J., Franco, K., Cardenes, E. (2005). Telemedicine Intelligent Learning. Ontology for Agent Technology. *The IPSI BgD Transactions on Advanced Research*, 46-54.

Ferrer-Roca, O., & Sosa-Iudicissa, M. (Eds.). (1998). *Handbook of Telemedicine* (*Vol. 54*). Netherlands: IOS Press, Ohmsha.

GS1- Where Standards Get Down to Business. Retrieved August 20, 2009 from http://www.gs1us.org/

Galarraga, M., Serrano, L., Martínez, I., & de Toledo, P. (2006). Standards for Medical Device Communication: X73 PoC-MDC . In Bos, L., Roa, L., Yogesan, K., O'Connell, B., Marsh, A., & Blobel, B. (Eds.), *Medical and Care Compunetics 3* (*Vol. 121*).

Galarraga, M., Serrano, L., Martinez, I., de Toledo, P., & Reynolds, M. (2007). *Telemonitoring systems interoperability challenge: an updated review of the applicability of ISO/IEEE 11073 standards for interoperability in telemonitoring*. Paper presented at the 29th Annual International Conference of the IEEE Engineering in Medicine and Biology Society.

Gantenbein, R. E., & Robinson, B. J. (2008). Decoding CODECs. *Journal of Telemedicine and Telecare*, *14*(2), 59–61. doi:10.1258/jtt.2007.070810

International Standards Organization. *International Standards in process*. Retrieved March 30, 2008 from http://www.iso.org/iso/isoupdate_march08.pdf

ISO RFID Standards. A complete list. Retrieved September 30, 2009 from http://rfidwizards.com/index.php?option=com_content&view=article&id=242:iso-rfid-standards-a-complete-list&catid=227:standards

Mdi Europa – The Medical Device Service-Management. Retrieved September 30, 2009 from http://www.mdi-europa.com/services.htm

Medical device standards Portal – USA. Retrieved September 30, 2009 from http://www.medicaldevicestandards.com/

NHS Connecting for Health. Retrieved September 30, 2009 from http://www.connectingforhealth.nhs.uk

Philips. Mobile Point of Care. Retrieved September 30, 2009 from http://www.fimi.philips.com/mobile-point-of-care/index.html

Standards, R. F. I. D. Retrieved September 30, 2009 from http://www.corerfid.com/technology/TechnologyIssues/IssuesStandards.aspx

Sutherland, L., Igras, E., Ulmer, R., Sargious, P. (2000). A laboratory for testing the interoperability of telehealth systems. *Journal of Telemedicine and Telecare*, 6- Suppl 2, S74-75.

Wail, M. O., & Taleb-Bendiab, A. (2006). *Service Oriented Architecture for E-health Support Services Based on Grid Computing Over*. Paper presented at the IEEE International Conference on Services Computing.

ENDNOTES

1 EC= Endoscopic capsule
2 CAS= Computer assistant surgery
3 PoC= Point of Care
4 GPS= Global positioning systems
5 PAN= Personal area networks
6 PoR= Point of Reception
7 POCs= Points of contact (Disaster mitigation and relief operations)
8 AEP= Assisted Electronic Prescription
9 PUI= Patient Unique Identifier;
10 TCI= Telemedicine Center Identifier
11 LOINC= Logical Observation Identifiers names and codes
12 DES= Data Encryption Standards
13 DID= Doctor ID
14 QoS= Quality of Service
15 NP= Network performance
16 QoE= Quality of Experience
17 CHA= Continua Health Alliance

18 PLC= Power Line Communications.

19 Electronic healthcare record communication

20 Systems of Concepts to Support Continuity of Care

21 A syntax to represent the content of medical classification systems

22 General purpose information components

23 CCR = Continuity Care Record (ASTM E 2369)

24 NCPSP= National Council for Prescription Drug Programs (e-prescription)

25 CCHIT= Certification Commission for Healthcare Information Technology

26 CDA-CCD=Clinical document architecture-Continuity of Care document

27 RIM= Reference information model

28 AQL=Archetype query language.

29 CTS= Common terminology Services

30 OMG-HSSP= Object management group-Healthcare Services Specification Project.

31 CCOW= Clinical Context Management Specification

32 Common Message Element Types

33 Context Management Standard

34 RADT= Reservation/Registration - Admission, Discharge, Transfer

35 UHID= Universal Healthcare Identifier

36 CCR= Continuity of Care Record

37 EUA= Enterprise User Authentication

38 SSVS= Small size virtual slides

39 DIM= Domain information model

40 CLSI=Clinical Laboratory standard Institute

41 SMBG= Self Monitoring blood glucosae

42 NIST-CAB is integrated by Becton Dickinson Advanced Diagnostics, Ciba-Corning Diagnostics,
Dow Chemical Co., E.I. duPont de Nemours and Co., Miles Inc. And Ohmicron Corp.

43 eEHIC= electronic European Health Insurance Card

44 IoT= Internet of Things

45 MIIM=Mobile item identification and management

46 UH-OCT= Ultra high resolution Optical coherence tomography;

47 US = Ultrasound

48 PAM= Photoacustic microscopy

49 DOT= Diffuse optical tomography

50 CE= Confocal Endoscopy

51 EMMA= Extensive multimodal annotation mark up language

52 FIPA= Foundations for Intelligent physical agents

53 ADL=Archetype definition language

54 CDA= Clinical Document Architecture

55 LOINC= Logical Observation Identifiers Names and Codes

56 EQMS= Electronic quality management system

57 EBTm= Evidence Based Telemedicine

58 OCS= Open Cloud Standard

59 OGSI= Open Grid Service Infrastructure

60 MPQF= Mpeg query function

61 RAI=Registration Authority Identifier

62 ISMS= Information Security Management systems

63 CMMI= Capability Maturity Model Integrated

64 EPC= Electronic Product Code standards

65 UI= Unique Identifiers

66 CUA= Cost Utility Analysis

67 CVA= Cost Validity Analysis

68 QALY= Quality adjusted life years

69 DALY= Disability adjusted life years

70 HALY= Health Adjusted life years

71 CEA= Cost Effectivity Analysis

72 CBA= Cost Benefit Analysis

73 ERP= Enterprise Resource Planning

74 Electronic Product Code™/Radio Frequency Identification

75 IaaS= Infraestructure as a service

76 DaaS= Data Base as a services

77 PaaS= Platform as a service

78 SLA= Service Level Agreedments

79 EPC = Electronic Product Code

Chapter 18
Standards and Guidelines Development in the American Telemedicine Association

Elizabeth A. Krupinski
University of Arizona, USA

Nina Antoniotti
Marshfield Clinic Telehealth Network, USA

Anne Burdick
University of Miami Miller School of Medicine, USA

ABSTRACT

The American Telemedicine Association (ATA) was established in 1993 to promote access to medical care for consumers and health professionals via telecommunications technology. The ATA Standards and Guidelines Committee has been charged by the Board of Directors with identifying, overseeing, and assisting work groups to develop individual standards and guidelines for specific technical, clinical and administrative areas. This chapter will review the mission of the ATA Standards and Guidelines Committee, the process by which standards and guidelines documents are produced, and report on its progress to date in providing the telehealth community with standards and guidelines for the practicing medicine at a distance.

INTRODUCTION

The American Telemedicine Association was established in 1993 as a non-profit organization to bring together a variety of groups from medicine, academia, technology and telecommunications companies, e-health, m-health, medical societies, government and others to overcome barriers to the advancement of telemedicine. The Association works to achieve this goal through a variety of mission-related activities. One of its main activities is to educate government and the public about telemedicine in order to validate its role as an essential component in the delivery of modern medical care. The ATA also serves as a resource for information and services related to telemedicine. Its 2009 Annual Meeting in Las Vegas, NV had an attendance of over 2700 people – a 12% increase

DOI: 10.4018/978-1-61692-843-8.ch018

over the previous year, attesting to its role as a leader in telemedical information and resources. The ATA website (www.americantelemed.org) is a leading source for telemedicine news. In its effort to foster networks and collaboration, the ATA sponsors 14 Special Interest and Discussion Groups and has two Regional Chapters (Latin America & Caribbean and Pacific Islands). Each of the groups meets regularly and discusses critical issues related to their interest focus (e.g., Business & Finance, Teledermatology). The ATA also promotes research and education by sponsoring the Annual Meeting with its associated scientific program and exhibition showcase, and periodically forming task forces to develop vision papers on a specific telemedicine topic (Krupinski et al., 2006). Finally, the ATA is creating the basis for assuring uniform quality in the delivery of remote healthcare services, particularly via the Standards and Guidelines Committee efforts.

BACKGROUND

There have been efforts towards establishing standards and guidelines for telemedicine practice prior to the formal establishment of the ATA Standards and Guidelines Committee. For example, radiology has a number of technical and practice guidelines in place for digital image acquisition, storage, transfer and display via Picture Archiving and Communications Systems (PACS) and teleradiology (Seibert, et al., 2004; Van Moore, et al., 2005; Siegel, et al., 2006; Williams et al., 2007; Krupinski et al., 2007); and the Society of American Gastrointestinal and Endoscopic Surgeons has guidelines for the Surgical Practice of Telemedicine (SAGES, 2004). The first set of guidelines from the ATA actually pre-dated the formation of the Standards and Guidelines Committee, and was created for Telepathology in 1999 (ATA, 1999).

In 2004 Richard Bakalar, MD and the ATA Ocular Telehealth Special Interest Group developed and published the first truly formal set of ATA practice guidelines. The guidelines specifically addressed diabetic retinopathy telehealth clinical and administrative issues and provided guidelines for designing and implementing a diabetic retinopathy ocular telehealth care program (ATA, 2004). This document established the general framework for future efforts in terms of addressing technical, administrative and clinical aspects associated with a particular clinical specialty using telemedicine as a means to deliver patient care. A very important precedence was established in the creation of these guidelines. Early in the development process the decision was made to contact the National Institute of Standards and Technology (NIST) for help and guidance regarding the accepted means by which standards and guidelines are produced and approved. Since then, NIST and the ATA have collaborated extensively in the guideline development process.

The formal effort to create a standing committee and establish a process for developing standards and guidelines within the ATA was initiated by Hon Pak, MD when he was Vice President of the Association in 2005-2006. As a practicing tele-dermatologist, he recognized the need for quality and consistency in the practice of teledermatology, so the first practice guidelines developed by the Standards and Guidelines Committee were the Practice Guidelines for Teledermatology (Krupinski, et al., 2007). This document followed the general format established in the diabetic retinopathy guidelines and addressed technical, administrative and clinical aspects of teledermatology.

Under guidance from NIST, the teledermatology guidelines were the first to incorporate the idea that practice recommendations could have different levels of importance and that the guidelines are required whenever *feasible and practical* as determined by the referring clinician practicing under local conditions. Thus, there are Guidelines that "shall" be implemented in order to meet a basic minimum level of operation in order to provide quality telehealth care. At the next level are Recommendations for Best Practices that "should" be adopted for optimal practice if possible. Finally, there are optional or permissible actions indicated by "may/attempt to" that can be adopted to further optimize the teleconsults process.

The Teledermatology guidelines were also the first to incorporate a preamble that broadly stated the intent of the document and the manner in which it should be used. A number of specific points were included that continue to be incorporated into current and future guideline documents. Three of these points are worth mentioning. The first is that compliance with the guidelines does not guarantee accurate diagnosis or successful outcomes. The goal of the guidelines is to assist the clinical practitioner in pursuing a sound course of action to provide effective and safe medical care founded on current information, available resources, and patient needs. The second point follows from the first and states that the primary care practitioner is responsible for all decisions regarding the appropriateness of a specific procedure or course of action. They must consider all presenting circumstances, and if they choose to use an approach that differs from the guideline it does not imply that the approach varied from the standard of care. Reasonable judgment based on local circumstances and the assessment of what is feasible and practical should be used at all times. Finally, the preamble notes that the guidelines are not designed nor meant to be unyielding requirements of practice and are not meant to serve as or be used to establish a legal standard of care.

CORE STANDARDS

Telemedicine is a very broad field, encompassing nearly every clinical sub-specialty being practiced today. Thus it is impractical, and likely not necessary, to develop standards and guidelines for every possible clinical specialty or telemedicine application. Recognizing this, the ATA Standards and Guidelines Committee decided early on to focus initially on a core set of principles that could guide telemedicine practice in general. The first part of this effort was to create a Telemedicine/Telehealth Glossary of Terms (ATA, 2006). The list is composed of terms and definitions that are commonly used in telemedicine/telehealth. It was assembled for the purpose of encouraging consistency in employing these terms in ATA related documents and resource materials, including standards and guidelines. The list is not all-inclusive and is designed to be augmented as specific groups develop practice guidelines for particular clinical applications.

The Core Standards for Telemedicine Operations document was completed in 2008 (ATA, 2008). This document covers broad policies and procedures that should be used by institutions providing remote medical services, interactive patient encounters, and any other electronic communications between patients and practitioners for the purposes of health care delivery. In order to define more precisely who the document was addressing, it noted that the standards apply to individual practitioners, group practices, health care systems, and other providers of health related services where there are telehealth interactions between patients and service providers for the purposes of health care delivery. As with the earlier ATA standards documents, this one provides guidance with respect to administrative, clinical and technical aspects of telemedicine practice.

The Administrative Standards section is divided into three parts, one directed at Organizations one at Health Professionals, and the third covers Telemedicine Ethics. The Organization and Health Professionals sections address those providing services via telehealth and covers primarily issues of responsibility and standard operating procedures. Briefly it notes that organizations and providers shall follow the standard operating policies and procedures of the governing institution especially with respect to: human resource management;

privacy and confidentiality; federal, state and other credentialing and regulatory agency requirements; fiscal management; ownership of patient records; documentation; patient rights and responsibilities; network security; telehealth equipment use; and research protocols. Quality improvement and assessment procedures are required to be place as are all other aspects of patient care that require adherence to federal, state and local regulatory bodies (i.e., patient consent, protection of health information, patient rights and responsibilities, integration of telemedicine into a practice, collaborative agreements/contracts). Health professionals in particular shall be fully licensed and registered, aware of credentialing requirements, aware of their locus of accountability, cognizant of when a provider-patient telehealth relationship has been established, and shall have the necessary education and training to insure safe provision of health services. Clearly, none of these administrative guidelines differ from the standard operating procedures that organizations and health professionals follow without involving telemedicine. They are meant in a sense to reiterate and emphasize that the practice of telemedicine needs to be carried out with the same high standards of patient care and safety that are normally followed.

Of particular importance in this document is the section on telemedicine practice ethics. It notes that although telemedicine is not a practice in and of itself, practicing at a distance does create a unique relationship with the patient. This requires attention to and adherence to professional ethical principles that may be new to most healthcare practitioners. Specifically, the ethics section states that an organization or healthcare professional shall (1) incorporate organizational values and ethics statements into the administrative policies and procedures for telemedicine; (2) be aware of medical and other professional discipline codes of ethics when using telemedicine; (3) inform the patient of their rights and responsibilities when receiving care at a distance (through telemedicine) including to influence decisions made about, for, or with patients who receive care via telemedicine. These Administrative Standards are applicable to all telemedicine encounters and thus are referred to in any specialty practice guidelines developed.

The Clinical Standards section of the Core document is rather brief, as clinical practice guidelines will be different to some degree for every clinical specialty and are thus more fully dealt with in the specialty guidelines. In the Core document, only two points are noted. One is that the organization and health professional shall be satisfied that health professionals providing care via telehealth are aware of their professional discipline standards and that those standards shall be upheld in telemedicine. The second point is that health professionals shall be guided by existing professional discipline and national practice guidelines when practicing telehealth and if modifications exist specifically for telehealth they shall be followed.

Finally, the Technical Standards deal with broad equipment and technology issues. Again, certain specialties will utilize equipment unique to their specialty and thus more specific technical standards are provided in each specialty set of practice guidelines. For example, the Diabetic Retinopathy guidelines provide technical guidelines for non-mydriatic devices and image acquisition, while the teledermatology guidelines provide technical specifications for store-forward digital cameras used to acquire images of the skin. In the Core document, technical standards include such aspects as insuring the equipment used is available and properly functioning; that the technology meets all relevant laws, regulations and codes for safety; that infection control policies and procedures are in place; patient information is safe and complies with local and federal legislation and rules regarding privacy and confidentiality; that systems have appropriate redundancies in place especially for network connectivity; that published technical standards are met for safety and efficacy of devices used with patients; and that equipment is properly maintained.

THE DEVELOPMENT PROCESS

The ATA has clearly evolved over the years in terms of the way it approaches the development of standards and guidelines for telemedicine. In recent years, the Committee has established a more formal process for guideline development. One of the main reasons for this has been the increased interest and need of the ATA Special Interest Groups (SIGs) in creating practice guidelines. Although many members of the SIGs are members of specialty societies, in general telemedicine seems to be a relatively low priority focus area for these societies and thus practice guideline development for telemedicine is rarely an activity they initiate. Thus, the ATA has become the go to organization for standards and guidelines development.

In order to deal with the increased demand and the number of groups seeking to develop guidelines documents, the Committee developed a standard operating procedure. In part, the goal is to ensure success and be in compliance with federal anti-trust regulations. Therefore, it was deemed critical that the process for implementing guidelines development be clear and open. At the core of process is the Standards and Guidelines Committee, which is appointed by the President of ATA in consultation with the ATA Executive Committee. The Committee has a Chair and Vice-Chair and a committee of interested members who all serve on a voluntary basis. The Committee meets by phone once a month and at the Annual Meeting. This Committee is charged with provided overall guidance in the following.

First it identifies Working Groups to be charged with developing individual standards and guidelines and then recommends the relative priority for each specific area to the Board of Directors for approval. The Working Groups typically emerge from the SIGs. SIGs that are interested in initiating development of standards and guidelines prepare a petition to the Standards Committee that includes suggestions for who will lead the effort, the names of people who will participate on the working group, and the purpose, objectives, and area(s) or general scope of the effort. The area or scope of effort to be addressed is determined by consensus among the members of the SIG in consultation with the ATA Staff and the Committee. In general, we have found that it is possible to work on an average of three sets of guidelines per year, so priority areas are chosen based on interest by ATA members, the relative level of current clinical activity compared to other areas in telemedicine, the availability of sufficient member support, the interest and willingness of allied organizations to contribute to the effort, and the availability of any established and recognized gold standards within the specialty area.

Once a Working Group is established, the ATA determines when the official commencement of activities will begin and what timeframe will be followed. Members and chairs of each Working Group are appointed by the Chair of Standards Committee with the approval by the full Committee. In recruiting members, it is encouraged highly that they achieve a balanced representation from clinical, industry, government and other potentially affected parties, both from within and outside the ATA membership. In particular, the involvement of NIST representatives is encouraged. Once the Working Group is established, a notice is circulated publicly noting that the ATA is forming a Working Group and information about its purpose, process, timelines and proposed products is described. If anyone not officially recruited to be a member chooses to be involved, they can attend future meetings, but only officially appointed members have a voice or a vote. Prior to any formal meetings, all participants are required to fully disclose any potential conflicts and this information is shared with the Working Group and is made public.

After the Working Group is established, there is a Suggested Work Plan encompassing 10 steps towards the development of a final document. A timeline is provided to help keep the momentum of the initial enthusiasm going. The first step is a Preparation Workshop in which the Document Scope and Definition are established (1 day kickoff meeting). During this meeting, the Working Group is expected to review standards and guidelines policy and guidance documents and the Telemedicine/Telehealth Glossary of Terms. They should then develop consensus on scope and definitions; identify and catalogue any existing clinical benchmark references or "as is" gold standards; identify stakeholder and committee membership; and develop one or more appropriate use cases. The second step is a Stakeholder Forum/ Component Workshop. Depending on the Working Group needs this may be a single or multiple Forum/Workshop. This should take place within 300 days of the process kickoff and is designed to collect information and knowledge based on the agenda established in the Preparation Workshop. The assigning of authors should also take place at this meeting, and it is recommended to split the writing responsibilities into three sections – administrative, technical and clinical.

Once the author teams have been created, they have 30 days to develop drafts of their respective document sections. Following this stage, the drafts are made available for 30 days for an on-line comment period open only to internal stakeholders. At the end of this period, the document sections must be incorporated into a single document that takes into account the stakeholder comments as deemed appropriate. Various working groups carry this step out in different ways, but typically the Chair and Vice-Chair of the Working Group or a designated Editorial Board create the final document version (45 days). The final draft document is then posted on the ATA web site for an on-line comment period of 90 days. This comment period is for external stakeholders and the general public. At the end of this period, the Working Group Chair and Vice-chair or Editorial Board reviews the comments and decides which, if any, should be incorporated into the document. At this point it is considered final and the Working Group submits it to the ATA Chair of the Standards and Guidelines Committee who then presents it to the ATA Board of Directors for final approval within 30 days. Endorsement by external societies can also be sought and is highly recommended. As noted, the Working Groups are encouraged to have representatives from external societies on board during the development process, with one goal being to facilitate the adoption by these societies.

The final document is posted on the ATA web site and is available for purchase by interested parties. The Working Group is also encouraged to publish the document in a relevant peer-reviewed journal. At this point the Working Group should also consider development of an Education and Implementation Strategy, and possibly a Certification Program. For example, the Teledermatology SIG has already published their standards document (Krupinski et al., 2007) and based on feedback from the dermatology community has initiated a two-pronged education effort. The original document was very comprehensive and included a detailed set of guidelines. Although thorough and complete, it is a rather dense document that is daunting to many healthcare providers. In response, the Teledermatology SIG is creating a modified version of the guidelines directed primarily at the healthcare provider that gives a clear description of the minimum set of clinically relevant recommended guidelines needed to practice safe and effective teledermatology. The second education effort is creating a "Teledermatology 101" on-line course with two levels of difficulty. The first level will serve more as an introduction to teledermatology and again provide a clear description of the minimum set of clinically relevant recommended guidelines needed to practice safe and effective teledermatology. The second level course will more closely parallel the original practice guidelines document, reviewing the administrative, technical and clinical guidelines in more detail with specific reference to the actual guideline language and recommendations (shall, should and may).

ISSUES, CONTROVERSIES, PROBLEMS

As already noted previously, one of the issues the ATA Standards and Guidelines Committee has faced in the past couple of years has been the increased demand for practice guidelines for specific areas within telemedicine. This is not a problem per se since the development of practice guidelines is precisely what the Committee has been charged with doing. Additionally, such guidelines are needed in the telemedicine community to help educate practitioners about the technology, procedures, benefits and limitations of practicing telemedicine. Having practice guidelines in place that are approved by the ATA Board of Directors and endorsed or approved by other professional also provides a source of data and information that can be used to develop public policy, lobby to the government for reducing limitations on the practice of telemedicine, and lobby to payors for increased telemedicine reimbursement.

A related issue is how to develop practice guidelines for clinical areas that in themselves are quite diverse and in the past typically have not had clear and/or published practice guidelines. For example, rehabilitation covers a broad spectrum of services from physical therapy, to occupational therapy, speech therapy, audiology and other related services. The challenge being faced is whether it is more appropriate to develop broad tele-practice guidelines that cover an entire specialty but at a more superficial level perhaps, or do we develop focused sets of practice guidelines for each sub-specialty? Unfortunately there is no one-size-fits-all solution and the ATA Committee currently decides this on a case by case basis.

One final issue is whether the ATA should or even can enforce the practice guidelines it develops. As described previously, the goal of the guidelines is to assist the clinical practitioner in pursuing a sound course of action to provide effective and safe medical care founded on current information, available resources, and patient needs. The guidelines specifically note that compliance does not guarantee accurate diagnosis or successful outcomes, and that the primary care practitioner is responsible for all decisions regarding the appropriateness of a specific procedure or course of action, using reasonable judgment based on local circumstances and the assessment of what is feasible and practical. The guidelines are not designed or meant to be unyielding requirements of practice and are not meant to serve as or be used to establish a legal standard of care. Currently the ATA does not have any certification or enforcement policies or procedures in place. The practice guidelines are developed, approved and disseminated as already described. It then becomes the responsibility of the individual practitioner to decide how and whether to implement them. The ATA is not a credentialing or certifying body and to become one would require the Association to set up a separate incorporated body specifically designed to take on this responsibility and function. At this point in time, the ATA has not seen the need for this level of regulation regarding the practice standards developed to date, and thus has not initiated any efforts to devise enforcement strategies.

SOLUTIONS AND RECOMMENDATIONS

In order to deal with the increased demand for developing telemedicine standards and guidelines, one of the first things the Committee did was to standardize the process as detailed above. In order to initiate a request to start the development process, the SIG leading the effort is required to complete an official request form to be submitted to the Committee. This form requires the SIG to designate a project chair and committee, a description of the project and its deliverables, the scope of the project, and an estimated timeline. In order to complete this document and prepare for the initial Preparation Workshop, it is expected that the SIG has already reviewed the literature and the field in general to determine existing guidelines are available and whether they are appropriate for telemedicine. In other words, the need for a new set of guidelines must be established. If there are existing, appropriate guidelines available, the SIG may choose to work on getting them endorsed by the ATA Board of Directors "as is", or they may choose to get permission from the body that created them to adapt them to the particular telemedicine application under consideration.

In general, the ATA Standards and Guidelines Committee encourages incorporation of existing standards and guidelines into telemedicine practice guidelines whenever appropriate. For example, the Core Standards for Telemedicine Operations document was amended in 2009 to include a new section on electronic health information security. As such guidelines already exist in a number of forms, the amendment was not a detailed description of all of the possible measures one should take to keep electronic health information secure. Instead, it noted that such standards do exist and that practitioners of telemedicine should be aware of them and incorporate them into their practice whenever feasible and appropriate. In the Standards and Guidelines section of the ATA web site, there is a list with links to existing guidelines and position statements developed by other organizations, as well as a list and links to various technical standards (e.g., International Telecommunications Union (ITU) and the Digital Imaging and Communications in Medicine (DICOM) standards) that are typically used in the telemedicine.

FUTURE DIRECTIONS

The ATA currently has four completed practice guidelines – Core Standards, Telepathology, Diabetic Retinopathy, and Teledermatology. During 2009, at least two new sets of guidelines will be completed - Evidence Based Practice for Telemental Health and Telepresenting. Two new groups are initiating the development process – Telerehabilitation and Home Telehealth and Remote Monitoring. The Committee also recognizes that any set of guidelines created is dynamic rather than static. Technology changes, clinical practices change, and new diagnostic methods and tools are developed. Practice guidelines developed even a couple of years ago can quickly become outdated and need to be revised to reflect the current state-of-the-art. Therefore, the Ocular Telehealth SIG is currently updating the Diabetic Retinopathy document and expanding it to include additional ocular conditions amenable to telemedicine. The Teledermatology SIG, as noted previously, is working on developing a more concise and easy to read version of its original practice guideline document. In the future, the Committee intends to develop approximately three practice guidelines per year as well as update and revise older guidelines as appropriate.

CONCLUSION

The development of guidelines and standards for telemedicine is an important and valuable process to help insure effective and safe delivery of quality healthcare. The ATA has made the development of standards and guidelines a priority within the Association and over the past five years has significantly streamlined and formalized the development process. The practice guidelines developed so far have been well received by the telemedicine community and are being adopted in numerous practices as attested to by the feedback we have received. It is interesting to note that the practice guidelines that are available are appearing in the research literature. For instance, Rudnisky et al., (2007) carried out a study to validate a teleophthalmology system and incorporated the Diabetic Retinopathy Practice Guidelines into their study both in terms of acquisition and display of the images, and in terms of grading them into diagnostic categories. Studies that utilize the published guidelines not only help bring them into grater public awareness, but they also provide the evidence needed to validate the existing guidelines and guide the revision of future versions.

As telemedicine continues to grow and be adopted by more healthcare practitioners as a regular part of their clinical practice, the ATA practice guidelines will be adopted as well. As dynamic documents, they will continue to evolve to reflect the changes in the way that telemedicine is practiced, and the ATA will continue to draw on the expertise and experience of representatives from medicine, industry, government and other potentially affected parties, both from within and outside the ATA membership.

REFERENCES

American Telemedicine Association. (1999). *Guidelines for Telepathology*. Retrieved May 13, 2009, from http://www.americantelemed.org/i4a/ams/amsstore/category.cfm?category_id=2

American Telemedicine Association. (2004). Telehealth practice recommendations for diabetic retinopathy. *Telemedicine and e-Health, 10*(4), 469-482.

American Telemedicine Association. (2006). *Telemedicine/Telehealth Terminology*. Retrieved May 13, 2009, from http://www.americantelemed.org/files/public/standards/glossaryofterms.pdf

American Telemedicine Association. (2008). *Core Standards for Telemedicine Operations*. Retrieved May 13, 2009, from http://www.americantelemed.org/i4a/pages/index.cfm?pageID=3311

Krupinski, E., Burdick, A., & Pak H. (2007). American Telemedicine Association's Practice Guidelines for Teledermatology. *Telemedicine and e-Health, 14*(3), 289-302.

Krupinski, E., Dimmick, S., & Grigsby, J. (2006). Research recommendations for the American Telemedicine Association. *Telemedicine and e-Health, 12*(5), 579-589.

Krupinski, E. A., Williams, M. B., & Andriole, K. (2007). Digital radiography image quality: image processing and display. *Journal of the American College of Radiology, 4*(6), 389–400. doi:10.1016/j.jacr.2007.02.001

Rudnisky, C. J., Tennant, M. T. S., & Weis, E. (2007). Web-based grading of compressed stereoscopic digital photography versus standard film photography for the diagnosis of diabetic retinopathy. *Ophthalmology, 114*(9), 1748–1754. doi:10.1016/j.ophtha.2006.12.010

SAGES (Society of American Gastrointestinal and Endoscopic Surgeons). (2004). *Guidelines for the Surgical Practice of Telemedicine*. Retrieved May 13, 2009, from http://www.sages.org/sagespublication.php?doc=21

Seibert, J. A., Kent, J. S., & Geiss, R. A. (2004). *Practice guideline for electronic medical information privacy and security*. Retrieved May 13, 2009, from http://www.acr.org/SecondaryMainMenuCategories/quality_safety/guidelines/med_phys/electronic_medical_info.aspx

Siegel, E., Krupinski, E., & Samei, E. (2006). Digital mammography image quality: image display. *Journal of the American College of Radiology, 3*(8), 615–627. doi:10.1016/j.jacr.2006.03.007

Van Moore, A., Allen, B., & Campbell, S. C. (2005). Report of the ACR task force on international teleradiology. *Journal of the American College of Radiology, 2*(2), 121–125. doi:10.1016/j.jacr.2004.08.003

Williams, M. B., Krupinski, E. A., & Strauss, K. J. (2007). Digital radiography image quality: image acquisition. *Journal of the American College of Radiology, 4*(6), 371–388. doi:10.1016/j.jacr.2007.02.002

Chapter 19
Telepaediatrics in Queensland: Evidence for Quality, Reliability and Sustainability

Sisira Edirippulige
The University of Queensland, Australia

Anthony C. Smith
The University of Queensland, Australia

ABSTRACT

Telemedicine has been shown to be an effective alternative technique to provide health services to rural and remote communities. Although the interest in telemedicine is growing, there is little evidence to show the quality and reliability of telemedicine techniques. This chapter describes the telepaediatric service in Queensland, Australia outlining some evidence for quality, reliability and sustainability.

INTRODUCTION

The provision of health care at distance using information and communication technologies (ICT) i.e. e-health (telemedicine) is believed to be an effective alternative way of providing health services to rural and remote communities (Edirippulige, Smith, Bensink et al., 2009). However, there is little evidence available on the quality and reliability of this technique. Similarly, there is no much evidence about the sustainability. This paper provides an overview of telemedicine services established by the University of Queensland Centre for Online Health (COH) to provide care to children and adolescent in rural Queensland. The chapter will provide some evidence on the quality and reliability of this program while examine the factors related to the design and development of these services that helped for the sustainability of this service.

DOI: 10.4018/978-1-61692-843-8.ch019

BACKGROUND

Health Care in Rural Queensland

Substandard healthcare in rural and remote communities is not a new phenomenon. Rural communities have less health facilities and a lack of health workforce, particularly specialist health professionals. This is true to both developed and developing countries. Geographical isolation and restricted access to specialist health services are main contributing factors to the inequality of health care around the world. This is more relevant to countries like Australia where communities are scattered across huge land-mass. A recent report by the Australian Institute of Health and Welfare indicated that the people in regional and remote areas are at greater risk of cancer, chronic diseases, alcohol and drug addiction and obesity. The report also noted that the life expectancy in regional areas is one to two years lower and in remote areas up to 7 years lower compared to their urban counterparts. There is a significant difference in the health status of indigenous people – the majority live in regional and remote Australia – compared to the non-indigenous population (Australian Institute of Health and Welfare, 2008).

Queensland is the second largest state in Australia with a population of about 4.2 million. Whilst two-thirds of the Queensland population lives in the south-east region of the state, the remainder is spread in major towns along the east coast (18%) or in remote townships (15%). The distances separating these communities with urban centres are vast. Because most specialist health centres are located in Brisbane, patients living in rural and remote communities usually have to travel to see the specialist if a referral is made.

Delivering specialist care to children living in the regional Queensland is challenging. Often these children are required to travel to tertiary centres for specialist consultations. In some circumstances, specialists travel to regional hospitals to conduct outreach clinics. These traditional methods of providing services are associated with numerous negative consequences including cost for health services and families, stress and discomfort for patients, families and providers.

To mitigate some of these difficulties, the health department in Queensland subsidises the travel costs incurred by regional patients through a patient travel subsidy scheme (PTSS) funded by the State government. This is the conventional model of delivering specialist health services to patients living in non-metropolitan areas. Doctors in regional areas are able to refer patients to a specialist, which then makes them eligible for support through the scheme. In 2007, the travel scheme cost the Queensland health department approximately $32 million (Queensland Health, 2008).

Specialist outreach clinics are also arranged for groups of patients in selected rural and remote communities. These clinics involve specialist teams who travel out to communities to see patients periodically throughout the year. These clinics are well received in these areas and offer specialist staff valuable insight into the needs and resources available within these communities. Nonetheless, the cost, travel time and inconvenience involved in these outreach clinics are considerable.

What is Telemedicine?

The use of information and communication technologies to deliver health services at distance is known as telemedicine (Edirippulige & Wootton, 2006). A number of different terms such as telemedicine, telehealth, online health and e-health are often used interchangeably. In this chapter, we will use telemedicine to denote this mode of health delivery.

Telemedicine services may be categorised according to method used – i.e. either real-time or store and forward. Parties involved in a real-time telemedicine consultation communicate synchronously via a telecommunication network. Telephone discussions or videoconferencing sessions are examples of real-time applications. The primary advantage of real-time telemedicine is that there is usually no detectable time delay between the information being transmitted and received, that is the parties concerned can interact as though they were present in the same room.

Store and forward telemedicine involves the transmission of stored information from one site to another over a period of time. Store and forward telemedicine, which is sometimes referred to as asynchronous or pre-recorded, involves information being captured and then transmitted to the other party for specialist opinion. Common examples include communication via email or facsimile. The main advantage of this method of working is that the parties involved can work independently from one another; i.e. they do not have to be present at a pre-arranged time. The choice between real-time or store-and-forward telemedicine is often dependant on the type of information which is being shared, the facilities/ telecommunications available and the urgency.

Telemedicine can be more applicable to countries such as Australia where communities are scattered across large distances,. In Australia, there are small townships, which are located thousands of kilometers away from metropolitan regions. Access to health services and health facilities in such distant locations is often restricted. The difficulty of accessing health and medical services (particularly specialist care) in rural Australia is well documented (Judd & Humphreys, 2001; Humphreys, 1990; Longsdale & Holms, 1981). Consequently, rural communities often have poor health outcomes compared to their urban counterparts. A report by the Australian Institute of Health and Welfare (AIHW) suggested that people living in remote communities have a higher mortality rate due to burns, fall, stroke, asthma, diabetes, homicide, suicide, and cancers. The studies have also found that there is a significant increase in injury, mortality, hospital separation and socio-economic disadvantages in rural and remote locations compared to capital cities (Australian Institute of Health and Welfare, 2008). The problems related to health status of indigenous communities - one of the main population-segments living in rural locations – have also been reported (Bulleting of World Health Organisations, 2006).

Telepaediatrics

In November 2000, a trial was initiated by the University of Queensland (UQ) Centre for Online Health (COH) in close partnership with the Royal Children's Hospital (RCH) in Brisbane and selected regional hospitals in Queensland. Given that the conventional method of sending patients to the specialist was well established, a central referral centre for telemedicine referrals was introduced as an alternative referral method. The basic tenet of this initiative was to try to make telemedicine a convenient option rather than a burden for the referring clinician.

The telepaediatric service gives regional clinicians a single point of contact for referring patients for a specialist consultation. A dedicated 1800 toll-free telephone number is available - which provides the referrer with contact with a telepaediatric coordinator who has an instrumental role in collecting referral information and arranging a response by an appropriate specialist. The telepaediatric coordinator plays an important role making sure all requests are managed with a minimal waiting time. All referrals have a guaranteed response time of 24 hours.

Since the telepaediatric service began, over 7000 consultations have been conducted for thousands of children in Queensland. The COH currently delivers telepaediatric services to 82 regional hospitals in Queensland and several health centres in northern New South Wales. The communication modes used are email, telephone and videoconferencing. The majority (approximately 85%) of all referrals made to the telepaediatric service result in a videoconference. The COH have installed a number of dedicated videoconference systems at selected sites for paediatric work but predominantly relies on the large network of videoconferencing systems available in public hospitals and health centres throughout Queensland. To date, more than 550 videoconferencing units have been installed and are managed by the Queensland Health department.

Since the trial began in 2000, the telepaediatric service has now grown into a routine service at the RCH. Most of the telepaediatric clinics are scheduled 12 months in much the same way as the specialist outpatient department at the RCH. The telepaediatric services cover 37 different subspecialist areas and involve more than 240 medical, nursing and allied health staff (Smith & Gray, 2009). Some of the sub-specialties include cardiology, dermatology, diabetes, general paediatrics, neurology, oncology, orthopaedics, post-acute burns care, psychiatry and surgery (Smith, Batch, Lang & Wootton, 2003; Justo, Smith, Williams et al, 2004; Smith, Youngberry, Mill et al, 2004).

Single Point of Contact

One unique feature of this service is the centralized referral centre. Based in Brisbane, this centralized referral centre is available to selected regional sites throughout Queensland. Telepaediatric referrals are easily made by calling a toll-free 1800 telephone number, which provides a direct link to the duty telepaediatric coordinator. Once a referral is made to the service, a specialist response is guaranteed within 24hrs. telepaediatric coordinators employ a rang of communication technologies, including the telephone, email and videoconferencing. About 90% of all telepaediatric referrals result in a consultation via videoconference.

Routine clinics are scheduled 12 months in advance, in a similar fashion to the conventional outpatient department. Regional patients who need to see a paediatric specialist can be easily referred to one of the weekly clinics available. More than 35 different paediatric subspecialties are offered by the telepaediatric service. One of the leading areas is post-acute burns care, where 17% of all paediatric burns outpatients are now managed via videoconference.

Technology Used

Telepaediatric consultations are conducted using a range of technologies. Telephone, email and videoconferencing are some of the widely used methods. However, a large number of consultations are conducted using videoconference. The COH is based with the children's hospital in Brisbane, which is the capital city of Queensland. COH has two specially equipped videoconference studios, which are used for the delivery of telepaediatric services.

Figure 1. Specialist consultation via videoconference (Centre for Online Health)

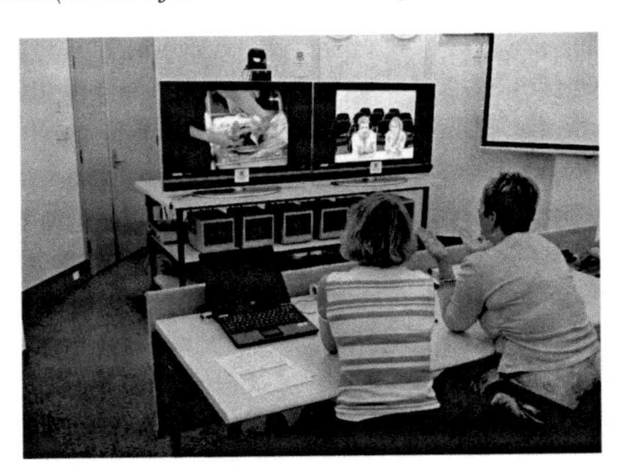

The studios contain commercial videoconferencing equipment; video document camera, laptop computer and DVD recorder. ISDN and IP connectivity allows the COH to connect to other videoconference systems when required. Depending on the type of consultation and the information which is being transmitted, bandwidth requirements can vary. However, the majority of connections are done at a transmission speed ranging from 128 to 384 kbit/s.

In addition to fixed telemedicine systems, the services are also provided using mobile and wireless telemedicine units. The mobile telemedicine units give regional clinicians the opportunity to consult with RCH specialists during their ward rounds at patients' bedside. The first mobile unit was stationed at a regional hospital in Gladstone where there has been no paediatrician for some years. To ensure that the videoconference facilities were child friendly, the COH developed a mobile videoconference system in the shape of a robot (Smith, Coulthard et al, 2005). During ward rounds, the unit was wheeled to patients' bedside for the consultation.

Figure 2. Robot consultation at the bedside

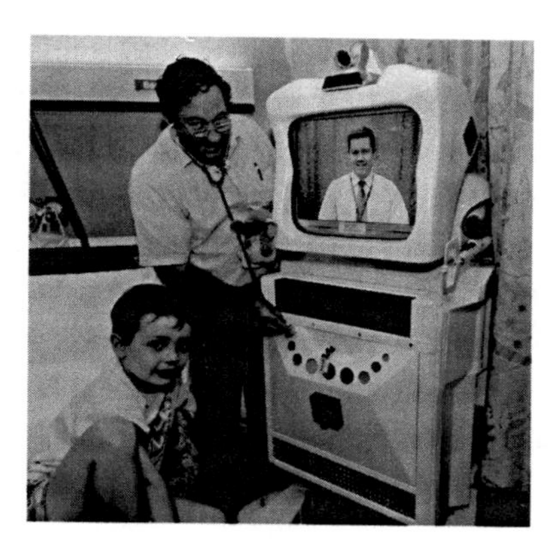

The specialist in Brisbane is able to communicate directly with the local staff, patient and family. Once the feasibility of these systems was demonstrated further funding was obtained to expand the network of mobile (robot) systems to five regional hospitals in Queensland.

One important feature of the mobile units is the remote management capability. These systems are fully maintained by telepaediatrics coordinators in Brisbane. All connections to the mobile systems are managed remotely including call connections and daily quality tests.

Another significant telemedicine activity of the telepaeditatric program is mobile health screening program. A combination of factors has led to the need for more innovative methods of providing specialist health services to Indigenous children in central and far north Queensland. These factors include the large distances, the logistics of sending specialists to remote regions and the high incidence of chronic disease (such as otitis media) amongst patients in these areas.

In 2008, the COH commenced a trial of a mobile health screening service (www.healthescreen4kids.org) which would allow health workers to travel to surrounding communities and provide routine screening of children. Regardless of where screening takes place, health workers can collect patient information and digital images of the eyes and ears, together with a clinical history of the patient, hearing assessment and health risk questionnaire. This information is stored on a computer and transmitted via the Internet to a secure database which can be routinely monitored by a team of specialists based in Brisbane. For example, children with suspected ear disease or hearing loss would have their records reviewed by an ENT specialist who will be able to view the images and data for diagnostic purposes and provide a recommended treatment plan for the primary care provider. If surgery is required, patients will be categorized according to urgency and scheduled in the next available clinic.

The need to address critical health issues of indigenous communities in Australia have been widely discussed (Bulletin of World Health Organisation, 2008). Improving health status of Aboriginal children has been one of the priority areas of the Government. The expectation is that the current trial will provide positive results to use this method to expand the services to other Aboriginal and Torres Strait Islander communities throughout the country which face similar challenges.

Quality and Reliability

Telemedicine services and research activities at the COH often overlap. While designing, developing and running telemedicine services, COH has been responsible for continuing evaluation of various aspects of these services. A number of qualitative and quantitative studies carried out by the COH have focused on various aspects including user satisfaction, efficacy of services, clinical outcomes and economics. In the following section, we will provide a brief summary of evidence from several studies.

Tele- ENT Program

Ear, nose and throat (ENT) disorders are common and represent a large proportion of healthcare problems in children. Lack of ENT specialists in rural and regional areas is a major problem for health systems to provide services to rural communities. There is a high rate of referrals to ENT specialty clinics in Queensland. For instance, in North Queensland the prevalence of childhood ENT problems, especially otitis media, is extremely high among aboriginal children (66%-95%).

Regional patients have to travel to urban centres to see a specialist which often involves several hours drive. The Royal Children's Hospital in Brisbane is one of the two major paediatric tertiary referral hospitals which provide ENT specialist services to Queensland population. Annually about 5000 ENT outpatient consultation and 2000 inpatient admissions are carried out by the RCH.

In early 2002, within the telepaediatric program COH initiated a tele-ENT service. Patients in selected regional areas were referred by their local primary healthcare providers to a telemedicine clinic at their local hospital. Instead of traveling to Brisbane to see the specialist, an ENT consultation was conducted via videoconference. During the videoconference appointment, an ENT examination was carried out using a video-otoscope connected to the videoconferencing system. The specialist was able to view real-time ENT images at a bandwidth of 384kbit/s. the consultant could also view the hearing test results, and x-rays transmitted via a document camera. During the consultation, consultant could discuss the history and clinical findings with the patient, family and the local paediatrician in order to make appropriate decisions on diagnosis and clinical management (Smith, Williams, Agnew et al, 2005).

Tele-ENT clinics have now become a regular service. Telehealth coordinator schedules the tele-ENT visits for the year in advance.

Several studies have examined the clinical outcomes of tele-ENT in comparison to out patient department (OPD-ENT) consultations. One study investigated the accuracy of pre-recorded digital ENT images and found over 80% concordance compared to follow-up and real time consultations (Smith, Perry, Agnew et al., 2006).

Another study was conducted to determine the agreement between diagnoses and management plans made during an initial videoconferencing appointment and subsequent face to face consultation in paediatric ENT surgery. Among the 68 patients seen via videoconference and in person, the recorded diagnosis was the same in 99% of cases. Surgical management decisions were the same in 93% of cases. The study concluded that the decision made about ENT surgical interventions for children during videoconference clinics are in close agreement with decisions made by the same surgeon at face to face consultation (Smith, Dowthwaite, Agnew et al., 2008).

Several studies have also been conducted to investigate the cost-effectiveness of tele-ENT service. One study found that from the health provider's perspective, the tele-ENT service is less expensive than the conventional OPD service. The tele-ENT service was cheaper when the workloads exceeded 100 consultations per year. The selected regional sites such as Bundaberg already had exceeded the threshold point making tele-ENT a cost-effective service (Xu, Smith, Scuffham et al., 2008).

Telepaediatric Burns Consultations

There is only one specialist paedatric burns centre in Queensland which is located at the Royal Children's Hospital. This means many patients those who need specialist burns consultation have to travel long distances to attend clinics in Brisbane.

Although telepaediatric is not likely to be useful for acute and urgent burns treatment, it is proven effective for burns follow-up consultations. Post acute burns consultations using videoconferencing, initiated by the Centre for Online Health envisaged to avoid long distance travels for patients, but provide a communication medium satisfactory to conduct clinical meetings. Since the outset, videoconference has become a routine technique for the post-acute burns care of children in Queensland. Telemedicine burns clinics are normally conducted using a single ISDN line at a bandwidth of 128 kbit/s. Audio and video quality are considered to be satisfactory for such consultations.

A study comparing the agreement between clinical assessments conducted via videoconference and assessments conducted in conventional face-to-face consultations showed a concordance of 85%. The study concluded that the quality of information collected during a videoconference appointment is comparable to that collected during a traditional, face-to-face appointment for a follow up burns consultation (Smith, Kimble et al., 2004).

Studies have also shown high satisfaction of consultants and patients using telemedicine techniques for burns follow-ups. Clinicians found that the telemedicine appointments were an adequate means for assessing the patient and formulating clinical decisions relating to management. Patients also agreed that their medical conditions could be adequately managed via telemedicine technique. Patients preferred the option of participating in a telemedicine consultation to travelling to Brisbane (Smith & Kimble, 2004).

Evidence shows that telemedicine has significantly reduced patients' travel time. A recent study found that over six years, 1000 videoconference consultations eliminated about 1.4 million km of patient travel (Smith, Patterson & Scott, 2009).

Paediatric Telecardiology

Traditionally, in Queensland, children born with congenital heart disease are managed by urgent transfer to a tertiary paediatric cardiology centres. Patients also attend in occasional outreach clinics for less urgent cases. Telepaediatric program at the Centre for Online Health was introduced to use telemedicine techniques to provide paediatric cardiology services to regional communities (Justo, Smith, Williams et al., 2004).

Figure 3. Telecardiology clinic at the Royal Children's Hospital

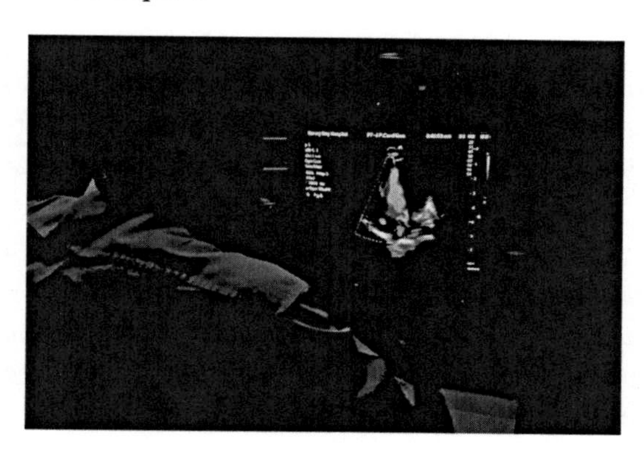

Basic concept of this system is to enable a paediatric cardiologist in Brisbane to examine the patient and view echo-cardiographic images real-time before making a decision to transfer the patient to Brisbane. The selected regional sites (for example, regional hospitals in Hervey Bay and Mackay) can link with a tertiary centre via telemedicine to have specialist consultation for patients. The service has enabled real-time communication of a team of carers such as ultrasonographer and paediatrician at the regional site, and the paediatric cardiologist at the tertiary referral centre. Since the service was established, hundreds of patients have been examined and provided services using the telecardiology system.

In the majority of cases, the telecardiology consultations have helped manage patients locally avoiding unnecessary transfer of patients to tertiary hospital. Telepaediatric cardiology clinics are now a routine service at the Royal Children's Hospital (Smith, Williams, & Justo, 2002).

A study has shown that simultaneous audio and video transmission including echocardigraphic images using ISDN lines at a bandwidth of 384 kbit/s was in general adequate for accurate diagnosis. This study also found that there were no major discrepancies in the diagnoses using echocardiographic image assessment via videoconference and onsite (Justo, Smith, Williams et al., 2004).

Impact of Telemedicine

The telepaediatric service in Queensland has resulted in a major change in the way traditional outpatient services are managed. Firstly, the service has shown that there are alternative ways to referring a patient to specialist clinics in tertiary hospitals. Referrals are still being made when a patient needs specialist care. But with the introduction of telepaediatric service, patient or the specialist do not need to travel a long and time consuming trip. Telemedicine has proven to be a useful and convenient way to provide specialist care to those patients.

The introduction of telepaediatric service has made a significant change in the traditional use of information and communication technologies and network available in Queensland. Prior to telepaediatric service was introduced, the equipment and network facilities available in hospitals in Queensland were mainly used for administrative and educational purposes. There was a very limited utility of the technology for clinical purposes. However, with the introduction of telepaediatric program the situation has significantly changed. For example, today nearly 17% of burns follow-up consultations are conducted via telemedicine at the RCH.

The telepaediatric service has also made significant changes to the way how clinicians work. There is a significant collaboration between the specialists and local clinicians. Telemedicine links have offered an opportunity for clinicians in two locations to discuss patients and make decisions collaboratively. From local clinicians' perspective, the opportunity to communicate closely with specialists has been educational.

Telepaediatric service has changed the attitudes and perceptions of clinicians and patients about telemedicine. Studies have shown a high satisfaction of this new technique in both groups. It is fair to say that there is a considerable enthusiasm among groups of clinicians about telemedicine. This change of attitude can prompt further expansion of telemedicine activities.

From policy makers' perspective, the telepaediatric service has offered some evidence for alternative ways of providing health services to rural communities. Evidence for telemedicine practices, particularly evidence for cost savings may encourage governments to invest more in telemedicine.

Unique Features

One common mistake made by telemedicine designers is giving priority to technology. This over-emphasis on the technology can often be misleading. While designing a telemedicine service, it is extremely important undertake a thorough needs analysis. One should carefully examine the pros and cons of existing health service (if applicable) with consideration of how telemedicine might be useful. The selection of all other components in the telemedicine program, including technology must then be determined in alliance with these goals.

Telemedicine programs developed at the COH are less technology focused and more tailored to the clinical needs and operational requirements. It is important that telemedicine systems are easy to use, present no hindrance to the clinicians and are conveniently accessible. It is also important that telemedicine services complement existing services (such as hospital outpatient services and travelling outreach clinics) provided by specialists.

This insight essentially comes as a result of the close interaction with clinicians who consequently use telemedicine. Successful telemedicine service cannot be developed in isolation from the clinicians. Understanding the needs of the clinicians and accommodating them is the key to a sustainable telemedicine service. It is also vital to give clinicians opportunity to play a leading role in designing, developing and running telemedicine projects.

CONCLUSION

Telemedicine has a potential for the delivery of health services, particularly for people living in rural and remote communities. The telepaediatrics in Queensland has proven effective. The service has provided services to thousands of kids in Queensland and gradually become an integral part of the health services at the Royal Children's Hospital. Both patients and providers have shown high level of satisfaction about the service. Evidence is also becoming available for quality, reliability and accuracy of the service.

REFERENCES

Australian Institute of Health and Welfare (AIHW). (2008). *Rural, Regional and Remote Health: Indicators of health status and determinants of health*, Australian Institute of Health and Welfare, Canberra, cat. no. PHE 97.

Bulletin of World Health Organisation. (2008). Australia's disturbing health disparities set Aboriginals apart. BWHO, 86(4): 241-320. Retrieved December 15, 2008, from http://www.who.int/bulletin/volumes/86/4/08-020408/en/index.html

Edirippulige, S., Smith, A. C., Bensink, M., Armfield, N., & Wootton, R. (2009). Nurses and Telehealth: current practice and future directions . In Staudinger, B., Hob, V., & Ostermann, H. (Eds.), *Nursing and Clinical Informatics: Socio-technical approaches* (pp. 94–409). New York: Medical Information Science Reference. doi:10.4018/978-1-60566-234-3.ch007

Edirippulige, S., & Wootton, R. (2006). Telehealth and Communication. In M. Conrick (Ed.). *Health Informatics, Transforming Health care with Technology*, 266-278, Melbourne, Thomson.

Humphreys, J. S. (1990). Super-clinics or a country practice? Contrasts in rural life and health service provision in northern NSW. D. J. Walmsley (Ed). *Change and Adjustment in Northern NSW*.(pp. 73-84). Armidale, ME: University of New England.

Judd, F., & Humphreys, J. (2001). Mental health issues for rural and remote Australia. *The Australian Journal of Rural Health*, *6*(5), 254–258. doi:10.1046/j.1440-1584.2001.00417.x

Justo, R., Smith, A. C., Williams, M., Westhuyzen, J. V., & der, ., Murray, J., Sciuto, G., & Wootton, R. (2004). Paediatric telecardiology services in Queensland: a review of three years' experience. *Journal of Telemedicine and Telecare*, *10*(Suppl 1), 57–60. doi:10.1258/1357633042614258

Lonsdale, R. E., & Holmes, J. H. (1981). *Settlement systems in sparsely populated regions: The United States and Australia*. New York: Pergamon Press.

Queensland Health. (2008). *Queensland Health Annual Report 2007-2008*. Brisbane, Queensland Government. Available at URL: http://www.health.qld.gov.au/publications/corporate/annual_reports/annualreport2008/default.asp

Smith, A. C., Batch, J., Lang, E., & Wootton, R. (2003). The use of online health techniques for the delivery of specialist paediatric diabetes services in Queensland . *Journal of Telemedicine and Telecare*, *9*(Suppl. 2), 54–57. doi:10.1258/135763303322596273

Smith, A. C., Coulthard, M., Clark, R., Armfield, N., Taylor, S., & Mottarelly, I. (2005). Wireless telemedicine for the delivery of specialist paediatric services to the bedside. *Journal of Telemedicine and Telecare*, *11*(Suppl 2), 81–85. doi:10.1258/135763305775124669

Smith, A. C., Dowthwaite, S., Agnew, J., & Wootton, R. (2008). Concordance between real-time telemedicine assessments and face-to-face consultations in paediatric otolaryngology. *The Medical Journal of Australia*, *188*(8), 457–460.

Smith, A. C., & Gray, L. C. (2009). Telemedicine across the ages. *The Medical Journal of Australia, 190*(1), 15–19.

Smith, A. C., Kimble, R., Bailey, D., Mill, J., & Wootton, R. (2004). Diagnostic accuracy of and patient satisfaction with telemedicine for the follow-up of paediatric burns patients. *Journal of Telemedicine and Telecare, 10*(4), 193–198. doi:10.1258/1357633041424449

Smith, A. C., Patterson, V., & Scott, R. E. (2007). Reducing your carbon footprint: How telemedicine helps? *British Medical Journal, 335*, 1060. doi:10.1136/bmj.39402.471863.BE

Smith, A. C., Perry, C., Agnew, J., & Wootton, R. (2006). Accuracy of pre-recorded video images for the assessment of rural indigenous children with ear, nose and throat conditions. *Journal of Telemedicine and Telecare, 12*(Suppl. 3), 76–80. doi:10.1258/135763306779380138

Smith, A. C., Williams, J., Agnew, J., Sinclair, S., Youngberry, K., & Wootton, R. (2005). Real-time telemedicine for paediatric otolaryngology pre-admission screening . *Journal of Telemedicine and Telecare, 11*(Suppl 2), 86–89. doi:10.1258/135763305775124821

Smith, A. C., Williams, M., & Justo, R. (2002). The multidisciplinary management of a paediatric cardiac emergency. *Journal of Telemedicine and Telecare, 8*, 112–114. doi:10.1258/1357633021937578

Smith, A. C., Youngberry, K., Mill, J., Kimble, R., & Wootton, R. (2004). A review of three years experience using email and videoconferencing for delivery of post-acute burns care to children in Queensland. *Burns, 30*(3), 248–252. doi:10.1016/j.burns.2003.11.003

Xu, C., Smith, A. C., Scuffham, P. A., & Wootton, R. (2008). A cost minimisation analysis of a telepaediatric otolaryngology service. *BMC Health Services Research, 8*, 30. doi:10.1186/1472-6963-8-30

Chapter 20
Evaluation Considerations for E-Health Systems

Anastasia N. Kastania
Biomedical Research Foundation of the Academy of Athens, Greece & Athens University of Economics and Business, Greece

ABSTRACT

E-health evaluation, which involves different dimensions, has increased. In traditional healthcare, quality dimensions exist but these are not sufficiently exploited for e-health. Reliability is often examined regarding technology, software, demand and survival. This chapter reviews the reasons that e-health systems need to be evaluated, the methods followed for conducting e-health evaluation studies and the main points that characterize an evaluation procedure as successful. Many researchers have presented evaluation considerations for e-health. Herein, the emphasis is on analyzing a series of ideas mined from the scientific literature that allows drawing up practical considerations for e-health evaluation. These considerations focus both on quality and reliability assurance as well as on quality and reliability improvement.

INTRODUCTION

Quality assurance and quality control are different both in the meaning and nature. Quality assurance consists of activities undertaken before data collection to ensure the data are of the highest possible quality at the time of collection (Arts et al., 2002). It involves techniques used to assure the quality requirements and should include prevention, detection and action (Arts et al., 2002). Selecting and training the workforce and designing a data collection method are essential aspects of prevention. Detection of data errors can be achieved through routinely recording the data, which means comparison with data in another independent data source. Finally, action implies correction of data errors and determination of their causes (Arts et al., 2002). Quality control takes place during and after data collection. It aims at identifying and correcting sources of data errors (Arts et al., 2002). Quality control involves activities, which ensure that the product will reach its

DOI: 10.4018/978-1-61692-843-8.ch020

quality requirements. Overall, quality measurements include (1) performance measurement, (2) outcome evaluation based in the standards, and (3) performance improvement if the standards are not satisfied (Donabedian, 1988).

However, traditional retrospective methods of quality assessment are not enough to meet the needs of current health care, especially those that involve the practice of medicine in an electronic environment (Kangarloo et al., 1999). Nevertheless, the standard measurements of quality assurance can be strengthened applying process models in a telehealth environment (Kangarloo et al., 1999). Product manufacturing has much bibliography for Total Quality Management (TQM) with the beginnings, directives and techniques on product quality (Wang, 1998). Therefore, in order to acquire the highest benefit from the new e-health services it is essential to establish an explicit method to describe the Quality of Service (QoS) requirements for the transferred information and the network management (Fortino & Nigro, 2000). Applications for electronic payment transactions, telemedicine, computerized medical records and open line access about newer treatments and prevention can help in quality improvement, access expansion and expenses management (AMIA, 1997).

On the other hand, reliability analysis in telemedicine networks requires theoretical knowledge and practical experience from the field of reliability engineering. A summary of reliability modeling in telemedicine networks includes various reliability assessment issues such as network, system, software and diagnosis (Kastania et al., 2008a). The robustness is also useful in determining the effectiveness during a reliability analysis (Dellaca et al., 2009).

Finally, Health Technology Assessment is necessary for quality improvement and for assuring the effectiveness in the health care (Leys, 2003; Stevens et al., 2004; Gagnon et al., 2006). Evaluation of existing interfaces and standards is complex and complicates the research questions related to adaptivity, safety and quality-preserving integration (Ras et al., 2007).

Therefore, the chapter collects and analyzes a series of ideas mined from current scientific literature related to quality and reliability in e-health. Another goal is to use these ideas to develop frameworks for evaluation purposes. These frameworks are expected to be useful for quality and reliability assessment in e-health.

BACKGROUND

Quality Assurance

Information technologies improve health care access and lower cost (Bashshur et al., 2000; Perednia & Allen, 1995; Kastania & Papadhmhtriou, 2008b) but increase risk. Overall, e-health technologies place serious questions for quality assurance. Therefore, in the e-health discourse, prominent questions include access and quality assurance.

Quality assurance depends on anyone practicing medicine as well its demand from the patients, the pharmaceutical companies and the health insurers. Moreover, quality assurance of clinical coding (including vocabularies and classifications) includes: simple data requirements, automated testing for cohesion, human inspections and field-testing (Schulz, et al., 1998). Service quality is also crucial (Hu, 2003; Pitt et al., 1995). Finally, the traditional definition of software quality relates quality to "fitness for use". In this context, the formal methods for requirements analysis (Fraser & Vaishnavi, 1997) demonstrate three software quality indices: correctness, maintainability, and integrity (Troster et al., 1993).

On the other hand, the inadequacy of traditional qualitative measurements has led scientists to seek new methods for improving the quality of care (Kangarloo et al., 1999; Hebert, 2001). They concluded that two components form the quality of medical care: quality of medical personnel and the technical quality about equipment (Sanazaro,

1980). Finally, the qualitative management of medical information on the Internet requires evaluation, labeling, and filtering of information (Cabrera et al., 2004).

It is worthwhile mentioning that process modeling is a quality management strategy appropriate for telemedicine/telehealth services (Kangarloo et al., 1999) while the SERVQUAL approach, which consists of five dimensions (Tangibles, Reliability, Responsiveness, Assurance and Empathy), can be used for the evaluation of healthcare services and for designing service improvements (Kastania & Zimeras, 2008c).

Reliability Assurance

An assessment tool is reliable if its repeated use produces the same results (Field, 1996). Moreover, reliability is the probability for a system to adequately achieve its purpose under specific operating conditions and predefined time (Reibman & Veeraraghavan, 1991; Klinger et al., 1989). The main reliability analysis technique for electronics is life testing (Reibman & Veeraraghavan, 1991) while software reliability is the failure-free operation for a predefined time in a specific context (Reussner et al., 2003; Lyu, 1996). Reliability analysis involves identification of the most critical components or states of the services (Spyrou et al., 2008). For example, telediagnostic systems are validated against gold standards (Holle & Zahlmann, 1999), which are defined by expert opinion, and are subject to inter-rater reliability problems that have to be clarified in the study design and analysis (Holle & Zahlmann, 1999).

Health outcomes are better the last few years as methodologists and researchers have tested and improved the validity and reliability, relevance, and usability of specific measures in clinical practice (Field, 1996). The Institute of Medicine (Field, 1996) drew attention to issues of validity and reliability of these test instruments. For several of the evaluation attributes (including reliability and validity) and certain kinds of clinical measures, a controlled vocabulary (that is, a precise, common clinical terminology) is crucial (Field, 1996). Moreover, services should conform to high standards for reliability and the quality of service (QoS) (Graschew et al., 2006). Finally, in evaluating the acceptability of telemedicine from patients and clinicians written questionnaires are used (Health Canada, 2000).

Evaluation Research

E-health services furnish challenges for the evaluators. Evaluating health information systems is a complex and controversial project focused on two parallel approaches: the framework, the process and content as well as the structure, the process and the outcomes (Klecun-Dabrowska & Cornford, 2001). Other researchers (May et al., 2003) have used qualitative inquiring methods to collect formative processes for the design and materialization of the new systems and their evaluation by their users.

Evaluation questions the clinical practice of care, the patient status, the health outcome, the access possibility, the cost and the acceptance when compared with different strategies of health care. It also requires a descriptive approach to be carried out (Klecun-Dabrowska & Cornford, 2001).

User satisfaction should be part of the evaluation procedure. However, evaluation often degrades to the satisfaction with the technical performance. Furthermore, stakeholder expectations affect the assessment outcome (O'Keefe, 1989; Remenyi & Money, 1991) while medical roots in the content and methods of assessment are feasibility, clinical outcome and safety (Lobley, 1997; Wallace, 1998).

An evaluation requirement for telemedicine includes results of patient care and social profits (Taylor, 1998a; Taylor, 1998b). The Institute of Medicine presented eleven definitions of telemedicine (Field, 1996) related to service benefit (Grigsby, 1998; Grigsby et al., 1995). Other related issues are teaching and administration (Lipson & Henderson, 1995).

Technology assessment for medical devices focuses on the risks, the costs, benefits and the clinical effectiveness. There are also other technologies and applications that should be evaluated based on specific criteria (Grigsby & Barton, 1998). Common assessment instruments include (Hu, 2003; DeChant et al., 1996): communication theory (Shannon, 2001), theory of information influence (Mason, 1978) and different dimensions of information system success (DeLone & McLean, 1992; DeLone & McLean, 2002).

Overall, a proposal for e-health success should take into consideration and compare doctor's opinions (Mairinger et al., 1996).

Fundamental Ideas for E-Health Quality Assurance

The first goal of quality is to ensure that a developed product or a service is effective and based on standards (Averill, 1994; Kastania & Zimeras, 2008b). Fundamental characteristics in the development of applications, which ensure system quality, are reliability, accuracy, ease of use, ease of integration, flexibility and functionality (Hu, 2003). However, they do not include estimates on the use or access.

A literature mining on the references concerning e-health quality assurance results to the dimensions of Figure 1.

Information System

The researchers of information systems should pay attention to controlling and measuring success considerations taking into account their interdependence (LeRouge et al., 2002). Overall, there are six key dimensions for information systems success (DeLone & McLean, 1992): system quality, information quality, quality of use, user satisfaction, individual impact and organizational impact. The information systems success models (DeLone & McLean, 1992; Hu, 2003) evaluate quality (May et al., 2000) based on the usefulness, effectiveness and acceptance of new systems (Buxton & Hanney, 1998). Security is (LeRouge et al., 2002; LeRouge et al., 2004) a quality concern for access (who can use) and location (to prevent equipment damage) while e-health codes of conduct and computer mediated data quality solutions should be also evaluated (Hu, 2003).

Data quality in electronic patient records can be quantified using availability and concordance (Aronsky & Haug, 2000). Availability is the percentage of observations from the reference standard recorded in the electronic patient record (Aronsky & Haug, 2000). Concordance is the percentage of observations that are identically recorded in the electronic patient record and the reference standard (Aronsky & Haug, 2000). The nature and the cause of medical errors can be analyzed depending on the source and the form of clinical variables. However, there is a software requirement, which involves data cleaning and data integration in order to allow refinement of usefulness and accuracy of electronic medical records (De Lusignan et al., 2002).

Various indicators describe satisfaction in e-health: quality of service, convenience, communication, and human connection (Thurmond & Boyle, 2002). Network monitoring can be used to control and track remote hosts, network traffic, routing table configurations, and service quality (Thai et al., 2001). Knowledge management within the context of evidence-based health care provides the potential to improve the quality of service provided to practitioners, who seek evidence (Fennessy, 2002). Finally, new professional roles may be needed for those who teach about data quality and searching (Kaplan & Flatley Brennan, 2001).

Telemedicine

Data quality is necessary in telemedicine while data transmission is an essential part of system quality (Hu, 2003). This involves bandwidth

Figure 1. Ideas involved in e-health quality assurance

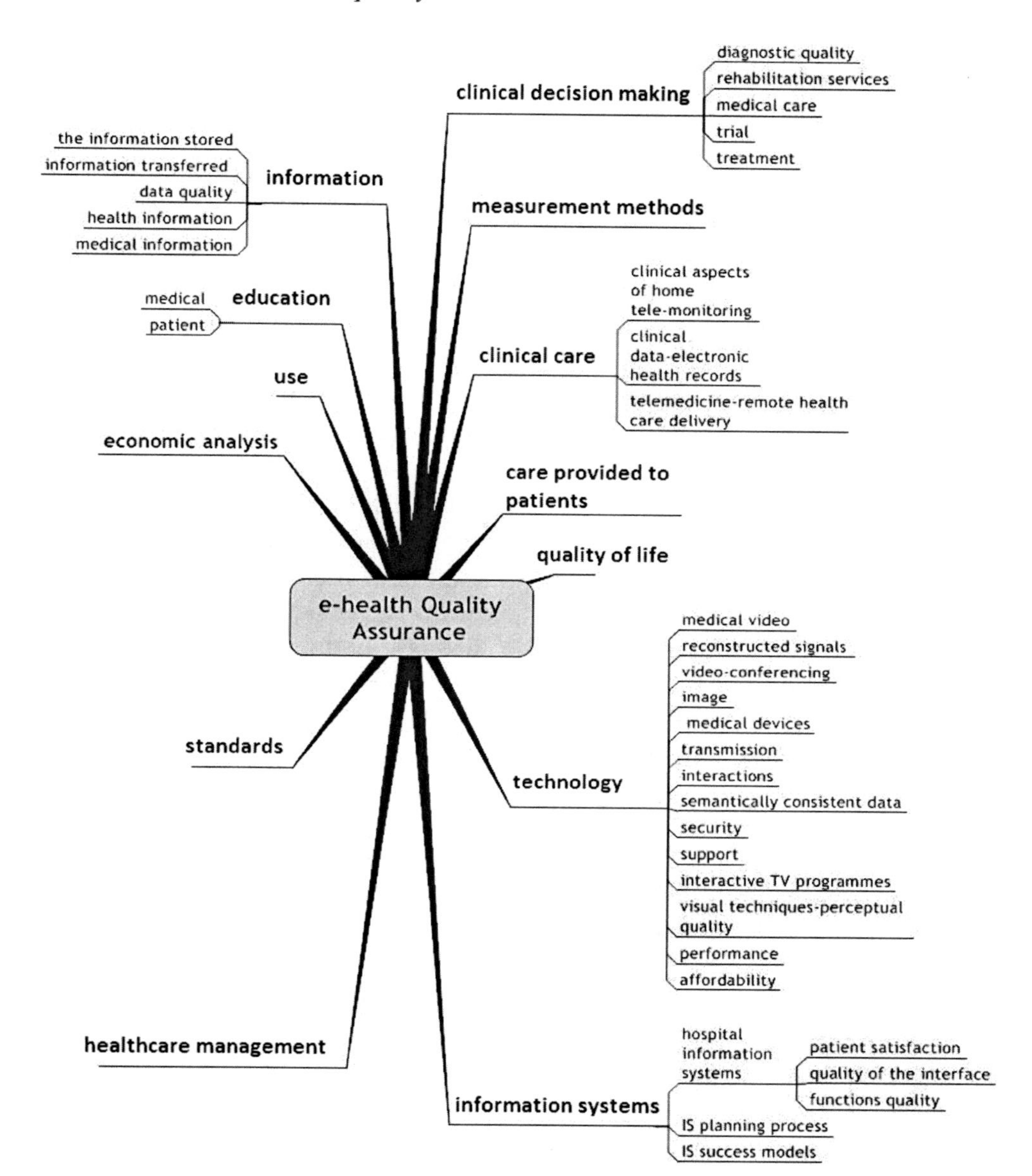

requirements, support of different formats, applications, infrastructure, delivery tools, setting and purpose, use and user satisfaction (Tulu et al., 2005). The construction of a qualitative infrastructure should include videoconferencing equipment, medical sensors/ devices and telecommunications (Dhillon & Forducey, 2006). Four quality features comprise a model developed for quality assured videoconferencing (LeRouge et al., 2002): technical, usability, physical environment, and the human element. The dimensions include (LeRouge et al., 2002): diagnostic accuracy, diagnostic impact, therapeutic impact and patient outcome.

Telemedicine transfer models are also noteworthy (Kifle et al., 2008) while the effectiveness of health care also depends on the quality of interaction between the equipment and users (Grigsby & Barton, 1998). Finally, quality modeling in telemedicine requires: (1) a quality framework for the service, (2) determination of differences, between the patient and the supplier, used to examine the qualitative attributes and (3) understanding of the service aspects that are more valuable in each attribute (LeRouge et al., 2004). The outcome is service quality (Hu, 2003).

Continuous Quality Improvement

An electronic infrastructure provides the opportunity to carry out a program of continuous quality improvement while effective and high quality medical practice in an electronic environment should support personalized approaches (Kangarloo et al., 1999). The immediate recognition of changes in patient's condition, in order to provide personalized services, is the ideal for continuous quality improvement (Laffel & Blumenthal, 1989). Finally, any telemedicine application should concurrently bring forward a program of outcome assessment (Grigsby, 1998; Ohinmaa et al., 1999).

Quality Assessment

Traditionally, the evaluation of health information systems has focused on the technical characteristics, which influence use, cost-benefit, user acceptance and patient outcomes (Health Canada, 2003). Furthermore, the assessment approaches have incorporated diffusion, change and innovation (Health Canada, 2003; Straub et al., 2004). Evaluation includes formal or informal mechanisms to describe the process and the results with emphasis on user acceptance, costs and clinical outcomes. It also explores the possibility of utilization, the quality of care, organizational, economic, technical, clinical, and moral or legal issues (May, 2006). Official or informal negotiations are performed during the assessment for adjustments in existing systems and practices to reduce risk (data risks, techniques risk, risks within networks).

Health Care Information Technology (Paré & Sicotte, 2001) develops tools that can be used to evaluate functional, technological, and psychometric and integration improvement (Jaana et al., 2009). Overall, evaluation in biomedical informatics should be realized as a running, strategically programmed approach (Miller, 2002). A systematic evaluation should be based on various existing prospects (clinical, technical, economic, social, legal), procedural and technical questions. Procedural questions include (Sang Kim, 2008) confidentiality, consent, protection and safety, cost of services, maintenance, electronic protocols for medical documents, responsibility and patient preferences (teleservices compared to traditional services). Technical questions include (Sang Kim, 2008) communication/ networking, latent circumstances because of time delay, bandwidth, transmission priorities and telesurgery environments for teleworkers. Apart from the quality of services, the impact of telemedicine on the system should also be evaluated from the prospects of satisfaction, efficiency and effectiveness of services (May et al., 2000). The market conditions and the health care providers' opinions should also be considered (Hu, 2003). Patients choose therapeutic strategies from several alternative solutions, accept treatment and evaluate the results (Flatley Brennan & Starren, 2006). Finally, moral issues in the evaluation studies should answer the wider questions of the ethical perspectives of the information society taking into account that ethics have a strong legal status in the medical delivery (Conford & Klecun-Dabrowska, 2001).

Overall, it is clear that the techniques of evaluation that were in effect for other technologies are difficult to be in effect for e-health, despite the rapid technological progress and the pressure (and from) the hospital doctors, the directors of services and institutions. Landmarks in the evaluation landscape are the observations and the recommendations of recognized evaluation researchers (The Lewin Group. Inc., 2002; Bashshur et al., 2005; Reardon, 2005). Lessons learned in e-health assessment (Glasgow, 2007) include health promotion and interactive technology (Street et al.,

Figure 2. Conceptual framework for quality assessment derived mining the scientific literature

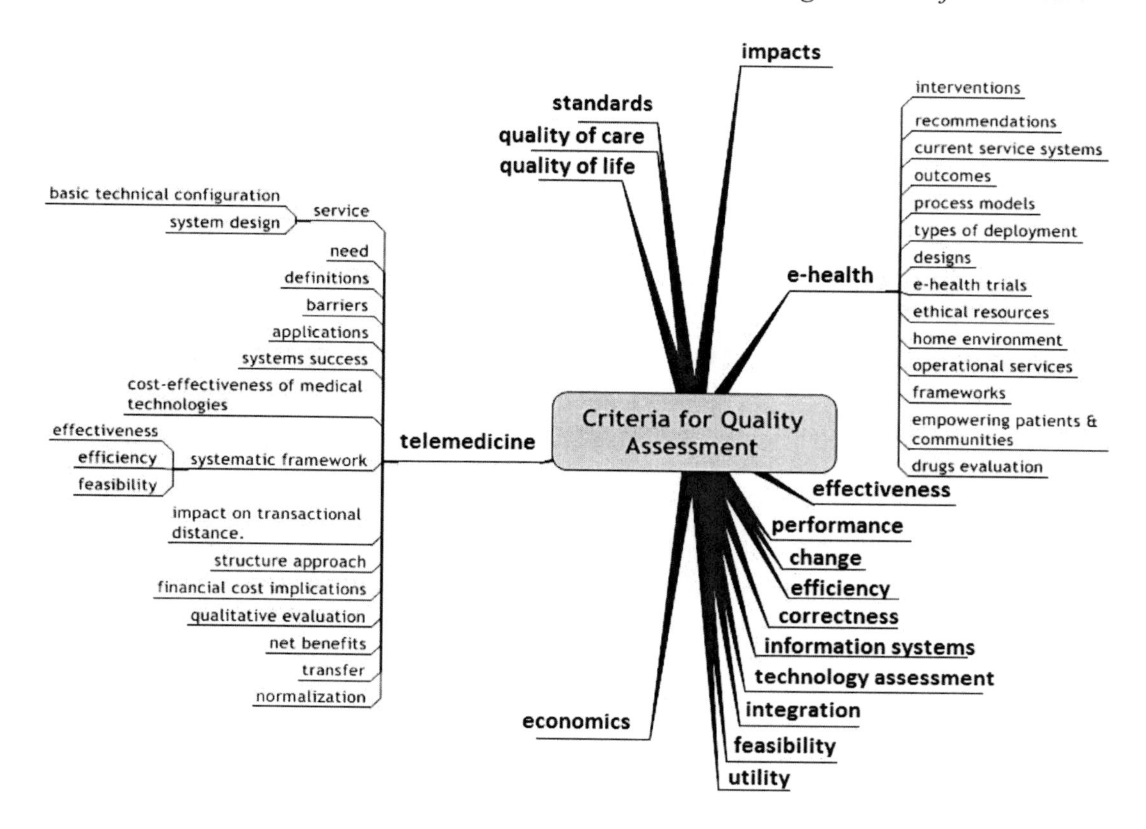

1997), empirical studies assessing the quality of health information for consumers on the World Wide Web (Eysenbach et al., 2002), impact of a patient-centered, computer-based health information/support (Gustafson et al., 1999), impact of automated calls (Piette et al., 2001), use of Internet technology (Tate et al., 2001; Tate et al., 2003; Dillman, 2000; Bull et al., 2005), patient compliance with paper and electronic diaries (Stone et al., 2003) and the future of health behavior change research (Glasgow et al., 2004). There are different translation and diffusion frameworks for e-health developers and evaluators including the RE-AIM model that focuses on both personal and setting level factors (Glasgow, 2002; Klesges et al., 2005; Glasgow, 2007), the diffusion of innovation theory (Rogers, 2003), the CURRES approach (Rotheram-Borus & Flannery, 2004), the PRECEDE-PROCEED model that outlines principles of patient and community-centered research (Green & Kreuter, 2005) and models of practical clinical and behavioral trials (Glasgow et al., 2005; Glasgow et al., 2006).

Overall, literature mining on the quality evaluation references results to the framework of Figure 2.

RELIABILITY ASSESSMENT

Multimedia and network modeling (Martínez & García, 2005a; Martínez & García, 2005b; Bala & Goyal, 2000) incorporates the service characterization (QoS basic), the application communication model (QoS application) and behavior analysis (QoS network) of the interconnection devices, buffers and links. The first step in Telemedicine network design is the theoretic analysis of hospital

Figure 3. Conceptual framework for reliability assessment derived mining the scientific literature

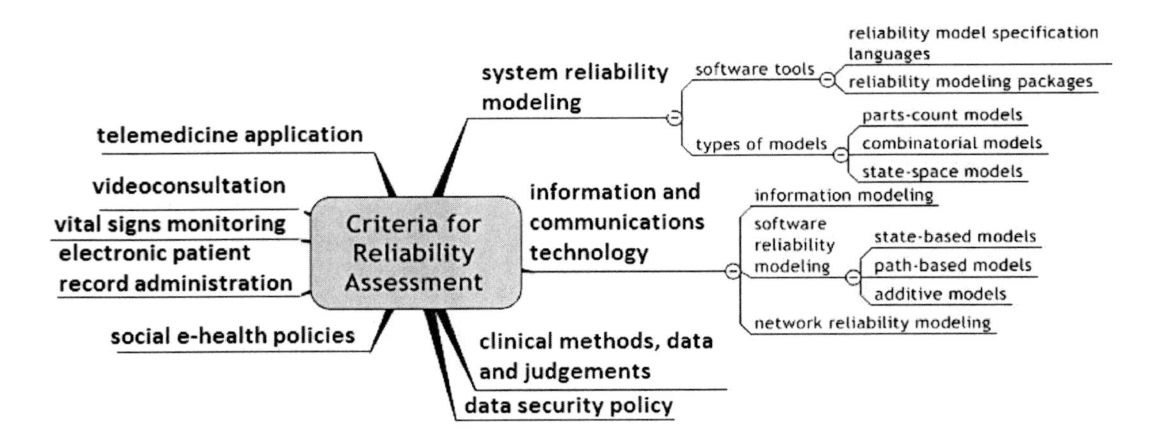

communications traffic (Martínez et al., 2003) using models for the communication features (sizes and rates) and configuration (bandwidth and delay). The urgent nature of medical applications and the bandwidth requirements (Vergados, 2007) indicate the need for QoS support in medical networks. Overall, network reliability, for data delivery, is a serious issue especially in emergency care where packet losses during medical information transferring may have devastating impacts on a patient's diagnosis.

Reliability models (Reibman & Veeraraghavan, 1991) help: (1) set and interpret system-reliability requirements, (2) predict the reliability of different configurations and (3) identify system-reliability weak points or reliability bottlenecks. Metrics include system reliability (depends on the length of time considered), meantime to failure, availability and expected number of failures while error analysis detects faults caused by the simplifying assumptions that underlie the model. Common errors include modeling, specification, parametric, and execution errors. An acceptable practice to reduce errors is sensitivity analysis (Blake et al., 1988).

Conclusively, software reliability depends on the characteristics of the product, and the development process (Spyrou et al., 2008) while software reliability engineering (Lyu, 1996; Goševa-Popstojanova & Trivedi, 2001) specifies the general form of failure.

The reliability of clinical methods, data and judgments involves reproducibility assessment (Last, 2000). Reproducibility quantifies the propagation of computation results (McConnochie et al., 2006), using an evaluation process (that is, telemedicine vs. in person), which affects acquisition of diagnostic information.

Literature mining of reliability evaluation references results to the framework of Figure 3.

FUTURE RESEARCH DIRECTIONS

There are two main categories of measurement methods, the objective or quantitative methods, and the subjective or qualitative methods. Therefore, future research directions should focus on deciding the features linked with each idea for quantitative or qualitative measurement. Furthermore, we have to identify a combination of features and their metrics in order to achieve a rational approach for quality and reliability assessment in e-health.

CONCLUSION

The complexity of the e-health environment complicates any e-health evaluation overview. However, the chapter considers the main ideas involved in evaluating e-health emphasizing on quality and reliability, and reviewing existing practices and methods. As a result, it provides considerations for the evaluation of quality and reliability in e-health environments interrelating studies and ideas, which draw the map of quality and reliability assessment in e-health.

REFERENCES

AMIA. (1997). The Practice of Informatics. A Proposal to Improve Quality, Increase Efficiency, and Expand Access in the U.S. Health Care System. *Journal of the American Medical Informatics Association*, *4*(5), 340–341.

Aronsky, D., & Haug, P. J. (2000). Assessing the Quality of Clinical Data in a Computer-based Record for Calculating the Pneumonia Severity Index. *Journal of the American Medical Informatics Association*, *7*(1), 55–65.

Arts, D. G. T., De Keizer, N. F., & Scheffer, G.-J. (2002). Defining and Improving Data Quality in Medical Registries: A Literature Review, Case Study, and Generic Framework. *Journal of the American Medical Informatics Association*, *9*(6), 600–611. doi:10.1197/jamia.M1087

Averill, E. (1994). Reference models and standards. *StandardView*, *2*(2), 96–109. doi:10.1145/202949.202959

Bala, V., & Goyal, S. (2000). A strategic analysis of network reliability. *Review of Economic Design*, *5*(3), 205–228. doi:10.1007/s100580000019

Bashshur, R., Shannon, G., Sapei H. (2005). Telemedicine Evaluation. *Telemedicine and e-Health*, *11*(3), 296-316.

Bashshur, R. L., Reardon, T. G., & Shannon, G. W. (2000). Telemedicine: A new health care delivery system. *Annual Review of Public Health*, *21*, 613–637. doi:10.1146/annurev.publhealth.21.1.613

Blake, J., Reibman, A., & Trivedi, K. (1988). Sensitivity Analysis of Reliability and Performability Measures for a Multiprocessor System. *ACM SIGMETRICS Performance Evaluation Review*, *16*(1), 177–186. doi:10.1145/1007771.55616

Bull, S. S., McKay, H. G., Gaglio, B., & Glasgow, R. E. (2005). Harnessing the potential of the Internet to promote diabetes self-management: how well are we doing? *Chronic Illness*, *1*(2), 143–155.

Buxton, M., & Hanney, S. (1998). Evaluating the NHS research and development programme: will the programme give value for money? *Journal of the Royal Society of Medicine*, *91*(Suppl 35), 2–6.

Cabrera, M., Burgelman, J-C., Boden, M., da Costa, O. and Rodríguez, C. (2004). eHealth in 2010: Realising a Knowledge-based Approach to Healthcare in the EU, Challenges for the Ambient Care System *Technical Report EUR 21486 EN*: European Commission, Directorate General Joint Research Centre, Institute for Prospective Technological Studies.

Conford, T., & Klecun-Dabrowska, E. (2001). Ethical Perspectives in Evaluation of Telehealth. *Cambridge Quarterly of Healthcare Ethics*, *10*(2), 161–169. doi:10.1017/S0963180101002079

De Lusignan, S. S., P.N., Adal, N., Majeed, A. (2002). Does Feedback Improve the Quality of Computerized Medical Records in Primary Care? *Journal of the American Medical Informatics Association*, *9*(4), 395–401. doi:10.1197/jamia.M1023

Dechant, H. K., Tohme, W. G., Mun, S. K., Hayes, W. S., & Schulman, K. A. (1996). Health Systems Evaluation of Telemedicine: A Staged Approach. *Telemedicine Journal*, *2*(4), 303–312.

Dellaca, R. L., Gobbi, A., Govoni, L., & Nevajas, D. Pedotti, A., Farré, R. (2009). *A Novel Simple Internet-Based System for Real Time Monitoring and Optimizing Home Mechanical Ventilation.* Paper presented at the 2009 International Conference on eHealth, Telemedicine, and Social Medicine.

DeLone, W. H., & McLean, E. R. (1992). Information Systems Success: The Quest for the Dependent Variable. *Information Systems Research*, *3*(1), 60–95. doi:10.1287/isre.3.1.60

DeLone, W. H., & McLean, E. R. (2002). *Information Systems Success Revisited.* Paper presented at the 35th Annual Hawaii International Conference on System Sciences.

Dhillon, H., & Forducey, P. G. (2006). *Implementation and Evaluation of Information Technology in Telemedicine.* Paper presented at the 39th Annual Hawaii International Conference on System Sciences.

Dillman, D. A. (2000). *Mail and Internet surveys: the tailored design method.* New York: Wiley, John & Sons, Incorporated.

Donabedian, A. (1988). The quality of care: how can it be assessed? *Journal of the American Medical Association*, *260*(12), 1743–1748. doi:10.1001/jama.260.12.1743

Eysenbach, G., Powell, J., Kuss, O., & Eun-Ryoung, S. (2002). Empirical studies assessing the quality of health information for consumers on the world wide web: a systematic review. *Journal of the American Medical Association*, *287*(20), 2691–2700. doi:10.1001/jama.287.20.2691

Fennessy, G. (2002). *Understanding and selecting knowledge management systems for a health information provider.* Paper presented at the 35th Annual Hawaii International Conference on System Sciences.

Field, M. J. (Ed.). (1996). *Telemedicine A Guide to Assessing Telecommunications in Health Care.* Institute of Medicine, National Academy Press.

Flatley Brennan, P., & Starren, J. B. (2006). Consumer Health Informatics and Telehealth . In Shortliffe, E. H., & Cimino, J. J. (Eds.), *Biomedical Informatics*. New York: Springer. doi:10.1007/0-387-36278-9_14

Fortino, G., & Nigro, L. (2000). *A Methodology Centered on Modularization of QoS Constraints for the Development and Performance Evaluation of Multimedia Systems.* Paper presented at the 33rd Annual Simulation Symposium.

Fraser, M. D., & Vaishnavi, V. K. (1997). A formal specifications maturity model. *Communications of the ACM*, *40*(12), 95–103. doi:10.1145/265563.265577

Gagnon, M.-P., Sánchez, E., & Pons, J. M. V. (2006). Integration of health technology assessment recommendations into organizational and clinical practice: A case study in Catalonia. *International Journal of Technology Assessment in Health Care*, *22*(2), 169–176. doi:10.1017/S0266462306050987

Glasgow, R. (2002). Evaluation of theory-based interventions: the RE-AIM model . In Glanz, K., Lewis, F. M., & Rimer, B. K. (Eds.), *Health behavior and health education* (3rd ed., pp. 531–544). San Francisco, CA: John Wiley & Sons.

Glasgow, R. E. (2007). eHealth Evaluation and Dissemination Research. *American Journal of Preventive Medicine*, *32*(Suppl 5), S119–S126. doi:10.1016/j.amepre.2007.01.023

Glasgow, R. E., Davidson, K. W., Dobkin, P. L., Ockene, J., & Spring, B. (2006). Practical behavioral trials to advance evidence-based behavioral medicine. *Annals of Behavioral Medicine*, *31*(1), 5–13. doi:10.1207/s15324796abm3101_3

Glasgow, R. E., Klesges, L. M., Dzewaltowski, D. A., Bull, S. S., & Estabrooks, P. (2004). The future of health behavior change research: what is needed to improve translation of research into health promotion practice? *Annals of Behavioral Medicine*, *27*(1), 3–12. doi:10.1207/s15324796abm2701_2

Glasgow, R. E., Magid, D. J., Beck, A., Ritzwoller, D., & Estabrooks, P. A. (2005). Practical clinical trials for translating research to practice: design and measurement recommendations. *Medical Care*, *43*(6), 551–557. doi:10.1097/01.mlr.0000163645.41407.09

Goševa-Popstojanova, K., & Trivedi, K. S. (2001). Architecture-based approach to reliability assessment of software systems. *Performance Evaluation*, *45*(2-3), 179–204. doi:10.1016/S0166-5316(01)00034-7

Graschew, G., Roelofs, T., Rakowsky, A., Schlag, P.M. (2006). Digital medicine in the virtual hospital of the future. *International Journal of Computer Assisted Radiology and Surgery*, *1*(Supp/1), 119-120.

Green, L. W., & Kreuter, M. W. (2005). *Health promotion planning: an educational and ecological approach* (4th ed.). Boston, MA: McGraw Hill.

Grigsby, J. (1998). *Evaluating Technologies for Providing Health Services at a Distance: Outcome-Driven Quality Improvement.* Paper presented at the Pacific Medical Technology Symposium.

Grigsby, J., & Barton, P. L. (1998). *Telecommunications Technology, Health Services, and Technology Assessment.* Paper presented at the Proceedings of the Symposium on Pacific Medical Technology.

Grigsby, J., Kaehny, M. M., Sandberg, E. J., Schlenker, R. E., & Shaughnessy, P. W. (1995). Effects and effectiveness of telemedicine . In Weisgrau, S. (Ed.), *Access to Health Care Services in Rural Areas: Delivery & Financial Issues*. Collingdale, PA: Diane Publishing Co.

Gustafson, D. H., Hawkins, R., Boberg, E., Pingree, S., Serlin, R. E., Graziano, F., & Chan, C. L. (1999). Impact of a patient-centered, computer-based health information/support system. *American Journal of Preventive Medicine*, *16*(1), 1–9. doi:10.1016/S0749-3797(98)00108-1

Health Canada (2000). Evaluating Telehealth 'Solutions' A Review and Synthesis of the Telehealth Evaluation Literature: Office of Health and the Information Highway.

Health Canada (2003). Toward an Evaluation Framework for Electronic Health Records Initiatives: Health and the Information Highway Division.

Hebert, M. (2001). *Telehealth Success: Evaluation Framework Development.* Paper presented at the 10th World Congress on Medical Informatics.

Holle, R., & Zahlmann, G. (1999). Evaluation of Telemedical Services. *IEEE Transactions on Information Technology in Biomedicine*, *3*(2), 84–91. doi:10.1109/4233.767083

Hu, P. J. H. (2003). *Evaluating Telemedicine Systems Success: A Revised Model.* Paper presented at the 36th Hawaii International Conference on System Sciences.

Jaana, M., Paré, G., & Sicotte, C. (2009). *IT Capacities Assessment Tool: A Survey of Hospitals in Canada.* Paper presented at the 42nd Hawaii International Conference on System Sciences.

Kangarloo, H., Dionisio, J. D. N., Sinha, U., Johnson, D., & Taira, R. K. (1999). *Process models for telehealth: an industrial approach to quality management of distant medical practice.* Paper presented at the American Medical Informatics Association Annual Symposium.

Kaplan, B., & Flatley Brennan, P. (2001). Consumer Informatics Supporting Patients as Co-Producers of Quality. *Journal of the American Medical Informatics Association*, *8*(4), 309–316.

Kastania, A., Zimeras, S., Papadhmhtriou, K., & Rizos, E. (2008a). *Reliability Assessment of Telemedicine Networks.* Paper presented at the 6th International Conference on Information and Communication Technologies in Health.

Kastania, A. N., & Papadhmhtriou, K. (2008b). An Evalution Model of Telemedicine Services in a Primary Care Setting. *The Journal on Information Technology in Healthcare*, *6*(3), 197–203.

Kastania, A. N., & Zimeras, S. (2008c). Quality and Reliability Aspects in Telehealth Systems . In Lazakidou, A., & Siassiakos, K. (Eds.), *Handbook of Research on Distributed Medical Informatics and E-Health* (pp. 425–441). Hershey, PA: IGI Global.

Kifle, M., Mbarika, V. W. A., Tsuma, C., Wilkerson, D., & Tan, J. (2008). *A TeleMedicine Transfer Model for Sub-Saharan Africa.* Paper presented at the 41st Annual Hawaii International Conference on System Sciences.

Klecun-Dabrowska, E., & Cornford, T. (2001). *Evaluation and Telehealth – an Interpretative Study.* Paper presented at the 34th Annual Hawaii International Conference on System Sciences.

Klesges, L. M., Estabrooks, P. A., Glasgow, R. E., & Dzewaltowski, D. (2005). Beginning with the application in mind: designing and planning health behavior change interventions to enhance dissemination. *Annals of Behavioral Medicine*, *29*(2), 66–75. doi:10.1207/s15324796abm2902s_10

Klinger, D., Nakada, Y., & Menendez, M. (Eds.). (1989). *AT&T Reliability Manual*. New York: Springer.

Koran, L. (1975a). The reliability of clinical methods, data and judgments (second of two parts). *The New England Journal of Medicine*, *293*(14), 695–701. doi:10.1056/NEJM197510022931405

Koran, L. M. (1975b). The reliability of clinical methods, data and judgments (first of two parts). *The New England Journal of Medicine*, *293*(13), 642–646. doi:10.1056/NEJM197509252931307

Laffel, G., & Blumenthal, D. (1989). The case for using industrial quality management science in health organizations. *Journal of the American Medical Association*, *262*(20), 2869–2873. doi:10.1001/jama.262.20.2869

Last, J. M. (Ed.). (2000). *A Dictionary of Epidemiology* (4th ed.). Oxford, UK: Oxford University Press.

LeRouge, C., Garfield, M. J., & Hevner, A. R. (2002). *Quality Attributes in Telemedicine Video Conferencing.* Paper presented at the 35th Annual Hawaii International Conference on System Sciences.

LeRouge, C., Hevner, A., Collins, R., Garfield, M., & Law, D. (2004). *Telemedicine Encounter Quality: Comparing Patient and Provider Perspectives of a Socio-Technical System.* Paper presented at the 37th Annual Hawaii International Conference on System Sciences.

Leys, M. (2003). Healthcare policy: Qualitative evidence and health technology assessment. *Health Policy (Amsterdam)*, *65*(3), 217–226. doi:10.1016/S0168-8510(02)00209-9

Lipson, L. R., & Henderson, T. M. (1995). State initiatives to promote telemedicine. *Telemedicine Journal*, *2*(2), 109–121.

Lobley, D. (1997). The economics of telemedicine. *Journal of Telemedicine and Telecare*, *3*(3), 117–125. doi:10.1258/1357633971930977

Lyu, M. R. (Ed.). (1996). *Handbook of Software Reliability Engineering*. Washington, DC: IEEE Computer Society Press and McGraw-Hill Book Company.

Mairinger, T., Gabl, C., Derwan, P., Mikuz, G., & Ferrer-Roca, O. (1996). What Do Physicians Think of Telemedicine? A Survey in Different European Regions. *Journal of Telemedicine and Telecare*, *2*, 50–56. doi:10.1258/1357633961929169

Martínez, I., & García, J. (2005a). *QoS Evaluation for Multimedia Telemedicine Services based on TCP/UDP cross-traffic.* Paper presented at the International Conference on Computer Communications and Networks.

Martínez, I., & García, J. (2005b). *SM3 – Quality Of Service (QoS) Evaluation Tool For Telemedicine-Based New Healthcare Services.* Paper presented at the II International Conference on Computational Bioengineering.

Martínez, I., Salvador, J., Fernández, J., & García, J. (2003). *Traffic Requirements Evaluation for a Telemedicine Network.* Paper presented at the International Congress on Computational Bioengineering.

Mason, R. O. (1978). Measuring information output: a communication systems approach. *Information & Management*, *1*(5), 219–234. doi:10.1016/0378-7206(78)90028-9

May, C. (2006). A rational model for assessing and evaluating complex interventions in health care. *BMC Health Services Research*, *6*, 86. doi:10.1186/1472-6963-6-86

May, C., Harrison, R., Finch, T., MacFarlane, A., Mair, F., & Wallace, P. (2003). Understanding the Normalization of Telemedicine Services through Qualitative Evaluation. *Journal of the American Medical Informatics Association*, *10*(6), 596–604. doi:10.1197/jamia.M1145

May, C., Mort, M., Mair, F., Ellis, N. T., & Gask, L. (2000). Evaluation of new technologies in healthcare systems: what's the context? *Health Informatics Journal*, *6*, 67–70. doi:10.1177/146045820000600203

McConnochie, K. M., Conners, G. P., Brayer, A. F., Goepp, J., Herendeen, N. E., & Wood, N. E. (2006). Differences in Diagnosis and Treatment Using Telemedicine Versus In-Person Evaluation of Acute Illness. *Ambulatory Pediatrics*, *6*(4), 196–197. doi:10.1016/j.ambp.2006.03.002

Miller, R. A. (2002). Reference Standards in Evaluating System Performance, Editorial comments. *Journal of the American Medical Informatics Association*, *9*(1), 87–91.

O'Keefe, R. M. (1989). The evaluation of decision-aiding systems: guidelines and methods. *Information & Management*, *17*, 217–226. doi:10.1016/0378-7206(89)90045-1

Ohinmaa, A., Hailey, D., & Roine, R. (1999). *The Assessment of Telemedicine- General principles and a systematic review*. Helsinki: Finnish Office for Health Care Technology Assessment and Alberta Heritage Foundation for Medical Research.

Paré, G., & Sicotte, C. (2001). Information Technology Sophistication in Health Care: An Instrument Validation Study among Canadian Hospitals. *International Journal of Medical Informatics*, *63*(3), 205–223. doi:10.1016/S1386-5056(01)00178-2

Perednia, D. A., & Allen, A. (1995). Telemedicine Technology and Clinical Applications. *Journal of the American Medical Association*, *273*(6), 483–488. doi:10.1001/jama.273.6.483

Piette, J. D., Weinberger, M., Kraemer, F. B., & McPhee, S. J. (2001). The impact of automated calls with nurse follow-up on diabetes treatment outcomes in a Veterans Affairs health care system. *Diabetes Care*, *24*(2), 202–208. doi:10.2337/diacare.24.2.202

Pitt, L. F., Watson, R. T., & Kavan, C. B. (1995). Service Quality: A Measure of Information Systems Effectiveness. *Management Information Systems Quarterly*, *19*(2), 173–187. doi:10.2307/249687

Ras, E., Becker, M., & Koch, J. (2007). *Engineering Tele-Health Solutions in the Ambient Assisted Living Lab.* Paper presented at the Proceedings of the 21st International Conference on Advanced Information Networking and Applications Workshops.

Reardon, T. (2005). Research Findings and Strategies for Assessing Telemedicine Costs. *Telemedicine and e-Health, 11*(3), 348-369.

Reibman, A. L., & Veeraraghavan, M. (1991). Reliability Modeling: An Overview for Svstem Designers. *Computer, 24*(4), 49–57. doi:10.1109/2.76262

Remenyi, D. S. J., & Money, A. (1991). A user-satisfaction approach to IS effectiveness measurement. *Journal of Information Technology, 6*, 162–175. doi:10.1057/jit.1991.30

Reussner, R. H., Schmidt, H. W., & Poernomo, I. H. (2003). Reliability prediction for component-based software architectures. *Journal of Systems and Software, 66*(3), 241–252. doi:10.1016/S0164-1212(02)00080-8

Rogers, E. M. (2003). *Diffusion of innovations* (5th ed.). Washington, DC: Free Press.

Rotheram-Borus, M. J., & Flannery, N. D. (2004). Interventions that are CURRES: costeffective, useful, realistic, robust, evolving, and sustainable . In Remschmidt, H., Belfer, M. L., & Goodyer, I. (Eds.), *Facilitating Pathways. Care, Treatment and Prevention in Child and Adolescent Mental Health* (pp. 235–244). New York: Springer.

Sanazaro, P. (1980). Quality Assessment and Quality Assurance in Medical Care. *Annual Review of Public Health, 1*, 37–68. doi:10.1146/annurev.pu.01.050180.000345

Sang Kim, Y. (2008). *Surgical Telementoring Initiation of a Regional Telemedicine Network: Projection of Surgical Expertise in the WWAMI Region.* Paper presented at the Third International Conference on Convergence and Hybrid Information Technology.

Schulz, E. B., Barret, J. W., & Price, C. (1998). Read Code Quality Assurance From Simple Syntax to Semantic Stability. *Journal of the American Medical Informatics Association, 5*(4), 337–346.

Shannon, C. E. (2001). A mathematical theory of communication. *ACM SIGMOBILE Mobile Computing and Communications Review, Special issue dedicated to Claude E. Shannon, 5*(1), 3–55.

Spyrou, S., Bamidis, P. D., Maglaveras, N., Pangalos, G., & Pappas, C. (2008). A methodology for reliability analysis in health networks. *IEEE Transactions on Information Technology in Biomedicine, 12*(3), 377–386. doi:10.1109/TITB.2007.905125

Stevens, A., & Milne, R. (2004). Health technology assessment in England and Wales. *International Journal of Technology Assessment in Health Care, 20*(1), 11–24. doi:10.1017/S0266462304000741

Stone, A. A., Shiffman, S., Schwartz, J. E., Broderick, J. E., & Hufford, M. R. (2003). Patient compliance with paper and electronic diaries. *Controlled Clinical Trials, 24*(2), 182–199. doi:10.1016/S0197-2456(02)00320-3

Straub, D. W., Boudreau, M.-C., & Gefen, D. (2004). Validation Guidelines for IS Positivist Research. *Communications of the Association for Information Systems, 13*, 380–427.

Street, R. L., Gold, W. R., & Manning, T. R. (Eds.). (1997). *Health Promotion and Interactive Technology. Theoretical Applications and Future Directions*. New York: Routledge, Taylor & Francis Group.

Tate, D. F., Jackvony, E. H., & Wing, R. R. (2003). Effects of Internet behavioral counseling on weight loss in adults at risk for type 2 diabetes: a randomized trial. *Journal of the American Medical Association, 289*, 1833–1836. doi:10.1001/jama.289.14.1833

Tate, D. F., Wing, R. R., & Winett, R. A. (2001). Using Internet technology to deliver a behavioral weight loss program. *Journal of the American Medical Association, 285*(9), 1172–1177. doi:10.1001/jama.285.9.1172

Taylor, P. (1998a). A survey of research in telemedicine. 1: Telemedicine systems. *Journal of Telemedicine and Telecare, 4*, 1–17. doi:10.1258/1357633981931227

Taylor, P. (1998b). A survey of research in telemedicine. 2: Telemedicine services. *Journal of Telemedicine and Telecare*, *4*, 63–71. doi:10.1258/1357633981931948

Thai, J., Pekilis, B., Lau, A., & Seviora, R. (2001). *Aspect-Oriented Implementation of Software Health Indicators.* Paper presented at the Eighth Asia-Pacific Software Engineering Conference.

The Lewin Group. Inc. (2002). Assessment of Approaches to Evaluating Telemedicine, Final Report: Prepared for Department of Health and Human Services Contract Number HHS-10-97-0012.

Thurmond, V. A., & Boyle, D. K. (2002). An integrative review of patients' perceptions regarding telehealth used in their health care. *The Online Journal of Knowledge Synthesis for Nursing*, *E9*(1), 12–32.

Troster, J., Henshaw, J., & Buss, E. (1993). *Filtering for quality.* Paper presented at the Proceedings of the 1993 conference of the Centre for Advanced Studies on Collaborative research: software engineering.

Tulu, B., Chatterjee, S., & Laxminarayan, S. (2005). *A Taxonomy of Telemedicine Efforts with Respect to Applications, Infrastructure, Delivery Tools, Type of Setting and Purpose.* Paper presented at the 38th Annual Hawaii International Conference on System Sciences.

Vergados, D. D. (2007). Simulation and Modeling Bandwidth Control in Wireless Healthcare Information Systems. *Simulation*, *83*(4), 347–364. doi:10.1177/0037549707083114

Wallace, S., Wyatt, J., & Taylor, P. (1998). Telemedicine in the NHS for the millennium and beyond. *Postgraduate Medical Journal*, *74*(878), 721–728. doi:10.1136/pgmj.74.878.721

Wang, R. Y. (1998). A product perspective on Total Data Quality Management. *Communications of the ACM*, *41*(2), 58–65. doi:10.1145/269012.269022

Chapter 21
Quality Issues in Personalized E-Health, Mobile Health and E-Health Grids

Anastasia N. Kastania
Biomedical Research Foundation of the Academy of Athens, Greece & Athens University of Economics and Business, Greece

Sophia Kossida
Biomedical Research Foundation of the Academy of Athens, Greece

ABSTRACT

The electronic healthcare in the modern society has the possibility of converting the practice of delivery of health care. Currently, chaos of information is characterizing the public health care, which leads to inferior decision-making, increasing expenses and even loss of lives. Technological progress in the sensors, integrated circuits, and the wireless communications have allowed designing low cost, microscopic, light, and smart sensors. These smart sensors are able to feel, transport one or more vital signals, and they can be incorporated in wireless personal or body networks for remote health monitoring. Sensor networks promise to drive innovation in health care allowing cheap, continuous, mobile and personalized health management of electronic health records with the Internet. The e-health applications imply an exciting set of requirements for Grid middleware and provide a rigorous testing ground for Grid. In the chapter, the authors present an overview of the current technological achievements in the electronic healthcare world combined with an outline of the quality dimensions in healthcare.

INTRODUCTION

E-health offers an optimistic vision of how computer and communication technology can help and improve healthcare provision at a distance. Health care provision is an environment that has presented remarkable improvement in the computing technology. For example, mobile e-health includes information and telecommunications technologies, which provide health care to patients that are at a distance from the supplier, and provide reinforcing tools for mobile health care. Recently, health care has embraced the mobile technology in electronic applications (Panteli et al., 2007). Various initiatives (public and private) have examined the different mobile applications

DOI: 10.4018/978-1-61692-843-8.ch021

of electronic health focusing on the mobility of doctors, the mobility of the patients, up to the Web based data access (Germanakos et al., 2005).

Moreover, personalized electronic health care provision through autonomous and adaptive Web applications is noteworthy (American College of Physicians, 2008). The growth of high bandwidth wireless networks, such as GPRS and UMTS, combined with miniaturized sensors and the computers will create applications and new services that will change the daily life of citizens. The citizens will be able to get medical advice from a distance but will also be in a position to send, from any place, complete and accurate vital signs measurements (Van Halteren et al., 2004). However, grid technologies and standards, currently examined in health care, will be adopted if they prove that they face all the valid concerns of security and follow the ethical guidelines (Stell, et al., 2007).

In this chapter, an overview of the existing personalized, mobile and Grid applications in electronic healthcare is presented. Further, quality aspects, which have successfully been applied in traditional health care quality assessment, are presented. A future challenge is to examine how these quality aspects can be successfully applied in electronic healthcare.

BACKGROUND

To realize the potential of electronic health, future electronic health should be able to support patient information management and medical decision support in an open and mobile medical environment. Such an environment will be strong in knowledge, sensitive and flexible in the needs of patients, and will allow collaboration of virtual teams that work in different geographic areas. Context-specific services to each individual are defined as personalized services. These are provided by agents usually with autonomy playing the role of personal assistant (Panayiotou & Samaras, 2004; Delicato et al., 2001). Personalization is a technique used to explore both interaction and information. It allows doctors to search personalized information about the health state of each patient (Nikolidakis, et al., 2008).

Since the number and the use of wireless connection and portable devices are increasing, the complexity of designing and setting up adaptive e-health systems is also increasing. The current improvement in physiologic sensors allows realizing future mobile computing environments that can impressively strengthen health care that is provided to the community, and individuals with chronic problems. Finally, there is interest from the academic and industrial world to assess the challenge of e-health automation management of mobile Grid infrastructures (Lupu et al., 2008).

PERSONALIZED E-HEALTH

The current tendency towards ubiquitous computing, the new sensor technologies, the powerful mobile devices and the wearable computers support different types of personalized electronic health applications. Telemonitoring applications have adopted this new technology to improve the quality of care and the quality of treatment for the sick and the elderly using questions and actions based on user preferences. The personalized application collects user activities and begins interpreting them to act according to user's wishes. The study of user activities also allows individualization of content. Reproduction of user experience, emotions, sentiments, thoughts, behavior and their actions is also performed (Lugmayr et al., 2009).

The textile products and computers are combined to create a recent model in the individualized mobile data processing. To create a programmable device, as part of clothes, design and implementation of a 'wearable' motherboard architecture is needed to embody clothing items, hardware and software. This type of information processing should not only provide high bandwidth but

Figure 1. Current aspects involved in personalized e-health

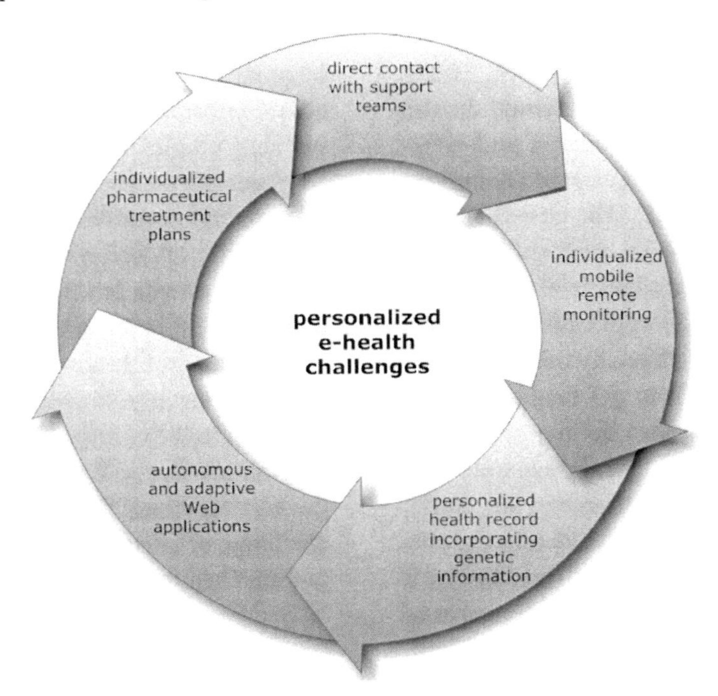

should also have the capability of seeing, feeling, thinking, and acting (Park et al., 2002).

A picture of remote health management supports the use of an individual cell phone, as a mediator that transfers multiple data streams from multiple wearable sensors in a response infrastructure (Mohomed et al., 2008). Autonomous and adaptive Web applications encourage individual 'participation' in the medical decision-making and self-management (American College of Physicians, 2008). The personalization is based on adapting information content that is returned as an answer to a user request based on who is the end user (Figure 1). Internet-based applications allow individuals to shape the application based on their individual needs because patients require timely access to high quality personalized health care (Nijland et al., 2009). Using websites of health risk calculation, the users of the Internet can receive personalized predictions for their health (Harle et al., 2009). Life assistance protocols, determined by medical experts, are based on evidence-based medicine and have been proved acceptable practice that is applied in one population group. Developing a life assistance protocol in different user groups will provide, in the long run, enormous volumes of information on health risk, and documentation on different healthcare paths (Meneu et al., 2009). Moreover, it will allow creating diverse and personalized snapshots and adaptations of the life assistance protocol (Meneu, et al., 2009).

The electronic health record (EHR) used in health administration reports and in clinical decision-making is an electronic record of patient history produced from personal health monitoring (Dong et al., 2009). Case-based reasoning has been used for the individualized production and delivery of health information to extract a personalized health record from the individual health profile (Abidi, 2002). Transport-independent personal-health data and protocol standards are defined by the ISO 11073/IEEE 1073 (known also as X73) for interoperability with the different sensors (Yusof et al., 2006; de Toledo et al., 2006).

Finally, an emerging opportunity for artificial intelligence researchers is to develop technologies that would check continuously 'healthy' in their houses and constantly direct them to healthy behavior (Intille et al., 2002). The use of intelligent techniques to analyze user satisfaction ensures the medical accuracy of the dynamically created patient empowerment form (Abidi et al., 2001).

Overall, the term context-awareness refers to the ability to obtain context information that describes the user environment and adjusts according to this context. Such an adaptation clearly leads to individualized services, but the sensitive information handling causes various privacy concerns (Chorianopoulos, 2008). Context-awareness is a promising model for flow control. The context is any information that characterizes the environment and the state of the user (for example setting and time) and any other component relative to the interaction between the user and the service (Wac et al., 2006). The personal user data and preferences are the main 'exploitation points' for finding ways to add value to user experience.

Therefore, essential areas of future e-health research should be personalization, the exchange of secure messages and the mobile services incorporating genetic information in electronic health applications (Carlsson & Walden, 2002). This will improve the medical practice, research and the convergence between the bioinformatics and the medical informatics (Oliveira et al., 2003). Integrating enormous sums of genetic information in the clinical setting will 'inspire' modern clinical practices where the clinical diagnosis and treatment will be supported by information on molecular level. Gene therapy provides the opportunity of hereditary illnesses minimization while molecular medicine requires an increasing exchange of knowledge between the clinicians and the biologists. The information that is available in biology and in medicine is so impressive that requires specific tools for information management. However, tools are needed to effectively connect the genetic and clinical information, electronic health applications and existing genetic databases. The usage of evolutionary algorithms opens many prospects for treatment optimization to combine biological and medical traits in the decision support.

Mobile Health

In the mobile health world, we conduct clinical data collection, healthcare information delivery, direct provision of care and real time monitoring of vital signs using mobile devices and other wireless devices. Moreover, in order to ensure that we deliver care of high quality at any time and space, access to patient records is necessary as well as additional information from distant sources such as consultation with experts and direct contact with databases. The mobile, wireless technology can offer this support but there are few medical devices on the market, which can be adapted and personalized according to patient needs (Riva, 2003; Joshi, 2000). Finally, classifying medical devices is critical because their effects can fluctuate from no threat to life threat.

On the other hand, we might integrate electronic health services in cell phones and connect biosensors with cell phones (Han et al., 2007). The necessary information is organized to establish an ontology for mobile electronic health services (Han, et al., 2007).

Furthermore, mobile health applications introduce new mobile services in health care based on the technologies 2.5 (GPRS) and 3G (UMTS). This can be achieved by integrating sensors and activators to continuously measure and transmit vital signs, with sound and video, to suppliers of health care in a Wireless Body Area Network (BAN) (Konstantas et al., 2002). These sensors and the activators are improving the life of patients while introducing new services in disease prevention and diagnostics, remote support, recording of normal conditions and the clinical research. The

Wireless Body Area Network will help the fast and reliable implementation of distant-aid services for sending reliable information from the place of accidents. Finally, the ubiquitous computing is a promising model for creating information systems. Databases improve data management for the patients, public health, drugstores and the workforce (Milenković et al., 2006).

The field of mobile healthcare requires continuous planning, solutions, decision-making and intelligent support technology that will reduce both the number of faults and their range. In our wireless world, the mobile devices use various networking installations. The existing context - aware applications are benefited from the user context (for example positioning information), nevertheless, few question the network quality of service (Wac, 2005; Broens et al., 2007; Hanak et al., 2007).

However, the services of electronic health share several distinctive features concerning the structure of services, the component services and the data requirements. Therefore, the ideal is to develop electronic health services in a common platform using standard features and services. Finally, various fundamental questions can affect the successful implementation of a mobile electronic health application. However, portable wireless applications at the point of care, based on information and connected with the clinical data, can reduce these problems. Interoperability of the existing applications of health care and/or databases is essential. The mobile technology of health care has the solution on not only supporting health care but also on easier management of mobile patients. The mobile applications can reduce faults and delays in creating accessible digital data (Archer, 2005).

GRID COMPUTING

Grid computing is a term that involves a 'hot' model of distributed computing. This model embraces various architectures and forms but is restricted by detailed operational and behavior rules. Its precise definition is a difficult task because of the model nature and the large number of its different implementations.

As a result, there are several misunderstandings of what the Grid is and what architectures can be called that way. Therefore, a clarification of the meaning of the Grid is needed. The computational Grid is practically a network of various types of heterogeneous computational engines and resources. Its size can vary from a small collection of stand-alone computers to a global network of thousands of interconnected units sharing distributed resources and working in parallel to establish a dominant global supercomputer. It involves computing, storage, application, coordination, and sharing. This architecture could be implemented at a local area network or the Internet to provide services to individuals or organizations all over the world.

A Grid should include mechanisms for dividing a specific task into a subset of smaller ones, scheduling and dynamic resource provisioning in order to perform parallel computation and merging the results. Overall, there are three basic principles that ought to be followed for a system to be called Computational Grid:

- The shared resources should not have centralized management, and there should be a successful coordination and service provision to users within different domains and geographical locations.
- A Grid should use standard, open and general-purpose protocols and interfaces for all its operations, such as authentication, resource sharing, and internode communication to avoid being an application-specific system.
- It should provide a competent service to the users about the collection of services, response time, computational performance and resource utilization to produce better

resource utilization and performance rates than stand-alone units.

Grid computing is often confused with utility computing, cluster computing or P2P computing. Utility computing involves trade on-demand supply of various resources that are charged as services. Utility computing, although it is limited to the service providers' network, resembles the Grid or can follow the Grids specifications. Cluster computing is a technology similar to the Grid computing but not quite the same. Clusters usually involve interconnected processors inside the restricted area networks. It is likely to be distributed and manage different resources, but they almost always require centralized control, which is the essential feature that distinguishes them from the Grid. Peer-to-peer applications, on the other hand, have remarkably similar infrastructure with the Grid since they use grid-like services for manipulating files. The main difference is based on the fact that P2P focus on services to be delivered to as many users as possible and these services are detailed and restrained while the Grid model is set on other priorities such as resource integration, performance, reliability, quality of service and security.

Grid computing is considered as the computing of the future. There is already an enormous amount of research around it, and new Grid applications are constantly emerging or take advantage of it. It already has a broad social value since it can be used by medical, biological and scientific research centers to handle resources and time-consuming calculations and tasks. However, there are issues under investigation for the Grid since it is a system of multiple objectives, a lot of which are difficult to be met. There is also a lot of research on the Quality of Service of the Grid, the performance, the effective coordination of users and resources and the serious issue of security at various levels and areas with attention to the remote computation and data integrity. Grid architecture makes extensive use of the Internet and the remote and distributed resources to create a global supercomputer that can perform complex tasks. It embraces the best features of many other distributed models, such as utility, cluster or P2P computing but its capacity and persistence to generalizing protocols, lack of centralized control, quality of service and failure tolerance make it unique and most probable 'partner' of the Semantic Web, which is the future of the Web. Its social and scientific contribution is incredible, and is expected to succeed in the future as its security, resource coordination and quality of service techniques will overcome the drawbacks of the present.

Furthermore, the questions of data management in the Grids become more and more serious. From the side of data management, the Grid allows many replicated data objects, which allow a high-level of availability, reliability and performance to assure the user and application needs. A breakdown of communication happens when (Voicu et al., 2009): (1) a message is degraded during the communication between two regions (2) a message is lost because of dysfunction of the network connection or (3) two regions cannot communicate because a network path is unavailable. In the first two cases, network protocols are used to maintain reliability (Voicu et al., 2009).

Incorporating mobile devices in the Grid can lead to uncertainty and to under performance because of the inherent restrictions of mobile devices and the wireless communication connections. For the future generation of ubiquitous Grids, we have to find ways to rectify the restrictions that are innate in these devices and combine them in the Grid, so that the available resources are strengthened and the field of provided services is extended (Isaiadis & Getov, 2005).

Tools and environments are available for simulation, data mining, knowledge discovery and collaborative work. There are various requirements for the Grid resource management strategies and its components (resource allocation, reservation management, job scheduling) since they should be in a position to react to failure of network connections (Volckaert et al., 2004).

Health Grids are computing environments of distributed resources in which diverse and scattered biomedical data are accessed, and knowledge discovery and computations are performed. The growth of the information technology allows the biomedical researchers to capitalize in ubiquitous and transparent distributed systems and in a broad collection of tools for resource distribution (computation, storage, data, replication, security, semantic interoperability, and distribution of software as services) (Kratz et al., 2007). Electronic health records in collaboration with the Grid technologies and the increasing interdisciplinary collaborations offer the opportunity to participate in advanced scientific and prestigious medical discoveries. Medical Informatics based on a Grid can be extended to support the entire spectrum of health care: screening, diagnosis, treatment planning, epidemiology and public health. Health Grid was the first that determined the need for a particular middleware layer, between the global grid infrastructure, the middleware and the medical or health applications (Breton et al., 2006). The Grid technology can support healthcare services integration but is usually unavailable at the point of care (for example in the house of the patient) (Koufi et al., 2008).

The Share Project is a European Union financed research to establish a road map for future health grid research, giving priority to the opportunities, the obstacles and the likely difficulties (Olive et al., 2007a; Olive et al., 2007b). The primary technical road map has produced a series of technologies, models and essential growth points, development of a reference implementation for grid services, and has concluded with expanding a knowledge grid for medical research. In the Share Project, to create knowledge from data requires complex data integration, data mining and image processing applications and includes the use of artificial intelligence techniques to build relations between data from different sources and frameworks (Olive et al., 2007a; Olive et al., 2007b).

Even if certain key pharmaceutical companies have established powerful Grid extensions for drug discovery, the specific skepticism remains for the value of Grid Computing in the sector. Therefore, in the Health Grid road map, particular attention should be given to the security and the choice of standards for the HealthGrid operating system and technologies. The security is an issue in all the technical levels: the networks should provide the protocols for secure data transfer, the Grid infrastructure should support secure mechanisms for Access, Authentication and Authorization, and the establishments should provide mechanisms for secure data storage (Breton et al., 2006). Computer systems should be autonomous (Sterritt & Hinchey, 2005a), where autonomicity implies self-management that often becomes visible in the frameworks of self-configuring, self-healing, self-optimizing, self-protecting and self-awareness. The autonomous computation is intended to improve the widespread utilization and computation possibilities of systems to assist the computer users. Since for most of the users access to computation is by personal devices, research on autonomous computation focuses on this field (Sterritt & Bantz, 2004). The autonomous computing and other initiatives on the self-management systems are a powerful new vision for constructing complex computer systems. They provide the ability of complexity control by implementing self-governance (autonomy) and self-management (autonomicity) (Sterritt & Hinchey, 2005b). The principal emerging strategies to achieve this requirement are the 'autonomic networks' and the 'autonomic communications'. The autonomicity vision is incorporated into the existing efforts that aim to the advanced automation including artificial intelligence research. This implies (Sterritt & Hinchey, 2005b) that all the processes should be designed effectively with autonomicity and self-managing capabilities. Adding semantics in the Grid using semantic services and the support of self-organization will allow creating more flexible and heterogeneous Grids (Beckstein et al., 2006). Proposals for the support of reliable electronic health business systems deal with adopting of the autonomic Grid computing and the Services-Oriented Architecture (SOA) (Omar & Taleb-Bendiab, 2006). This improvement provides the benefit of high quality of services and on-demand health monitoring (ubiquitously and on-line) (Omar & Taleb-Bendiab, 2006).

Overall, the wireless Grid allows the user mobility to share underused available resources in a network that is required for e-health applications. The applications of wireless Grid contain (Benedict et al., 2008) patient monitoring, multimedia, wireless devices, etc. Incorporating mobile devices in Grid technologies and server applications can provide (Ozturk & Altilar, 2007) the potential to control the state of supercomputers with mobile devices and allow applications to access valuable data ubiquitously (for example, the production of positioning information from GPS mobile devices). Moreover, integrating mobile, wireless devices in the Grid has recently (Jan et al., 2009) drawn the attention of the research community since this initiative has led to new challenges. Mobile ad hoc grid is a new approach of Grid computing (Jan et al., 2009) where appealing real scenarios can be applied. Finally, Knowledge Grid is an intelligent and realistic environment of Internet applications that allow operation from people or virtual roles to capture, publish and share explicit knowledge resources (Anya, et al., 2009).

However, handling situations that result from emergencies requires semantic information about the environment and one flexible self-organizing information technology infrastructure to provide services that can be used (Beckstein et al., 2006). For example, intelligent services can achieve personalized and proactive management of individual patients (Omar et al., 2006).

Quality Dimensions in Healthcare

During the last decades extensive efforts were focused on improvement of the provided products and services and quality improvement theories were adopted (Deming, 2000; Juran, 1988). The meaning of quality and the quality management strategies are much more complex in the health sector, compared to the industrial sector, where initially the theories for the quality were applied (Deming, 2000; Juran, 1988). Avedis Donabedian defined the following three dimensions of quality in healthcare: (1) structure, (2) process and (3) outcome (Donabedian, 1980a; Donabedian, 1980b). Given these quality dimensions, Donabedian formulated the following definition for quality in health care: this nature of health care that is expected to maximize the well-being of the patient, considering the balance of benefits but also losses that follow the health care process (Donabedian, 1980a; Donabedian, 1980b).

In Figure 2, the essential quality dimensions both for products and services, as these have been defined by distinguished researchers are presented (Donabedian, 1982; Donabedian, 1983; Donabedian, 1985; Donabedian, 1991; Donabedian, 2001; Garvin, 1988; Maxwell, 1984; Maxwell, 1992). Quality assessment and measurement in traditional health care systems is feasible through these dimensions.

FUTURE RESEARCH DIRECTIONS

The Semantic Grid applies Semantic Web technologies to raising the technical challenges we have to overcome. With the available data flow and handling, these issues are of utmost importance. Nowadays, when we think about amounts of data produced by simulations, experiments and sensors it becomes apparent that we have to automate the discovery. Therefore, we need automatic data management. This, in turn, calls

Figure 2. Quality dimensions as defined by Donabedian, Maxwell and Garvin

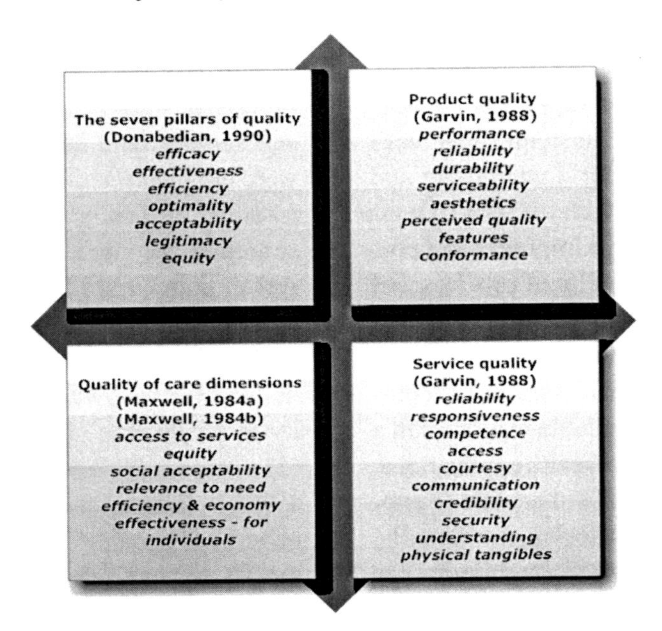

for automatic annotation of data with metadata describing attractive features of both of data storage and management. Lastly, we have to try to move towards automatic knowledge management. Producing data are one issue; preserving data is a separate issue. This process involves automated, semi-automated and manual annotation and data cleaning. Overall, there are many technical challenges to be resolved to ensure the information created today can undergo changes in storage media, devices and digital formats.

Furthermore, we should focus on utilizing the previously presented quality dimensions in healthcare by developing mathematical models, which will be useful for the quality assessment of public e-health systems and services.

CONCLUSION

E-health is an ambitious idea. It expects to set up a novel and powerful middleware that encourages a novel way of providing ubiquitous, personalized, intelligent and proactive health care services at a distance. The three promising visions embrace the three corners of the 'Semantic-Pervasive-Grid Triangle'. Exploring all these three visions together requires working across at least three communities. The proponents of this 'holistic' approach argue that only through exploring the combined world (the entire triangle) we will make a comprehensive infrastructure for the vision of ambient intelligence and e-Medicine. If crowned with success, the e-health approach will unite different communities creating reliable, virtual organizations, which tackle new challenges, utilize a wide range of distributed resources for improving the quality of care and quality of life. Issues of quality assurance in e-health should consider the dimensions already used for quality assessment in the traditional health care.

REFERENCES

Abidi, S. S. R. (2002). *A Case Base Reasoning Framework to Author Personalized Health Maintenance Information.* Paper presented at the 15th IEEE Symposium on Computer-Based Medical Systems.

Abidi, S. S. R., Han, C. Y., & Abidi, S. R. (2001). *An Intelligent Info-Structure for Composing and Pushing Personalised Healthcare Information Over the Internet.* Paper presented at the 14th IEEE Symposium on Computer-Based Medical Systems.

American College of Physicians (2008). E-health and its impact on Medical Practice. *Position paper.*

Anya, O., Tawfik, H., & Nagar, A. Amin, S. (2009). *E-workbench: A Case for Collaborative Decision Support in E-health.* Paper presented at the 11th International Conference on Computer Modelling and Simulation.

Archer, N. (2005). *Mobile eHealth: Making the Case. Euromgov2005.* Mobile Government Consortium International.

Beckstein, C., Dittrich, P., Erfurth, Ch., Fey, D., Konig-Ries, B., Mundhenk, M., & Sack, H. (2006). *SOGOS - A Distributed Meta Level Architecture for the Self-Organizing Grid of Services.* Paper presented at the 7th International Conference on Mobile Data Management.

Benedict, S., Rejitha, R. S., & Vasudevan, V. (2008). *Threshold Accepting Scheduling algorithm for scientific workflows in Wireless Grids.* Paper presented at the Fourth International Conference on Networked Computing and Advanced Information Management.

Breton, V., Blanquer, I., Hernandez, V., Legré, Y., & Solomonides, T. (2006). Proposing a roadmap for HealthGrids. *Studies in Health Technology and Informatics, 120*, 319–329.

Broens, T., van Halteren, A., van Sinderen, M., & Wac, K. (2007). Towards an application framework for context-aware m-health applications. *International Journal of Internet Protocol Technology, 2*(2), 109–116. doi:10.1504/IJIPT.2007.012374

Carlsson, C., & Walden, P. (2002). *Further Quests for Value-Added Products and Services in Mobile Commerce.* Paper presented at the The Xth European Conference on Information Systems.

Chorianopoulos, K. (2008). Personalized and mobile digital TV applications. *Multimedia Tools and Applications, 36*(1-2), 1–10. doi:10.1007/s11042-006-0081-8

de Toledo, P., Galarraga, M., Martínez, I., Serrano, L., Fernández, J., & Del Pozo, F. (2006). *Towards e-Health Device Interoperability: The Spanish Experience in the Telemedicine Research Network.* Paper presented at the Annual International Conference of the IEEE Engineering in Medicine and Biology Society.

Delicato, F., Pirmez, L., & Carmo, L. (2001). Fenix – personalized information filtering system for WWW pages. *Internet Research: Electronic Networking Applications and Policy, 11*(1), 42–48. doi:10.1108/10662240110365706

Deming, W. E. (2000). *Out of the crisis.* Cambridge, MA: The MIT Press.

Donabedian, A. (1980a). *The definition of quality and approaches to its assessment.* Ann Arbor, MI: Health Administration Press.

Donabedian, A. (1980b). *Explorations in quality assessment and monitoring* (*Vol. 6*). Ann Arbor, MI: Health Administration Press.

Donabedian, A. (1982). *The criteria and standards of quality.* Ann Arbor, MI: Health Administration Press.

Donabedian, A. (1983). Quality Assessment and Monitoring Retrospect and Prospect. *Evaluation & the Health Professions, 6*(3), 363–375. doi:10.1177/016327878300600309

Donabedian, A. (1985). *The methods and findings of quality assessment and monitoring.* Ann Arbor, MI: Health Administration Press.

Donabedian, A. (1991). *Striving for quality in health care.* Ann Arbor, MI: Health Administration Press.

Donabedian, A. (2001). *An Introduction to Quality Assurance in Health Care.* New York: Oxford University Press.

Dong, J. C., Hu, X. P., Zhang, Z.-M., Zhou, D., & Jiang, K. (2009). *Analysis and Design on Standard System of Electronic Health Records.* Paper presented at the First International Workshop on Education Technology and Computer Science.

Garvin, D. A. (1988). *Managing Quality: The strategic and competitive edge.*

Germanakos, P., Mourlas, C., & Samaras, G. (2005). *A Mobile Agent Approach for Ubiquitous and Personalized eHealth Information Systems.* Paper presented at the 10th International Conference on User Modeling.

Han, D., Park, S., & Kurkuri, S. (2007). *An Evolving Mobile E-Health Service Platform.* Paper presented at the International Conference on Consumer Electronics.

Hanak, D., Szijarto, G., & Takacs, B. (2007). *A mobile approach to ambient assisted living.* Paper presented at the IADIS Wireless Applications and Computing.

Harle, C. A., Padman, R., & Downs, J. S. (2009). *Design, Implementation, and Preliminary Evaluation of a Web-Based Health Risk Calculator.* Paper presented at the 42nd Hawaii International Conference on System Sciences.

Intille, S. S., Larson, K., & Kukla, C. (2002). *Just-In-Time Context-Sensitive Questioning for Preventative Health Care.* Paper presented at the AAAI 2002 Workshop on Automation as Caregiver: The Role of Intelligent Technology in Elder Care.

Isaiadis, S., & Getov, V. (2005). *Integrating Mobile Devices into the Grid: Design Considerations and Evaluation. Euro-Par 2005* (*Vol. 3648*). Berlin: Springer Berlin / Heidelberg.

Jan, S., Shah, I. A., & Al-Raweshidy, H. S. (2009). *Performance Analysis of Proactive and Reactive Routing Protocols for Mobile Ad-hoc Grid in ehealth Applications.* Paper presented at the International Conference on Communication Software and Networks.

Joshi, A. (2000). On proxy agents, mobility, and web access. *Mobile Networks and Applications, 5*(4), 233–241. doi:10.1023/A:1019120915034

Juran, J. (1988). *Juran on Planning for Quality.* Washington, DC: Free Press.

Konstantas, D., Jones, V., & Herzog, R. (2002). *MobiHealth –innovative 2.5 / 3G mobile services and applications for healthcare.* Paper presented at the Eleventh Information Society Technologies (IST) Mobile and Wireless Telecommunications.

Koufi, V., Malamateniou, F., & Vassilacopoulos, G. (2008). *A Medical Diagnostic and Treatment Advice System for the Provision of Home Care.* Paper presented at the 1st international conference on Pervasive Technologies Related to Assistive Environments.

Kratz, M., Silverstein, J., & Dev, P. (2007). HealthGrid: Grid Technologies for Biomedicine. Fort Detrick, Maryland: Telemedicine & Advanced Technology Research Center, U.S. Army Medical Research and Materiel Command.

Lugmayr, A., Risse, T., Stockleben, B., Kaario, J., & Laurila, K. (2009). Special issue on semantic ambient media experience. *Multimedia Tools and Applications*, 331–335. doi:10.1007/s11042-009-0283-y

Lupu, E., Dulay, N., Sloman, M., Sventek, J., Heeps, S., & Strowes, S. (2008). AMUSE: autonomic management of ubiquitous e-Health systems. *Concurrency and Computation, 20*(3), 277–295. doi:10.1002/cpe.1194

Maxwell, R. J. (1984). Quality assessment in health. *British Medical Journal, 288*(6428), 1470–1472. doi:10.1136/bmj.288.6428.1470

Maxwell, R. J. (1992). Dimensions of quality revisited: from thought to action. *Quality in Health Care, 1*, 171–177. doi:10.1136/qshc.1.3.171

Meneu, T., Traver, V., Fernández, C., Serafin, R., Domínguez, D., & Guillén, S. (2009). *Life Assistance Protocols (LAP) – A Model for the Personalization of Lifestyle Support for Health and Wellbeing.* Paper presented at the International Conference on eHealth, Telemedicine, and Social Medicine.

Milenković, A., Otto, C., Jovanov, E. (2006). Wireless Sensor Networks for Personal Health Monitoring: Issues and an Implementation. *Computer Communications (Special issue: Wireless Sensor Networks: Performance, Reliability, Security, and Beyond), 29*(13-14), 2521-2533.

Mohomed, I., Misra, A., Ebling, M., & Jerome, W. (2008). *Context-Aware and Personalized Event Filtering for Low-Overhead Continuous Remote Health Monitoring.* Paper presented at the International Symposium on a World of Wireless, Mobile and Multimedia Networks.

Nijland, N., Seydel, E. R., van Gemert-Pijnen, J. E. W. C., Brandenburg, B., Kelders, S. M., & Will, M. (2009). *Evaluation of an Internet-Based Application for Supporting Self-Care of Patients with Diabetes Mellitus Type 2.* Paper presented at the International Conference on eHealth, Telemedicine, and Social Medicine.

Nikolidakis, S., Vergados, D. D., & Anagnostopoulos, I. (2008). *Health Care Information Systems and Personalized Services for Assisting Living of Elderly People at Nursing Home.* Paper presented at the Third International Workshop on Semantic Media Adaptation and Personalization.

Olive, M., Rahmouni, H., & Solomonides, T. (2007a). From HealthGrid to SHARE: A Selective Review of Projects. *Studies in Health Technology and Informatics, 126*, 306–313.

Olive, M., Rahmouni, H., Solomonides, T., Breton, V., Legre, Y., & Blanquer, I. (2007b). SHARE Roadmap 1: Towards a Debate. *Studies in Health Technology and Informatics, 126*, 164–173.

Oliveira, I. C., Oliveira, J. L., Santos, M., Martin-Sanchez, F., & Sousa Pereira, A. (2003). *On the requirements of biomedical information tools for health applications: the INFOGENMED case study.* Paper presented at the 7th Protuguese Conference on Biomedical Engineering.

Omar, W. M., Ahmad, B. A., & Taleb-Bendiab, A. (2006). *Grid Overlay for Remote e-Health Monitoring.* Paper presented at the IEEE International Conference on Computer Systems and Applications.

Omar, W. M., & Taleb-Bendiab, A. (2006). *Service Oriented Architecture for e-Health Support Services Based on Grid Computing Overlay.* Paper presented at the Proceedings of the IEEE International Conference on Services Computing.

Ozturk, E., & Altilar, D. T. (2007). *IMOGA: An Architecture for Integrating Mobile Devices into Grid Applications.* Paper presented at the Fourth Annual Conference on Mobile and Ubiquitous Systems: Networking & Services.

Panayiotou, C., & Samaras, G. (2004). mPERSONA: Personalized Portals for the Wireless User: An Agent Approach. *Mobile Networks and Applications, 9*(6), 663–677. doi:10.1023/B:MONE.0000042505.07003.e6

Panteli, N., Pitsillides, B., Pitsillides, A., & Samaras, G. (2007). An E-healthcare Mobile application: A Stakeholders' analysis: Experience of Reading . In Al-Hakim, L. (Ed.), *Web Mobile-Based Applications for Healthcare Management.* Hershey, PA: IGI Global.

Park, S., Mackenzie, K., & Jayaraman, S. (2002). *The wearable motherboard: a framework for personalized mobile information processing (PMIP).* Paper presented at the 39th Design Automation Conference.

Riva, G. (2003). Ambient Intelligence in Health Care. *Cyberpsychology & Behavior, 6*(3), 295–300. doi:10.1089/109493103322011597

Stell, A., Sinnott, R., Ajayi, O., & Jiang, J. (2007). *Security Oriented e-Infrastructures Supporting Neurological Research and Clinical Trials.* Paper presented at the Proceedings of the The Second International Conference on Availability, Reliability and Security.

Sterritt, R., & Bantz, D. F. (2004). *PAC-MEN: Personal Autonomic Computing Monitoring Environment.* Paper presented at the Database and Expert Systems Applications, 15th International Workshop.

Sterritt, R., & Hinchey, M. (2005a). *Autonomicity – An Antidote for Complexity?* Paper presented at the Proceedings of the 2005 IEEE Computational Systems Bioinformatics Conference - Workshops.

Sterritt, R., & Hinchey, M. (2005b). *Why Computer-Based Systems Should be Autonomic.* Paper presented at the Proceedings of the 12th IEEE International Conference and Workshops on Engineering of Computer-Based Systems.

Van Halteren, A., Konstantas, D., Bults, R., Wac, K., Dokovsky, N., & Koprinkov, G. (2004). MobiHealth: Ambulant Patient Monitoring Over Next Generation Public Wireless Networks . In Demiris, G. (Ed.), *E-Health: Current Status and Future Trends* (*Vol. 106*). Amsterdam: IOS Press.

Voicu, L. C., Schuldt, H., Breitbart, Y., & Schek, H. J. (2009). *Replicated Data Management in the Grid: The Re:GRIDiT Approach.* Paper presented at the 1st ACM workshop on Data grids for eScience.

Volckaert, B., Thysebaert, P., De Leenheer, M., De Turck, F., Dhoedt, B., & Demeester, P. (2004). Grid computing: the next network challenge! *Journal of the Communications Network*, *3*, 159–165.

Wac, K. (2005). *Towards QoS-awareness of Context-aware Mobile Applications and Services.* Paper presented at the On the Move to Meaningful Internet Systems 2005: OTM Workshops, Ph.D. Student Symposium.

Wac, K., van Halteren, A., & Konstantas, D. (2006). *QoS-Predictions Service: Infrastructural Support for Proactive QoS- and Context-Aware Mobile Services (Position Paper) On the Move to Meaningful Internet Systems 2006: OTM 2006 Workshops*. Berlin: Springer Berlin / Heidelberg.

Yusof, M. M., Paul, R. J., & Stergioulas, L. K. (2006). *Towards a Framework for Health Information Systems Evaluation.* Paper presented at the 39th Annual Hawaii International Conference on System Sciences.

Chapter 22
E-Health as the Realm of Healthcare Quality:
A Mental Image of the Future

Anastasius Moumtzoglou
Hellenic Society for Quality & Safety in Healthcare & European Society for Quality in Healthcare, Greece

ABSTRACT

E-health has widely revolutionized medicine, creating subspecialties that include medical image technology, computer aided surgery, and minimal invasive interventions. New diagnostic approaches, treatment, prevention of diseases, and rehabilitation seem to speed up the continual pattern of innovation, clinical implementation and evaluation up to industrial commercialization. The advancement of e-health in healthcare derives large quality and patient safety benefits. Advances in genomics, proteomics, and pharmaceuticals introduce new methods for unraveling the complex biochemical processes inside cells. Data mining detects patterns in data samples, and molecular imaging unites molecular biology and in vivo imaging. At the same time, the field of microminiaturization enables biotechnologists to start packing their bulky sensing tools and medical simulation bridges the learning divide by representing certain key characteristics of a physical system.

INTRODUCTION

There is a worldwide increase in the use of health information technology (IT), which holds promise of health system breakthroughs. Emerging information and communication technologies promise groundbreaking solutions for healthcare problems. Moreover, a global e-health consensus framework is beginning to take shape in IT discourse, which includes stakeholders, policy, funding, coordination, standards and interoperability (Gerber, 2009). However, in an unprecedented technological innovation, many aspects of health care systems require careful consideration due to error and inefficiency although e-health bridges clinical and nonclinical sectors.

The endorsement of information technology in the health sector is spreading slowly. Few companies focus on population-oriented e-health tools partly because of perceptions about the viability

DOI: 10.4018/978-1-61692-843-8.ch022

and extent of the market segment. Moreover, developers of e-health resources are a highly diverse group with differing skills and resources while a common problem for developers is finding the balance between investment and outcome. According to recent surveys, one of the most severe restraining factors for the proliferation of e-health is the lack of security measures. Therefore, a large number of individuals are not willing to engage in e-health (Katsikas et al., 2008). E-health presents risks to patient health data that involve not only technology and appropriate protocols but also laws, regulations and professional security cultures. Furthermore, breaches of network security and international viruses have elevated the public awareness of online data and computer security. Although the overwhelming majority of security breaches do not directly involve health-related data, the notion that online data are exposed to security threats is widespread. Moreover, as we understand the clinical implications of the genetic components of disease, we expect a remarkable increase in the genetic information of clinical records. As a result, there is likely to be considerable pressure in favor of specific laws protecting genetic privacy (Magnusson, 2002). Therefore, secure e-health requires not only national standardization of professional training and protocols but also global interoperability of regulations and laws. Professional health information organizations must take the lead in professional certification, security protocols and applicable codes of ethics on a global basis ((Kluge, 2007; Moor & Claerhoutb, 2004).

On the other hand, clinicians have moved toward the Internet within the last few years while purchasers seek higher quality and lower costs. The Internet offers an unprecedented opportunity to integrate various health-related sectors while some Internet-related trends and technologies will have a substantial impact on the design, content, functionality, dissemination, and use of future e-health tools. Moreover, quality assurance and improvement are key issues for the e-health sector while strategic planning could provide an insightful view of the impacts (Asoh et al., 2008). However, the accessibility and confidentiality of electronic resources does not guarantee quality access (West and E. A. Miller, 2006) and the current quality assurance strategies do not address the dynamic nature of e-health technologies. Furthermore, the contribution of various socio-economic factors to 'the digital divide', which refers to the difference in computer and Internet access between population groups segmented by various parameters, is controversial. However, recent data suggests that the digital divide may be closing in some aspects, due to access to PCs, and the Internet. Access, however, is only one facet of the digital divide, as health literacy (Bass, 2005), and relevant content are also key elements.

Moreover, there are overlapping and gaps in e-health content due to the uncoordinated and essentially independent efforts. Current market forces are driving e-health development in clinical care support, and health care transactions, but they do not provide population health-related functions. Therefore, increased information exchange and collaboration among developers may result in efficient use of resources. The challenge is to foster collaborative e-health development in the context of fair competition. Greater collaboration presents new communication challenges, which include a standardized communication and information flow (Lorence & R. Churchill, 2008), which will enhance:

- social support
- cognitive functioning
- clinical decision-making
- cost-containment

Many observers believe that a picture of interoperable clinical, laboratory, and public health information systems, will provide unprecedented opportunities for improving individual and community health care (Godman, 2008; Lorence & Sivaramakrishnan, 2008; Toledo et al., 2006).

Interoperable electronic medical records (EMRs) contain the potential to improve efficiency and reduce cost (James, 2005). Moreover, semantic interoperability is essential for sound clinical care (Goodenough, 2009) although electronic prescribing does not increase steadily (Friedman et al., 2009).

The lack of integration in health care also carries over into the online world. Therefore, universal data exchange requires a translating software and the development of data exchange standards (Friedman et al., 2009). There is also need to integrate the various features and functions of e-health tools to provide a seamless continuum of care, which might include:

- health data
- processing of transactions
- electronic health records
- clinical health information systems
- disease management programs
- behavior modification and health promotion

Finally, as the complexity and amount of genetic information expand, new e-health tools, which support clinicians and consumers decision-making in genetics will be in considerable demand. Moreover, once nanotechnology applications become available, we have to establish nanoethics as a new sub-discipline of applied ethics (Godman, 2008). Overall, although we have to understand care in a renewed dimension (Nord, 2007), we might consider e-health as a method to improve the health status of the population. The promise of applying emerging e-health technologies to improve health care is substantial. However, it is crucial to build partnerships among healthcare providers, organizations, and associations to ensure its continued development (Harrison & Lee, 2006).

Thus, the perspective of the chapter is to examine the prospects of e-health to become the realm of healthcare quality.

BACKGROUND

The term e-health has evolved through prolonged periods of time, which include the era of discovery (1989-1999), acceptance (1999-2009), and deployment (2009-). Each period has distinctive features, and critical applications. For example, in the age of discovery, we denounced traditional approaches to realize during the era of acceptance that we need a collaboration model. Key application areas of this period of time include electronic medical records (including patient records, clinical management systems, digital imaging & archiving systems, e-prescribing, e-booking), telemedicine and telecare services, health information networks, decision support tools, Internet-based technologies and services. E-health also covers virtual reality, robotics, multimedia, digital imaging, computer assisted surgery, wearable and portable monitoring systems, health portals. Finally, the distinctive features of the era of deployment might involve community care, evidence based medicine, collaborative care, and self-management. Furthermore, centrifugal or centripetal mobility will contribute to a new service integrating e-health and quality.

However, the term e-health is a common neologism, which lacks precise definition (Oh et al., 2005). The European Commission defines e-health as 'the use of modern information and communication technologies to meet needs of citizens, patients, healthcare professionals, healthcare providers, as well as policy makers' while the World Health Organization offers a more precise definition. Specifically, e-health is 'the cost-effective and secure use of information and communications technologies in support of health and health-related fields, including health-care services, health surveillance, health literature, and health education, knowledge and research'. Eysenbach, in the most frequently cited definition, defines e-health as 'an emerging field in the intersection of medical informatics, public health and business, referring to health services and information delivered or enhanced through the Internet and related technologies. In a broader sense, the term characterizes not only a technical development, but also a state-of-mind, a way of thinking, an attitude, and a commitment for networked, global thinking, to improve health care locally, regionally, and worldwide by using information and communication technology. Finally, Pagliari et al., (2005) in a highly detailed analysis provide a definition, which covers human and organizational factors.

E-health is not the only sector, which lacks a clear definition. A literature review reveals a multitude of definitions of quality of care (Banta, 2001). The World Health Organization has defined the quality of health systems as 'the level of attainment of a health system's intrinsic goals for health improvement and responsiveness to the legitimate expectations of the population' (WHO, 2000). W. Edward Deming argued that 'a product or service possesses quality if it helps somebody and enjoys a good and sustainable market', Juran (1974) stated that 'quality is fitness for use', and Crosby (1979) 'quality means conformance to requirements'. Still, the most widely cited definition of healthcare quality was formulated by the Institute of Medicine (IOM) in 1990. According to the IOM, quality consists of the 'degree to which health services for individuals and populations increase the likelihood of desired health outcomes and are consistent with current professional knowledge'.

Overall, the meaning of quality is complex, elusive, and uncertain (Burhans, 2007), and its meaning is an optimal balance between possibilities and the framework of norms and values (Harteloh, 2004). Nevertheless, the concept of healthcare quality involves the standardization and national endorsement of performance measures, the evaluation of outcomes, reporting for accountability, and technological innovation (Smith, 2007). Furthermore, we might distinguish three levels of quality, which include conformance quality, requirements quality, and quality of kind.

Even so, the present and future healthcare systems demonstrate a quality chasm, formed by a large number of different factors. Medical science and advanced technology have advanced at an unprecedented rate but have also contributed to a growing complexity. Faced with such rapid changes, the healthcare system has fallen considerably short in its ability to refine theoretical knowledge into professional practice and to use modern technology. The healthcare needs have changed quite dramatically as well. Individuals are living longer, due to fundamental advances in medical science. Subsequently, the aging population translates into an exponential growth in the prevalence of chronic conditions. In addition, today's complex health system overly deals with acute, episodic care needs and cannot consistently deliver today's science and technology. It is less prepared to respond to the tremendous advances that surely will appear in the near future. Healthcare delivery cannot face the various challenges and is overly complicated and uncoordinated. Therefore, complex processes waste resources and lead to excessive loss of useful information. Eventually, healthcare organizations, hospitals, and physicians operate without the added value of information. As a result, state-of-the-art care requires a fundamental and extensive redesign. The health system should avoid injuries, provide responsive services based on scientific knowledge, reduce waits and delays, avoid waste, and eliminate differences in quality. Overall, according to the Institute of Medicine 'Crossing the Quality Chasm: A New Health System for the 21st Century' report, the health system should be safe, effective, patient-centered, timely, efficient, and equitable (IOM, 2001). To achieve these improvement aims, we should adopt ten simple statements (IOM, 2001):

- patients should receive care or access to care whenever they need it
- the entire system should meet the most frequent types of needs and preferences
- empower the patient

- allow information flow freely and share knowledge
- decision-making is evidence-based
- patient safety is a system property
- transparency is necessary
- anticipate needs
- decrease waste
- enhance cooperation

Furthermore, redesigning the healthcare delivery system involves changing the structure and administrative processes of healthcare organizations. Such changes need to appear in four key areas (IOM, 2001):

- application of evidence to healthcare delivery
- information technology
- alignment of payment policies with quality improvement
- preparation of the future workforce

Finally, we should not underestimate the importance of adequately preparing the future workforce to undergo the transition into a new healthcare system. There are three contrasting approaches, which we might use (IOM, 2001):

- redesign the educational approach (Hasman et al., 2006)
- change the way we accredit or regulate health professionals
- define and ensure accountability among health professionals and professional organizations

Conclusively, the Institute of Medicine's 'Crossing the Quality Chasm: A New Health System for the 21st Century' report, implies:

- to improve physician-patient interaction beyond encounter-oriented care (Leong et al., 2005)
- to introduce a partnership approach to clinical decision-making (Coulter & Ellins, 2006)
- to improve health literacy and encourage full disclosure of adverse events (Gallagher et al., 2007)
- to revolutionize patient safety by providing clinicians with clinical decision support and by involving patients (Coulter & Ellins, 2006)
- to raise public accountability by measuring the quality of care at the provider level
- to improve patient care on the basis of ongoing evaluation, lifetime learning, systems-based practice and interpersonal skills of clinicians

Although groundbreaking, IOM's approach raises several limitations:

- the evidence on health literacy demonstrates that there are substantial gaps in what we know about how to raise its standards (Coulter & Ellins, 2006)
- the implementation of innovations, which improve clinical decision-making and promote greater patient involvement, has yet to occur (Coulter & Ellins, 2006; Billings 2004; Graham et al., 2003)
- safety improvement, through patient involvement, should be enhanced
- patient feedback, provider choice, complaints, and advocacy systems should be carefully assessed

E-health holds enormous potential for transforming the quality aspect of healthcare by supporting the delivery of care, improving transparency and accountability, aiding evidence-based practice and error reduction, improving diagnostic accuracy and treatment appropriateness, facilitating patient empowerment, and improving cost-efficiency.

THE QUALITY PERSPECTIVE OF E-HEALTH

E-health has its roots in physics, engineering, informatics, mathematics and chemistry and links with biosciences, especially biomedical physics, biomedical engineering, biomedical computing and medicine. Therefore, the improvement in science and technology accelerate its tremendous growth the last few decades. Furthermore, e-health has widely revolutionized medicine, creating sub-specialties that include medical image technology, computer aided surgery, and minimal invasive interventions. New diagnostic approaches, treatment, prevention of diseases, and rehabilitation seem to speed up the continual pattern of innovation, clinical implementation and evaluation up to industrial commercialization. Some of the current technologies are the electronic patient record, a routine for a few countries, the patient data card, health professional card, e-prescription, e-reporting, networking and tele-consulting. BioMEMOS, imaging technology, minimally invasive surgery, and computer-assisted diagnosis, therapy and treatment monitoring, e-health/telemedicine/ networking, and medical engineering for regenerative medicine are the fields of e-health technologies, which have emerged in recent years. For example, tissue engineering combines specific medical disciplines with cell and molecular biology, material sciences, physics and engineering aiming at developing methods for regenerating, repairing or replacing human tissue. Specifically, it uses in situ stem cell control focusing specifically on stem cells of the central nervous system for neurogeneration (Nusslin, 2006). Finally, beyond the boundaries of the medical field, at least in the highly industrialized countries, e-health has a substantial impact on the economy, the whole society and the ethical system.

The advancement of e-health in healthcare derives large quality and patient safety benefits. Health information technology holds enormous potential to improve outcomes, and efficiency within the health care system. Electronic health records, decision support systems, computerized physician order entry systems, computerized adverse events systems, automatic alerts, national or regional incident or event reporting systems improve administrative efficiency, adherence to guideline-based care, and reduce medication errors. Electronic health records, which store information electronically, provide the opportunity to find patients with certain conditions, and look for specific issues (Honigman et al., 2001a; Honigman et al., 2001b).The IOM (2001) argued that an electronic based patient record system would be the single action that would most improve patient safety. Coiera et al., (2006) argued that the use of decision support systems, comprehensive solutions often incorporated in a variety of e-health applications, can improve patient outcomes and make clinical services more effective. Tierney et al (2003) found that the intervention had no effect on physicians' adherence to care suggestions while Kawamoto et al (2005), in a meta-analysis of seventy studies, concluded that decision support systems significantly improve clinical practice. Computerized physician order entry systems, a process whereby physicians file electronically instructions to individuals responsible for patient care, improve the quality of care by increasing clinician compliance. It is an outstanding application (Sittig & Stead, 1994), which reduces preventable adverse drug events (Kaushal & Bates, 2003). Computerized adverse event systems have shown a notable increase in the number of reported adverse drug events, and automatic alerts reduce the time until treatment of patients with critical laboratory tests (2001). Many studies have shown that prevention guidelines and the reminder computerization improve adherence (Balas et al., 2000) while reminders are noteworthy in the care of chronic conditions, which constitute a large quotient of expenditures (Lobach & Hammond, 1994). Furthermore, national or regional incident or event reporting systems, which collect data from local sources, lead to remarkable changes at the community and national level (Runciman, 2002). Finally, a particularly compelling reason for promoting the adoption of e-health is its potential to improve the processes of health care. E-Health improves the likelihood that the processes will be successful; strengthens the distribution of evidence-based decision support to providers, narrows the gaps between evidence and practice, and might lead to exceptional savings in administrative costs.

On the other hand, electronic clinical knowledge support systems have decreased barriers to answering clinical questions (Bonis et al., 2008), and organizational learning at the system level fosters improvement (Rivard et al., 2006). However, e-health is not just a technology but a complex technological and relational process (Metaxiotis et al., 2004). Therefore, the Internet, a platform available to remote areas, constitutes a radical change, which empowers patients.

Patient-centered care is an emerging approach, which the Picker Institute defines as informing and involving patients, eliciting and respecting their preferences; responding quickly, effectively and safely to patients' needs and wishes; ensuring that patients are treated in an ennobled and caring manner; delivering well coordinated and integrated care. Patient empowerment, which means that patients play a more active role in partnership with health professionals, and relates to strategies for education and e-health information (Pallesen et al., 2006), is increasingly being seen as a essential component of a modern patient-centered health system. Kilbridge (2002) suggested that technologies, which allow access to general and specific health care information, technologies capable to conduct data entry and tracking of personal self-management, empower patients. These technologies included Personal Health Records, Patient Access to Hospital Information Systems, Patient Access to General Health Information, Electronic Medical Records (EMRs), Pre-Visit Intake, Inter-Hospital Data Sharing, Information for Physicians to Manage Patient Populations, Patient-Physician Electronic Messaging, and Patient Access to Tailored Medical Information, Online Data Entry and Tracking, Online Scheduling, Computer-Assisted Telephone Triage and Assistance, and Online Access to Provider Performance Data. Moreover, handheld devices increasingly allow expansion of desktop systems and capture vital signs or administer medications while much of the quality improvement revolves around refinement of processes.

It is worthwhile mentioning that telemedicine, a branch of e-health that uses communication networks and it is deployed to overcome uneven distribution and lack of infrastructural and human resources, provides a category by itself (Sood et al., 2007). Finally, the sciences of chaos and complexity are generating considerable interest within the domains of healthcare quality and patient safety (Benson, 2005), and clinical narratives has the potential to improve healthcare quality and safety (Brown et al., 2008; Baldwin, 2008). Still, there is a lack of interoperability, which makes the provision of clinical decision support and the extracting of pertinent information vastly more complicated (Schiff & Rucker, 1998; Schiff et al., 2008), and risks to patient health data (Kluge, 2007).

Issues, Controversies, Problems

Notwithstanding the e-health potential for contributing to improved processes of health care, greater efficiency and enhanced understanding of clinically-effective care, financial and other barriers persist that result in comparatively low penetration rates of e-health. These barriers include acquisition and implementation costs, the lack of interoperability standards, skepticism about the business case for investment, uncertainty about system longevity, and psychological barriers related to uncertainty and change. E-health systems are expensive and providers face problems making the investment. Even if they can handle the initial acquisition and implementation costs, still must remain confident that an e-health system will improve efficiency or cover its upfront and ongoing costs to make the investment. In addition, some providers' reluctance to adopt e-health may be a rational response to skewed financial incentives since the health care system provides little financial incentive for quality improvement (Blumenthal & Glaser, 2007). Perhaps the most controversial barrier to adoption of quality-related information technology is the lack of incentives for change. Therefore, non-governmental groups might play an extremely pivotal role in developing incentives, and regulatory agencies can ask for valid, standardized, and more easily gathered quality measurement data.

Additional barriers to the spread of e-health include legal and regulatory concerns and technological issues (Davenport, 2007). Legal challenges include privacy of identifiable health information, reliability and quality of health data and tort-based liability while recommendations for legal reform include (Hodge et al., 1999):

- sensitivity of health information
- privacy safeguards
- patient empowerment
- data and security protection

Technological barriers to e-health stem from the evolutionary nature of these systems but also rapid obsolescence, and the lack of standards or criteria for interoperability. Without the technical specifications that enable interoperability, data exchange between providers who use different e-health systems is severely limited. Moreover, security and confidentiality in information technology represent a serious matter (Anderson, 2007).

Finally, implementation and dissemination issues are decipherable. The effects of e-health tools on patient behavior, the patient-clinician relationship, the legal and ethical implications of using health information technologies and clinical decision support systems are unclear. Furthermore, potential health inequalities resulting from the digital divide have to restrain within bounds. Overall, key questions include clinical decision support, refinement of guidelines for local implementation, implementation and dissemination of clinical information systems, patient involvement and the role of the Internet.

On the other hand, the variation in the quality strategies is the effect of different levels of political commitment and/or available financial resources (Legido-Quigley, 2008; Lombarts, et al., 2009; Spencer & Walshe, 2008; Spencer & Walshe, 2009; Sunol et al., 2009). The most eminent drivers of policy have been governments, professional organizations, scientific societies, and media. Governments are the key players in developing and implementing quality improvement policies, and setting quality standards and targets. However, the lack of quality incentives, lack of funding for quality improvement and absence of professional training and education in quality improvement are the key barriers to progress. We might also argue that funding and financing cause conflict of interest. Furthermore, in the current economic crisis, governments are less inclined to invest in the development of quality strategies as they will not provide adequate financial return in the short or medium terms. Additionally, the existence of a statutory legal requirement to implement quality improvement strategies for healthcare systems and organizations is an overriding motivation for supporting progress in the development of quality improvement initiatives. Nevertheless, patient and service user organizations have the least impact on the development of quality improvement strategy. The preponderance of governments and health professions makes difficult for patient and user groups to set the limits of quality improvement policies and strategies. This means that the quality improvement activities reflect a professional and provider perspective.

Another issue concerns evaluation and implementation strategies. Little information is available about the effects of the strategies. As a consequence, investing in quality strategies appears expensive and inefficient, and education and training in quality improvement constitutes a barrier to progress. Therefore, there is a role for quality improvement training in education and institutional development of healthcare professionals.

Finally, quality improvement requires strong, engaged and informed professional leadership, which develops if healthcare professionals have access to appropriate training in healthcare quality improvement. However, such training is usually not available, the development of clinical guidelines, accreditation schemes, auditing of standards, and quality management are optional, and evaluation of quality improvement is not available to patients.

SOLUTIONS AND RECOMMENDATIONS

The integration of e-health into the existing work flow is increasingly difficult due to the complexity of the clinical setting. Consequently, strong leadership within the clinical setting is essential in the successful implementation. Leadership should work in conjunction with the staff in order to mitigate any apprehensions (Iakovidis, 1998; Burton et al., 2004). With this internal backing and commitment, healthcare professionals will become involved and integrate e-health into their daily practice. Moreover, there is a critical relationship between organizational and technological change (Berg, 2001), which providers should understand prior to implementation because they constitute the driving force behind changes within the clinical setting. Conclusively, the successful implementation of e-health requires a thoughtful integration of routine procedures and information technology elements. E-health integration is a process, which is determined by the uniqueness of each setting (Berg, 2001) and social and human variables. Immediate policy changes, which promote e-health adoption, might include standards for interoperability, privacy protection, clinical effectiveness research, and amelioration of parallel working by software developers and health services researchers (Pagliari, 2007).

Quality, access and efficiency are the general key issues for the success of e-health (Vitacca et al., 2009). However, a realistic definition of the dimensions of quality care is insufficient to accomplish the goal of continuous improvement. Therefore, healthcare quality improvement is a work in progress. Nonetheless, we might argue that quality improvement relates with leadership, measurement, reliability, practitioner skills and the marketplace. Kotter (1996) provides an eight-stage process to cope with change, which is necessary for the effective leadership. The eight processes include:

- establish a sense of urgency
- set up the guiding coalition
- develop a vision and strategy
- spread the change perspective
- empower broad-based events
- trigger short-term wins
- consolidate gains and provide more change
- harbor new approaches in the culture

Change acceleration is also the issue of the ADKAR psychological model, which rates on a scale of 1 to 5 the following elements (Hiatt & Creasey, 2003):

- awareness of the need to change
- desire to participate and continue change
- understanding of how to change
- means to implement change
- support to keep change in place

Quality measurement involves the outcome or the process (Auerbach, 2009). However, process measurement is the commonest because we can easily measure changes in processes (Davis & Barber, 2004) that in the patient health status. There is also resistance although change has spawned a number of trends in the assessment of doctors' competence (Norcini & Talati, 2009), when we recommend practicing medicine in a predictable and reliable way. Reliability revolves around command and control, risk appreciation, quality, metrics, and reward (Rochlin et al., 1987). However, a highly reliable organization must include mechanisms, which support flexibility, constrained improvisation, and cognition management (Bigley & Roberts, 2001). The problem in creating reliable processes is reducing variability, which interprets into high-quality decision making and high-quality performance of the practitioners. Finally, taking into account that quality is a vital component of healthcare business model, we have to understand the role it plays in the market. So far, quality has a tough time demonstrating its business case because of the complexity of care and the difficulty in capturing the actual fixed and variable cost of patient treatment (Leatherman et al., 2003; Sachdeva & Jain, 2009).

FUTURE RESEARCH DIRECTIONS

To substantiate the argument that e-health is the future realm of healthcare quality, we identify emerging scientific fields, and assess their impact on quality and patient safety.

- Biobanks, formally known as biological resource centers (BRCs), are depositories of 'biological standards'. Haga & Beskow (2008) estimated that the U.S. store more than 270 million tissue samples, with a growth rate of approximately 20 million samples annually. There are many types of BRC, which differ in their functional role and the kinds of material they hold. Public and private entities have developed them in order to provide researchers the opportunity to explore collections of human biospecimen. However, we believe that all BRCs have the potential to unravel the causes of complex diseases, as well as the interaction between biological and environmental factors.

Biobanking is an emerging discipline (Riegman et al., 2008), which follows the continuing expansion of new techniques and scientific goals. Overall, it constitutes a device, which facilitates the understanding of the genetic basis of disease (Ormond et al., 2009) and holds taxonomic strains (Day et al., 2008).

However, its establishment and maintenance is a skill-rich activity, which requires careful attention to the implementation of preservation technologies. Moreover, biobanking represents a challenge to informed consent (Ormond et al., 2009) while only appropriate quality assurance ensures that recovered cultures and other biological materials behave in the same way as the originally isolated culture.

- A biochip is a series of microarrays arranged on a solid substrate which permits to perform various tests at the same time (Fan et al., 2009; Cady, 2009). It replaces the typical reaction platform and produces a patient profile, which we use in disease screening, diagnosis and monitoring disease progression. The development of biochips is a considerable thrust of the rapidly growing biotechnology industry, which encompasses a diverse range of research efforts. Advances in genomics, proteomics, and pharmaceuticals introduce new methods for unraveling the complex biochemical processes inside cells. At the same time, the field of microminiaturization enables biotechnologists to start packing their bulky sensing tools. These biochips are essentially miniaturized laboratories, which allow researchers to produce hundreds or thousands of simultaneous biochemical reactions, and rapidly screen large numbers of biological analyses. Reproducibility and standardization of biochip processes is, therefore, essential to ensure quality of results and provide the best tool for the elucidation of complex relationships between different proteins in detrimental conditions (Molloy et al., 2005).

- As traditional clinical investigation evolves, different needs have emerged, which require data integration. Data mining is the process of extracting patterns from data. It supports workflow analysis (Lang et al., 2007) and saves time and energy leading to less hassle for clinicians. While data mining can be used to detect patterns in data samples, it is crucial to understand that non-representative samples may cause non-indicative results. Therefore, we sometimes use the term in a negative sense. As a result, in order to avoid confusion, we recently mention the negative perception of data mining as data dredging and data snooping.

Some people believe that data mining is ethically neutral. However, the way we might use data mining can raise questions regarding privacy, legality, and ethics. Specifically, data mining may compromise confidentiality and privacy obligations through data aggregation.

Data mining is rarely applied to healthcare, although it can facilitate the understanding of patient healthcare preferences (Liu et al., 2009). However, as we gather more data, data mining is becoming an increasingly indispensable tool in mining a wide selection of health records (Norén et al., 2008). Moreover, we might complement it with semantics-based reasoning in the management of medicines.

Finally, data mining can support quality assurance (Jones, 2009), simplify the automation of data retrieval, facilitate physician quality improvement (Johnstone et al., 2008), and accurately capture patient outcomes if combined with simulation (Harper, 2005). Recently, there is interest in switching to algorithms and database development for microarray data mining (Cordero et al., 2008).

- Disease modeling, the mathematical representation of a clinical condition, summarizes the knowledge of disease epidemiology, and requires computational modeling, which follows two different approaches. The bottom-up approach accentuates complex intracellular molecular models while the top-down modeling strategy identifies key features of the disease.

However, despite ongoing efforts, there are complex issues regarding the use of computational modeling. A key question concerns the handling of model uncertainty since the selection of a computational model has to take into account the additional interactions and components beyond those of a discursive model. Therefore, a successful strategy is the identification of minimal models or search for parameter dimensions that are indispensable for the model performance. However, we cannot select competing structures on the basis of their relative fitness. As a result, a high priority for future disease modeling is model selection and hierarchical modeling (Tegnér et al., 2009).

- Genomics, the study of the genomes of living entities, encompasses considerable efforts to determine the complete DNA sequence of organisms through fine-scale genetic mapping efforts. It also includes studies of intragenomic phenomena and interactions between loci and alleles within the genome. However, it does not deal with the functions of individual genes, a primary focus of molecular biology or genetics. Research of individual genes does not fall into the meaning of genomics unless the purpose of the research is to clarify its impact on the networks of the genome.

Technology development has played a vital role in structural genomics (Terwilliger et al., 2009). Nowadays, we can quantify the difficulties of determining a pattern of a single protein. Moreover, the systems approach, which the post-genomics follow, interprets into a greater responsibility for artificial intelligence and robotics. Overall, many disciplines turn on the issue of automating the different stages in post-genomic research with a view to developing high-dimensional data of high quality (Laghaee et al., 2005).

- Molecular Imaging unites molecular biology and in vivo imaging while enabling the visualization of the cellular function and the follow-up of the molecular process (Weissleder & Mahmood, 2001). It differs from conventional imaging in that we use biomarkers to image specific reference points. Biomarkers and their surroundings interact chemically altering the image according to molecular changes, which occur within the point of interest. This method is markedly different from previous methods of imaging which typically image differences in qualities.

The accomplishment to image sheer molecular changes opens up an impressive number of exciting possibilities for medical attention. These include the optimization of preclinical and clinical tests of new medication and early detection and treatment of disease. Molecular imaging imparts a greater degree of fairness to quantitative tests, and numerous potentialities to the diagnosis of cancer, neurological and cardiovascular diseases. Therefore, it has a substantial economic impact due to earlier and more accurate diagnosis.

- Nanotechnology is the study of the atomic and molecular matter. Although, we might think that it only develops materials of the size of 100 nanometers or smaller, nanotechnology is extremely diverse. It encompasses the extensions of conventional device physics, different approaches based upon molecular self-assembly, and new materials with nanoscale dimensions.

Nanomedicine, the medical practice of nanotechnology, encompasses the use of nanomaterials and nanoelectronic biosensors and seeks to provide a valuable collection of research and tools (Wagner et al., 2006; Freitas, 2005a). New applications in the pharmaceutical industry include advanced drug delivery systems, alternative therapies, and in vivo imaging. Moreover, molecular nanotechnology, a preliminary subfield of nanotechnology, deals with the engineering of molecular assemblers. So far, it is highly speculative seeking to predict what inventions nanotechnology might produce. However, we already know that we will need nanocomputers to lead molecular assemblers and expect nanorobots to join the medical armamentarium (Cavalcanti et al., 2008; Freitas, 2005b).

Finally, neuro-electronic interfacing, a visionary project dealing with the creation of nanodevices, will connect computers to the nervous system while nanonephrology will play a role in the management of patients with kidney disease. However, advances in nanonephrology require nano-scale information on the cellular molecular mechanism involved in kidney processes.

There has been much discussion in which reasons are advanced for and against nanotechnology. However, nanotechnology has the inherent capacity to provide many different materials in medicine, electronics, and energy production. In contrast, it raises concerns about its ecological effects of nanomaterials, and their potential effects on international economics (Allhoff & Lin, 2008). These concerns have led to a dialogue among advocacy groups and governments on whether particular regulation of nanotechnology is warranted.

- Ontology is the philosophical study of the nature of an entity, which also examines the main categories of reality. As a part of the metaphysics philosophy, ontology deals with questions concerning the entity existence and their grouping according to similarities and differences. However, in computer science, ontology is a formal representation of a set of concepts and their relationships.

Ontologies have become a mainstream issue in biomedical research (Pesquita et al., 2009) since we can explain biological entities by using annotations. This type of comparability, which we call semantic similarity, assesses the length of connectedness between two entities using annotations similarity. The implementation of semantic similarity to biomedical ontologies is new. Nevertheless, semantic similarity is a valuable tool for the validation of gene clustering results, molecular interactions, and disease gene prioritization (Pesquita et al., 2009).

However, the capacity to assure the quality of ontologies or evaluate their eligibility is limited (Rogers, 2006). Therefore, we need a combination of existing methodologies and tools to support a comprehensive quality assurance scheme. However, an ontology of superlative quality is not verifiable and might not be useful since a 'perfect' ontology, which complies with all current philosophical theories, might be too complex (Rogers, 2006).

- Proteomics, a term coined in 1997 to make an analogy with genomics, is the comprehensive study of proteins, their structures and functions (Anderson & Anderson, 1998; Blackstock & Weir, 1999). The term proteome, a combination of protein and genome (Wilkins et al., 1996) defines the full complement of proteins (Wilkins et al., 1996), and encompasses the modifications made to a single set of proteins. Therefore, proteome varies with time rendering proteomics, the next step in the study of biological systems, as more complicated than genomics.

One of the most promising developments from the study of human genes and proteins is the discovery of potential new drugs. This relies on the identification of proteins associated with a disease, and involves computer software which uses proteins as targets for new drugs. For example, virtual ligand screening is a computer technique which attempts to fit millions of small molecules to the three-dimensional structure of a protein. The computer assigns a rank of quality matching to various sites in the protein, enhancing or disabling the role of the protein in the cell.

In the last ten years, the field of proteomics has expanded at a rapid rate. Nevertheless, it appears that we have underestimated the level of stringency required in proteomic data generation and analysis. As a result, several published findings require additional evidence (Wilkins et al., 2006). However, clinical proteomics certify that the majority of errors occur in the preanalytical phase. Therefore, before introducing complex proteomic analysis into the clinical setting, we need standardization of the preanalytical phase.

- Modern health systems have focused their attention on micro issues, which include the minimization of diagnostic, treatment, and medication errors. However, safety culture, a macro issue, requires our attention. Safety culture is a sub-set of the organizational culture (Olive et al., 2006). Although an overriding concern in recent years, we need additional work to identify and soundly measure the key dimensions of patient safety culture (Ginsburg et al., 2009; Singer et al., 2008) and understand its relationship with the leadership.

A key finding of research is that efforts to improve culture may not succeed if hospital managers perceive patient safety differently from frontline workers. Research shows the pivotal role of managers in the promotion of employees' safe behavior, both through their attitudes, and by developing a safety management system (Fernandez-Muniz et al., 2007). Senior managers perceive patient safety climate more positively than non senior managers while it has proved difficult to engage frontline staff with the concept (Hellings et al., 2007).

Therefore, the agenda should move from rhetoric to converting the concept into observable behavior. A prerequisite for the realization of this perspective is the collection, analysis, and dissemination of information deriving from incidents and near misses as well as the adoption of the reporting, just, flexible and learning cultures (Ruchlin et al., 2004).

- As patients become increasingly concerned about safety, clinical medicine focuses more on quality (Simmons & Wagner, 2009) than on bedside teaching and education. Educators react to these challenges by restructuring curricula, developing small-group sessions, and increasing self-directed education and independent research (Okuda et al., 2009). Nevertheless, there is a disconnect between the classroom and the clinical setting, resulting in medical students feeling that they are inadequately trained.

Medical simulation bridges the learning divide by representing certain key characteristics of a physical system. Historically, the first medical simulators were unsophisticated models of human patients (Meller, 1997). Later on, active models seemed to imitate living anatomy and more recently interactive models respond to actions taken by a student or physician. These are two dimensional computer programs, which constitute a textbook, and demonstrate the edge of allowing a student to fix errors.

Quality improvement, patient safety, and the actual assessment of clinical skills have impelled medical simulation into the clinical arena (Carroll & Messenger, 2008). Still, there is convincing evidence that simulation training improves provider self-efficacy and effectiveness (Nishisaki et al., 2007) and increases patient safety. Finally, the process of iterative learning creates a much stronger learning environment and computer simulators are an ideal tool for evaluation of students' clinical skills (Murphy et al., 2007)..

On the contrary, there is no evidence that simulation training improves patient outcome. Therefore, we need ongoing academic research in order to evaluate the teaching effectiveness of simulation, and determine its impact on quality of care, patient safety (Cherry & Ali, 2008), and retention of knowledge. Even so, there is a plausible belief that medical simulation is the training device of the future.

CONCLUSION

E-health, which already supports outstanding advances in healthcare quality, has the potential to become its realm, if we make a representation of the cognitive and social factors related to its design and use and associate them with the clinical practice.

REFERENCES

Allhof, F., & Lin, P. (Eds.). (2008). *Nanotechnology & Society: Current and Emerging Ethical Issues*. New York: Springer.

Anderson, J. G. (2007). Social, ethical and legal barriers to e-health. *International Journal of Medical Informatics*, *76*(5-6), 480–483. doi:10.1016/j.ijmedinf.2006.09.016

Anderson, N. L., & Anderson, N. G. (1998). Proteome and proteomics: new technologies, new concepts, and new words. *Electrophoresis*, *19*(11), 1853–1861. doi:10.1002/elps.1150191103

Auerbach, A. (2009). Healthcare quality measurement in orthopaedic surgery: current state of the art. *Clinical Orthopaedics and Related Research*, *467*(10), 2542–2547. doi:10.1007/s11999-009-0840-8

Balas, E. A., Weingarten, S., Garb, C. T., Blumenthal, D., Boren, S. A., & Brown, G. D. (2000). Improving preventive care by prompting physicians. *Archives of Internal Medicine*, *160*, 301–308. doi:10.1001/archinte.160.3.301

Baldwin, K. B. (2008). Evaluating healthcare quality using natural language processing. *Journal for Healthcare Quality*, *30*(4), 24–29.

Bass, L. (2005). Health literacy: Implications for teaching the adult patient. *Journal of Infusion Nursing*, *28*(1), 15–22. doi:10.1097/00129804-200501000-00002

Benson, H. (2005). Chaos and complexity: applications for healthcare quality and patient safety. *Journal for Healthcare Quality*, *27*(5), 4–10.

Berg, M. (2001). Implementing Information Systems in Health Care Organizations: Myths and Challenges. *International Journal of Medical Informatics*, *64*, 143–156. doi:10.1016/S1386-5056(01)00200-3

Bigley, G. A., & Roberts, K. H. (2001). Structuring Temporary Systems for High Reliability . *Academy of Management Journal*, *44*, 1281–1300. doi:10.2307/3069401

Blackstock, W. P., & Weir, M. P. (1999). Proteomics: quantitative and physical mapping of cellular proteins. *Trends in Biotechnology*, *17*(3), 121–127. doi:10.1016/S0167-7799(98)01245-1

Blumenthal, D., & Glaser, J. (2007). Information technology comes to medicine. *The New England Journal of Medicine*, *356*(24), 2527–2534. doi:10.1056/NEJMhpr066212

Bonis, P. A., Pickens, G. T., Rind, D. M., & Foster, D. A. (2008). Association of a clinical knowledge support system with improved patient safety, reduced complications and shorter length of stay among Medicare beneficiaries in acute care hospitals in the United States. *International Journal of Medical Informatics*, *77*(11), 745–753. doi:10.1016/j.ijmedinf.2008.04.002

Brown, S. H., Elkin, P. L., Rosenbloom, S. T., Fielstein, E., & Speroff, T. (2008). eQuality for all: Extending automated quality measurement of free text clinical narratives. *AMIA Annual Symposium Proceedings,* 71-75.

Burhans, L. D. (2007). What is quality? Do we agree, and does it matter? *Journal for Healthcare Quality*, *29*(1), 39–44, 54.

Burton, L. C., Anderson, G. F., & Kues, I. W. (2004). Using Health Records to Help Coordinate Care. *The Milbank Quarterly*, *82*(3), 457–481. doi:10.1111/j.0887-378X.2004.00318.x

Cady, N. C. (2009). *Microchip-based PCR Amplification Systems. Lab-on-a-Chip Technology: Biomolecular Separation and Analysis*. Norwich, UK: Caister Academic Press.

Carroll, J. D., & Messenger, J. C. (2008). Medical simulation: the new tool for training and skill assessment. *Perspectives in Biology and Medicine*, *51*(1), 47–60. doi:10.1353/pbm.2008.0003

Cavalcanti, A., Shirinzadeh, B., Freitas, RA Jr., Hogg, T. (2008). Nanorobot architecture for medical target identification. *Nanotechnology, 19* (1), 015103(15pp).

Cherry, R. A., & Ali, J. (2008). Current concepts in simulation-based trauma education. *The Journal of Trauma*, *65*(5), 1186–1193. doi:10.1097/TA.0b013e318170a75e

Coiera, E., Westbrook, J. I., & Wyatt, J. C. (2006). The Safety and Quality of Decision Support Systems . In Haux, R., & Kulikowski, C. (Eds.), *IMIA Yearbook of Medical Informatics*.

Cordero, F., Botta, M., & Calogero, R. A. (2007). Microarray data analysis and mining approaches. *Briefings in Functional Genomics & Proteomics*, *6*(4), 265–281. doi:10.1093/bfgp/elm034

Davenport, K. (2007). Navigating American Health Care: How Information Technology Can Foster Health Care Improvement. *Center for American Progress*. Retrieved April 24, 2009, from www. americanprogress.com

Davis, K., Otwell, R., & Barber, J. (2004). Managing costs through clinical quality improvement. *Healthcare Financial Management*, *58*(4), 76–82.

Day, J. G., & Stacey, G. N. (2008). Biobanking. *Molecular Biotechnology*, *40*(2), 202–213. doi:10.1007/s12033-008-9099-7

Eysenbach, G. (2001). What is e-health?In Keith E. Herold, K., & Rasooly, A. (Eds.) *Journal of Medical Internet Research, 3*(2), e20.

Fan, Z. H., Das, C., & Chen, H. (2009). Two-Dimensional Electrophoresis in a Chip. In Keith E. Herold, K., & Rasooly, A. (Ed.), *Lab-on-a-Chip Technology: Biomolecular Separation and Analysis.* (pp. 122-138). Norfolk: Caister Academic Press.

Fernandez-Muniz, B., Montes-Peon, J. M., & Vazquez-Ordas, C. J. (2007). Safety culture: analysis of the causal relationships between its key dimensions. *Journal of Safety Research*, *38*(6), 627–641. doi:10.1016/j.jsr.2007.09.001

Freitas, R. A. Jr. (2005a). What is Nanomedicine? *Nanomedicine; Nanotechnology, Biology, and Medicine*, *1*(1), 2–9. doi:10.1016/j.nano.2004.11.003

Freitas, R. A. Jr. (2005b). Current Status of Nanomedicine and Medical Nanorobotics. *Journal of Computational and Theoretical Nanoscience*, *2*, 1–25.

Gandhi, T. K., & Bates, D. W. (2001). Computer Adverse Drug Event (ADE) Detection and Alerts. Chapter 8 in: University of California at San Francisco – *Stanford University Evidence based Practice Center Making Health Care Safer: A Critical Analysis of Patient Safety Practices* (pp 81).

Ginsburg, L., Gilin, D., Tregunno, D., Norton, P. G., Flemons, W., & Fleming, M. (2009). Advancing measurement of patient safety culture. *Health Services Research*, *44*(1), 205–224. doi:10.1111/j.1475-6773.2008.00908.x

Haga, S. B., & Beskow, L. M. (2008). Ethical, legal, and social implications of biobanks for genetics research. *Advances in Genetics*, *60*, 505–544. doi:10.1016/S0065-2660(07)00418-X

Harper, P. (2005). Combining data mining tools with health care models for improved understanding of health processes and resource utilisation. *Clinical and Investigative Medicine. Medecine Clinique et Experimentale*, *28*(6), 338–341.

Harteloh, P. (2004). The Meaning of Quality in Health Care: A Conceptual Analysis Health Care Analysis . *Health Care Analysis*, *11*(3), 259–267. doi:10.1023/B:HCAN.0000005497.53458.ef

Hellings, J., Schrooten, W., Klazinga, N., & Vleugels, A. (2007). Challenging patient safety culture: survey results. *International Journal of Health Care Quality Assurance*, *20*(7), 620–632. doi:10.1108/09526860710822752

Hiatt, J. M., & Creasey, T. J. (2003). *Change Management*. Loveland, CO: Prosci Research.

Hodge, J. G. Jr, Gostin, L. O., & Jacobson, P. D. (1999). Legal issues concerning electronic health information: privacy, quality, and liability. *Journal of the American Medical Association, 282*(15), 1466–1471. doi:10.1001/jama.282.15.1466

Honigman, B., Lee, J., Rothschild, J., Light, P., Pulling, R. M., Yu, T., & Bates, D. W. (2001). Using computerized data to identify adverse drug events in outpatients. *Journal of the American Medical Informatics Association, 8*, 254–266.

Honigman, B., Light, P., Pulling, R. M., & Bates, D. W. (2001). A computerized method for identifying incidents associated with adverse drug events in outpatients. *Journal of the American Medical Informatics Association, 61*, 21–32.

Iakovidis, I. (1998). Towards Personal Health Record: Current Situation, Obstacles, and Trends in Implementation of Electronic Healthcare Record in Europe. *International Journal of Medical Informatics, 52*, 105–115. doi:10.1016/S1386-5056(98)00129-4

Johnstone, P. A., Crenshaw, T., Cassels, D. G., & Fox, T. H. (2008). Automated data mining of a proprietary database system for physician quality improvement. *International Journal of Radiation Oncology, Biology, Physics, 70*(5), 1537–1541. doi:10.1016/j.ijrobp.2007.08.056

Jones, A. R. (2009). Data mining can support quality assurance. *Journal of the Royal Society of Medicine, 102*(9), 358–359. doi:10.1258/jrsm.2009.090216

Kluge, E. H. (2007). Secure e-Health: managing risks to patient health data. *International Journal of Medical Informatics, 76*(5-6), 402–406. doi:10.1016/j.ijmedinf.2006.09.003

Kuperman, G. J., Teich, J., Bates, D. W., Hilz, F. L., Hurley, J., Lee, R. Y., et al. (1996). Detecting alerts, notifying the physician, and offering action items: a comprehensive alerting system. *Proceedings of AMIA Annual Fall Symposium,* (pp. 704-708).

Laghaee, A., Malcolm, C., Hallam, J., & Ghazal, P. (2005). Artificial intelligence and robotics in high throughput post-genomics. *Drug Discovery Today, 10*(18), 1253–1259. doi:10.1016/S1359-6446(05)03581-6

Lang, M., Kirpekar, N., Burkle, T., Laumann, S., & Prokosch, H. U. (2007). Results from data mining in a radiology department: the relevance of data quality. *Studies in Health Technology and Informatics, 129*(Pt 1), 576–580.

Leatherman, S., Berwick, D., Iles, D., Lewin, L., Davidoff, F., Nolan, T., Bisognano, M. (2003). The Business Case for Quality: Case Studies and an Analysis. *Health Affairs, 22* (2),17–30, 18.

Legido-Quigley, H., McKee, M., Walshe, K., Suñol, R., Nolte, E., & Klazinga, N. (2008). How can quality of care be safeguarded across the European Union? *British Medical Journal, 336*, 920–923. doi:10.1136/bmj.39538.584190.47

Liu, S. S., & Chen, J. (2009). Using data mining to segment healthcare markets from patients' preference perspectives. *International Journal of Health Care Quality Assurance, 22*(2), 117–134. doi:10.1108/09526860910944610

Lobach, D. F., & Hammond, W. E. (1994). Development and evaluation of a computer-assisted management protocol (CAMP): improved compliance with care guidelines for diabetes mellitus. *Proceedings of the Annual Symposium on Computer Applications in Medical Care,* 787-791

Lombarts, M. J. M. H., Rupp, I., Vallejo, P., Suñol, R., & Klazinga, N. (2009). Application of quality improvement strategies in 389 European hospitals: results of the MARQuIS project. *Quality & Safety in Health Care, 18*, 28–37. doi:10.1136/qshc.2008.029363

Meller, G. (1997). A Typology of Simulators for Medical Education. *Journal of Digital Imaging, 10*, 194–196. doi:10.1007/BF03168699

Metaxiotis, K., Ptochos, D., & Psarras, J. (2004). E-health in the new millennium: a research and practice agenda. *International Journal of Electronic Healthcare*, *1*(2), 165–175. doi:10.1504/IJEH.2004.005865

Molloy, R. M., Mc Connell, R. I., Lamont, J. V., & FitzGerald, S. P. (2005). Automation of biochip array technology for quality results. *Clinical Chemistry and Laboratory Medicine*, *43*(12), 1303–1313. doi:10.1515/CCLM.2005.224

Murphy, D., Challacombe, B., Nedas, T., Elhage, O., Althoefer, K., Seneviratne, L., & Dasgupta, P. (2007). Equipment and technology in robotics (in Spanish; Castilian). *Archivos Espanoles de Urologia*, *60*(4), 349–355.

Nishisaki, A., Keren, R., & Nadkarni, V. (2007). Does Simulation Improve Patient Safety?: Self-Efficacy, Competence, Operational Performance, and Patient Safety. *Anesthesiology Clinics*, *25*(2), 225–236. doi:10.1016/j.anclin.2007.03.009

Norcini, J., & Talati, J. (2009). Assessment, surgeon, and society. *International Journal of Surgery*, *7*(4), 313–317. doi:10.1016/j.ijsu.2009.06.011

Norén, G. N., Bate, A., Hopstadius, J., Star, K., & Edwards, I. R. (2008). Temporal Pattern Discovery for Trends and Transient Effects: Its Application to Patient Records. In *Proceedings of the Fourteenth International Conference on Knowledge Discovery and Data Mining SIGKDD 2008* (pp. 963-971). Las Vegas NV.

Nusslin, F. (2006). Current status of medical technology. *Acta Neurochirurgica*, *98*, 25–31. doi:10.1007/978-3-211-33303-7_5

Okuda, Y., Bryson, E. O., DeMaria, S Jr., Jacobson, L., Quinones, J., Shen, B., & Levine, A. I. (2009). The utility of simulation in medical education: what is the evidence? *Mount Sinai Journal of Medicine: A Journal of Translational and Personalized Medicine, 76*(4), 330-343.

Olive, C., O'Connor, T. M., & Mannan, M. S. (2006). Relationship of safety culture and process safety. *Journal of Hazardous Materials*, *130*(1-2), 133–140. doi:10.1016/j.jhazmat.2005.07.043

Ormond, K. E., Cirino, A. L., Helenowski, I. B., Chisholm, R. L., & Wolf, W. A. (2009). Assessing the understanding of biobank participants. *American Journal of Medical Genetics*, *149A*(2), 188–198. doi:10.1002/ajmg.a.32635

Pagliari, C. (2007). Design and evaluation in eHealth: challenges and implications for an interdisciplinary field. *Journal of Medical Internet Research*, *9*(2), e15. doi:10.2196/jmir.9.2.e15

Pallesen, B., Engberg, A., & Barlach, A. (2006). Developing e-health information by empowerment strategy. *Studies in Health Technology and Informatics*, *122*, 776.

Pesquita, C., Faria, D., Falcao, A. O., Lord, P., & Couto, F. M. (2009). Semantic similarity in biomedical ontologies. *PLoS Computational Biology*, *5*(7), e1000443. doi:10.1371/journal.pcbi.1000443

Riegman, P. H., Morente, M. M., Betsou, F., de Blasio, P., & Geary, P. (2008). Biobanking for better healthcare. *Molecular Oncology*, *2*(3), 213–222. doi:10.1016/j.molonc.2008.07.004

Rivard, P. E., Rosen, A. K., & Carroll, J. S. (2006). Enhancing patient safety through organizational learning: Are patient safety indicators a step in the right direction? *Health Services Research*, *41*(4 Pt 2), 1633–1653. doi:10.1111/j.1475-6773.2006.00569.x

Rochlin, G. I., La Porte, T.R., & Roberts, K. H., K.H. (1987). The Self-Designing High-Reliability Organization: Aircraft Carrier Flight Operations at Sea. *Naval War College Review*, *40*(4), 76–90.

Rogers, J. E. (2006). Quality assurance of medical ontologies. *Methods of Information in Medicine*, *45*(3), 267–274.

Ruchlin, H. S., Dubbs, N. L., & Callahan, M. A. (2004). The role of leadership in instilling a culture of safety: lessons from the literature. *Journal of Healthcare Management*, *49*(1), 47–58.

Runciman, W. B. (2002). Lessons from the Australian Patient Safety Foundation: setting up a national patient safety surveillance system – is this the right model? *Quality & Safety in Health Care*, *11*, 246–251. doi:10.1136/qhc.11.3.246

Sachdeva, R. C., & Jain, S. (2009). Making the case to improve quality and reduce costs in pediatric health care. *Pediatric Clinics of North America*, *56*(4), 731–743. doi:10.1016/j.pcl.2009.05.013

Schiff, G. D., Aggarwal, H. C., Kumar, S., & McNutt, R. A. (2000). Prescribing potassium despite hyperkalemia: medication errors uncovered by linking laboratory and pharmacy information systems. *The American Journal of Medicine*, *109*, 494–497. doi:10.1016/S0002-9343(00)00546-5

Schiff, G. D., & Rucker, T. D. (1998). Computerized prescribing: building the electronic infrastructure for better medication usage. *Journal of the American Medical Association*, *279*, 1024–1029. doi:10.1001/jama.279.13.1024

Simmons, B., & Wagner, S. (2009). Assessment of continuing interprofessional education: lessons learned . *The Journal of Continuing Education in the Health Professions*, *29*(3), 168–171. doi:10.1002/chp.20031

Singer, S. J., Falwell, A., Gaba, D. M., & Baker, L. C. (2008). Patient safety climate in US hospitals: variation by management level. *Medical Care*, *46*(11), 1149–1156. doi:10.1097/MLR.0b013e31817925c1

Sittig, D. F., & Stead, W. W. (1994). Computer-based physician order entry: the state of the art. *Journal of the American Medical Informatics Association*, *1*, 108–123.

Smith, Moore T., Francis, M. D., & Corrigan, J. M. (2007). Health care quality in the 21st century. *Clinical and Experimental Rheumatology*, *25*, 3–5.

Sood, S., Mbarika, V., Jugoo, S., Dookhy, R., Doarn, C. R., Prakash, N., & Merrell, R. C. (2007). What is telemedicine? A collection of 104 peer-reviewed perspectives and theoretical underpinnings. *Telemedicine journal and e-health: the official journal of the American Telemedicine Association, 13*(5), 573-590.

Spencer, E., & Walshe, K. (2008). Quality and safety in healthcare in Europe. A growing challenge for policymakers. *Harvard Health Policy Review*, *1*, 46–54.

Spencer, E., & Walshe, K. (2009). National quality improvement policies and strategies in European Healthcare Systems. *Quality & Safety in Health Care*, *18*, 22–27. doi:10.1136/qshc.2008.029355

Suñol, R., Vallejo, P., Thompson, A., Lombarts, M. J. M. H., Shaw, C. D., & Klazinga, N. (2009). Impact of quality strategies on hospital outputs. *Quality & Safety in Health Care*, *18*, 57–63. doi:10.1136/qshc.2008.029439

Tegnér, J. N., Compte, A., Auffray, C., An, G., Cedersund, G., & Clermont, G. (2009). Computational disease modeling - fact or fiction? *BMC Systems Biology*, *3*, 56. doi:10.1186/1752-0509-3-56

Terwilliger, T. C., Stuart, D., & Yokoyama, S. (2009). Lessons from structural genomics. *Annual Review of Biophysics*, *38*, 371–383. doi:10.1146/annurev.biophys.050708.133740

Vitacca, M., Mazzu, M., & Scalvini, S. (2009). Socio-technical and organizational challenges to wider e-Health implementation. *Chronic Respiratory Disease*, *6*(2), 91–97. doi:10.1177/1479972309102805

Wagner, V., Dullaart, A., Bock, A. K., & Zweck, A. (2006). The emerging nanomedicine landscape. *Nature Biotechnology*, *24*(10), 1211–1217. doi:10.1038/nbt1006-1211

Weissleder, R., & Mahmood, U. (2001). Molecular imaging . *Radiology*, *219*, 316–333.

Wilkins, M., Pasquali, C., Appel, R., Ou, K., Golaz, O., & Sanchez, J. C. (1996). From Proteins to Proteomes: Large Scale Protein Identification by Two-Dimensional Electrophoresis and Arnino Acid Analysis. *Nature Biotechnology*, *14*(1), 61–65. doi:10.1038/nbt0196-61

Wilkins, M. R., Appel, R. D., Van Eyk, J. E., Chung, M. C., Gorg, A., & Hecker, M. (2006). Guidelines for the next 10 years of proteomics. *Proteomics*, *6*(1), 4–8. doi:10.1002/pmic.200500856

ADDITIONAL READING

Elger, B., Biller-Andorno, N., Mauron, A., Capron, A., & Morgan Capron, A. (2008). *Ethical Issues in Governing Biobanks*. Hampshire, UK: Ashgate Publishing Limited.

Gottweis, H. (2008). *Biobanks: Governance in Comparative Perspective*. New York: Roputledge.

Kewal, J. (2009). *The Handbook of Nanomedicine*. Totwa, New Jersey: Humana Press.

Nisbet, R., Elder, J., & Miner, G. (2009). *Handbook of Statistical Analysis and Data Mining Applications*. Cambridge, MA: Elsevier.

Pevsner, J. (2009). *Bioinformatics and Functional Genomics*. New Jersey: Wiley & Sons. doi:10.1002/9780470451496

Pisanelli, D. M. (2004). *Ontologies in Medicine*. Amsterdam: IOS Press.

Riley, R. (2008). *A Manual of Simulation in Healthcare*. Oxford, UK: Oxford University Press.

Xing, W. L., & Cheng, J. (2006). *Frontiers in Biochip Technology*. New York: Springer. doi:10.1007/b135657

Compilation of References

AABB. (2003). *American Association of Blood Banks, Standards for Blood Banks and Transfusion Services* (22nd ed). Bethesda, MD. Retrieved from www.aabb.org

Abidi, S. S. R. (2002). *A Case Base Reasoning Framework to Author Personalized Health Maintenance Information.* Paper presented at the 15th IEEE Symposium on Computer-Based Medical Systems.

Abidi, S. S. R., Han, C. Y., & Abidi, S. R. (2001). *An Intelligent Info-Structure for Composing and Pushing Personalised Healthcare Information Over the Internet.* Paper presented at the 14th IEEE Symposium on Computer-Based Medical Systems.

Adams, J., Edgar, L., & Mounib, A. P. (2006). Healthcare 2015: Win-win or lose-lose? *IBM Institute for business value,* Retrieved May 10, 2009, from http://www.ibm.com/healthcare/hc2015

Adibi, S., & Agnew, G. B. (2008). On the diversity of eHealth security systems and mechanisms. *Conference Proceedings; ... Annual International Conference of the IEEE Engineering in Medicine and Biology Society. IEEE Engineering in Medicine and Biology Society. Conference*, 1478–1481.

Agency for Healthcare Research and Quality and National Institute of Mental Health. (2001). *Patient-centered care: customizing care to meet patients' needs*. Retrieved April 24, 2009, from http://grants.nih.gov/grants/guide/pa-files/PA-01-124.html.

Aiello, M., & Dustdar, S. (2008). Are our homes ready for services? A domotic infrastructure based on the Web service stack. *Pervasive and Mobile Computing*, *4*(4), 506–525. doi:10.1016/j.pmcj.2008.01.002

Alexa Internet. (2007a). *Three-month traffic statistics for wikipedia.org*. Retrieved from http://www.alexa.com/data/details/main?q=&url=wikipedia.org

Alexa Internet. (2007b). *Top Sites United States*. Retrieved from http://www.alexa.com/site/ds/top_sites?cc=US&ts_mode=country&lang=none

Allhof, F., & Lin, P. (Eds.). (2008). *Nanotechnology & Society: Current and Emerging Ethical Issues*. New York: Springer.

Ally, M. (2004). Foundations of Educational Theory for Online Learning. In Anderson T. & Elloumi F. (Eds.), *Theory and Practice of Online Learning.* Athabasca University. Retrieved January 30, 2009 from http://cde.athabascau.ca/online_book/.

Altman, D. G., Schltz, K. F., Mohler, D., & al. (2001). The revised CONSORT statement for reporting randomized trials: Explanation and elaboration. *Annals of Internal Medicine,* 134, 663-694. See also [http://www.annals.org/cgi/content/abstract/134/8/663] and associated Web site [www.consort-statement.org].

American College of Physicians (2008). E-health and its impact on Medical Practice. *Position paper*.

American Library Association. (1989). *Presidential Committee on Information Literacy - Final Report*. Retrieved from http://www.ala.org/ala/acrl/acrlpubs/whitepapers/presidential.htm

American National Standards Institute – HITSP Specifications. Retrieved September 30, 2009 from http://wiki.hitsp.org/docs/

American Telemedicine Association. (1999). *Guidelines for Telepathology*. Retrieved May 13, 2009, from http://www.americantelemed.org/i4a/ams/amsstore/category.cfm?category_id=2

American Telemedicine Association. (2004). Telehealth practice recommendations for diabetic retinopathy. *Telemedicine and e-Health, 10*(4), 469-482.

American Telemedicine Association. (2006). *Telemedicine/Telehealth Terminology*. Retrieved May 13, 2009, from http://www.americantelemed.org/files/public/standards/glossaryofterms.pdf

American Telemedicine Association. (2008). *Core Standards for Telemedicine Operations*. Retrieved May 13, 2009, from http://www.americantelemed.org/i4a/pages/index.cfm?pageID=3311

AMIA. (1997). The Practice of Informatics. A Proposal to Improve Quality, Increase Efficiency, and Expand Access in the U.S. Health Care System. *Journal of the American Medical Informatics Association*, *4*(5), 340–341.

Anand, S., Feldman, M., Geller, D., Bisbee, A., & Bauchner, H. (2005). A content analysis of e-mail communication between primary care providers and parents. *Pediatrics*, *115*, 1283–1288. doi:10.1542/peds.2004-1297

Andersen, S. K., Klein, G. O., Schulz, S., Aarts, J., & Mazzoleni, M. C. (Eds.). (2008). *eHealth Beyond the Horizon – Get IT There. Proceedings of MIE2008*. Amsterdam: IOS Press.

Anderson, J. G., Rainey, M., & Eysenbach, G. (2003). The impact of cyberHealthcare on the physician-patient relationship. *Journal of Medical Systems*, *27*, 67–84. doi:10.1023/A:1021061229743

Anderson, J. G., Jay, S. J., Anderson, M., & Hunt, T. J. (2002). Evaluating the capability of information technology to prevent adverse drug events: a computer simulation approach. *Journal of the American Medical Informatics Association*, *9*, 479–490. doi:10.1197/jamia.M1099

Anderson, J. G. (2007). Social, ethical and legal barriers to e-health. *International Journal of Medical Informatics*, *76*(5-6), 480–483. doi:10.1016/j.ijmedinf.2006.09.016

Anderson, N. L., & Anderson, N. G. (1998). Proteome and proteomics: new technologies, new concepts, and new words. *Electrophoresis*, *19*(11), 1853–1861. doi:10.1002/elps.1150191103

Anderson, J.G. (2007). Social, ethical, and legal barriers to e-health. *International Journal of Medical Information, 76* (5, 6), 480 – 483.

Andrews, D. C. (2002). Audience-specific online community design. *Communications of the ACM*, *45*(4), 64–68. doi:10.1145/505248.505275

Ansani, N. T., Vogt, M., & Henderson, B. A., McKaVeney, T. P., Weber, R. J., Smith, R. B., Burda, M., Kwoh, C. K., Osial, T. A., & Starz, T. (2005). Quality of arthritis information on the Internet. *American Journal of Health-System Pharmacy*, *62*, 1184–1189.

Antman, E., Lau, J., Kupelnick, B., Mosteller, F., & Chalmers, T. (1992). A comparison of results of meta-analyses of randomized control trials and recommendations of clinical experts. *Journal of the American Medical Association*, *268*, 240–248. doi:10.1001/jama.268.2.240

Anya, O., Tawfik, H., & Nagar, A. Amin, S. (2009). *E-workbench: A Case for Collaborative Decision Support in E-health.* Paper presented at the 11th International Conference on Computer Modelling and Simulation.

Apostolakis, I., Varlamis, I., & Papadopoulou, A. (2008). *Virtual learning communities*. Athens: Papazisis Publishers.

Archer, N. (2005). *Mobile eHealth: Making the Case. Euromgov2005*. Mobile Government Consortium International.

Argyris, C. (1994, July-August). Good communication that blocks learning. *Harvard Business Review*, 77–85.

Argyris, C. (2005). Double-loop learning in organizations: A theory of action perspective . In Smith, K. G., & Hitt, M. A. (Eds.), *Great minds in management: The process of theory development* (pp. 261–279). Oxford, UK: Oxford University Press.

Aronsky, D., & Haug, P. J. (2000). Assessing the Quality of Clinical Data in a Computer-based Record for Calculating the Pneumonia Severity Index. *Journal of the American Medical Informatics Association*, *7*(1), 55–65.

Aronson, A. (2001). Effective mapping of biomedical text to the UMLS Metathesaurus: The MetaMap program. In *Proceedings of the 2001 AMIA Symposium* (pp. 17-21).

Arts, D. G. T., De Keizer, N. F., & Scheffer, G.-J. (2002). Defining and Improving Data Quality in Medical Registries: A Literature Review, Case Study, and Generic Framework. *Journal of the American Medical Informatics Association*, *9*(6), 600–611. doi:10.1197/jamia.M1087

Athanasiou, G. S., Maris, N. I., & Apostolakis, I. A. (2008). Evaluation of Virtual Learing Communities for Supporting e-Learing in Health Care Domain. In *Proceedings of 6th ICICTH* (pp 287-293), Samos, Greece.

Atkins, D., Best, D., & Briss, P. A. (2004). Grading quality of evidence and strength of recommendations. *British Medical Journal*, *328*(7454), 1490. doi:10.1136/bmj.328.7454.1490

Atkins, D. (2008). *The limits of evidence based medicine.* Retrieved January 15, 2009, from http://www.dbskeptic.com/2008/08/17/the-limits-of-evidence-based-medicine/

Auerbach, A. (2009). Healthcare quality measurement in orthopaedic surgery: current state of the art. *Clinical Orthopaedics and Related Research*, *467*(10), 2542–2547. doi:10.1007/s11999-009-0840-8

Austin, C. J., & Boxerman, S. B. (1998). *Information systems for health services administration* (5th ed.). Chicago, IL: Health Administration Press.

Austin, J. L. (1962). *How to do things with words*. Cambridge, MA: Harvard University Press.

Australian Institute of Health and Welfare (AIHW). (2008). *Rural, Regional and Remote Health: Indicators of health status and determinants of health*, Australian Institute of Health and Welfare, Canberra, cat. no. PHE 97.

Averill, E. (1994). Reference models and standards. *StandardView*, *2*(2), 96–109. doi:10.1145/202949.202959

Ávila de Tomás, J. F., Portillo Boyero, B. E., & Pajares Izquierdo, J. M. (2001). Calidad en la información biomédica existente en Internet. *Atencion Primaria*, *28*, 674–679.

Aydin, C., Anderson, J., Rosen, P., Felitti, V. J., & Weng, H. (2004). *Computers in the Consulting Room: A Case Study of Clinician and Patient Perspectives.* In JG. Anderson & CE. Aydin (Eds.), *Evaluating the Organizational Impact of Healthcare Information Systems, Second Edition*, (pp.225-47).

Bacsich, P. (2005). *Benchmarks for e-learning in UK HE - adaptation of existing good practice*. Presented at the e-Learning workshop of the Association for Learning Technology Conference. Retrieved September 10, 2009 from http://www.matic-media.co.uk/pubsandpres-2005.htm.

Bakavos, I., & Apostolakis, I. (2007). *Model of the certification procedure for internet health related websites*. In Proceedings of 5th ICICTH (pp 164-169), Samos, Greece.

Baker, M., Quignard, M., Lund, K., & van Amelsvoort, M. (2002). Designing a computer-supported collaborative learning situation for broadening and deepening understanding of the space of debate. In *Proceedings of the Fifth Conference of the International Society for the Study of Argumentation, 25-28 June 2002* (pp. 55-61). Amsterdam, Netherlands.

Bala, V., & Goyal, S. (2000). A strategic analysis of network reliability. *Review of Economic Design*, *5*(3), 205–228. doi:10.1007/s100580000019

Balas, E. A., Weingarten, S., Garb, C. T., Blumenthal, D., Boren, S. A., & Brown, G. D. (2000). Improving preventive care by prompting physicians. *Archives of Internal Medicine*, *160*, 301–308. doi:10.1001/archinte.160.3.301

Baldwin, K. B. (2008). Evaluating healthcare quality using natural language processing. *Journal for Healthcare Quality*, *30*(4), 24–29.

Ball, C., Sackett, D., Phillips, B., Straus, S., & Haynes, B. (1998). *Levels of evidence and grades of recommendations*. Retrieved January 17, 2009, from http://www.cebm.net/levels_of_evidence.asp

Barach, P., & Small, S. (2000). Reporting and preventing medical mishaps: lessons from non-medical near miss reporting systems. *British Medical Journal*, *320*, 759–763. doi:10.1136/bmj.320.7237.759

Bashshur, R. L., Reardon, T. G., & Shannon, G. W. (2000). Telemedicine: A new health care delivery system. *Annual Review of Public Health*, *21*, 613–637. doi:10.1146/annurev.publhealth.21.1.613

Bashshur, R., Shannon, G., Sapei H. (2005). Telemedicine Evaluation. *Telemedicine and e-Health, 11*(3), 296-316.

Bass, L. (2005). Health literacy: Implications for teaching the adult patient. *Journal of Infusion Nursing*, *28*(1), 15–22. doi:10.1097/00129804-200501000-00002

Bates, D. (2005a). Computerized Physician Order entry and medication errors: finding a balance. *Journal of Biomedical Informatics*, *38*(4), 250–261. doi:10.1016/j.jbi.2005.05.003

Bates, D. W. (2005b). Physicians and ambulatory electronic health records. *Health Affairs*, *24*(5), 1180–1189. doi:10.1377/hlthaff.24.5.1180

Bates, D. W., Leape, L. L., Cullen, D. J., & Laird, N. (1998). Effect of computerized physician order entry and a team intervention on prevention of serious medical errors. *Journal of the American Medical Association*, *280*, 1311–1316. doi:10.1001/jama.280.15.1311

Bates, D. W., Cohen, M., Leape, L. L., Overhage, J. M., Shabot, M. M., & Sheridan, T. (2001). Reducing the frequency of errors in medicine using information technology. *Journal of the American Medical Informatics Association*, *8*, 299–308.

Bates, D. W., Evans, R. S., Murff, H., Stetson, P. D., Pizziferri, L., & Hripcsak, G. (2003). Detecting adverse events using information technology. *Journal of the American Medical Informatics Association*, *10*, 115–128. doi:10.1197/jamia.M1074

Bates, D. W. (2002). The quality case for information technology in healthcare. *Medical Informatics and Decision Making, 2*(7), Retrieved May 2, 2009, from http://www.pubmedcentral.nih.gov/articlerender.fcgi?artid=137695

Bauer, K. A. (2002). Using the Internet to empower patients and to develop partnerships with clinicians. *World Hospitals and Health Services*, *38*(2), 2–10.

Baughman, K., Logue, E., Sutton, K., Capers, C., Jarjoura, D., & Smucker, W. (2003). Biopsychosocial characteristics of overweight and obese primary care patients: do psychosocial and behavior factors mediate sociodemographic effects? *Preventive Medicine*, *37*(2), 129–137. doi:10.1016/S0091-7435(03)00095-1

Beagon, M. (1992). *Roman Nature: The Thought of Pliny the Elder. Oxford Classical Monographs*. Oxford, UK: Clarendon Press.

Beckstein, C., Dittrich, P., Erfurth, Ch., Fey, D., Konig-Ries, B., Mundhenk, M., & Sack, H. (2006). *SOGOS - A Distributed Meta Level Architecture for the Self-Organizing Grid of Services*. Paper presented at the 7th International Conference on Mobile Data Management.

Benedict, S., Rejitha, R. S., & Vasudevan, V. (2008). *Threshold Accepting Scheduling algorithm for scientific workflows in Wireless Grids*. Paper presented at the Fourth International Conference on Networked Computing and Advanced Information Management.

Bennett, S., Harper, B., & Hedberg, J. (2002). Designing real life cases to support authentic design activities. *Australian Journal of Educational Technology*, *18*(1), 1–12.

Benson, H. (2005). Chaos and complexity: applications for healthcare quality and patient safety. *Journal for Healthcare Quality*, *27*(5), 4–10.

Benton, S., & Manning, B. R. M. (2006). Assistive Technology - Behaviourally Assisted . In Bos, L., Roa, L., Yogesan, K., O'Connell, B., Marsh, A., & Blobel, B. (Eds.), *Medical and Care Compunetics* (*Vol. 3*, pp. 7–14). Amsterdam: IOS Press.

Berg, M. (2001). Implementing Information Systems in Health Care Organizations: Myths and Challenges. *International Journal of Medical Informatics*, *64*, 143–156. doi:10.1016/S1386-5056(01)00200-3

Bernard, R., Abrami, P. L., Lou, Y., & Borokhovski, E. (2004). How does distance education compare with classroom instruction? A meta-analysis of the empirical literature. *Review of Educational Research*, *74*, 379–439. doi:10.3102/00346543074003379

Berner, E. (Ed.). (2007). *Clinical Decision Support Systems: Theory & Practice*. New York, NY: Springer. doi:10.1007/978-0-387-38319-4

Bernstein, M., McCreless, T., & Côté, M. (2007, Winter). 2007). Five constants of information technology adoption in healthcare. [from Academic Search Complete database]. *Hospital Topics*, *85*(1), 17–25. Retrieved May 3, 2009. doi:10.3200/HTPS.85.1.17-26

Bessell, T., McDonald, S., Silagy, Ch., Anderson, J., & Hiller, J., & Sansom, Ll. (2002). Do Internet interventions for consumers cause more harm than good? A systematic review. *Health Expectations*, *5*, 28–37. doi:10.1046/j.1369-6513.2002.00156.x

Bigley, G. A., & Roberts, K. H. (2001). Structuring Temporary Systems for High Reliability . *Academy of Management Journal*, *44*, 1281–1300. doi:10.2307/3069401

Billings, J. (2004). Promoting the dissemination of decision aids: an odyssey in a dysfunctional health care financing system. *Health Affairs*, (Supplement Web Exclusive), 128–132.

Bishop, A. P., Bruce, B. C., & Jones, M. C. (2006). Community inquiry and informatics: Collaborative learning through ICT. *The Journal of Community Informatics*, *2*(2), 3–5.

Black, M. E., Yamada, J., & Mann, V. (2002). A systematic literature review of the effectiveness of community-based strategies to increase cervical cancer screening. *Canadian Journal of Public Health*, *93*(5), 386–393.

Blackstock, W. P., & Weir, M. P. (1999). Proteomics: quantitative and physical mapping of cellular proteins. *Trends in Biotechnology*, *17*(3), 121–127. doi:10.1016/S0167-7799(98)01245-1

Blake, J., Reibman, A., & Trivedi, K. (1988). Sensitivity Analysis of Reliability and Performability Measures for a Multiprocessor System. *ACM SIGMETRICS Performance Evaluation Review*, *16*(1), 177–186. doi:10.1145/1007771.55616

Blobel, B. (2007). Comparing approaches for advanced e-health security infrastructures. *International Journal of Medical Informatics*, *76*(5-6), 454–459. doi:10.1016/j.ijmedinf.2006.09.012

Blobel, B., Pharow, P., & Nerlich, M. (Eds.). (2008). *eHealth: Combining Health Telematics, Telemedicine, Biomedical Engineering and Bioinformatics to the Edge. Global Experts Summit Textbook*. Amsterdam: IOS Press.

Blumenthal, D., & Glaser, J. (2007). Information Technology Comes to Medicine. *The New England Journal of Medicine*, *356*(24), 2527–2534. doi:10.1056/NEJMhpr066212

Bodie, G.D., & Dutta, M. J. (2008). Understanding health literacy for strategic health marketing; eHealth disparities, and the digital divide. *Health Marketing Quarterly*, *25*(1/2), p175-203, 29p. Retrieved August 23, 2009 from Academic Search complete.

Bolon, D. S. (1997). Organizational citizenship behavior among hospital employees: a multidimensional analysis involving job satisfaction and organizational commitment. *Hospital & Health Services Administration*, *42*(2), 221–241.

Bonis, P. A., Pickens, G. T., Rind, D. M., & Foster, D. A. (2008). Association of a clinical knowledge support system with improved patient safety, reduced complications and shorter length of stay among Medicare beneficiaries in acute care hospitals in the United States. *International Journal of Medical Informatics*, *77*(11), 745–753. doi:10.1016/j.ijmedinf.2008.04.002

Bossuyt, P. M., Reitsma, J. B., & Bruns, D. E., & al. (2003). Towards complete and accurate reporting of studies of diagnostic accuracy. *Clinical Chemistry*, *49*, 1–6. doi:10.1373/49.1.1

Bourek, A., Tůma, P., & Bourková, A. (2008, July). *Indicators as signals for assuring living and healthy health care organizations*. Paper presented at the WHO Vienna Public Healthcare Conference Performance Assessment in Healthcare Delivery PATH II, Vienna, Austria.

Bourková, A., & Bourek, A. (2007). Týmová spolupráce – Techniky týmové spolupráce, process týmové spolupráce, definice pojmu teamwork, zavádění týmové spolupráce do zdravotnického prostředí, klinické protokoly . In Forýtková, L., & Bourek, A. (Eds.), *Programy kvality a standardy léčebných postupů* (pp. 1–12). Praha, Czech Republic: Verlag-Dashofer.

Bradley, V. M., Steltenkamp, C. L., & Hite, K. B. (2006). Evaluation of reported medication errors before and after implementation of computerized practitioner order entry. *Journal of Healthcare Information Management*, *20*(4), 46–53.

Brandenburg, D. C., & Binder, C. (1992). Emerging trends in human performance interventions . In Stolovitch, H. D., & Keeps, E. J. (Eds.), *Handbook of human performance technology: A comprehensive guide for analyzing and solving performance problems in organizations*. San Francisco, CA: Jossey-Bass Publishers.

Bravo, J., & Merino, M. (2001). Pediatría e Internet. *Atencion Primaria*, *27*, 574–578.

Brerider-Jr-McNai, P. (1996). User requirements on the future laboratory information systems. *Computer Methods and Programs in Biomedicine*, *50*(2), 87–93. doi:10.1016/0169-2607(96)01738-Q

Breton, V., Blanquer, I., Hernandez, V., Legré, Y., & Solomonides, T. (2006). Proposing a roadmap for HealthGrids. *Studies in Health Technology and Informatics*, *120*, 319–329.

Brewer, T., & Colditz, G. A. (1999). Postmarketing surveillance and adverse drug reactions: current perspectives and future needs. *Journal of the American Medical Association*, *281*, 824–829. doi:10.1001/jama.281.9.824

Briss, P, Rimer, B, Reilley, B, Coates, RC, Lee, NC, Mullen, P, Corso, P, Hutchinson, AB, Hiatt, R, Kerner, J, George, P, White, C, Gandhi, N, Saraiya, M, Breslow, R, Isham, G, Teutsch, SM, Hinman, AR, & Lawrence, R, & Task Force on Community Preventive Services. (2004). Promoting informed decisions about cancer screening in communities and healthcare systems. *American Journal of Preventive Medicine*, *26*(1), 67–80. doi:10.1016/j.amepre.2003.09.012

Broens, T., van Halteren, A., van Sinderen, M., & Wac, K. (2007). Towards an application framework for context-aware m-health applications. *International Journal of Internet Protocol Technology*, *2*(2), 109–116. doi:10.1504/IJIPT.2007.012374

Bromme, R., Jucks, R., & Wagner, T. (2005). How to refer to 'diabetes'? Language in online health advice. *Applied Cognitive Psychology*, *19*(5), 569–586. doi:10.1002/acp.1099

Brown, H. C., & Smith, H. J. (2004). Giving women their own case notes to carry during pregnancy. *Cochrane Database of Systematic Reviews*, *CD002856*(2). doi:10.1002/14651858.CD002856.pub2

Brown, C., Hofer, T., Johal, A., Thomson, R., Nicholl, J., & Franklin, B. D. (2008). An epistemology of patient safety research: a framework for study design and interpretation. Part 3. End points and measurement. *Quality & Safety in Health Care*, *17*, 170–177. doi:10.1136/qshc.2007.023655

Brown, J. F., & Marshall, B. L. (2008). Continuous quality improvement: An effective strategy of program outcomes in a higher education setting. *Nursing Education Perspectives*, *29*(4), 205–211.

Brown, S. H., Elkin, P. L., Rosenbloom, S. T., Fielstein, E., & Speroff, T. (2008). eQuality for all: Extending automated quality measurement of free text clinical narratives. *AMIA Annual Symposium Proceedings,* 71-75.

Buchtela, D., Peleška, J., Veselý, A., & Zvárová, J. (2008). Medical Knowledge Representation System . In Andersen, S. K. (Eds.), *eHealth Beyond the Horizon-Get It There* (pp. 377–382). Amsterdam: IOS Press.

Buchtela, D., Peleška, J., Veselý, A., Zvárová, J., & Zvolský, M. (2009). Guideline Knowledge Representation Model. *European Journal for Biomedical Informatics.* Retrieved April 28, 2009, from http://www.ejbi.eu/

Bull, S. S., McKay, H. G., Gaglio, B., & Glasgow, R. E. (2005). Harnessing the potential of the Internet to promote diabetes self-management: how well are we doing? *Chronic Illness, 1*(2), 143–155.

Bulletin of World Health Organisation. (2008). Australia's disturbing health disparities set Aboriginals apart. BWHO, 86(4): 241-320. Retrieved December 15, 2008, from http://www.who.int/bulletin/volumes/86/4/08-020408/en/index.html

Burger, A., Romano, P., Paschke, A., & Splendiani, A. (2009). Semantic Web Applications and Tools for Life Sciences, 2008-preface. *BMC Bioinformatics, 10*(Suppl 10), S1. doi:10.1186/1471-2105-10-S10-S1

Burgers, J. S., Bailey, J. V., & Klazinga, N. S., & al. (2002). Inside Guidelines: Comparative analysis of recommendations and evidence in diabetes guidelines from 13 countries. *Diabetes Care, 25,* 1933–1939. doi:10.2337/diacare.25.11.1933

Burgers, J. S., Cluzeau, F. A., & Hanna, S. E., & al, & the AGREE Collaboration. (2003). Characteristics of high quality guidelines: evaluation of 86 clinical guidelines developed in ten European countries and Canada. *International Journal of Technology Assessment in Health Care, 19*(1), 148–157.

Burhans, L. D. (2007). What is quality? Do we agree, and does it matter? *Journal for Healthcare Quality, 29*(1), 39–44, 54.

Burnett, G., & Buerkle, H. (2004, January). Information exchange in virtual communities: A comparative study. *Journal of Computer-mediated Communication, 9* (2). Retrieved August 19, 2009 from http://jcmc.indiana.edu/vol9/issue2/.

Burton, L. C., Anderson, G. F., & Kues, I. W. (2004). Using Health Records to Help Coordinate Care. *The Milbank Quarterly, 82*(3), 457–481. doi:10.1111/j.0887-378X.2004.00318.x

Buxton, M., & Hanney, S. (1998). Evaluating the NHS research and development programme: will the programme give value for money? *Journal of the Royal Society of Medicine, 91*(Suppl 35), 2–6.

Byrne, S., Cooper, Z., & Fairburn, C. G. (2004). Psychological predictors of weight regain in obesity. *Behaviour Research and Therapy, 42*(11), 1341–1356. doi:10.1016/j.brat.2003.09.004

C., & Bates, DW. (2000). Incidence and preventability of adverse drug events in nursing homes. *American Journal of Medicine,* 109, 87-94.

Cabrera, M., Burgelman, J-C., Boden, M., da Costa, O. and Rodríguez, C. (2004). eHealth in 2010: Realising a Knowledge-based Approach to Healthcare in the EU, Challenges for the Ambient Care System *Technical Report EUR 21486 EN*: European Commission, Directorate General Joint Research Centre, Institute for Prospective Technological Studies.

Cady, N. C. (2009). *Microchip-based PCR Amplification Systems. Lab-on-a-Chip Technology: Biomolecular Separation and Analysis.* Norwich, UK: Caister Academic Press.

Cafazzo, J. A., Trbovich, P. L., Cassano-Piche, A., Chagpar, A., Rossos, P. G., Vicente, K. J., & Easty, A. C. (2009). Human factors perspectives on a systemic approach to ensuring a safer medication delivery process. *Healthcare Quarterly (Toronto, Ont.)*, 70–74.

Campbell, H. S., Phaneuf, M. R., & Deane, K. (2004). Cancer peer support programs - do they work? *Patient Education and Counseling, 55*, 3–15. doi:10.1016/j.pec.2003.10.001

Campbell, G.S., Sherry, D., Sternberg, D J. (2002). A hospital Web site that works. *Marketing Health Services, 22*(2), 40-2. Retrieved February 26, 2009, from ABI/INFORM Global database. (Document ID: 121772167).

Canadian Task Force. (1979). Canadian Task Force on the Periodic Health Examination: The periodic health examination. *Canadian Medical Association Journal, 121*, 1193–1254.

Cappuccio, F. P., Kerry, S. M., Forbes, L., & Donald, A. (2004). Blood pressure control by home monitoring: metaanalysis of randomised trials. *British Medical Journal, 329*(7458), 145. doi:10.1136/bmj.38121.684410.AE

Capra, F. (n.d.). *Management.* Retrieved May 4, 2009, from http://www.fritjofcapra.net/management.html

Car, J., & Sheikh, A. (2004). E-mail consultations in health care: scope and effectiveness. *British Medical Journal, 329*, 435–438. doi:10.1136/bmj.329.7463.435

Car, J., & Sheikh, A. (2004). Email consultations in health care: 2—acceptability and safe application. *British Medical Journal, 329*, 439–442. doi:10.1136/bmj.329.7463.439

Carlson, C. (2003). Information overload, retrieval strategies and Internet user empowerment . In Haddon, L. (Ed.), *The Good, the Bad and the Irrelevant (COST 269)* (*Vol. 1*, pp. 169–173). Helsinki, Finland.

Carlsson, C., & Walden, P. (2002). *Further Quests for Value-Added Products and Services in Mobile Commerce.* Paper presented at the The Xth European Conference on Information Systems.

Carrasco, G. (2002). Medicina basada en la evidencia "electrónica" (e-MBE): metodología, ventajas y limitaciones. *Revista Calidad Asistencial, 17*, 113–125.

Carroll, J. D., & Messenger, J. C. (2008). Medical simulation: the new tool for training and skill assessment. *Perspectives in Biology and Medicine, 51*(1), 47–60. doi:10.1353/pbm.2008.0003

Carruthers, A., & Jeacocke, D. (2000). Adjusting the balance in health-care quality. *Journal of Quality in Clinical Practice, 20*(4), 158-160. http://tiger.spc.alamo.edu:2052

Cavalcanti, A., Shirinzadeh, B., Freitas, RA Jr., Hogg, T. (2008). Nanorobot architecture for medical target identification. *Nanotechnology, 19* (1), 015103(15pp).

CEBM. (2007). *Why the sudden interest in EBM?* Retrieved from http://www.cebm.utoronto.ca/intro/interest.htm

CEN/ISSS. (2003). *Workshop Learning Technologies. Quality Assurance Standards*. Brussels: CEN.

CEN/ISSS. (2005). *Learning Technologies Workshop, Project Team "Accessibility properties for Learning Resources"*. Retrieved January 25, 2009 from http://www2.ni.din.de/sixcms/detail.php?id=5984.

Center for Drug Evaluation and Research. (2005). Adverse event reporting system. Retrieved from http://www.fda.gov/cder/aers/default.htm

Cerchiairi, D. (2007). Revolutionising patient care – medical technology of the future. Thought-provoking ideas for policymaking. In Health First Europe (Ed), *2050: A Health Odyssey* (pp. 24-27). Brussels: Health First Europe.

Certification Commission for Health Information Technology. Retrieved September 30, 2009 from http://www.cchit.org/media

Chadwick, P. E. (2007). *Regulations and standards for wireless applications in eHealth.* Paper presented at the 29th Annual International Conference of the IEEE Engineering in Medicine & Biology Society.

Chang, H. H., & Chang, C. S. (2008). An assessment of technology-based service encounters & network security on the e-health care systems of medical centers in Taiwan. *BMC Health Services Research, 8*, 87. doi:10.1186/1472-6963-8-87

Chaudhry, B., Jerome, W., Shinyi, W., Maglione, M., Mojica, W., & Roth, E. (2006). Systematic Review: Impact of Health Information Technology on Quality, Efficiency, and Costs of Medical Care. *Annals of Internal Medicine, 144*(10), E12–W18. http://search.ebscohost.com.

Cherry, R. A., & Ali, J. (2008). Current concepts in simulation-based trauma education. *The Journal of Trauma, 65*(5), 1186–1193. doi:10.1097/TA.0b013e318170a75e

Chorianopoulos, K. (2008). Personalized and mobile digital TV applications. *Multimedia Tools and Applications, 36*(1-2), 1–10. doi:10.1007/s11042-006-0081-8

Chumley-Jones, H. S., Dobbie, A., & Alford, C. L. (2002). Web-based learning: sound educational method or hype? A review of the evaluation literature. *Academic Medicine, 77*(10suppl), S86–S93. doi:10.1097/00001888-200210001-00028

Clarke, M., Bogia, D., Hassing, K., Steubesand, L., Chan, T., & Ayyagari, D. (2007). *Developing a standard for personal health devices based on 11073.* Paper presented at the 29th Annual International Conference of the IEEE Engineering in Medicine & Biology Society. Committee for Healthcare eStandards. Retrieved September 30, 2009 from http://www.chestandards.org/

Classen, D. C., Pestotnik, S. L., Evans, R. S., & Burke, J. P. (1991). Computerized surveillance of adverse drug events in hospital patients. *Journal of the American Medical Association, 266*, 2847–2851. doi:10.1001/jama.266.20.2847

CLSI publication GP22-A2. (2004). *Continuous Quality Improvement: Integrating Five Key Quality System Components; Approved Guideline* (2nd ed.). Wayne, Pennsylvania, USA: CLSI.

CLSI publication HS1-A2. (2004). *Quality Management System Model for Health Care; Approved Guideline* (2nd ed.). Wayne, Pennsylvania, USA: CLSI.

CLSI publication HS6-A. (2004). *Studies to Evaluate Patients Outcomes; Approved Guideline.* Wayne, Pennsylvania, USA: CLSI.

Cluzeau, F. A., Burgers, J. S., & Brouwers, M., & al. (2003). Development and validation of an international appraisal instrument for assessing the quality of clinical practice guidelines: the AGREE project. *Quality & Safety in Health Care, 12*(1), 18–23. doi:10.1136/qhc.12.1.18

Codex Gigas. ff. 240r-243v. Retrieved February 7, 2009, from http://www.kb.se/codex-gigas/eng/Browse-the-Manuscript/Ars-medicinae/

Cohen, M. M., Kimmel, N. L., Benage, M. K., Cox, M. J., Sanders, N., Spence, D., & Chen, J. (2005). Medication safety program reduces adverse drug events in a community hospital. *Quality & Safety in Health Care, 14*, 169–174. doi:10.1136/qshc.2004.010942

Coiera, E., Westbrook, J. I., & Wyatt, J. C. (2006). The Safety and Quality of Decision Support Systems . In Haux, R., & Kulikowski, C. (Eds.), *IMIA Yearbook of Medical Informatics.*

Coile, R. (2000). E-health: Reinventing healthcare in the information age. *Journal of Healthcare Management, 45*(3), 206–210.

Colen, H., Neuenschwander, M., Neef, C., Krabbendam, K. (2006). Using Automated Dispensing Machines to improve medication safety. *Journal of the European Association of Hospital Pharmacists, 12*(5), 71-73-1.

Collins, P. M., Golembeski, S. M., Selgas, M., & al. (2007). Clinical Excellence Through Evidence-Based Practice - A Model to Guide Practice Changes. *Topics in Advanced Practice Nursing eJournal. 7*(4), Medscape, Posted 01/25/2008. Retrieved from [http://www.medscape.com/viewarticle].

Commission of the European Communities. (2004). e-Health - making healthcare better for European citizens: An action plan for a European e-Health Area. Brussels: Commission of the European Communities.

Commission of the European Communities. (2007). *A lead market initiative for Europe.* Brussels: Commission of the European Communities.

Commission of the European Communities. (2007). *Together for Health: A Strategic Approach for the EU 2008-2013*. White Paper 23.10.2007. Brussels: Author.

Commission of the European Communities. (2007). *White Paper 'Together for Health: A Strategic Approach for the EU 2008-2013*. Retrieved November 2009 from http://ec.europa.eu/health/ph_overview/Documents/strategy_wp_en.pdf.

Computing in the Physician's Practice. (2000). Retrieved from http://www.harrisinteractive.com/harris_poll/index.asp?PID=58

Conford, T., & Klecun-Dabrowska, E. (2001). Ethical Perspectives in Evaluation of Telehealth. *Cambridge Quarterly of Healthcare Ethics*, *10*(2), 161–169. doi:10.1017/S0963180101002079

Contribution to the implementation of relevant Quality approaches in the European Higher Education Retrieved January 15, 2009 from http://www.enpc.fr/fr/formations/ecole_virt/nte/rencontresGEVP/index.htm

Cordero, F., Botta, M., & Calogero, R. A. (2007). Microarray data analysis and mining approaches. *Briefings in Functional Genomics & Proteomics*, *6*(4), 265–281. doi:10.1093/bfgp/elm034

Cornbleet, MA, Campbell, P, Murray, S, Stevenson, M, & Bond, S, & Joint Working Party of the Scottish Partnership Agency for Palliative and Cancer Care and National Council for Hospice and Specialist Palliative Care Services. (2002). Patient-held records in cancer and palliative care: a randomized, prospective trial. *Palliative Medicine*, *16*(3), 205–212. doi:10.1191/0269216302pm541oa

Coster, S., Gulliford, M. C., Seed, P. T., Powrie, J. K., & Swaminathan, R. (2000). Monitoring blood glucose control in diabetes mellitus: a systematic review. *Health Technology Assessment*, *4*(12).

Coulter, A., & Ellins, J. (2006). *Patient-focused interventions: A review of the evidence*. London: The Health Foundation.

Council of Europe. (2004). *Recommendation Rec (2006)7 of the Committee of Ministers to member states on management of patient safety and prevention of adverse events in health care*. Retrieved November 2009 from https://wcd.coe.int/ViewDoc.jsp?id=1005439&BackColorInternet=9999CC&BackColorIntranet=FFBB55&BackColorLogged=FFAC75.

Council of Europe. (2009). *COUNCIL RECOMMENDATION of 9 June 2009 on patient safety, including the prevention and control of healthcare associated infections (2009/C 151/01)*. Retrieved November 2009 from http://eur-lex.europa.eu/LexUriServ/LexUriServ.do?uri=OJ:C:2009:151:0001:0006:EN:PDF.

Crawford, W. (2006). *Why aren't ebooks more successful?* Retrieved from http://www.econtentmag.com/Articles/ArticleReader.aspx?ArticleID=18144

Croft, D., & Peterson, M. (2002). An Evaluation of the Quality and Contents of Asthma Education on the World Wide Web. *CHEST, 121*(4), 1301. http://tiger.spc.alamo.edu:2052

Cronin, C. (2004). *Patient-Centered Care: An overview of Definitions and Concepts*. Washington, DC: National Health Council.

Crowe, J., Hayes-Gill, B., Sumner, M., Barratt, C., Palethorpe, B., Greenhalgh, C., et al. (2004). *Modular Sensor Architecture for Unobtrusive Routine Clinical Diagnosis*. Paper presented at the Proceedings of the 24th International Conference on Distributed Computing Systems Workshops.

Currell, R., & Urquhart, C. (2003). Nursing record systems: effects on nursing practice and health care outcomes. *Cochrane Database of Systematic Reviews*, *CD002099*(3). doi:10.1002/14651858.CD002099

Curro, V., Buonuomo, P. S., Onesimo, R., de Rose, P., Vituzzi, A., di Tanna, G. L., & D'Atri, A. (2004). A quality evaluation methodology of health web-pages for non-professionals. *Medical Informatics and the Internet in Medicine*, *29*, 95–107. doi:10.1080/14639230410001684396

D'Alessandro, D. M., Kingsley, P., & Johnson-West, J. (2001). The readability of pediatric patient education materials on the World Wide Web. *Archives of Pediatrics & Adolescent Medicine*, *155*, 807–812.

Damberg, C., Ridgely, M., Shaw, R., Meili, R., Sorbero, M., Bradley, L., et al. (2009, April 15). Adopting Information Technology to Drive Improvements in Patient Safety: Lessons from the Agency for Healthcare Research and Quality Health Information Technology Grantees. *Health Services Research, 44*(2p2), 684-700. Retrieved September 30, 2009, doi:10.1111/j.1475-6773.2008.00928.x

Davenport, K. (2007). Navigating American Health Care: How Information Technology Can Foster Health Care Improvement. Center for American Progress, Retrieved April 24, 2009, from www. americanprogress.com

Davis, D., Thomson, M., Oxman, A., & Haynes, R. (1997). Changing physician performance: A systematic review of the effect of continuing medical education strategies. *Journal of the American Medical Association*, *274*, 700–705. doi:10.1001/jama.274.9.700

Davis, K., Otwell, R., & Barber, J. (2004). Managing costs through clinical quality improvement. *Healthcare Financial Management*, *58*(4), 76–82.

Day, J. G., & Stacey, G. N. (2008). Biobanking. *Molecular Biotechnology*, *40*(2), 202–213. doi:10.1007/s12033-008-9099-7

De, Meyer F., & De, Moor G., & Reed-Fourquet, L. (2008). Privacy Protection through pseudonymisation in eHealth. *Studies in Health Technology and Informatics*, *141*, 111–118.

De Lusignan, S. S., P.N., Adal, N., Majeed, A. (2002). Does Feedback Improve the Quality of Computerized Medical Records in Primary Care? *Journal of the American Medical Informatics Association*, *9*(4), 395–401. doi:10.1197/jamia.M1023

de Toledo, P., Galarraga, M., Martínez, I., Serrano, L., Fernández, J., & Del Pozo, F. (2006). *Towards e-Health Device Interoperability: The Spanish Experience in the Telemedicine Research Network.* Paper presented at the Annual International Conference of the IEEE Engineering in Medicine and Biology Society.

de Vries, E. N., Ramrattan, M. A., Smorenburg, S. M., Gouma, D. J., & Boermeester, M. A. (2008). The incidence and nature of in-hospital adverse events: a systematic review. *Quality & Safety in Health Care*, *17*, 216–223. doi:10.1136/qshc.2007.023622

Dechant, H. K., Tohme, W. G., Mun, S. K., Hayes, W. S., & Schulman, K. A. (1996). Health Systems Evaluation of Telemedicine: A Staged Approach. *Telemedicine Journal*, *2*(4), 303–312.

Deepwell, F. (2007). Embedding Quality in e-Learning Implementation through Evaluation. *Journal of Educational Technology & Society*, *10*(2), 34–43.

Delicato, F., Pirmez, L., & Carmo, L. (2001). Fenix – personalized information filtering system for WWW pages. *Internet Research: Electronic Networking Applications and Policy*, *11*(1), 42–48. doi:10.1108/10662240110365706

Dellaca, R. L., Gobbi, A., Govoni, L., & Nevajas, D. Pedotti, A., Farré, R. (2009). *A Novel Simple Internet-Based System for Real Time Monitoring and Optimizing Home Mechanical Ventilation.* Paper presented at the 2009 International Conference on eHealth, Telemedicine, and Social Medicine.

DeLone, W. H., & McLean, E. R. (1992). Information Systems Success: The Quest for the Dependent Variable. *Information Systems Research*, *3*(1), 60–95. doi:10.1287/isre.3.1.60

DeLone, W. H., & McLean, E. R. (2002). *Information Systems Success Revisited.* Paper presented at the 35th Annual Hawaii International Conference on System Sciences.

Deming, W. E. (2000). *Out of the crisis*. Cambridge, MA: The MIT Press.

Demiris, G. (2006). The diffusion of virtual communities in health care: Concept and challenges. *Patient Education and Counseling*, *62*(2), 178–188. doi:10.1016/j.pec.2005.10.003

Demiris, G. (Ed.). (2004). *eHealth: Current Static and Future Trends*. Amsterdam: IOS Press.

Detsky, A. S., Naglie, G., & Krahn, M. D., & al. (1997). Primer on Medical Decision Analysis. *Medical Decision Making*, *17*, 123–233. doi:10.1177/0272989X9701700201

Dhillon, H., & Forducey, P. G. (2006). *Implementation and Evaluation of Information Technology in Telemedicine*. Paper presented at the 39th Annual Hawaii International Conference on System Sciences.

Diamond, C., & Shirky, C. (2008). Health Information Technology: A Few Years Of Magical Thinking? *Health Affairs*, *27*(5), w383–w390. http://search.ebscohost.com, doi:10.1377/hlthaff.27.5.w383. doi:10.1377/hlthaff.27.5.w383

Dillman, D. A. (2000). *Mail and Internet surveys: the tailored design method*. New York: Wiley, John & Sons, Incorporated.

DIN. (2005). Deutsches Institut für Normung e.V. (ed.). *e-Learning. Qualitätssicherung und Qualitätsmanagement im e-Learning*. Berlin: Beuth.

Dixon, N. (2000). *Common Knowledge: How companies thrive by sharing what they know*. Boston: Harvard Business School Press.

Dobrev, P., Famolari, D., Kurzke, C., Miller, B. A., Dobrev, P., & Famolari, D. (2002). Device and service discovery in home networks with OSGi. *IEEE Communications Magazine*, *40*(8), 86–92. doi:10.1109/MCOM.2002.1024420

Dolmans, D.H.J.M., Wolfhagen, H.A.P., & Scherpbier, A.J.J.A (2003, July). From Quality Assurance to Total Quality Management: How Can Quality Assurance Result in Continuous Improvement in Health Professions Education?. *Education for Health: Change in Learning & Practice (Taylor & Francis Ltd)*, *16*(2), 210. Retrieved September 28, 2009, from Health Source: Nursing/Academic Edition database.

Donabedian, A. (2005, December). Evaluating the Quality of Medical Care. *The Milbank Quarterly*, *83*(4), 691–729. Retrieved August 30, 2009. .doi:10.1111/j.1468-0009.2005.00397.x

Donabedian, A. (1982). *Explorations in Quality Assessment and Monitoring*. Chicago: Health Administration Press.

Donabedian, A. (1988). The quality of care: how can it be assessed? *Journal of the American Medical Association*, *260*(12), 1743–1748. doi:10.1001/jama.260.12.1743

Donabedian, A. (1980a). *The definition of quality and approaches to its assessment*. Ann Arbor, MI: Health Administration Press.

Donabedian, A. (1980b). *Explorations in quality assessment and monitoring* (*Vol. 6*). Ann Arbor, MI: Health Administration Press.

Donabedian, A. (1982). *The criteria and standards of quality*. Ann Arbor, MI: Health Administration Press.

Donabedian, A. (1983). Quality Assessment and Monitoring Retrospect and Prospect. *Evaluation & the Health Professions*, *6*(3), 363–375. doi:10.1177/016327878300600309

Donabedian, A. (1985). *The methods and findings of quality assessment and monitoring*. Ann Arbor, MI: Health Administration Press.

Donabedian, A. (1991). *Striving for quality in health care*. Ann Arbor, MI: Health Administration Press.

Donabedian, A. (2001). *An Introduction to Quality Assurance in Health Care*. New York: Oxford University Press.

Donelly, L., & Shaw, R., & van der Akker. (2008). eHealth as a challenge to 'expert' power: a focus group study of internet use for health information and management. *Journal of the Royal Society of Medicine*, *101*, 501-506. Drury, M., Yudkin, P., Harcourt, J., Fitzpatrick, R., Jones, L., Alcock, C. & Minton, M. (2000). Patients with cancer holding their own records: a randomised controlled trial. *The British Journal of General Practice*, *50*(451), 105–110.

Dong, J. C., Hu, X. P., Zhang, Z.-M., Zhou, D., & Jiang, K. (2009). *Analysis and Design on Standard System of Electronic Health Records.* Paper presented at the First International Workshop on Education Technology and Computer Science.

Dostálová, T., Seydlová, M., Zvárová, J., Hanzlíček, P., & Nagy, M. (2007). Computer-Supported Treatment of Patients with the TMF Parafunction. In B. Blobel, P. Pharow, J. Zvarova, & D. Polez (Eds.), *eHealth: Combining Health Telematics, Telemedicine, Biomedical Engineering and Bioinformatics to the Edge* (pp. 171-178). Berlin: CEHR Conference Proceedings 2007, AKA. ehealth(AT)ec.europa.eu. (2009). *Europe's Information Society. Thematic Portal.* Retrieved July 21, 2009, from http://ec.europa.eu/information_society/activities/health/whatis_ehealth/index_en.htm

Doupi, P., Ruotsalainen, P., & Pohjonen, H. (2005). Implementing interoperable secure health information systems. *Studies in Health Technology and Informatics, 115*, 187–214.

Drummond, M., Sculpher, M., Torrance, G., O'Brien, B., & Stoddart, G. (2005). *Methods for the Economic Evaluation of Health Care Programmes.* Oxford, UK: Oxford University Press.

Eco, U. (2004). *Theory of semiotics.*

Edirippulige, S., Smith, A. C., Bensink, M., Armfield, N., & Wootton, R. (2009). Nurses and Telehealth: current practice and future directions . In Staudinger, B., Hob, V., & Ostermann, H. (Eds.), *Nursing and Clinical Informatics: Socio-technical approaches* (pp. 94–409). New York: Medical Information Science Reference. doi:10.4018/978-1-60566-234-3.ch007

Edirippulige, S., & Wootton, R. (2006). Telehealth and Communication. In M. Conrick (Ed.). *Health Informatics, Transforming Health care with Technology*, 266-278, Melbourne, Thomson.

Ehlers, U. D., & Pawlowski, J. M. (2006). Quality in European e-learning: An introduction . In Ehlers, U.-D., & Pawlowski, J. M. (Eds.), *Handbook on Quality and Standardization in E-Learning* (pp. 1–8). New York: Springer-Verlag. doi:10.1007/3-540-32788-6_1

Ehlers, U. D. (2003a). Quality in E-Learning – The Learner as a key quality assurance category. *Vocational Training European Journal, 2003/II.*

Ehlers, U. D. (2003b). *Qualität beim E-Learning.* Retrieved January 15, 2009 from http://www.lernqualitaet.de/qualität ehlers.pdf (15/1/2009).

Ellaway, R., & Masters, K. (2008). AMEE Guide 32: e-Learning in medical education Part 1: Learning, teaching and assessment. *Medical Teacher, 30*(5), 455–473. http://tiger.spc.alamo.edu:2052, doi:10.1080/01421590802108331. doi:10.1080/01421590802108331

Engel, K., Blobel, B., & Pharow, P. (2006). Standards for enabling health informatics interoperability. *Studies in Health Technology and Informatics, 124*, 145–150.

ENISA. (European Network and Information Security Agency)-Cloud computing Risk Assessment. Retrieved September 30, 2009 from http://www.enisa.europa.eu/act/rm/files/deliverables/cloud-computing-risk-assessment/

EPCglobal Inc. EPC™ Radio-Frequency Identity Protocols Class-1 Generation-2 UHF RFID Protocol for Communications at 860 MHz – 960 MHz, Retrieved March 30, 2005 from http://www.epcglobalinc.org/standards/uhfc1g2/uhfc1g2_1_0_9-standard-20050126.pdf

EQO. (2004). French-European workshop. *Comparing Quality models adequacy to the needs of clients in e-learning.* Retrieved January 15, 2009 from http://www.eqo.info/?fuseaction=news.extraspecial_062004

European Commission Enterprise and Industry European Standards. Retrieved September 30, 2009 from http://ec.europa.eu/enterprise/policies/european-standards/documents/harmonised-standards-legislation/list-references/

EuroRec: European Institute for Health Records. Retrieved September 30, 2009 from http://www.eurorec.org/services/standards/standards.cfm

Evans, R., Edwards, A., Brett, J., Bradburn, M., Watson, E., Austoker, J., & Elwyn, G. (2005). Reduction in uptake of PSA tests following decision aids: systematic review of current aids and their evaluations. *Patient Education and Counseling*, *58*(1), 13–26. doi:10.1016/j.pec.2004.06.009

Evans, R. S., Pestotnik, S. L., Classen, D. C., Bass, S. B., & Burke, J. P. (1992). Prevention of adverse drug events through computerized surveillance. *Proceedings- The Annual Symposium on Computer Applications in Medical Care*. 437-41.

Evidence-Based Medicine Working Group. (1992). Evidence-Based Medicine Working Group: Evidence-based medicine. A new approach to teaching the practice of medicine. *Journal of the American Medical Association*, *268*, 2420–2425. doi:10.1001/jama.268.17.2420

Eysenbach, G. (2000). Consumer health informatics. *BMJ (Clinical Research Ed.)*, *320*, 1713–1716. doi:10.1136/bmj.320.7251.1713

Eysenbach, G. (2001). What is e-health? *Journal of Medical Internet Research*, *3*, E20. doi:10.2196/jmir.3.2.e20

Eysenbach, G., & Köhler, C. (2002). How do consumers search for and appraise health information on the world wide web? Qualitative study using focus groups, usability tests, and in-depth interviews. *British Medical Journal*, *324*, 573–577. doi:10.1136/bmj.324.7337.573

Eysenbach, G., & Köhler, C. (2004). Health-Related Searches on the Internet. *Journal of the American Medical Association*, *291*, 2946. doi:10.1001/jama.291.24.2946

Eysenbach, G., Powell, J., Kuss, O., & Sa, E. R. (2002). Empirical studies assessing the quality of health information for consumers on the World Wide Web: a systematic review. *Journal of the American Medical Association*, *287*, 2691–2700. doi:10.1001/jama.287.20.2691

Eysenbach, G. (2001). What is e-health? *Journal of Medical Internet Research*, *3*(2), e20. doi:10.2196/jmir.3.2.e20

Eysenbach, G., Powell, J., Englesakis, M., Rizo, C., & Stern, A. (2004). Health related virtual communities and electronic support group: systematic review of the effects of online peer to peer interactions. *British Medical Journal*, *328*, 1166–1172. doi:10.1136/bmj.328.7449.1166

Eysenbach, G., Powell, J., Kuss, O., & Eun-Ryoung, S. (2002). Empirical studies assessing the quality of health information for consumers on the world wide web: a systematic review. *Journal of the American Medical Association*, *287*(20), 2691–2700. doi:10.1001/jama.287.20.2691

Eysenbach, G. (2001). What is e-health? *Journal of Medical Internet Research*, 3(2). Retrieved March 4, 2009 from http://www.jmir.org/2001/2/e20/

Eysenbach, G., & Köhler C. (2002). Does the internet harm health? Database of adverse events related to the internet has been set up. *British Medical Journal*, 324-239. Retrieved September 23, 2008 from 10.1136/bmj.324.7337.573.

Eysenbach, G., & Thomson, M. (2007). The FA4CT Algorithm: A New Model and Tool for Consumers to Assess and Filter Health Information on the Internet. Studies in Health Technology and Informatics.In Klaus A. Kuhn, James R. Warren, Tze-Yun Leong, (Eds.), MEDINFO 2007 - *Proceedings of the 12th World Congress on Health (Medical) Informatics – Building Sustainable Health Systems. (vol.* 129).

Fahey, T., Schroeder, K., Ebrahim, S., & Glynn, L.(2006). Interventions used to improve control of blood pressure in patients with hypertension. *Cochrane.Database.of SystematicReviews*, CD005182 (1).

Fan, Z. H., Das, C., & Chen, H. (2009). Two-Dimensional Electrophoresis in a Chip. In Keith E. Herold, K., & Rasooly, A. (Ed.), *Lab-on-a-Chip Technology: Biomolecular Separation and Analysis*. (pp. 122-138). Norfolk: Caister Academic Press.

Farmer, A., Gibson, OJ., Tarassenko, L., & Neil A. (2005). A systematic review of telemedicine interventions to support blood glucose self-monitoring in diabetes. *Diabetic medicine:A journal of the British Diabetic Association, 22* (10), 1372-1378.

Farris, K. B., Kumbera, P., Halterman, T., & Fang, G. (2002). Outcomes-based pharmacist reimbursement: reimbursing pharmacists for cognitive services. *Journal of Managed Care Pharmacy*, *5*(8), 383–393.

Fennessy, G. (2002). *Understanding and selecting knowledge management systems for a health information provider.* Paper presented at the 35th Annual Hawaii International Conference on System Sciences.

Ferguson, T., & Frydman, G. (2004). The first generation of e-patients. *British Medical Journal*, *328*, 1148–1149. doi:10.1136/bmj.328.7449.1148

Ferlie, E., Pettigre, A., Ashburner, L., & Fitzgerald, L. (1996). *The New Public Management in Action*. Oxford: Oxford University Press.

Fernandez-Muniz, B., Montes-Peon, J. M., & Vazquez-Ordas, C. J. (2007). Safety culture: analysis of the causal relationships between its key dimensions. *Journal of Safety Research*, *38*(6), 627–641. doi:10.1016/j.jsr.2007.09.001

Ferrer-Roca, O. (2009). Control de calidad y patoinformatica. *Rev Española Patologia*, *42*(2), 85–95. doi:10.1016/S1699-8855(09)70161-8

Ferrer-Roca, O., & Sosa-Iudicissa, M. (Eds.). (1998). *Handbook of Telemedicine* (*Vol. 54*). Netherlands: IOS Press, Ohmsha.

Ferrer-Roca, O., Figueredo, J., Franco, K., Cardenes, E. (2005). Telemedicine Intelligent Learning. Ontology for Agent Technology. *The IPSI BgD Transactions on Advanced Research*, 46-54.

Field, M. J. (Ed.). (1996). *Telemedicine A Guide to Assessing Telecommunications in Health Care*. Institute of Medicine, National Academy Press.

Finkelstein, J., O'Connor, G., & Friedmann, R. H. (2001). Development and Implementation of the home asthma telemonitoring (HAT) system to facilitate asthma self-care. *Studies in Health Technology and Informatics*, *84*, 810–814.

Fisher, S., & Bryant, S. G. (1990). Postmarketing surveillance: accuracy of patient drug attribution judgments. *Clinical Pharmacology and Therapeutics*, *48*, 102–107.

Fisher, S., & Bryant, S. G. (1992). Postmarketing surveillance of adverse drug reactions: patient self-monitoring. *The Journal of the American Board of Family Practice*, *5*, 17–25.

Fisher, S., Bryant, S. G., & Kent, T. A. (1993). Postmarketing surveillance by patient self-monitoring: trazodone versus fluoxetine. *Journal of Clinical Psychopharmacology*, *13*, 235–242. doi:10.1097/00004714-199308000-00002

Fisher, S., Bryant, S. G., Kent, T. A., & Davis, J. E. (1994). Patient drug attributions and postmarketing surveillance. *Pharmacotherapy*, *14*, 202–209.

Fisher, S., Bryant, S. G., Solovitz, B. L., & Kluge, R. M. (1987). Patient-initiated postmarketing surveillance: a validation study. *Journal of Clinical Pharmacology*, *27*, 843–854.

Fisher, S., Kent, T. A., & Bryant, S. G. (1995). Postmarketing surveillance by patient self-monitoring: preliminary data for sertraline versus fluoxetine. *The Journal of Clinical Psychiatry*, *56*, 288–296.

Fitzgerald, L., Ferlie, E., & Hawkins, C. (2003). Innovation in healthcare: How does credible evidence influence professionals? *Health & Social Care in the Community*, *11*(3), 219–228. doi:10.1046/j.1365-2524.2003.00426.x

Fitzmaurice, D., Murray, E., Gee, K., Allan, T., & Hobbs, F. (2002). A randomised controlled trial of patient self management of oral anticoagulation treatment compared with primary care management. *Journal of Clinical Pathology*, *55*(11), 845–849. doi:10.1136/jcp.55.11.845

Flatley Brennan, P., & Starren, J. B. (2006). Consumer Health Informatics and Telehealth . In Shortliffe, E. H., & Cimino, J. J. (Eds.), *Biomedical Informatics*. New York: Springer. doi:10.1007/0-387-36278-9_14

Flood, A. B., Zinn, J. S., Shortell, S. M., & Scott, W. R. (2000). Organizational performance: Managing for success . In Shortell, S. M., & Kaluzny, A. D. (Eds.), *Health care management: Organization design and behavior* (4th ed., pp. 356–389). Albany, NY: Delmar.

Fontanarosa, P., Rennie, D., & DeAngelis, C. (2004). Postmarketing surveillance — Lack of vigilance, lack of trust. *Journal of the American Medical Association, 292*(21). doi:10.1001/jama.292.21.2647

Food & Drug Administration. (2002). *FDA Clears Computer-Connected Glucose Meters*. Retrieved July 31, 2009 from http://www.accessdata.fda.gov/scripts/cdrh/cfdocs/psn/transcript.cfm?show=7#2

Food & Drug Administration. (2004). *Warning on Counterfeit Contraceptive Patches*. Retrieved July 31, 2009 from http://www.accessdata.fda.gov/scripts/cdrh/cfdocs/psn/transcript.cfm?show=26#2

Food & Drug Administration. (2005). *How to Evaluate Health Information on the Internet*, Retrieved July 31, 2009 from http://www.fda.gov/Drugs/EmergencyPreparedness/BioterrorismandDrugPreparedness/ucm134620.htm

Food & Drug Administration. (2006). *Drug Name Confusion: Salagen and Selegiline*. Retrieved July 31, 2009 from http://www.accessdata.fda.gov/scripts/cdrh/cfdocs/psn/transcript.cfm?show=48#9

Food & Drug Administration. (2006). *FDA/ISMP Campaign to Eliminate Dangerous Abbreviations*. Retrieved July 31, 2009 from http://www.accessdata.fda.gov/scripts/cdrh/cfdocs/psn/transcript.cfm?show=53#8

Food & Drug Administration. (2008). *Mixups between Insulin U-100 and U-500*. Retrieved July 31, 2009 from http://www.accessdata.fda.gov/scripts/cdrh/cfdocs/psn/transcript.cfm?show=79#1

Food and Drug Administration. (1996). The clinical impact of adverse event reporting. Retrieved from http://www.fda.gov/downloads/Safety/MedWatch/UCM168505.pdf

Fortino, G., & Nigro, L. (2000). *A Methodology Centered on Modularization of QoS Constraints for the Development and Performance Evaluation of Multimedia Systems*. Paper presented at the 33rd Annual Simulation Symposium.

Fox, J., Patkar, V., & Thomson, R. (2006). Decision Support for Healthcare: the PROforma evidence base. *Informatics in Primary Care, 14*, 49.

Fox, N. J., Ward, K. J., & O'Rourke, A. J. (2005). The 'expert patient': Empowerment or medical dominance? The case of weight loss, pharmaceutical drugs and the Internet. *Social Science & Medicine, 60*(6), 1299–1309. doi:10.1016/j.socscimed.2004.07.005

Fox, S. & Fallows, D. (2003, July 16). *Internet health resources*. Pew Internet & American Life Project.

Fox, S. Online Health Search 2006. Pew Internet & American Life Project. Retrieved October 23, 2008 from http://www.pewinternet.org/PPF/r/190/report_display.asp

Fraser, M. D., & Vaishnavi, V. K. (1997). A formal specifications maturity model. *Communications of the ACM, 40*(12), 95–103. doi:10.1145/265563.265577

Freeman, A. C., & Sweeney, K. (2001). Why General Practitioners Do Not Implement Evidence: Guidelines for Reading Literature Reviews. *British Medical Journal, 323*(7321), 1100–1104. doi:10.1136/bmj.323.7321.1100

Freitas, R. A. Jr. (2005a). What is Nanomedicine? *Nanomedicine; Nanotechnology, Biology, and Medicine, 1*(1), 2–9. doi:10.1016/j.nano.2004.11.003

Freitas, R. A. Jr. (2005b). Current Status of Nanomedicine and Medical Nanorobotics. *Journal of Computational and Theoretical Nanoscience, 2*, 1–25.

Fridman, S. (2000). *Doctors lag when it comes to computer use - Industry trend or event*. Retrieved from http://www.findarticles.com/p/articles/mi_m0HDN/is_2000_March_28/ai_60907019

Fried, M., Quigley, E. M., Hunt, R. H., & al. (2008). Is an Evidence-Based Approach to Creating Guidelines Always the Right one? *National Clinical Practice in Gastroenterology and Hepatology, 5*(2), 60-61. Nature Publishing Group. Posted 03/10/2008.

Friedman, M. (1967). *A Theory of Consumption Function*. Princeton, NJ: Princeton University Press.

Friedman, D. B., Hoffman-Goetz, L., & Arocha, J. F. (2004). Readability of cancer information on the internet. *Cancer Education, 19*, 117–122. doi:10.1207/s15430154jce1902_13

Friedman, M. A., Schueth, A., & Bell, D. S. (2009). Interoperable electronic prescribing in the United States: a progress report. *Health Affairs (Project Hope), 28*(2), 393–403. doi:10.1377/hlthaff.28.2.393

Friedman, L. S., & Richter, E. D. (2004). *Relationship between conflicts of interest and research results*. Retrieved January 18, 2009, from http://www.ncbi.nlm.nih.gov/entrez/query.fcgi?cmd=Retrieve&db=pubmed&dopt=Abstract&list_uids=14748860&itool=iconabstr

Furukawa, M. F., Raghu, T. S., Spaulding, T. J., & Vinze, A. (2008). Adoption of Health Information Technology for Medication Safety in U.S. Hospitals, 2006. *Health Affairs, 27*(3), 865–875. doi:10.1377/hlthaff.27.3.865

Gagnon, M.-P., Sánchez, E., & Pons, J. M. V. (2006). Integration of health technology assessment recommendations into organizational and clinical practice: A case study in Catalonia. *International Journal of Technology Assessment in Health Care, 22*(2), 169–176. doi:10.1017/S0266462306050987

Galarraga, M., Serrano, L., Martínez, I., & de Toledo, P. (2006). Standards for Medical Device Communication: X73 PoC-MDC . In Bos, L., Roa, L., Yogesan, K., O'Connell, B., Marsh, A., & Blobel, B. (Eds.), *Medical and Care Compunetics 3* (*Vol. 121*).

Galarraga, M., Serrano, L., Martinez, I., de Toledo, P., & Reynolds, M. (2007). *Telemonitoring systems interoperability challenge: an updated review of the applicability of ISO/IEEE 11073 standards for interoperability in telemonitoring*. Paper presented at the 29th Annual International Conference of the IEEE Engineering in Medicine and Biology Society.

Gandhi, T. K., Burstin, H. R., Cook, E. F., Puopolo, A. L., Haas, J. S., Brennan, T. A., & Bates, D. W. (2000). Drug complications in outpatients . *Journal of General Internal Medicine, 15*(3), 207–208. doi:10.1046/j.1525-1497.2000.04199.x

Gandhi, T. K., Weingart, S. N., Borus, J., Seger, A. C., Peterson, J., & Burdick, E. (2003). Adverse drug events in ambulatory care. *The New England Journal of Medicine, 348*(16), 1556–1564. doi:10.1056/NEJMsa020703

Gandhi, T. K., & Bates, D. W. (2001). Computer Adverse Drug Event (ADE) Detection and Alerts. Chapter 8 in: University of California at San Francisco – *Stanford University Evidence based Practice Center Making Health Care Safer: A Critical Analysis of Patient Safety Practices* (pp 81).

Gantenbein, R. E., & Robinson, B. J. (2008). Decoding CODECs. *Journal of Telemedicine and Telecare, 14*(2), 59–61. doi:10.1258/jtt.2007.070810

Gardois, P., Grillo, G., Lingua C., & al. (2004). Assessing the efficacy of EBM teaching in a clinical setting Santander 9 EAHIL Conference,September 24,2004.

Garvin, D. A. (1988). *Managing Quality: The strategic and competitive edge*.

Gaston, C. M., & Mitchell, G. (2005). Information giving and decision-making in patients with advanced cancer: A systematic review. *Social Science & Medicine, 61*(10), 2252–2264. doi:10.1016/j.socscimed.2005.04.015

Geliebter, A., & Aversa, A. (2003). Emotional eating in overweight, normal weight, and underweight individuals. *Eating Behaviors, 3*(4), 341–347. doi:10.1016/S1471-0153(02)00100-9

Georgiou, A., & Westbrook, J. I. (2007). Computerized order entry systems and pathology services — a synthesis of the evidence. *The Clinical Biochemist. Reviews / Australian Association of Clinical Biochemists*, *27*, 79–87.

Gerber, B. S., Brodsky, I. G., Lawless, K. A., Smolin, L. I., Arozullah, A. M., & Smith, E. V. (2005). Implementation and evaluation of a low-literacy diabetes education computer multimedia application. *Diabetes Care*, *28*(7), 1574–1580. doi:10.2337/diacare.28.7.1574

Gerhardus, D. (2003). Robot-Assisted Surgery: The Future Is Here. *Journal of Healthcare Management*, *48*(4), 242–251.

Germanakos, P., Mourlas, C., & Samaras, G. (2005). *A Mobile Agent Approach for Ubiquitous and Personalized eHealth Information Systems.* Paper presented at the 10th International Conference on User Modeling.

Gibbons, A., & Fairweather, P. (2000). Computer-based instruction. InTobias, S., Fletcher, J. (Eds), *Training & Retraining: A Handbook for Business, Industry, Government, and the Military* (pp 410-422). New York: Macmillan.

Giles, J. (2005). *Internet encyclopedias go head to head.* Retrieved from http://www.nature.com/news/2005/051212/full/438900a.html

Ginsburg, L., Gilin, D., Tregunno, D., Norton, P. G., Flemons, W., & Fleming, M. (2009). Advancing measurement of patient safety culture. *Health Services Research*, *44*(1), 205–224. doi:10.1111/j.1475-6773.2008.00908.x

Ginter, P. M., Swayne, L. E., & Duncan, W. J. (1998). *Strategic management of health care organizations* (3rd ed.). Malden, MA: Blackwell Publishers, Inc.

Glance, L. G., Osler, T. M., Mukamel, D. B., & Dick, A. W. (2008). Impact of the present-on-admission indicators on hospital quality measurement experiance with the Agency for Healthcare Research and Quality. (AHRQ) Inpatient Quality Indicators. *Medical Care*, *46*(2), 112–119. doi:10.1097/MLR.0b013e318158aed6

Glasgow, R. E. (2007). eHealth Evaluation and Dissemination Research. *American Journal of Preventive Medicine*, *32*(Suppl 5), S119–S126. doi:10.1016/j.amepre.2007.01.023

Glasgow, R. E., Davidson, K. W., Dobkin, P. L., Ockene, J., & Spring, B. (2006). Practical behavioral trials to advance evidence-based behavioral medicine. *Annals of Behavioral Medicine*, *31*(1), 5–13. doi:10.1207/s15324796abm3101_3

Glasgow, R. E., Klesges, L. M., Dzewaltowski, D. A., Bull, S. S., & Estabrooks, P. (2004). The future of health behavior change research: what is needed to improve translation of research into health promotion practice? *Annals of Behavioral Medicine*, *27*(1), 3–12. doi:10.1207/s15324796abm2701_2

Glasgow, R. E., Magid, D. J., Beck, A., Ritzwoller, D., & Estabrooks, P. A. (2005). Practical clinical trials for translating research to practice: design and measurement recommendations. *Medical Care*, *43*(6), 551–557. doi:10.1097/01.mlr.0000163645.41407.09

Glasgow, R. (2002). Evaluation of theory-based interventions: the RE-AIM model . In Glanz, K., Lewis, F. M., & Rimer, B. K. (Eds.), *Health behavior and health education* (3rd ed., pp. 531–544). San Francisco, CA: John Wiley & Sons.

Godin, B. (1997). The rhetoric of a health technology: The microprocessor patient card. *Social Studies of Science*, *27*(6), 865–902. doi:10.1177/030631297027006002

Goodenough, S. (2009). Semantic interoperability, e-health and Australian statistics. *Health Information Management Journal*, *38*(2), 41–45.

Google. (2007). *Search returned "GI Motility."* Retrieved from http://www.google.com/search?hl=en&q=GI+Motility

Gore, A. (1992). Infrastructure for the global village. *Scientific American*, *265*, 150–153.

Goševa-Popstojanova, K., & Trivedi, K. S. (2001). Architecture-based approach to reliability assessment of software systems. *Performance Evaluation*, *45*(2-3), 179–204. doi:10.1016/S0166-5316(01)00034-7

Graber, M. A., Roller, C. M., & Kaeble, B. (1999). Readability levels of patient education material on the world wide web. *The Journal of Family Practice*, *48*, 58–61.

Grabinder, R. S., Jonassen, D., & Wilson, B. G. (1992). The use of expert systems . In Stolovitch, H. D., & Keeps, E. J. (Eds.), *Handbook of human performance technology: A comprehensive guide for analyzing and solving performance problems in organizations*. San Francisco, CA: Jossey-Bass Publishers.

Graham, I. D., Logan, J., O'Connor, A., Weeks, K. E., Aaron, S., & Cranney, A. (2003). A qualitative study of physicians' perceptions of three decision aids. *Patient Education and Counseling*, *50*, 279–283. doi:10.1016/S0738-3991(03)00050-8

Graschew, G., Roelofs, T., Rakowsky, A., Schlag, P.M. (2006). Digital medicine in the virtual hospital of the future. *International Journal of Computer Assisted Radiology and Surgery, 1*(Supp/1), 119-120.

Green, L. W., & Kreuter, M. W. (2005). *Health promotion planning: an educational and ecological approach* (4th ed.). Boston, MA: McGraw Hill.

Griffin, F. A., & Classen, D. C. (2008). Detection of adverse events in surgical patients using the Trigger Tool approach. *Quality & Safety in Health Care*, *17*, 253–258. doi:10.1136/qshc.2007.025080

Griffiths, K., & Christensen, H. (2005). Websites quality indicators for consumers. *Journal of Medical Internet Research*, *7*, e55. doi:10.2196/jmir.7.5.e55

Griffiths, C., Motlib, J., Azad, A., Ramsay, J., Eldridge, S., & Feder, G. (2005). Randomised controlled trial of a lay-led self-management programme for Bangladeshi patients with chronic disease. *The British Journal of General Practice*, *55*, 831–837.

Grigsby, J., Kaehny, M. M., Sandberg, E. J., Schlenker, R. E., & Shaughnessy, P. W. (1995). Effects and effectiveness of telemedicine . In Weisgrau, S. (Ed.), *Access to Health Care Services in Rural Areas: Delivery & Financial Issues*. Collingdale, PA: Diane Publishing Co.

Grigsby, J. (1998). *Evaluating Technologies for Providing Health Services at a Distance: Outcome-Driven Quality Improvement.* Paper presented at the Pacific Medical Technology Symposium.

Grigsby, J., & Barton, P. L. (1998). *Telecommunications Technology, Health Services, and Technology Assessment.* Paper presented at the Proceedings of the Symposium on Pacific Medical Technology.

Grilli, R., Ramsay, C., & Minozzi, S. (2002). Mass media interventions: effects on health services utilisation. *Cochrane.Database.of Systematic Reviews*, CD000389 (1).

Grimson, J., Stephens, G., Jung, B., Grimson, W., Berry, D., & Pardon, S. (2001). Sharing Health-Care Records over the Internet. *IEEE Internet Computing*, *5*(3), 49–58. doi:10.1109/4236.935177

Grin, O. W. (1994). Patient-centered care: Empowering Patients to Achieve Real Health Care Reform. *Michigan Medicine*, *93*, 25–29.

Groene, O., Lombarts, M., Klazinga, N., Alonso, J., Thompson, A., & Sunol, M. (2009). Is patient-centredness in European hospitals related to existing quality improvement strategies? Analysis of a cross-sectional survey (MARQuIS study). *Quality & Safety in Health Care*, *18*(Supplement I), i44–i50. doi:10.1136/qshc.2008.029397

Grunfeld, E., Urquhart, R., Mykhalovskiy, E., & al. (2008). Toward population-based indicators of quality end-of-life care: testing stakeholder agreement. *Cancer, 112*(10), 2301-8. (PreMedline Identifier: 18219238).

GS1- Where Standards Get Down to Business. Retrieved August 20, 2009 from http://www.gs1us.org/

Gurwitz, J. H., Field, T. S., Avorn, J., McCormick, D., Jain, S., Eckler, M., Benser, M., Edmondson, A.

Gustafson, D. H., Hawkins, R., Boberg, E., Pingree, S., Serlin, R. E., Graziano, F., & Chan, C. L. (1999). Impact of a patient-centered, computer-based health information/support system. *American Journal of Preventive Medicine*, *16*(1), 1–9. doi:10.1016/S0749-3797(98)00108-1

Gutiérrez, U., & Blanco, A. (2001). Información para pacientes en español en Internet. *Atencion Primaria*, *28*, 283–288.

Guyatt, G. H., Oxman, A. D., Kunz, R., Vist, G. E., Falck-Ytter, Y., & Schunemann, H. J.Grade Working Group. (2008). What is 'quality of evidence' and why is it important to clinicians? *British Medical Journal*, *336*(1), 995–998. doi:10.1136/bmj.39490.551019.BE

Guyatt, G. H., Schünemann, H., Cook, D., Pauker, S., Sinclair, J., Bucher, H., & Jaeschke, R. (2001). Grades of recommendation for antithrombotic agents. *Chest*, *119*(1), 3S–7S. doi:10.1378/chest.119.1_suppl.3S

Guyatt, G. H., Oxman, A. D., Vist, G. E., & al. (2008). Rating quality of evidence and strength of recommendations GRADE: an emerging consensus on rating quality of evidence and strength of recommendations. *British Medical Journal*, 336, 924-926 (26 April), for the GRADE Working Group doi: 10.1136/bmj.39489.470347.AD. Retrieved from [http://www.gradeworkinggroup.org/intro.htm]

Guyatt, G., Gutterman, D., Baumann, M. H., & al (2006). Grading Strength of Recommendations and Quality of Evidence in Clinical Guidelines Report from an American College of Chest Physicians. *Task Force Chest*, 129, 174-181. Retrieved March 16, 2009 from [http://www.chestjournal.org/content/129/1/174.full.pdf+html]

Haga, S. B., & Beskow, L. M. (2008). Ethical, legal, and social implications of biobanks for genetics research. *Advances in Genetics*, *60*, 505–544. doi:10.1016/S0065-2660(07)00418-X

Hakkarainen, K., Palonen, T., Paavola, S., & Lehtinen, E. (2004). *Communities of Networked Expertise*. Amsterdam: Elsevier.

Halamka, J. D., Mandl, K. D., & Tang, P. C. (2008). Early experiences with personal health records. *Journal of the American Medical Informatics Association*, *15*(1), 1–7. doi:10.1197/jamia.M2562

Hammond, W. E. (2008). eHealth interoperability. *Studies in Health Technology and Informatics*, *134*, 245–253.

Hampton, J. R. (2002). Evidence-based medicine, opinion-based medicine, and real-world medicine. *Perspectives in Biology and Medicine*, *45*, 549–568. doi:10.1353/pbm.2002.0070

Han, D., Park, S., & Kurkuri, S. (2007). *An Evolving Mobile E-Health Service Platform*. Paper presented at the International Conference on Consumer Electronics.

Hanak, D., Szijarto, G., & Takacs, B. (2007). *A mobile approach to ambient assisted living*. Paper presented at the IADIS Wireless Applications and Computing.

Harbour, R., & Miller, J. (2001). A new system for grading recommendations in evidence based guidelines. *British Medical Journal*, *323*(1), 334–336. doi:10.1136/bmj.323.7308.334

Harle, C. A., Padman, R., & Downs, J. S. (2009). *Design, Implementation, and Preliminary Evaluation of a Web-Based Health Risk Calculator*. Paper presented at the 42nd Hawaii International Conference on System Sciences.

Harmsen, H., Bernsen, R., Meeuwesen, L., Thomas, S., Dorrenboom, G., Pinto, D., & Bruijnzeels, M. (2005). The effect of educational intervention on intercultural communication: results of a randomised controlled trial. *The British Journal of General Practice*, *55*(514), 343–350.

Harper, P. (2005). Combining data mining tools with health care models for improved understanding of health processes and resource utilisation. *Clinical and Investigative Medicine. Medecine Clinique et Experimentale*, *28*(6), 338–341.

Harris, L., Adamson, B., & Hunt, A. (1998). Assessing quality in higher education: Criteria for evaluating programmes for allied health. *Assessment & Evaluation in Higher Education, 23*(3), 273. http://tiger.spc.alamo.edu:2052

Harrison, J., & Lee, A. (2006, November). The role of e-health in the changing health care environment. [from Academic Search Complete database.]. *Nursing Economics, 24*(6), 283–289. Retrieved May 2, 2009.

Hart, A., Henwood, F., & Wyatt, S. (2004). The role of the Internet in patient–practitioner relationships: findings from a qualitative research study. *Journal of Medical Internet Research, 6*, 36. doi:10.2196/jmir.6.3.e36

Harteloh, P. (2004). The Meaning of Quality in Health Care: A Conceptual Analysis Health Care Analysis . *Health Care Analysis, 11*(3), 259–267. doi:10.1023/B:HCAN.0000005497.53458.ef

Harvey, L., & Green, D. (2000). Qualität definieren. Fünf unterschiedliche Ansätze. *Zeitschrift fur Padagogik, 41*, 17–39.

Haughey, M., & Muirhead, B. (2005). The pedagogical and multimedia designs of learning objects for schools. *Australasian Journal of Educational Technology, 21*(4), 470–490.

Hawking, S. (2001). *The universe in a nutshell.* New York: Bantam Books.

Hay, M. C., Cadigan, R. J., Khanna, D., Strathmann, C., Lieber, E., & Altman, R. (2008). Prepared patients: internet information seeking by new rheumatology patients. *Arthritis and Rheumatism, 59*, 575–582. doi:10.1002/art.23533

Haynes, R. (1993). Where's the meat in clinical journals? [Editorial]. *ACP Journal Club, 119*, A22–A23.

Haythornthwaite, C. (2007). Social networks and online community . In Joinson, A., McKenna, K., Postmes, T., & Reips, U.-D. (Eds.), *The Oxford handbook of Internet psychology* (pp. 121–137). New York: Oxford University Press.

Haythornthwaite, C. (2006). The social informatics of elearning. Paper presented at *Information, Communication & Society (ICS) 10th Anniversary International Symposium, 20-22 September 2006*. Retrieved from the Illinois Digital Environment for Access to Learning and Scholarship (IDEALS) Web site: http://hdl.handle.net/2142/8959.

Health Canada (2000). Evaluating Telehealth 'Solutions' A Review and Synthesis of the Telehealth Evaluation Literature: Office of Health and the Information Highway.

Health Canada (2003). Toward an Evaluation Framework for Electronic Health Records Initiatives: Health and the Information Highway Division.

Health Level Seven, Inc. (2009). *Health Level Seven.* Retrieved July 21, 2009, from http://www.hl7.org/

Healthcare, R. A. N. D. (2006). *Health Information Technology: Can HIT Lower Costs and Improve Quality?* Santa Monica, CA: RAND Corporation.

Healy, J. C. (2007). The WHO eHealth resolution - eHealth for all by 2015? *Methods of Information in Medicine, 46*, 2–5.

Hebert, M. (2001). *Telehealth Success: Evaluation Framework Development.* Paper presented at the 10th World Congress on Medical Informatics.

Hellings, J., Schrooten, W., Klazinga, N., & Vleugels, A. (2007). Challenging patient safety culture: survey results. *International Journal of Health Care Quality Assurance, 20*(7), 620–632. doi:10.1108/09526860710822752

Heneghan, C. J., Glasziou, P. P., & Perera, R. (2006). Reminder packaging for improving adherence to self-administered long-term medications. *Cochrane Database of Systematic Reviews, (1)*, CD005025. Hess, R., Bryce, C., Paone, S., Fischer, G., McTigue, K., Olshansky, E., Zickmund, S., Fitzgerald, K., & Siminerio, L. (2007). Exploring challenges and potentials of personal health records in diabetes self-management: implementation and initial assessment. *Telemedicine and e-health, 13* (5), 509–18. Holmes-Rovner, M., Stableford, S., Fagerlin, A., Wei, J., Dunn, R., Ohene-Frempong, J., Blake, K., & Rovner, D. (2005). Evidence-based patient choice: a prostate cancer decision aid in plain language. *BMC Medical Informatics and Decision Making, 5*(1), 16.

Hiatt, J. M., & Creasey, T. J. (2003). *Change Management.* Loveland, CO: Prosci Research.

Hildebrand, C., Pharow, P., Engelbrecht, R., Blobel, B., Savastano, M., & Hovsto, A. (2006). BioHealth--the need for security and identity management standards in eHealth. *Studies in Health Technology and Informatics*, *121*, 327–336.

Hodge, J. G. Jr, Gostin, L. O., & Jacobson, P. D. (1999). Legal issues concerning electronic health information: privacy, quality, and liability. *Journal of the American Medical Association*, *282*(15), 1466–1471. doi:10.1001/jama.282.15.1466

Holle, R., & Zahlmann, G. (1999). Evaluation ofTelemedical Services. *IEEE Transactions on Information Technology in Biomedicine*, *3*(2), 84–91. doi:10.1109/4233.767083

Holmes, B., & Gardner, J. (2006). *E-Learning. Concepts and practice*. London: Sage Publications.

Holmes, B. (2006). Quality in a Europe of diverse systems and shared goals . In Ehlers, U. D., & Pawlowski, J. M. (Eds.), *Handbook on Quality and Standardization in E-Learning* (pp. 15–28). New York: Springer-Verlag. doi:10.1007/3-540-32788-6_2

HONcode. Retrieved November 25, 2008 from: http://www.hon.ch/HONcode/Conduct.html http://www.communities.gov.uk/publications/communities/understandingdigitalexclusion

Honigman, B., Lee, J., Rothschild, J., Light, P., Pulling, R. M., Yu, T., & Bates, D. W. (2001). Using computerized data to identify adverse drug events in outpatients. *Journal of the American Medical Informatics Association*, *8*, 254–266.

Honigman, B., Light, P., Pulling, R. M., & Bates, D. W. (2001). A computerized method for identifying incidents associated with adverse drug events in outpatients. *Journal of the American Medical Informatics Association*, *61*, 21–32.

Hu, P. J. H. (2003). *Evaluating Telemedicine Systems Success: A Revised Model.* Paper presented at the 36th Hawaii International Conference on System Sciences.

Hughes, J., & Humphrey, C. (1990). *Medical Audit in General Practice: Practice Guide to the literature*. London: King's Fund Centre.

Humphreys, J. S. (1990). Super-clinics or a country practice? Contrasts in rural life and health service provision in northern NSW. D. J. Walmsley (Ed). *Change and Adjustment in Northern NSW*.(pp. 73-84). Armidale, ME: University of New England.

Hwang, K. O., Farheen, K., Johnson, C. W., Thomas, E. J., Barnes, A. S., & Bernstam, E. V. (2007). Quality of weight loss advice on Internet forums. *The American Journal of Medicine*, *120*(7), 604–609. doi:10.1016/j.amjmed.2007.04.017

Iakovidis, I. (1998). Towards Personal Health Record: Current Situation, Obstacles, and Trends in Implementation of Electronic Healthcare Record in Europe. *International Journal of Medical Informatics*, *52*, 105–115. doi:10.1016/S1386-5056(98)00129-4

Iakovidis, I., Wilson, P., & Healy, J. C. (Eds.). (2004). *eHealth: Current Situation and Examples of Implemented and Beneficial eHealth Applications*. Amsterdam: IOS Press.

IMDB. (2007). *How/where do you get your information? How accurate/reliable is it?* Retrieved from http://imdb.com/help/show_leaf?infosource

Impicciatore, P., Pandolfini, C., Casella, N., & Bonati, M. (1997). Reliability of health information for the public on the world wide wed: systematic survey of advice on managing fever in children at home. *British Medical Journal*, *314*, 1875–1879.

Institute for Health Improvement. (2005). *Going Lean in Health Care*. Cambridge, MA: Institute for Health Improvement.

Institute of Medicine. (2001). *Crossing the Quality Chasm: A new health system for the 21st century*. Washington, DC: National Academy Press.

Institute of Medicine. (2006). *Preventing Medication Errors*. Washington, DC: The National Academies Press.

Instituto Nacional de Estadística (INE). (2003). Encuesta sobre equipamiento y uso de tecnologías de información y comunicación en las viviendas. Datos preliminares. Segundo trimestre de 2003. Press note. Retrieved October 11, 2005 from: http://www.ine.es/prensa/np1203.htm.

International Alliance of Patients' Organizations. (2007). *What is Patient-Centred Healthcare? A Review of Definitions and Principles.* London: International Alliance of Patients' Organizations.

International Standards Organization. *International Standards in process.* Retrieved March 30, 2008 from http://www.iso.org/iso/isoupdate_march08.pdf

Intille, S. S., Larson, K., & Kukla, C. (2002). *Just-In-Time Context-Sensitive Questioning for Preventative Health Care.* Paper presented at the AAAI 2002 Workshop on Automation as Caregiver: The Role of Intelligent Technology in Elder Care.

Isaiadis, S., & Getov, V. (2005). *Integrating Mobile Devices into the Grid: Design Considerations and Evaluation. Euro-Par 2005 (Vol. 3648).* Berlin: Springer Berlin / Heidelberg.

ISO 9000. (2000). Quality management systems - Fundamentals and vocabulary. Geneva: International Organization for Standardization.

ISO RFID Standards. A complete list. Retrieved September 30, 2009 from http://rfidwizards.com/index.php?option=com_content&view=article&id=242:iso-rfid-standards-a-complete-list&catid=227:standards

ISO/IEC. (2005). *Technical report about proposed standards concerning Participant Information data models.* Retrieved from http://jtc1sc36.org/doc/36N0965.pdf

Itagaki, M. W., Berlin, R. B., Bruce, R., & Schatz, B. R. (2002). The Rise and Fall of E-Health: Lessons From the First Generation of Internet Healthcare. *Medscape General Medicine 4*(2). Retrieved August, 6, 2009 from [http://www.medscape.com/viewarticle/431144] .

Jaana, M., Paré, G., & Sicotte, C. (2009). *IT Capacities Assessment Tool: A Survey of Hospitals in Canada.* Paper presented at the 42nd Hawaii International Conference on System Sciences.

Jadad, A. (2005). What will it take to bring the internet into the consulting room? We cannot remain oblivious to our patients' expectations. *Journal of General Internal Medicine, 20,* 787–788. doi:10.1111/j.1525-1497.2005.051359.x

Jadad, A. R., & Delamothe, T. (2003). From electronic gadgets to better health: where is the knowledge? *British Medical Journal, 327,* 300–301. doi:10.1136/bmj.327.7410.300

Jadad, A., & Gagliardi, A. (1998). Rating health information on the Internet. Navigating to knowledge or to Babel? *Journal of the American Medical Association, 279,* 611–614. doi:10.1001/jama.279.8.611

Jaffery, J. B., & Becker, B. N. (2004). Evaluation of e-Health web sites for patients with chronic kidney disease. *American Journal of Kidney Diseases, 44,* 71–76. doi:10.1053/j.ajkd.2004.03.025

James, B. (2005, January 2). E-health: Steps on the road to interoperability. *Health Affairs, 24,* 26–30. Retrieved March 4, 2009. doi:.doi:10.1377/hlthaff.W5.26

Jan, S., Shah, I. A., & Al-Raweshidy, H. S. (2009). *Performance Analysis of Proactive and Reactive Routing Protocols for Mobile Ad-hoc Grid in ehealth Applications.* Paper presented at the International Conference on Communication Software and Networks.

Jansen, J. P. (2006). Self-monitoring of glucose in type 2 diabetes mellitus: a Bayesian meta-analysis of direct and indirect comparisons. *Current Medical Research and Opinion, 22*(4), 671–681. doi:10.1185/030079906X96308

Jewell, S. F., & Jewell, D. O. (1992). Organization design . In Stolovitch, H. D., & Keeps, E. J. (Eds.), *Handbook of human performance technology: A comprehensive guide for analyzing and solving performance problems in organizations.* San Francisco, CA: Jossey-Bass Publishers.

Jha, A. K., Doolan, D., Grandt, D., Scott, T., & Bates, D. W. (2008). The use of health information technology in seven nations. *International Journal of Medical Informatics*, *77*(12), 848–854. doi:10.1016/j.ijmedinf.2008.06.007

Johnson, P. D., Tu, S. W., Booth, N., Sugden, B., & Purves, I. N. (2000). *Using scenarios in chronic disease management guidelines for primary care* (pp. 389–393). Proc. AMIA Annu. Fall Symp.

Johnson, J. W. (1995). Health care and higher education: A chilling parallel. *EDUCOM Review*, *28*(5), 42–45.

Johnson, C. E., Hurtubise, L. C., & Castrop, J. (2004). Learning management systems: technology to measure the medical knowledge competency of the ACGME. *Medical Education*, *38*, 599–608. doi:10.1111/j.1365-2929.2004.01792.x

Johnson, J. A., & Bootman, J. L. (1995). Drug-related morbidity and mortality. A cost-of-illness model.

Johnston, C. L., & Cooper, P. K. (1997). Patient-Focused Care. What is it? *Holistic Nursing Practice*, *11*, 1–7.

Johnstone, P. A., Crenshaw, T., Cassels, D. G., & Fox, T. H. (2008). Automated data mining of a proprietary database system for physician quality improvement. *International Journal of Radiation Oncology, Biology, Physics*, *70*(5), 1537–1541. doi:10.1016/j.ijrobp.2007.08.056

Jonassen, D. H., Peck, K., & Wilson, B. G. (1999). *Learning with Technology: A Constructivist Perspective*. Merril: Prentice-Hall.

Jones, A. R. (2009). Data mining can support quality assurance. *Journal of the Royal Society of Medicine*, *102*(9), 358–359. doi:10.1258/jrsm.2009.090216

Josefsson, U. (2007). Coping online – Patients' use of the Internet. Doctoral thesis, 37, Dep. of Applied Information Technology, IT-University of Göteborg, Sweden.

Joshi, A. (2000). On proxy agents, mobility, and web access. *Mobile Networks and Applications*, *5*(4), 233–241. doi:10.1023/A:1019120915034

Judd, F., & Humphreys, J. (2001). Mental health issues for rural and remote Australia. *The Australian Journal of Rural Health*, *6*(5), 254–258. doi:10.1046/j.1440-1584.2001.00417.x

Juran, J. (1988). *Juran on Planning for Quality*. Washington, DC: Free Press.

Justo, R., Smith, A. C., Williams, M., Westhuyzen, J. V., & der, ., Murray, J., Sciuto, G., & Wootton, R. (2004). Paediatric telecardiology services in Queensland: a review of three years' experience. *Journal of Telemedicine and Telecare*, *10*(Suppl 1), 57–60. doi:10.1258/1357633042614258

Kaisser, J. P. (2000). Patients, physicians, and the Internet. *Health Affairs (Project Hope)*, *19*, 115–123. doi:10.1377/hlthaff.19.6.115

Kaltenthaler, E., Shackley, P., Stevens, K., Beverley, C., Parry, G., & Chilcott, J. (2002). A systematic review and economic evaluation of computerised cognitive behaviour therapy for depression and anxiety. *Health Technology Assessment*, *6*(22), 1–89.

Kangarloo, H., Dionisio, J. D. N., Sinha, U., Johnson, D., & Taira, R. K. (1999). *Process models for telehealth: an industrial approach to quality management of distant medical practice.* Paper presented at the American Medical Informatics Association Annual Symposium.

Kaplan, B., & Flatley Brennan, P. (2001). Consumer Informatics Supporting Patients as Co-Producers of Quality. *Journal of the American Medical Informatics Association*, *8*(4), 309–316.

Kasper, D., Fauci, A., Longo, D., Braunwald, E., Hauser, S., & Jameson, J. (2005). *Harrison's principles of internal medicine* (16th ed.). New York: McGraw-Hill.

Kastania, A. N., & Papadhmhtriou, K. (2008b). An Evalution Model of Telemedicine Services in a Primary Care Setting. *The Journal on Information Technology in Healthcare*, *6*(3), 197–203.

Kastania, A. N., & Zimeras, S. (2008c). Quality and Reliability Aspects in Telehealth Systems . In Lazakidou, A., & Siassiakos, K. (Eds.), *Handbook of Research on Distributed Medical Informatics and E-Health* (pp. 425–441). Hershey, PA: IGI Global.

Kastania, A., Zimeras, S., Papadhmhtriou, K., & Rizos, E. (2008a). *Reliability Assessment of Telemedicine Networks.* Paper presented at the 6th International Conference on Information and Communication Technologies in Health.

Katsikas, S., Lopez, J., & Pernul, G. (2008). The challenge for security and privacy services in distributed health settings. *Studies in Health Technology and Informatics, 134*, 113–125.

Katz, E., Levin, M. L., & Hamilton, H. (1963). Traditions of research on the diffusion of innovations. *American Sociological Review, 28*(2), 237–252. doi:10.2307/2090611

Kawamoto, K., Houlihan, C., Andrew Balas, E., & Lobach, D. (2005). Improving clinical practice using clinical decision support systems: a systematic review of trials to identify features critical to success. *British Medical Journal, 330*, 765. doi:10.1136/bmj.38398.500764.8F

Kee, J. E., & Newcomer, K. E. (2008). Why do change efforts fail? [from ABI/INFORM Global database.]. *Public Management, 37*(3), 5–12. Retrieved December 18, 2008.

Kifle, M., Mbarika, V. W. A., Tsuma, C., Wilkerson, D., & Tan, J. (2008). *A TeleMedicine Transfer Model for Sub-Saharan Africa.* Paper presented at the 41st Annual Hawaii International Conference on System Sciences.

Kilbridge, P. (2002). *Crossing the Chasm with Information Technology: Bridging the Quality Gap in Health Care.* CA: California HealthCare Foundation.

Kim, P., Eng, T. R., Deering, M. J., & Maxfield, A. (1999). Published criteria for evaluating health related web sites [review]. *British Medical Journal, 318*, 647–649.

Klebl, M. (2006). Educational interoperability standards: IMS learning design and DIN didactical object model . In Ehlers, U.-D., & Pawlowski, J. M. (Eds.), *Handbook on Quality and Standardization in e-Learning* (pp. 225–250). New York: Springer-Verlag. doi:10.1007/3-540-32788-6_16

Klecun-Dabrowska, E., & Cornford, T. (2001). *Evaluation and Telehealth – an Interpretative Study.* Paper presented at the 34th Annual Hawaii International Conference on System Sciences.

Kleiner, K., Akers, R., Burke, B., & Werner, E. (2002). Parent and Physician Attitudes Regarding Electronic Communication in Pediatric Practices. *Pediatrics, 109*, 740–744. doi:10.1542/peds.109.5.740

Klesges, L. M., Estabrooks, P. A., Glasgow, R. E., & Dzewaltowski, D. (2005). Beginning with the application in mind: designing and planning health behavior change interventions to enhance dissemination. *Annals of Behavioral Medicine, 29*(2), 66–75. doi:10.1207/s15324796abm2902s_10

Kling, R. (2000). Learning about information technologies and social change: The contribution of social informatics. *The Information Society, 16*(3), 217–232. doi:10.1080/01972240050133661

Kling, R. (2001). Social informatics. *Encyclopedia of Lis.* Amsterdam: Kluwer Publishing. Retrieved from http://rkcsi.indiana.edu/.

Klinger, D., Nakada, Y., & Menendez, M. (Eds.). (1989). *AT&T Reliability Manual.* New York: Springer.

Kluge, E. H. (2007). Secure e-Health: managing risks to patient health data. *International Journal of Medical Informatics, 76*(5-6), 402–406. doi:10.1016/j.ijmedinf.2006.09.003

Koh, G., Budge, D., Butow, P., Renison, B., & Woodgate, P. G. (2005). Audio recordings of consultations with doctors for parents of critically sick babies. *Cochrane Database of Systematic Reviews*, (1): CD004502.

Kohn, L. T., Corrigan, J. M., & Donaldson, M. S. (Eds.). (2000). *To err is human: building a safer health system.* Washington, DC: National Academy Press.

Kohn, L. T. (2001). The Institute of Medicine report on medical error: Overview and implications for pharmacy. *American Journal of Health-System Pharmacy*, *58*(1), 63–66.

Kolbasuk, M., & McGree, N. (2009). Retrieved June 17, 2009, from http://www.docmemory.com/page/news/shownews.asp?num=11826

Komis, V. (2006). *Introduction to education of information technology*. Athens: Kleidarithmos Publishers.

Konference Biosémiotiků (anouncement). (n.d.). *Vesmír, 88*(139), 343.

Konstantas, D., Jones, V., & Herzog, R. (2002). *MobiHealth –innovative 2.5 / 3G mobile services and applications for healthcare.* Paper presented at the Eleventh Information Society Technologies (IST) Mobile and Wireless Telecommunications.

Koper, R., Olivier, B., & Anderson, T. (2003). *IMS Learning Design Information Model*. Retrieved January 25, 2009 from http://www.imsglobal.org/learningdesign/ldv1p0/imsld_infov1p0.html.

Koppel, R., Metlay, J., Cohen, A., Abaluck, B., Russell Localio, A., Kimmel, S., & Strom, B. (2005). Role of Computerized Physician Order Entry Systems in Facilitating Medication Errors. *Journal of the American Medical Association*, *293*(10), 1197–1203. doi:10.1001/jama.293.10.1197

Koran, L. (1975a). The reliability of clinical methods, data and judgments (second of two parts). *The New England Journal of Medicine*, *293*(14), 695–701. doi:10.1056/NEJM197510022931405

Koran, L. M. (1975b). The reliability of clinical methods, data and judgments (first of two parts). *The New England Journal of Medicine*, *293*(13), 642–646. doi:10.1056/NEJM197509252931307

Korp, P. (2006). Health on the internet: Implications for health promotion. *Health Education Research – Theory & Practice, 21*(1), 78-86.

Koster, M., Jurgensen, U., Spetz, C. L., & Rutberg, H. (2008). ["Standardized hospital mortality" as health quality indicator. An English method has been tested in Swedish patient registries]. *Lakartidningen*, *105*, 1391–1397.

Koufi, V., Malamateniou, F., & Vassilacopoulos, G. (2008). *A Medical Diagnostic and Treatment Advice System for the Provision of Home Care.* Paper presented at the 1st international conference on Pervasive Technologies Related to Assistive Environments.

Koukolík, F. (2006). *Sociální mozek.* Praha, Czech Republic: Karolinum.

Kratz, M., Silverstein, J., & Dev, P. (2007). HealthGrid: Grid Technologies for Biomedicine. Fort Detrick, Maryland: Telemedicine & Advanced Technology Research Center, U.S. Army Medical Research and Materiel Command.

Kristensen, S., Mainz, J., & Bartels, P. (2007). *Patient Safety. Establishing a set of Patient Safety Indicators* Aarhus: Sun-Tryk Aarhus University. Retrieved November 2009 from http://www.simpatie.org/Main/pf1175587453/wp1175588035/wp1176820943

Krupinski, E. A., Williams, M. B., & Andriole, K. (2007). Digital radiography image quality: image processing and display. *Journal of the American College of Radiology*, *4*(6), 389–400. doi:10.1016/j.jacr.2007.02.001

Krupinski, E., Burdick, A., & Pak H. (2007). American Telemedicine Association's Practice Guidelines for Teledermatology. *Telemedicine and e-Health, 14*(3), 289-302.

Krupinski, E., Dimmick, S., & Grigsby, J. (2006). Research recommendations for the American Telemedicine Association. *Telemedicine and e-Health, 12*(5), 579-589.

Kubono, K. (2004). Quality management system in the medical laboratory--ISO15189 and laboratory accreditation. *Rinsho Byori*, *2*(3), 274–278.

Kubono, K. (2007). Outline of the revision of ISO 15189 and accreditation of medical laboratory for specified health checkup. *Rinsho Byori, 55*(11), 1029–1036.

Kumar, A. (2005). *Ontology-driven access to biomedical information (ODABI)*. Undergraduate Thesis, University of Arizona.

Kunst, H., Groot, D., Latthe, P., & Khan, K. (2002). Accuracy of information on apparently credible websites: survey of five common health topics. *British Medical Journal, 324*, 581–582. doi:10.1136/bmj.324.7337.581

Kupchunas, W. R. (2007). Personal health record: new opportunity for patient education. *Orthopedic Nursing, 26*(3), 185–191. doi:10.1097/01.NOR.0000276971.86937.c4

Kuperman, G. J., Teich, J., Bates, D. W., Hilz, F. L., Hurley, J., Lee, R. Y., et al. (1996). Detecting alerts, notifying the physician, and offering action items: a comprehensive alerting system. *Proceedings of AMIA Annual Fall Symposium,* (pp. 704-708).

Laffel, G., & Blumenthal, D. (1989). The case for using industrial quality management science in health organizations. *Journal of the American Medical Association, 262*(20), 2869–2873. doi:10.1001/jama.262.20.2869

Laghaee, A., Malcolm, C., Hallam, J., & Ghazal, P. (2005). Artificial intelligence and robotics in high throughput post-genomics. *Drug Discovery Today, 10*(18), 1253–1259. doi:10.1016/S1359-6446(05)03581-6

Laine, C., & Davidoff, F. (1996). Patient-centered medicine. A professional evolution. *Journal of the American Medical Association, 275*(2), 152–156. doi:10.1001/jama.275.2.152

Laleci, G. B., Dogac, A., et al. (2009). *SAPHIRE: A Multi-Agent System for Remote Healthcare Monitoring through Computerized Clinical Guidelines*. Retrieved April 28, 2009, from http://www.srdc.metu.edu.tr/webpage/projects/saphire/

Lang, M., Kirpekar, N., Burkle, T., Laumann, S., & Prokosch, H. U. (2007). Results from data mining in a radiology department: the relevance of data quality. *Studies in Health Technology and Informatics, 129*(Pt 1), 576–580.

Lanktree, C., & Briere, J. (1991, January). *Early data on the Trauma Symptom Checklist for Children (TSC-C)*. Paper presented at the meeting of the American Professional Society on the Abuse of Children, San Diego, CA.

Last, J. M. (Ed.). (2000). *A Dictionary of Epidemiology* (4th ed.). Oxford, UK: Oxford University Press.

Lazarou, J., Pomeranz, B., & Corey, P. (1998). Incidence of adverse drug reactions in hospitalized patients. *Journal of the American Medical Association, 279*, 1200–1205. doi:10.1001/jama.279.15.1200

Leaffer, T., & Gonda, B. (2000). The Internet: an underutilized tool in patient education. *Computers in Nursing, 18*, 47–52.

Leape, L. L., & Berwick, D. M. (2005). Five years after To Err Is Human: what have we learned? *Journal of the American Medical Association, 293*, 2384–2390. doi:10.1001/jama.293.19.2384

Leatherman, S., Berwick, D., Iles, D., Lewin, L., Davidoff, F., Nolan, T., Bisognano, M. (2003). The Business Case for Quality: Case Studies and an Analysis. *Health Affairs, 22* (2),17–30, 18.

Lecouturier, J., Crack, L., Mannix, K., Hall, R. H., & Bond, S. (2002). Evaluation of a patient-held record for patients with cancer. *European Journal of Cancer Care, 11*(2), 114–121. doi:10.1046/j.1365-2354.2002.00301.x

Lee, M., Delaney, C., & Moorhead, S. (2007). Building a personal health record from a nursing perspective. *International Journal of Medical Informatics, 76*(Supplement 2), S308–S316. doi:10.1016/j.ijmedinf.2007.05.010

Legido-Quigley, H., McKee, M., Walshe, K., Suñol, R., Nolte, E., & Klazinga, N. (2008). How can quality of care be safeguarded across the European Union? *British Medical Journal, 336*, 920–923. doi:10.1136/bmj.39538.584190.47

Leimeister, J. M., Daum, M., & Krcmar, H. (2004). Towards mobile communities for cancer patients: the case of krebsgemeinschaft.de. [IJWBC]. *International Journal of Web Based Communities, 1*, 1–9.

Leisch, E., Sartzetakis, S., Tsiknakis, M., & Orphanoudakis, S. C. (1997). A framework for the integration of distributed autonomous healthcare information systems. *Informatics for Health & Social Care*, *22*(4), 325–335. doi:10.3109/14639239709010904

Leong, S., Gingrich, D., Lewis, P., Mauger, D., & George, J. (2005). Enhancing Doctor-Patient Communication Using Email: A Pilot Study. *The Journal of the American Board of Family Practice*, *18*(3), 180–188. doi:10.3122/jabfm.18.3.180

Leppisaari, I., & Vainio, L. (2006b). *Online mentoring - to Developing Teachers' Online Pedagogy Expertise in Content Producing Teams*. In C.M. Crawford (Ed.), *Proceedings 17th International Conference of Society for Information Technology and Teacher Education* (pp. 2314-2321), Orlando, Florida.

Leppisaari, I., & Vainio, L. (2007). Teachers as Peer Evaluators of Learning Object Pedagogical Quality in the Virtual Polytechnic. In *Proceedings of Educause Australasia*, Melbourne, Australia. Retrieved January 10, 2009 from http://www.caudit.edu.au/educauseaustralasia07/papers/Teachers%20as%20Peer%20Evaluators%20of%20Learning.pdf.

Leppisaari, I., Silander, P., & Vainio, L. (2006a). Autenttisuus ammattikorkeakoulun virtuaaliopetuksen haasteena. In M. Ylikarjula (Ed.) *Ihmettelya ja oppimista tutkimuksen aarella*: Opettaja oman tyonsa tutkijana – symposiumin III artikkelit (pp. 17-36). Keski-Pohjanmaan ammattikorkeakoulun julkaisuja.

LeRouge, C., Garfield, M. J., & Hevner, A. R. (2002). *Quality Attributes in Telemedicine Video Conferencing*. Paper presented at the 35th Annual Hawaii International Conference on System Sciences.

LeRouge, C., Hevner, A., Collins, R., & al. (2004). Telemedicine Encounter Quality: Comparing Patient and Provider Perspectives of a Socio-Technical System. *Proc. 37th Hawaii International Conference on System Sciences*. Retrieved March 25, 2009 from [http://www2.computer.org/portal/web/csdl/doi?doc=abs/proceedings/hicss/2004/2056/06/205660149a.abs.htm]

LeRouge, C., Hevner, A., Collins, R., Garfield, M., & Law, D. (2004). *Telemedicine Encounter Quality: Comparing Patient and Provider Perspectives of a Socio-Technical System*. Paper presented at the 37th Annual Hawaii International Conference on System Sciences.

Lester, H., Allan, T., Wilson, S., Jowett, S., & Roberts, L. (2003). A cluster randomised controlled trial of patient-held medical records for people with schizophrenia receiving shared care. *The British Journal of General Practice*, *53*(488), 197–203.

Letterie, G. S. (2003). Medical education as a science: the quality of evidence for computer-assisted instruction. *American Journal of Obstetrics and Gynecology*, *188*, 849–853. doi:10.1067/mob.2003.168

Lewin, S. A., Skea, Z. C., Entwistle, V., Zwarenstein, M., & Dick, J. (2001). Interventions for providers to promote a patient-centred approach in clinical consultations. *Cochrane Database of Systematic Reviews*, (4): CD003267.

Lewis, F., & Batey, M. (1982). Clarifying autonomy and accountability. Part 2. *The Journal of Nursing Administration*, 10–15.

Leys, M. (2003). Healthcare policy: Qualitative evidence and health technology assessment. *Health Policy (Amsterdam)*, *65*(3), 217–226. doi:10.1016/S0168-8510(02)00209-9

Liber, O. (2002). The revolutionary possibilities of eLearning standards . In Bachmann, G., Haefeli, O., & Kindt, M. (Eds.), *Die Virtuelle Hochschule in der Konsolidierungsphase* (pp. 197–208). Münster, New York, München, Berlin: Waxmann.

Liddell, C., Brown, T., Johnston, D., Coates, V., & Mallett, J. (2004). Giving patients an audiotape of their GP consultation: a randomised controlled trial. *The British Journal of General Practice*, *54*(506), 667–672.

Lindberg, D. (2003). *NIH: Moving research from the bench to the bedside*. Presentation to the Subcommittee on Health.

Lipson, L. R., & Henderson, T. M. (1995). State initiatives to promote telemedicine. *Telemedicine Journal*, *2*(2), 109–121.

Liu, S. S., & Chen, J. (2009). Using data mining to segment healthcare markets from patients' preference perspectives. *International Journal of Health Care Quality Assurance*, *22*(2), 117–134. doi:10.1108/09526860910944610

Loader, B. D., Hardey, M., & Keeble, L. (2008). Health informatics for older people: A review of ICT facilitated integrated care for older people. *International Journal of Social Welfare*, *17*(1), 46–53.

Loader, B. D., & Keeble, L. (2004). *Challenging the digital divide? – A literature review of community informatics initiatives*. York, England: Joseph Rowntree Foundation.

Lobach, D. F., & Hammond, W. E. (1994). Development and evaluation of a computer-assisted management protocol (CAMP): improved compliance with care guidelines for diabetes mellitus. *Proceedings of the Annual Symposium on Computer Applications in Medical Care,* 787-791

Lobley, D. (1997). The economics of telemedicine. *Journal of Telemedicine and Telecare*, *3*(3), 117–125. doi:10.1258/1357633971930977

Lombarts, M. J. M. H., Rupp, I., Vallejo, P., Suñol, R., & Klazinga, N. (2009). Application of quality improvement strategies in 389 European hospitals: results of the MARQuIS project. *Quality & Safety in Health Care*, *18*, 28–37. doi:10.1136/qshc.2008.029363

Lonsdale, R. E., & Holmes, J. H. (1981). *Settlement systems in sparsely populated regions: The United States and Australia*. New York: Pergamon Press.

Lorenzo, S., & Mira, J. J. (2004). Are Spanish physicians ready to take advantage of the Internet? *World Hospitals and Health Services*, *40*, 31–35.

Lorenzo, S. (2008). Toward new approaches to quality. The patient as coprotagonist. *Gaceta Sanitaria,* 22(Supl 1), 186-91.

Louro González, A., & González Guitián, C. (2001). Portales sanitarios para la atención primaria. *Atencion Primaria*, *27*, 346–350.

Lugmayr, A., Risse, T., Stockleben, B., Kaario, J., & Laurila, K. (2009). Special issue on semantic ambient media experience. *Multimedia Tools and Applications*, 331–335. doi:10.1007/s11042-009-0283-y

Luke, R., Walston, S., & Plummer, P. (2004). *Healthcare strategy: in pursuit of competitive advantage*. Chicago, IL: Health Administration Press.

Lundberg, G. D. (1992). Perspective from the editor of JAMA. *The JAMA Bulletin of the Medical Library Association*, *80*(2), 110–114.

Lupu, E., Dulay, N., Sloman, M., Sventek, J., Heeps, S., & Strowes, S. (2008). AMUSE: autonomic management of ubiquitous e-Health systems. *Concurrency and Computation*, *20*(3), 277–295. doi:10.1002/cpe.1194

Lyman, P., & Varian, H. (2003). *How much information?* Retrieved from http://www2.sims.berkeley.edu/research/projects/how-much-info-2003/index.htm

Lyu, M. R. (Ed.). (1996). *Handbook of Software Reliability Engineering*. Washington, DC: IEEE Computer Society Press and McGraw-Hill Book Company.

Maceratini, R., Rafanelli, M., & Ricci, F. L. (1995). Virtual Hospitalization: reality or utopia? *Medinfo*, *2*, 1482–1486.

Madsen, M. D., & Østergaard, D. (2004). *Udvikling af metode og værktøj til at måle sikkerhedskultur på sygehusafdelinger. Afrapportering af projekt om sikkerhedskultur og patientsikkerhed i Københavns Amt*. Retrieved November 2009 from http://www.risoe.dk/rispubl/SYS/syspdf/ris-r-1491.pdf.

Maheu, M. M., Whitten, P., Allen, A. (2001). *E-Health, Telehealth, and Telemedicine: A Guide to Start-up and Success: Jossey-Bass Health Series*. San Francisco. Retrieved June 15, 2009 from Academic Search complete.

Mainz, J. (2003a). Defining and classifying clinical indicators for quality improvement. *International Journal for Quality in Health Care*, *15*, 523–530. doi:10.1093/intqhc/mzg081

Mainz, J. (2003b). Developing evidence-based clinical indicators: a state of the art methods primer. *International Journal for Quality in Health Care*, *15*(Suppl 1), i5–i11. doi:10.1093/intqhc/mzg084

Mainz, J. (2004). Quality Indicators: Essential for Quality Improvement. *International Journal for Quality in Health Care*, *16*, 1–2. doi:10.1093/intqhc/mzh036

Mainz, J., & Bartels, P. D. (2006). Nationwide quality improvement--how are we doing and what can we do? *International Journal for Quality in Health Care*, *18*, 79–80. doi:10.1093/intqhc/mzi099

Mainz, J., Krog, B. R., Bjornshave, B., & Bartels, P. (2004). Nationwide continuous quality improvement using clinical indicators: the Danish National Indicator Project. *International Journal for Quality in Health Care*, *16*(Suppl 1), i45–i50. doi:10.1093/intqhc/mzh031

Mairinger, T., Gabl, C., Derwan, P., Mikuz, G., & Ferrer-Roca, O. (1996). What Do Physicians Think of Telemedicine? A Survey in Different European Regions. *Journal of Telemedicine and Telecare*, *2*, 50–56. doi:10.1258/1357633961929169

Malec, B. T. (1998). Administrative applications . In Austin, C. J., & Boxerman, S. B. (Eds.), *S.B. (1998). Information systems for health services administration* (5th ed.). Chicago, IL: Health Administration Press.

Mallett, J. (1996). Sense of Direction. *Nursing Times*, *92*, 40–42.

Mamdani, M., Ching, A., Golden, B., & al. (2008). Challenges to Evidence-Based Prescribing in Clinical Practice. Annals of Pharmacotherapy, 42(5), 704-707. Harvey Whitney Books Company. Posted 07/15/2008. Retrieved from [http://www.medscape.com/viewarticle/576145].

Mander, R. (1995). Where does the buck stop? In Watson, R. (Ed.), *Accountability in midwifery* (pp. 95–106). London: Chapman and Hall.

Manning, B. R. M. (2003). Clinical Process Maps as an indexing link to knowledge and Records. In *Healthcare Digital Libraries Workshop, 7th European Conference on Research and Advanced Technology for Digital Libraries*, Trondheim, Norway.

Marco, J., Barba, R., Losa, J. E., de la Serna, C. M., Sainz, M., & Lantigua, I. F. (2006). Advice from a medical expert through the Internet on queries about AIDS and hepatitis: Analysis of a pilot experiment. *PLoS Medicine*, *3*(7), 1041–1047. doi:10.1371/journal.pmed.0030256

Marcus, A. C., & Crane, L. A. (1998). A review of cervical cancer screening intervention research: implications for public health programs and future research. *Preventive Medicine*, *27*(1), 13–31. doi:10.1006/pmed.1997.0251

Marine, S., Embi, P. J., McCuistion, M., Haag, D., & Guard, J. R. (2005). NetWellness 1995-2005: Ten years of experience and growth as a non-profit consumer health information and Ask-an-Expert service. In *AMIA 2005 Symposium Proceedings, 22-26 October 2005*. Washington DC, USA.

Markin, R. S., & Whalen, S. A. (2000). Laboratory automation: trajectory, technology, and tactics. *Clinical Chemistry*, *46*, 764–771.

MARQuIS research project. Qual Saf Health Care, 18, i1-i74. (2009) *National Guideline Clearinghouse (NGC)*, Guideline Syntheses (accessed 17 October 2007). Retrieved from [http://www.ngc.org/compare/synthesis.aspx].

Marshall, S. J., & Mitchell, G. (2007). *Benchmarking International E-learning Capability with the E-Learning Maturity Model*. In Proceedings of EDUCAUSE Australasia, Melbourne, Australia. Retrieved January 10, 2009 from http://www.caudit.edu.au/educauseaustralasia07/authors_papers/Marshall-103.pdf.

Martínez, I., & García, J. (2005a). *QoS Evaluation for Multimedia Telemedicine Services based on TCP/UDP cross-traffic.* Paper presented at the International Conference on Computer Communications and Networks.

Martínez, I., & García, J. (2005b). *SM3 – Quality Of Service (QoS) Evaluation Tool For Telemedicine-Based New Healthcare Services.* Paper presented at the II International Conference on Computational Bioengineering.

Martínez, I., Salvador, J., Fernández, J., & García, J. (2003). *Traffic Requirements Evaluation for a Telemedicine Network.* Paper presented at the International Congress on Computational Bioengineering.

Mason, R. O. (1978). Measuring information output: a communication systems approach. *Information & Management*, *1*(5), 219–234. doi:10.1016/0378-7206(78)90028-9

Masum, H. (2002). TOOL: The Open Opinion Layer. *First Monday, 7*(7). Retrieved June 28, 2003 fromhttp://firstmonday.org/issues/issue7_7/masum/index.html

Maxwell, R. J. (1984). Quality assessment in health. *British Medical Journal*, *288*(6428), 1470–1472. doi:10.1136/bmj.288.6428.1470

Maxwell, R. J. (1992). Dimensions of quality revisited: from thought to action. *Quality in Health Care*, *1*, 171–177. doi:10.1136/qshc.1.3.171

May, C. (2006). A rational model for assessing and evaluating complex interventions in health care. *BMC Health Services Research*, *6*, 86. doi:10.1186/1472-6963-6-86

May, C., Harrison, R., Finch, T., MacFarlane, A., Mair, F., & Wallace, P. (2003). Understanding the Normalization of Telemedicine Services through Qualitative Evaluation. *Journal of the American Medical Informatics Association*, *10*(6), 596–604. doi:10.1197/jamia.M1145

May, C., Mort, M., Mair, F., Ellis, N. T., & Gask, L. (2000). Evaluation of new technologies in healthcare systems: what's the context? *Health Informatics Journal*, *6*, 67–70. doi:10.1177/146045820000600203

Mayer, M. A., Leis, A., & Ruiz, P. (2004). Navegando por Internet: los sellos de calidad y la web semántica pueden ser un camino para encontrar el oro que reluce. *Atencion Primaria*, *34*, 383. doi:10.1157/13067780

McConnochie, K. M., Conners, G. P., Brayer, A. F., Goepp, J., Herendeen, N. E., & Wood, N. E. (2006). Differences in Diagnosis and Treatment Using Telemedicine Versus In-Person Evaluation of Acute Illness. *Ambulatory Pediatrics*, *6*(4), 196–197. doi:10.1016/j.ambp.2006.03.002

McDermott, R. (2000). Knowing in community: 10 critical success factors in building communities of practice. *IHRIM Journal*, March 2000. Retrieved from http://www.a-i-a.com/capital-intelectual/KnowingInCommunity.pdf

McKeon Stosuy, M., Manning, B. R. M., & Layzell, B. R. (2005). *E-care co-ordination: An inclusive community-wide holistic approach*. Boston: Springer.

McManus, R. J., Mant, J., Roalfe, A., Oakes, R. A., Bryan, S., Pattison, H. M., & Hobbs, F. D. (2005). Targets and self monitoring in hypertension: randomised controlled trial and cost effectiveness analysis. *British Medical Journal*, *331*(7515), 493. doi:10.1136/bmj.38558.393669.E0

McMullan, M. (2006). Patients using the Internet to obtain health information: How this affects the patient–health professional relationship. *Patient Education and Counseling*, *63*, 24–28. doi:10.1016/j.pec.2005.10.006

McSherry, R., & Pearce, P. (Eds.). (2002). *Clinical Governance: A Guide to Implementation for Health Care Professionals*. Oxford: Blackwell Science.

Mdi Europa – The Medical Device Service-Management. Retrieved September 30, 2009 from http://www.mdi-europa.com/services.htm

Mead, N., & Bower, P. (2002). Patient-centred consultations and outcomes in primary care: a review of the literature. *Patient Education and Counseling*, *48*, 51–61. doi:10.1016/S0738-3991(02)00099-X

Mearian, L. (2009). Cost of Obama E-health Plan Could Reach $100B. *Computerworld, 43*(5), 12-14. http://tiger.spc.alamo.edu:2052

Mechaca, L. (2007). *Goodbye, Axim*. Message posted to http://direct2dell.com/one2one/archive/2007/04/11/11397.aspx

Medical device standards Portal – USA. Retrieved September 30, 2009 from http://www.medicaldevicestandards.com/

MedIEQ. Retrieved November 25, 2008 from: http://www.medieq.org/about

Medina-Mora, R., Winograd, T., Flores, R., & Flores, F. (1992). The Action Workflow Approach to workflow management technology. In *Proceedings from the 1992 ACM Conference on Computer-Supported Cooperative Work*, 281-288. Retrieved from http://portal.acm.org.

Medscape, L. L. C. Retrieved February 22 2009, from http://www.medscape.com/pages/features/hospitalcompare/hospitalcompare

Mehra, B., Merkel, C., & Bishop, A. P. (2004). The internet for empowerment of minority and marginalized users. *New Media & Society*, *6*(6), 781–802. doi:10.1177/146144804047513

Meller, G. (1997). A Typology of Simulators for Medical Education. *Journal of Digital Imaging*, *10*, 194–196. doi:10.1007/BF03168699

Menachemi, N., Burke, D., & Brooks, R. G. (2004). Adoption factors associated with patient safety-related information technology. *Journal for Healthcare Quality*, *26*(6), 39–44.

Meneu, T., Traver, V., Fernández, C., Serafin, R., Domínguez, D., & Guillén, S. (2009). *Life Assistance Protocols (LAP) – A Model for the Personalization of Lifestyle Support for Health and Wellbeing.* Paper presented at the International Conference on eHealth, Telemedicine, and Social Medicine.

Metaxiotis, K., Ptochos, D., & Psarras, J. (2004). E-health in the new millennium: a research and practice agenda. *International Journal of Electronic Healthcare*, *1*(2), 165–175. doi:10.1504/IJEH.2004.005865

Milenković, A., Otto, C., Jovanov, E. (2006). Wireless Sensor Networks for Personal Health Monitoring: Issues and an Implementation. *Computer Communications (Special issue: Wireless Sensor Networks: Performance, Reliability, Security, and Beyond)*, *29*(13-14), 2521-2533.

Milicevic, I., Gareis, K., & Korte, W. B. (2005). Making progress towards user-orientation in online public service provision in Europe . In Cunningham, P., & Cunningham, M. (Eds.), *Innovation and the Knowledge Economy: Issues, Applications, Case Studies*. Amsterdam, The Netherlands: IOS Press.

Miller, R. A. (2002). Reference Standards in Evaluating System Performance, Editorial comments. *Journal of the American Medical Informatics Association*, *9*(1), 87–91.

Mira, J. J., Pérez-Jover, V., & Lorenzo, S. (2004). Navegando en Internet en busca de información sanitaria: no es oro todo lo que reluce.... *Atencion Primaria*, *33*, 391–399. doi:10.1157/13060754

Mira, J. J., Llinás, G., Tomás, O., & Pérez-Jover, V. (2006). Quality of websites in Spanish public hospitals. *Medical Informatics and the Internet in Medicine*, *31*, 23–44. doi:10.1080/14639230500519940

Mira, J. J., Llinás, G., & Perez Jover, V. (2008). Habits of Internet users and usefulness of websites in Spanish for health education. *World Hospitals and Health Services*, *44*, 30–35.

MITC. Ministerio de Industria, Turismo y Comercio. Estudio sobre Actividades realizadas en Internet 2007. Red.es. Retrieved October 23, 2008 from: http://observatorio.red.es/estudios/documentos/actividades_internet_2007.pdf

Mitchell, J. (1999). *From telehealth to e-health: the unstoppable rise of e-health.* Canberra, Australia: National Office for the Information Technology.

Moberg, T. F., & Whitcomb, M. E. (1999). Educational technology to facilitate medical students' learning: background paper 2 of the medical school objectives project. *Academic Medicine*, *74*, 1146–1150. doi:10.1097/00001888-199910000-00020

Mohomed, I., Misra, A., Ebling, M., & Jerome, W. (2008). *Context-Aware and Personalized Event Filtering for Low-Overhead Continuous Remote Health Monitoring.* Paper presented at the International Symposium on a World of Wireless, Mobile and Multimedia Networks.

Molloy, R. M., Mc Connell, R. I., Lamont, J. V., & FitzGerald, S. P. (2005). Automation of biochip array technology for quality results. *Clinical Chemistry and Laboratory Medicine*, *43*(12), 1303–1313. doi:10.1515/CCLM.2005.224

Morales Rodriguez, M., Casper, G., & Brennan, P. F. (2007). Patient-centered design. The potential of user-centered design in personal health records. *Journal of American Health Information Management Association*, *78*(4), 44–46.

Morton, S., & Michael, S. (1991). *The Corporation of the 1990s: Information Technology and Organizational Transformation*. New York: Oxford University Press.

Murai, T. (2002). Future outlook for LAS, LIS. *Rinsho Byori*, *50*(7), 698–701.

Muramoto, M., Campbell, J., & Salazar, Z. (2003). Provider Training and Education in Disease Management: Current and Innovative Technology. *Disease Management & Health Outcomes*, McLeod, S., & Barbara, A. (2005). Online technology in rural health: Supporting students to overcome the tyranny of distance. *Australian Journal of Rural Health, 13*(5), 276-281. http://tiger.spc.alamo.edu:2052

Murff, H. J., Patel, V. L., Hripcsak, G., & Bates, D. W. (2003). Detecting adverse events for patient safety research: a review of current methodologies. *Journal of Biomedical Informatics*, *36*(1-2), 131–143. doi:10.1016/j.jbi.2003.08.003

Murphy, D., Challacombe, B., Nedas, T., Elhage, O., Althoefer, K., Seneviratne, L., & Dasgupta, P. (2007). Equipment and technology in robotics (in Spanish; Castilian). *Archivos Espanoles de Urologia*, *60*(4), 349–355.

Murray, E., Fitzmaurice, D., McCahon, D., Fuller, C., & Sandhur, H. (2004). Training for patients in a randomised controlled trial of self management of warfarin treatment. *British Medical Journal*, *328*(7437), 437–438. doi:10.1136/bmj.328.7437.437

Murray, M. D., Loos, B., Tu, W., Eckert, G. J., Zhou, X. H., & Tierney, W. M. (1998). Effects of computer-based prescribing on pharmacist work patterns. *Journal of the American Medical Informatics Association*, *5*(6), 585–586.

Murray, E., Burns, J., See Tai, S., Lai, R., & Nazareth, I. (2005). Interactive Health Communication Applications for people with chronic disease. *Cochrane.Database.of Systematic Reviews.*, CD004274 (4).

Murray, E., Lo, B., Pollack, L., Donelan, K., Catania, J., Lee, K., et al. (2003). The impact of health information on the internet on health care and the physician-patient relationship: national U.S. survey among 1,050 U.S. physicians. *Journal of Medical Internet Research,* 5:e17. Retrieved April 21 2009, from: http://www.jmir.org/2003/3/e17

National Health and Medical Research Council. (2000). *How to use the evidence: assessment and application of scientific evidence*. Retrieved January 18, 2009, from http://www.nhmrc.gov.au/publications/synopses/cp65syn.htm

National Institutes of Health. (2009). *SNOMED Clinical Terms®*. Retrieved July 21, 2009, from http://www.nlm.nih.gov/research/umls/Snomed/snomed_main.html

Navarro-Royo, C., Monteagudo-Piqueras, O., Rodríguez-Suárez, L., Valentín-López, B., & García-Caballero, J. (2002). Legibilidad de los documentos de consentimiento informado del Hospital La Paz. *Revista de Calidad Asistencial*, *17*, 331–336.

Negroponte, N. (1996). *Being digital*. New York: Random House.

Nelson, R. (2007). The personal health record. *American Journal of Nursing, 107 (9),* 27–8. O'Connor, A., Llewellyn-Thomas, H., & Barry Flood, A. (2004). Modifying unwarranted variations in health care: shared decision making using patient decision aids. *Health Affairs (Project Hope)*, (Supplement Web Exclusive), VAR63–VAR72.

Nesbit, J., Belfer, K., & Vargo, J. (2002). A Convergent Participation Model for Evaluation of Learning Objects. *Canadian Journal of Learning and Technology 28(3)*. Retrieved January 20, 2009 from http://www.cjlt.ca/index.php/cjlt/issue/view/11

New York State Department of Health. Retrieved February 22 2009, from: http://hospitals.nyhealth.gov/

NHS Connecting for Health. Retrieved September 30, 2009 from http://www.connectingforhealth.nhs.uk

Nijland, N., Seydel, E. R., van Gemert-Pijnen, J. E. W. C., Brandenburg, B., Kelders, S. M., & Will, M. (2009). *Evaluation of an Internet-Based Application for Supporting Self-Care of Patients with Diabetes Mellitus Type 2.* Paper presented at the International Conference on eHealth, Telemedicine, and Social Medicine.

Nikolidakis, S., Vergados, D. D., & Anagnostopoulos, I. (2008). *Health Care Information Systems and Personalized Services for Assisting Living of Elderly People at Nursing Home.* Paper presented at the Third International Workshop on Semantic Media Adaptation and Personalization.

Nishisaki, A., Keren, R., & Nadkarni, V. (2007). Does Simulation Improve Patient Safety?: Self-Efficacy, Competence, Operational Performance, and Patient Safety. *Anesthesiology Clinics*, *25*(2), 225–236. doi:10.1016/j.anclin.2007.03.009

Norcini, J., & Talati, J. (2009). Assessment, surgeon, and society. *International Journal of Surgery*, *7*(4), 313–317. doi:10.1016/j.ijsu.2009.06.011

Norén, G. N., Bate, A., Hopstadius, J., Star, K., & Edwards, I. R. (2008). Temporal Pattern Discovery for Trends and Transient Effects: Its Application to Patient Records. In *Proceedings of the Fourteenth International Conference on Knowledge Discovery and Data Mining SIGKDD 2008* (pp. 963-971). Las Vegas NV.

Nusslin, F. (2006). Current status of medical technology. *Acta Neurochirurgica*, *98*, 25–31. doi:10.1007/978-3-211-33303-7_5

OBHE (Observatory on Borderless Higher Education). (2008), Retrieved January 20, 2009 from http://www.obhe.ac.uk.

O'Connor, J., & McDermott, I. (1997). *The Art of Systems Thinking*. San Francisco: Thorsons.

Oh, H., Rizo, C., Enkin, M., & Jadad, A. (2005). What is eHealth?: a systematic review of published definitions. *World Hospitals and Health Services*, *41*(1), 32–40.

Oh, Y., McCombs, J. S., Cheng, R. A., & Johnson, K. A. (2002). Pharmacist time required for counseling in an outpatient pharmacy. *American Journal of Health-System Pharmacy*, *59*(23), 2346–2355.

Ohinmaa, A., Hailey, D., & Roine, R. (1999). *The Assessment of Telemedicine- General principles and a systematic review*. Helsinki: Finnish Office for Health Care Technology Assessment and Alberta Heritage Foundation for Medical Research.

Ohno-Machado, L., Gennari, J. H., Murphy, S. N., Jain, N. L., Tu, S. W., & Oliver, D. (1998). The GuideLine Interchange Format: A model for representing guidelines. *Journal of the American Medical Informatics Association*, 357–372.

Okada, M. (2002). Future of laboratory informatics. *Rinsho Byori*, *50*(7), 691–693.

O'Keefe, R. M. (1989). The evaluation of decision-aiding systems: guidelines and methods. *Information & Management*, *17*, 217–226. doi:10.1016/0378-7206(89)90045-1

Okuda, Y., Bryson, E. O., DeMaria, S Jr., Jacobson, L., Quinones, J., Shen, B., & Levine, A. I. (2009). The utility of simulation in medical education: what is the evidence? *Mount Sinai Journal of Medicine: A Journal of Translational and Personalized Medicine, 76*(4), 330-343.

Olive, M., Rahmouni, H., & Solomonides, T. (2007a). From HealthGrid to SHARE: A Selective Review of Projects. *Studies in Health Technology and Informatics*, *126*, 306–313.

Olive, M., Rahmouni, H., Solomonides, T., Breton, V., Legre, Y., & Blanquer, I. (2007b). SHARE Roadmap 1: Towards a Debate. *Studies in Health Technology and Informatics*, *126*, 164–173.

Olive, C., O'Connor, T. M., & Mannan, M. S. (2006). Relationship of safety culture and process safety. *Journal of Hazardous Materials*, *130*(1-2), 133–140. doi:10.1016/j.jhazmat.2005.07.043

Oliveira, I. C., Oliveira, J. L., Santos, M., Martin-Sanchez, F., & Sousa Pereira, A. (2003). *On the requirements of biomedical information tools for health applications: the INFOGENMED case study.* Paper presented at the 7th Protuguese Conference on Biomedical Engineering.

Oliver, R., Herrington, J., & Reeves, T. C. (2006). Creating authentic learning environments through blended learning approaches . In Bonk, J., & Graham, C. R. (Eds.), *The handbook of blended learning* (pp. 502–515). San Francisco: Pleiffer.

Olivier, B., & Tattersall, C. (2005). The Learning Design Specification . In Koper, R., & Tattersall, C. (Eds.), *Learning Design. A Handbook on Modeling and Delivering Networked Education and Training* (pp. 21–40). Berlin, Heidelberg, New York: Springer.

Omar, W. M., & Taleb-Bendiab, A. (2006). *Service Oriented Architecture for e-Health Support Services Based on Grid Computing Overlay.* Paper presented at the Proceedings of the IEEE International Conference on Services Computing.

Omar, W. M., Ahmad, B. A., & Taleb-Bendiab, A. (2006). *Grid Overlay for Remote e-Health Monitoring.* Paper presented at the IEEE International Conference on Computer Systems and Applications.

Ormond, K. E., Cirino, A. L., Helenowski, I. B., Chisholm, R. L., & Wolf, W. A. (2009). Assessing the understanding of biobank participants. *American Journal of Medical Genetics*, *149A*(2), 188–198. doi:10.1002/ajmg.a.32635

Ortendahl, M. (2008). Different time perspectives of the doctor and the patient reduce quality in health care. *Quality Management in Health Care*, *17*, 136–139.

Ozturk, E., & Altilar, D. T. (2007). *IMOGA: An Architecture for Integrating Mobile Devices into Grid Applications.* Paper presented at the Fourth Annual Conference on Mobile and Ubiquitous Systems: Networking & Services.

Pagliari, C., Detmer, D., & Singleton, P. (2007). Potential of electronic personal health records. *British Medical Journal*, *335*(7615), 330–333. doi:10.1136/bmj.39279.482963.AD

Pagliari, C. (2007). Design and evaluation in eHealth: challenges and implications for an interdisciplinary field. *Journal of Medical Internet Research*, *9*(2), e15. doi:10.2196/jmir.9.2.e15

Pallarés, A. (2000). Las nuevas tecnologías de la información desde la perspectiva de los ciudadanos: la paradoja de Internet. *Revista de Calidad Asistencial*, *15*, 221–222.

Pallesen, B., Engberg, A., & Barlach, A. (2006). Developing e-health information by empowerment strategy. *Studies in Health Technology and Informatics*, *122*, 776.

Palmieri, P., Peterson, L., & Ford, E. (2007). Technological iatrogenesis: New risks force heightened management awareness. *Journal of Healthcare Risk Management*, *27*(4), 19–24. doi:10.1002/jhrm.5600270405

Panayiotou, C., & Samaras, G. (2004). mPERSONA: Personalized Portals for the Wireless User: An Agent Approach. *Mobile Networks and Applications*, *9*(6), 663–677. doi:10.1023/B:MONE.0000042505.07003.e6

Pandolfini, Ch., & Bonati, M. (2002). Follow up of quality of public oriented health information on the world wide web: systematic re-evaluation. *British Medical Journal*, *324*, 582–583. doi:10.1136/bmj.324.7337.582

Panteli, N., Pitsillides, B., Pitsillides, A., & Samaras, G. (2007). An E-healthcare Mobile application: A Stakeholders' analysis: Experience of Reading . In Al-Hakim, L. (Ed.), *Web Mobile-Based Applications for Healthcare Management*. Hershey, PA: IGI Global.

Papadopoulou, A., Varlamis, I., & Apostolakis, I. (2007). Models and Practices for the development of e-learning communities in healthcare. In proceedings of the 5th ICICTH (pp. 170–174). Greece: Samos.

Paré, G., & Sicotte, C. (2001). Information Technology Sophistication in Health Care: An Instrument Validation Study among Canadian Hospitals. *International Journal of Medical Informatics*, *63*(3), 205–223. doi:10.1016/S1386-5056(01)00178-2

Park, S., Mackenzie, K., & Jayaraman, S. (2002). *The wearable motherboard: a framework for personalized mobile information processing (PMIP).* Paper presented at the 39th Design Automation Conference.

Patterson, E. S., Cook, R. I., & Render, M. L. (2002). Improving patient safety by identifying side effects from introducing bar coding in medication administration. *Journal of the American Medical Informatics Association*, *9*(5), 540–553. doi:10.1197/jamia.M1061

Pawlowski, J. M. (2006). Adopting quality standards for education and e-learning. In U.-D. Ehlers & J. M. Pawlowski (Eds.), Handbook on Quality and Standardization in E-Learning (pp. 65–77). New York: Springer-Verlag. doi:10.1007/3-540-32788-6_5doi:10.1007/3-540-32788-6_5

Pealer, L. N., & Dorman, S. M. (1997). Evaluating health-related Web sites. *The Journal of School Health*, *67*, 232–235. doi:10.1111/j.1746-1561.1997.tb06311.x

Pearlman, E., Wolfert, M., & Miele, R. (2001). Utilization management and information technology: adapting to the new era. *Clinical Leadership & Management Review*, *15*(2), 85–88.

Peleg, M., Ogunyemi, O., Tu, S., et al. (2001). Using features of Arden Syntax with object-oriented medical data models for guideline modeling. In *Proc AMIA Symp.* (pp. 523-7).

Perednia, D. A., & Allen, A. (1995). Telemedicine Technology and Clinical Applications. *Journal of the American Medical Association*, *273*(6), 483–488. doi:10.1001/jama.273.6.483

Pesquita, C., Faria, D., Falcao, A. O., Lord, P., & Couto, F. M. (2009). Semantic similarity in biomedical ontologies. *PLoS Computational Biology*, *5*(7), e1000443. doi:10.1371/journal.pcbi.1000443

Pew Internet and American Life Project. The Online Health Care Revolution: How the Web Helps Americans Take Better Care of Themselves. November 26, 2000. Retrieved November 23, 2008 from: http://www.pewinternet.org.

Pharow, P., & Blobel, B. (2008). Mobile health requires mobile security: challenges, solutions, and standardization. *Studies in Health Technology and Informatics*, *136*, 697–702.

Philips. Mobile Point of Care. Retrieved September 30, 2009 from http://www.fimi.philips.com/mobile-point-of-care/index.html

Picker Institute. (2004). *Patient-Centered Care 2015: Scenarios, Vision, Goals & Next Steps*. Camden, Maine: The Picker Institute.

Piemme, T. E. (1988). Computer-assisted learning and evaluation in medicine. Journal of the American Medical Association, 260, 367–372. PubMed doi:10.1001/jama.260.3.367doi:10.1001/jama.260.3.367

Piette, J. D., Weinberger, M., Kraemer, F. B., & McPhee, S. J. (2001). The impact of automated calls with nurse follow-up on diabetes treatment outcomes in a Veterans Affairs health care system. *Diabetes Care*, *24*(2), 202–208. doi:10.2337/diacare.24.2.202

Pirnejad, H., Bal, R., Stoop, A. P., & Berg, M. (2007). Infrastructures to support integrated care: connecting across institutional and professional boundaries: Inter-organisational communication networks in healthcare: centralised versus decentralised approaches. *International Journal of Integrated Care*, *7*, 14.

Pitsillides, A., Pitsillides, B., Samaras, G., Dikaikos, M., Christodoulou, E., Andreou, P., & Georgiadis, D. (2004). DITIS: A collaborative virtual medical team for home healthcare of cancer patients . In Istepanian, R., Laxminarayan, S., & Pattichis, C. (Eds.), *M-Health: emerging mobile health systems*. New York: Kluwer Academic/Plenum.

Pitt, L. F., Watson, R. T., & Kavan, C. B. (1995). Service Quality: A Measure of Information Systems Effectiveness. *Management Information Systems Quarterly*, *19*(2), 173–187. doi:10.2307/249687

Poon, E. G., Cina, J. L., Churchill, W., Patel, N., Featherstone, E., & Rothschild, J. M. (2006). Medication dispensing errors and potential adverse drug events before and after implementing bar code technology in the pharmacy. *Annals of Internal Medicine*, *145*(6), 426–434.

Preece, J. (2000). *Online communities – Designing usability, supporting sociability*. Chichester, UK: Wiley & Sons, Ltd.

Price, D. (2005, May). Continuing medical education, quality improvement, and organizational change: implications of recent theories for twenty-first-century CME. *Medical Teacher*, *27*(3), 259–268. doi:10.1080/01421590500046270

Privateer, P. M. (1999). Academic technology and the future of higher education: Strategic paths taken and not taken. *The Journal of Higher Education*, *70*(1), 60–79. doi:10.2307/2649118

Quaglini, S., Stefanelli, M., Lanzola, G., Caporusso, V., & Panzarasa, S. (2001). Flexible guideline-based patient careflow systems. *Artificial Intelligence in Medicine*, *22*, 65–80. doi:10.1016/S0933-3657(00)00100-7

Queensland Health. (2008). *Queensland Health Annual Report 2007-2008*. Brisbane, Queensland Government. Available at URL: http://www.health.qld.gov.au/publications/corporate/annual_reports/annualreport2008/default.asp

Rancaño, I., Rodrigo, J. A., Villa, R., Abdelsater, M., Díaz, R., & Alvarez, D. (2003). Evaluación de las páginas web en lengua española útiles para el médico de atención primaria. *Atencion Primaria*, *31*, 575–584. doi:10.1157/13048143

Ranci Ortigiosa, E. (2000). *La valutazione di qualità nei servizi sanitari*. Milano, Italy: Franco Angeli Edizioni.

Ras, E., Becker, M., & Koch, J. (2007). *Engineering Tele-Health Solutions in the Ambient Assisted Living Lab*. Paper presented at the Proceedings of the 21st International Conference on Advanced Information Networking and Applications Workshops.

Ravet, S. (2007). *From quality of eLearning to eQuality of learning*. Retrieved September 22, 2009 from http://www.qualityfoundation.org/index.php?m1=2&m2=28&page_id=34.

Ravitch, D. (1995). *National standards in American education: A citizen's guide*. Washington: Brookings Institution Press.

Reardon, T. (2005). Research Findings and Strategies for Assessing Telemedicine Costs. *Telemedicine and e-Health, 11*(3), 348-369.

Reddy, R., & Wladawsky-Berger, I. (co-chairs) (2001). *Transforming Health Care through Information Technology*. Arlington, VA: National Coordination Office for Information Technology Research & Development.

Regenstrief Institute, Inc. (2009). *Logical Observation Identifiers Names and Codes*. Retrieved July 21, 2009, from http://loinc.org/

Reibman, A. L., & Veeraraghavan, M. (1991). Reliability Modeling: An Overview for Svstem Designers. *Computer*, *24*(4), 49–57. doi:10.1109/2.76262

Remenyi, D. S. J., & Money, A. (1991). A user-satisfaction approach to IS effectiveness measurement. *Journal of Information Technology*, *6*, 162–175. doi:10.1057/jit.1991.30

Reussner, R. H., Schmidt, H. W., & Poernomo, I. H. (2003). Reliability prediction for component-based software architectures. *Journal of Systems and Software*, *66*(3), 241–252. doi:10.1016/S0164-1212(02)00080-8

Reuters. (2003) Consumer-targeted internet investment: online strategies to improve patient care and product positioning. Reuters Business Insight Report; May.

Richardson, R. (2003). eHealth for Europe. *Studies in Health Technology and Informatics*, *96*, 151–156.

Richardson, R., Schug, S., Bywater, M., & Lloyd-Williams, D. (2004). *Development of eHealth in Europe: Position Paper*. Brussels: European Health Telematics Association.

Riegman, P. H., Morente, M. M., Betsou, F., de Blasio, P., & Geary, P. (2008). Biobanking for better healthcare. *Molecular Oncology*, *2*(3), 213–222. doi:10.1016/j.molonc.2008.07.004

Rifkin, J. (2004). *The European Dream: How Europe's Vision of the Future is Quietly Eclipsing the American Dream*. Cambridge: Polity Press.

Riva, G. (2003). Ambient Intelligence in Health Care. *Cyberpsychology & Behavior*, *6*(3), 295–300. doi:10.1089/109493103322011597

Rivard, P. E., Rosen, A. K., & Carroll, J. S. (2006). Enhancing patient safety through organizational learning: Are patient safety indicators a step in the right direction? *Health Services Research*, *41*(4 Pt 2), 1633–1653. doi:10.1111/j.1475-6773.2006.00569.x

Rochlin, G. I., La Porte, T.R., & Roberts, K. H., K.H. (1987). The Self-Designing High-Reliability Organization: Aircraft Carrier Flight Operations at Sea. *Naval War College Review*, *40*(4), 76–90.

Rogers, W. A. (2004). Evidence based medicine and justice: a framework for looking at the impact of EBM upon vulnerable or disadvantaged groups. *Journal of Medical Ethics*, *30*(1), 141–145. doi:10.1136/jme.2003.007062

Rogers, E. M. (2003). *Diffusion of innovations* (5th ed.). Washington, DC: Free Press.

Rogers, J. E. (2006). Quality assurance of medical ontologies. *Methods of Information in Medicine*, *45*(3), 267–274.

Rong-Huang, Q. (2003). Creating informed consumers and achieving shared decisions making. *Family Physician*, *32*, 335–341.

Ross, S. E., Moore, L. A., Earnest, M. A., Wittevrongel, L., & Lin, C. T. (2004). Providing a web-based online medical record with electronic communication capabilities to patients with congestive heart failure: randomized trial. *Journal of Medical Internet Research*, *6*(2), e12. doi:10.2196/jmir.6.2.e12

Rossi Mori, A. (2008). *eHealth deployment roadmap and roll-out planning: Guiding design principles.* Paper presented at the eHealth Planning and Management Symposium, Copenhagen, Denmark.

Rotheram-Borus, M. J., & Flannery, N. D. (2004). Interventions that are CURRES: costeffective, useful, realistic, robust, evolving, and sustainable . In Remschmidt, H., Belfer, M. L., & Goodyer, I. (Eds.), *Facilitating Pathways. Care, Treatment and Prevention in Child and Adolescent Mental Health* (pp. 235–244). New York: Springer.

Rubiera, G., Arbizu, R., Alzueta, A., Agúndez, J. J., & Riera, J. J. (2004). La legibilidad de los documentos de consentimiento informado en los hospitales de Asturias. *Gaceta Sanitaria*, *18*, 153–158. doi:10.1157/13059288

Ruchlin, H. S., Dubbs, N. L., & Callahan, M. A. (2004). The role of leadership in instilling a culture of safety: lessons from the literature. *Journal of Healthcare Management*, *49*(1), 47–58.

Rudnisky, C. J., Tennant, M. T. S., & Weis, E. (2007). Web-based grading of compressed stereoscopic digital photography versus standard film photography for the diagnosis of diabetic retinopathy. *Ophthalmology*, *114*(9), 1748–1754. doi:10.1016/j.ophtha.2006.12.010

Runciman, W. B. (2002). Lessons from the Australian Patient Safety Foundation: setting up a national patient safety surveillance system – is this the right model? *Quality & Safety in Health Care*, *11*, 246–251. doi:10.1136/qhc.11.3.246

Sachdeva, R. C., & Jain, S. (2009). Making the case to improve quality and reduce costs in pediatric health care. *Pediatric Clinics of North America*, *56*(4), 731–743. doi:10.1016/j.pcl.2009.05.013

Sackett, D. (1997). Using evidence-based medicine to help physicians keep up-to-date. *The Journal for the Serials Community*, *9*, 178–181. doi:10.1629/09178

Sackett, D., & Straus, S. (1998). Finding and applying evidence during clinical rounds: The evidence cart. *Journal of the American Medical Association*, *280*, 1336–1338. doi:10.1001/jama.280.15.1336

Sackett, D. (2003). Evidence-based medicine. What is it and what it isn't. *The Origins and Aspirations of ACP Journal Club.* Retrieved January 20, 2009, from http://www.minervation.com/cebm/ebmisisnt.html

Sackett, D. L., Straus, S. E., Richardson, W. S., Rosenberg, W., & Haynes, R. B. (2000). Evidence-*Based Madicine. Now to Practice and Teach EBM.* Second Edition, Churcill Livingstone, Edinburg, London, New York & al., as well as in [http://www.library.utoronto.ca/medicine/ebm/].

SAGES (Society of American Gastrointestinal and Endoscopic Surgeons). (2004). *Guidelines for the Surgical Practice of Telemedicine*. Retrieved May 13, 2009, from http://www.sages.org/sagespublication.php?doc=21

Sanazaro, P. (1980). Quality Assessment and Quality Assurance in Medical Care. *Annual Review of Public Health*, *1*, 37–68. doi:10.1146/annurev.pu.01.050180.000345

Sang Kim, Y. (2008). *Surgical Telementoring Initiation of a Regional Telemedicine Network: Projection of Surgical Expertise in the WWAMI Region.* Paper presented at the Third International Conference on Convergence and Hybrid Information Technology.

Sanger, L. (2001). *Let's make a wiki.* Message posted to http://web.archive.org/web/20030414014355/http://www.nupedia.com/pipermail/nupedia-l/2001-January/000676.html

Santo, A., Laizner, A. M., & Shohet, L. (2005). Exploring the value of audiotapes for health literacy: a systematic review. *Patient Education and Counseling*, *58*(3), 235–243. doi:10.1016/j.pec.2004.07.001

Sarnikar, S., & Gupta, A. (2007). *A context-specific mediating schema approach for information exchange between heterogeneous hospital systems.* Forthcoming in International Journal of Healthcare Technology and Management.

Sarnikar, S., Zhao, J., & Gupta, A. (2005). Medical information filtering using content-based and rule-based profiles. In *Proceedings of the AIS Americas Conference on Information Systems (AMCIS 2005),* Omaha, NE.

Savage, J., & Morre, L. (2004). *Intrpreting Accountability: An ethnographic study of practice nurses, accountability and multidisciplinary team decision-making in the context of clinical governance*. London: RCN Institute.

Savastano, M., Hovsto, A., Pharow, P., & Blobel, B. (2008). Security, safety, and related technology - the triangle of eHealth service provision. *Studies in Health Technology and Informatics*, *136*, 709–714.

Schey, S. (2001). *Guidelines for Haemo-oncology Treatment Processes* [Internal Document]. London: Guys and St Thomas' Hospitals NHS Trust.

Schiff, G. D., Aggarwal, H. C., Kumar, S., & McNutt, R. A. (2000). Prescribing potassium despite hyperkalemia: medication errors uncovered by linking laboratory and pharmacy information systems. *The American Journal of Medicine*, *109*, 494–497. doi:10.1016/S0002-9343(00)00546-5

Schiff, G. D., & Rucker, T. D. (1998). Computerized prescribing: building the electronic infrastructure for better medication usage. *Journal of the American Medical Association*, *279*, 1024–1029. doi:10.1001/jama.279.13.1024

Schiffauerova, A., & Thomson, V. (2006). A review of research on cost of quality models and best practices. *International Journal of Quality & Reliability Management*, *23*(6), 647–669. doi:10.1108/02656710610672470

Schommer, J. C., Pedersen, C. A., Doucette, W. R., Gaither, C. A., & Mott, D. A. (2002). Community pharmacists' work activities in the United States during 2000. *Journal of the American Pharmacists Association*, *42*(3), 399–406. doi:10.1331/108658002763316815

Schulz, E. B., Barret, J. W., & Price, C. (1998). Read Code Quality Assurance From Simple Syntax to Semantic Stability. *Journal of the American Medical Informatics Association*, *5*(4), 337–346.

Schwartz, K. L., Roe, T., Northrup, J., Meza, J., Seifeldin, R., & Neale, A. V. (2006). Family medicine patients' use of the Internet for health information: a MetroNet study. *Journal of the American Board of Family Medicine*, *19*, 39–45. doi:10.3122/jabfm.19.1.39

Schwartz, B. (2004). *The paradox of choice*. New York: HarperCollins Publishers.

Sciacovelli, L., Secchiero, S., Zardo, L., D'Osualdo, A., & Plebani, M. (2007). Risk management in laboratory medicine: quality assurance programs and professional competence. *Clinical Chemistry and Laboratory Medicine*, *45*, 756–765. doi:10.1515/CCLM.2007.165

Scott, J. T., Harmsen, M., Prictor, M. J., Entwistle, V. A., Sowden, A. J., & Watt, I. (2003). Recordings or summaries of consultations for people with cancer. *Cochrane. Database.of Systematic Reviews*, *2*, CD001539.

Scrivens, E. (1997). *Accreditamento dei servizi sanitari: Esperienze internazionali a confronto*. Torino, Italy: Centro Scientifico Editore.

Seibert, J. A., Kent, J. S., & Geiss, R. A. (2004). *Practice guideline for electronic medical information privacy and security*. Retrieved May 13, 2009, from http://www.acr.org/SecondaryMainMenuCategories/quality_safety/guidelines/med_phys/electronic_medical_info.aspx

SEIS. Sistema de Información Esencial en Terapéutica y Salud. Retrieved October 23, 2008 from: http://www.icf.uab.es/informacion/Papyrus/

SEMFYC. Sociedad Española de Medicina Familiar y Comunitaria. Informatización en la Atención Primaria. Documento nº 13. Retrieved October 13, 2008 from: http://www.semfyc.es/es/actividades/publicaciones/documentos-semfyc/docum013.html.

Senge, P. (1994). *The fifth discipline: The art and practice of the learning organization*. New York: Doubleday/Currency.

Senge, P. M. (2004). The leader's New Work: Building learning organizations. In K. Starkey, S. Tempest, & A. McKinlay (Eds.), *How Organizations Learn: Managing the search for knowledge* (pp. 462-486), 2nd. London, UK: Thomson Learning.

Shahar, Y., Miksch, S., & Johnson, P. (1998). The Asgaard Project: a task-specific Framework for the application and critiquing of time-oriented clinical guidelines. *Artificial Intelligence in Medicine*, *14*, 29–51. doi:10.1016/S0933-3657(98)00015-3

Shannon, C. E. (2001). A mathematical theory of communication. *ACM SIGMOBILE Mobile Computing and Communications Review, Special issue dedicated to Claude E. Shannon*, *5*(1), 3–55.

Shapiro, G. T., & Frawley, W. J. (Eds.). (1991). *Knowledge Discovery in Databases*. San Francisco: AAAI/MIT Press.

Sharma, R. (2005). *Automatic integration of text documents in the medical domain.* Undergraduate Thesis, University of Arizona.

Shen, Z., & Yang, Z. (2001). The Problems and Strategy relevant to the Quality Management of Clinical Laboratories. *Clinical Chemistry and Laboratory Medicine*, *39*(12), 1216–1218. doi:10.1515/CCLM.2001.194

Sheppard, L., & Mackintosh, S. (1998). Technology in education: What is appropriate for rural and remote allied health professionals? *The Australian Journal of Rural Health*, *6*(4), 189–193. doi:10.1111/j.1440-1584.1998.tb00311.x

Shiffman, R. N., Michel, G., Essaihi, A., & Thornquist, E. (2004). Bridging the Guideline Implementation Gap: A Systematic, Document-Centered Approach to Guideline Implementation. *Journal of the American Medical Informatics Association*, *11*(5), 418–426. doi:10.1197/jamia.M1444

Shojania, K. G., & Forster, A. J. (2008). Hospital mortality: when failure is not a good measure of success. *Canadian Medical Association Journal*, *179*, 153–157. doi:10.1503/cmaj.080010

Siebenhofer, A., Berghold, A., & Sawicki, P. T. (2004). Systematic review of studies of self-management of oral anticoagulation. *Thrombosis and Haemostasis, 91* (2), 225-232. Smith, SP., Barefield, AC. (2007). Patients meet technology: the newest in patient-centered care initiatives. *The Health Care Manager*, *26*(4), 354–362.

Siegel, E., Krupinski, E., & Samei, E. (2006). Digital mammography image quality: image display. *Journal of the American College of Radiology*, *3*(8), 615–627. doi:10.1016/j.jacr.2006.03.007

Simmons, B., & Wagner, S. (2009). Assessment of continuing interprofessional education: lessons learned . *The Journal of Continuing Education in the Health Professions*, *29*(3), 168–171. doi:10.1002/chp.20031

Singer, S. J., Falwell, A., Gaba, D. M., & Baker, L. C. (2008). Patient safety climate in US hospitals: variation by management level. *Medical Care*, *46*(11), 1149–1156. doi:10.1097/MLR.0b013e31817925c1

Sittig, D. F., & Stead, W. W. (1994). Computer-based physician order entry: the state of the art. *Journal of the American Medical Informatics Association*, *1*, 108–123.

Slawson, D. C., & Shaughnessy, A. F. (2000). Becoming an information master: using POEMs to change practice with confidence. Patient-oriented evidence that matters. [Retrieved from]. *The Journal of Family Practice*, *49*, 63–67.

Slawson, D., Hauck, F., Strayer, S., & Rollins, L. (2007). *What is information master?* Retrieved from http://www.healthsystem.virginia.edu/internet/familymed/docs/info_mastery.cfm#Information

Slutsky, J. (2008). Session Current Care - G-I-N abstracts. Retrieved March, 27, 2009 from [http://www.g-i-n.net/download/files/G_I_N_newsletter_May_2008.pdf]

Smedberg, Å. (2007a). *How to combine the online community with Ask the expert system in a health care site – A comparison of online health systems usage.* IEEE Computer Society Press.

Smedberg, Å. (2008a). Learning conversations for people with established bad habits: A study of four health-communities. *International Journal of Healthcare Technology and Management*, *9*(2), 143–154. doi:10.1504/IJHTM.2008.017369

Smedberg, Å. (2004). Learning through online communities: A study of health-care sites in Europe . In Cunningham, P., & Cunningham, M. (Eds.), *eAdoption and the Knowledge Economy: Issues, Applications, Case Studies* (pp. 1333–1339). Amsterdam, The Netherlands: IOS Press.

Smedberg, Å. (2007b). To design holistic health service systems on the Internet. In *Proceedings of World Academy of Science, Engineering and Technology*, November 2007 (pp. 311-317). Retrieved from: http://www.waset.org/journals/waset/v31/v31-56.pdf.

Smedberg, Å. (2008b). Online health-communities on bad habits for preventive care. In *Proceedings of the 4th Kuala Lumpur International Conference on Biomedical Engineering (Biomed2008), 25-28 June 2008* (pp. 291-294). Kuala Lumpur, Malaysia.

Smith, A. C., Batch, J., Lang, E., & Wootton, R. (2003). The use of online health techniques for the delivery of specialist paediatric diabetes services in Queensland . *Journal of Telemedicine and Telecare*, *9*(Suppl. 2), 54–57. doi:10.1258/135763303322596273

Smith, A. C., Coulthard, M., Clark, R., Armfield, N., Taylor, S., & Mottarelly, I. (2005). Wireless telemedicine for the delivery of specialist paediatric services to the bedside. *Journal of Telemedicine and Telecare*, *11*(Suppl 2), 81–85. doi:10.1258/135763305775124669

Smith, A. C., Dowthwaite, S., Agnew, J., & Wootton, R. (2008). Concordance between real-time telemedicine assessments and face-to-face consultations in paediatric otolaryngology. *The Medical Journal of Australia*, *188*(8), 457–460.

Smith, A. C., & Gray, L. C. (2009). Telemedicine across the ages. *The Medical Journal of Australia*, *190*(1), 15–19.

Smith, A. C., Kimble, R., Bailey, D., Mill, J., & Wootton, R. (2004). Diagnostic accuracy of and patient satisfaction with telemedicine for the follow-up of paediatric burns patients. *Journal of Telemedicine and Telecare, 10*(4), 193–198. doi:10.1258/1357633041424449

Smith, A. C., Patterson, V., & Scott, R. E. (2007). Reducing your carbon footprint: How telemedicine helps? *British Medical Journal, 335*, 1060. doi:10.1136/bmj.39402.471863.BE

Smith, A. C., Perry, C., Agnew, J., & Wootton, R. (2006). Accuracy of pre-recorded video images for the assessment of rural indigenous children with ear, nose and throat conditions. *Journal of Telemedicine and Telecare, 12*(Suppl. 3), 76–80. doi:10.1258/135763306779380138

Smith, A. C., Williams, J., Agnew, J., Sinclair, S., Youngberry, K., & Wootton, R. (2005). Real-time telemedicine for paediatric otolaryngology pre-admission screening . *Journal of Telemedicine and Telecare, 11*(Suppl 2), 86–89. doi:10.1258/135763305775124821

Smith, A. C., Williams, M., & Justo, R. (2002). The multidisciplinary management of a paediatric cardiac emergency. *Journal of Telemedicine and Telecare, 8*, 112–114. doi:10.1258/1357633021937578

Smith, A. C., Youngberry, K., Mill, J., Kimble, R., & Wootton, R. (2004). A review of three years experience using email and videoconferencing for delivery of post-acute burns care to children in Queensland. *Burns, 30*(3), 248–252. doi:10.1016/j.burns.2003.11.003

Smith, Moore T., Francis, M. D., & Corrigan, J. M. (2007). Health care quality in the 21st century. *Clinical and Experimental Rheumatology, 25*, 3–5.

Smothers, V., Greene, P., Ellaway, R., & Detmer, D. (2008, March). Sharing innovation: the case for technology standards in health professions education. *Medical Teacher, 30*(2), 150–154. doi:10.1080/01421590701874082

Soller, A. (2001). Supporting social interaction in an intelligent collaborative learning system. *International Journal of Artificial Intelligence in Education, 12*(1), 40–62.

Soller, A., & Lesgold, A. (2000). Modeling the process of collaborative learning. In *Proceedings of the International Workshop on New Technologies in Collaborative Learning*. Awaji-Yumebutai, Japan. Retrieved from http://www.cscl-research.com/Dr/documents/Soller-Lesgold-NTCL2000.doc.

Sood, S., Mbarika, V., Jugoo, S., Dookhy, R., Doarn, C. R., Prakash, N., & Merrell, R. C. (2007). What is telemedicine? A collection of 104 peer-reviewed perspectives and theoretical underpinnings. *Telemedicine journal and e-health: the official journal of the American Telemedicine Association, 13*(5), 573-590.

Sowden, A. J., & Arblaster, L. (2000). Mass media interventions for preventing smoking in young people. *Cochrane.Database.of Systematic. Reviews, 2*, CD001006.

Spencer, E., & Walshe, K. (2008). Quality and safety in healthcare in Europe. A growing challenge for policymakers. *Harvard Health Policy Review, 1*, 46–54.

Spencer, E., & Walshe, K. (2009). National quality improvement policies and strategies in European Healthcare Systems. *Quality & Safety in Health Care, 18*, 22–27. doi:10.1136/qshc.2008.029355

Spyrou, S., Bamidis, P. D., Maglaveras, N., Pangalos, G., & Pappas, C. (2008). A methodology for reliability analysis in health networks. *IEEE Transactions on Information Technology in Biomedicine, 12*(3), 377–386. doi:10.1109/TITB.2007.905125

Stahl, L., & Spatz, M. (2003, January). Quality Assurance in eHealth for Consumers. [from Health Source: Nursing/Academic Edition database.]. *Journal of Consumer Health on the Internet, 7*(1), 33. Retrieved September 27, 2009. doi:10.1300/J381v07n01_03

Stalberg, P., Yeh, M., Ketteridge, G., Delbridge, H., & Delbridge, L. (2008). E-mail Access and Improved Communication Between Patient and Surgeon. *Archives of Surgery, 143*(2), 164–169. doi:10.1001/archsurg.2007.31

Standards, R. F. I. D. Retrieved September 30, 2009 from http://www.corerfid.com/technology/TechnologyIssues/IssuesStandards.aspx

Steel, N., Melzer, D., & Shekelle, P. G., & al. (2004). Developing quality indicators for older adults: transfer from the USA to the UK is feasible. *Quality & Safety in Health Care*, *13*(4), 260–264. doi:10.1136/qshc.2004.010280

Stell, A., Sinnott, R., Ajayi, O., & Jiang, J. (2007). *Security Oriented e-Infrastructures Supporting Neurological Research and Clinical Trials.* Paper presented at the Proceedings of the The Second International Conference on Availability, Reliability and Security.

Stephenson, K., Peloquin, S., Richmond, S., Hinman, M., & Christiansen, C. (2002). Changing Educational Paradigms to Prepare Allied Health Professionals for the 21st Century. *Education for Health: Change in Learning & Practice (Taylor & Francis Ltd), 15*(1), 37-49.

Sternberg, D. J. (2002). Seven steps to e-health success. [from ABI/INFORM Global.]. *Marketing Health Services*, *22*(2), 44–47. Retrieved August 23, 2009.

Sterritt, R., & Bantz, D. F. (2004). *PAC-MEN: Personal Autonomic Computing Monitoring Environment.* Paper presented at the Database and Expert Systems Applications, 15th International Workshop.

Sterritt, R., & Hinchey, M. (2005a). *Autonomicity – An Antidote for Complexity?* Paper presented at the Proceedings of the 2005 IEEE Computational Systems Bioinformatics Conference - Workshops.

Sterritt, R., & Hinchey, M. (2005b). *Why Computer-Based Systems Should be Autonomic.* Paper presented at the Proceedings of the 12th IEEE International Conference and Workshops on Engineering of Computer-Based Systems.

Stevens, A., & Milne, R. (2004). Health technology assessment in England and Wales. *International Journal of Technology Assessment in Health Care*, *20*(1), 11–24. doi:10.1017/S0266462304000741

Stiglitz, J. (2000). *Economics of the Public Sector*. New York: W. W. Norton & Co Inc.

Stone, E. G., Morton, S. C., Hulscher, M. E., Maglione, M. A., Roth, E. A., & Grimshaw, J. M. (2002). Interventions that increase use of adult immunization and cancer screening services: a meta-analysis. *Annals of Internal Medicine*, *136*(9), 641–651.

Stone, A. A., Shiffman, S., Schwartz, J. E., Broderick, J. E., & Hufford, M. R. (2003). Patient compliance with paper and electronic diaries. *Controlled Clinical Trials*, *24*(2), 182–199. doi:10.1016/S0197-2456(02)00320-3

Straub, D. W., Boudreau, M.-C., & Gefen, D. (2004). Validation Guidelines for IS Positivist Research. *Communications of the Association for Information Systems*, *13*, 380–427.

Street, R. L., Gold, W. R., & Manning, T. R. (Eds.). (1997). *Health Promotion and Interactive Technology. Theoretical Applications and Future Directions.* New York: Routledge, Taylor & Francis Group.

Suárez, J., Beltrán, C., Molina, T., & Navarro, P. (2005). Receta electrónica: de la utopía a la realidad. *Atencion Primaria*, *35*, 451–459. doi:10.1157/13075469

Sullivan, F., & Wyatt, J. (2005). Is a consultation needed? *British Medical Journal*, *331*, 625–627. doi:10.1136/bmj.331.7517.625

Suñol, R., Vallejo, P., Thompson, A., Lombarts, M. J. M. H., Shaw, C. D., & Klazinga, N. (2009). Impact of quality strategies on hospital outputs. *Quality & Safety in Health Care*, *18*, 57–63. doi:10.1136/qshc.2008.029439

Survey of states finds boom in e-health strategies. (2008, July). *State Health Watch*. Retrieved March 4, 2009, from Academic Search Complete database.

Sutherland, L., Igras, E., Ulmer, R., Sargious, P. (2000). A laboratory for testing the interoperability of telehealth systems. *Journal of Telemedicine and Telecare*, 6- Suppl 2, S74-75.

Swanwick, T., Ahluwalia, S., Rennison, T., & Talbot, T. (2007). The Quality and Outcomes Framework (QOF) and the assessment of training practices as learning organisations. *Education for Primary Care*, *18*(2), 173–179.

Tate, D. F., Jackvony, E. H., & Wing, R. R. (2003). Effects of Internet behavioral counseling on weight loss in adults at risk for type 2 diabetes: a randomized trial. *Journal of the American Medical Association, 289*, 1833–1836. doi:10.1001/jama.289.14.1833

Tate, D. F., Wing, R. R., & Winett, R. A. (2001). Using Internet technology to deliver a behavioral weight loss program. *Journal of the American Medical Association, 285*(9), 1172–1177. doi:10.1001/jama.285.9.1172

Taylor, P. (1998a). A survey of research in telemedicine. 1: Telemedicine systems. *Journal of Telemedicine and Telecare, 4*, 1–17. doi:10.1258/1357633981931227

Taylor, P. (1998b). A survey of research in telemedicine. 2: Telemedicine services. *Journal of Telemedicine and Telecare, 4*, 63–71. doi:10.1258/1357633981931948

Tegnér, J. N., Compte, A., Auffray, C., An, G., Cedersund, G., & Clermont, G. (2009). Computational disease modeling - fact or fiction? *BMC Systems Biology, 3*, 56. doi:10.1186/1752-0509-3-56

Terwilliger, T. C., Stuart, D., & Yokoyama, S. (2009). Lessons from structural genomics. *Annual Review of Biophysics, 38*, 371–383. doi:10.1146/annurev.biophys.050708.133740

Thai, J., Pekilis, B., Lau, A., & Seviora, R. (2001). *Aspect-Oriented Implementation of Software Health Indicators.* Paper presented at the Eighth Asia-Pacific Software Engineering Conference.

The Lewin Group. Inc. (2002). Assessment of Approaches to Evaluating Telemedicine, Final Report: Prepared for Department of Health and Human Services Contract Number HHS-10-97-0012.

The National Alliance for Health Information Technology. (2008). *Defining Key Health Information Technology Terms*. Washington, DC: Department of Health & Human Services.

Theodore, L., & Turocy, B. (2001). *Texas A&M University London School of Economics.* CDAM Research Report LSE-CDAM-2001-09.

Thompson, A. E., & Graydon, S. L. (2009). Patient oriented methotrexate information sites on the Internet: A review of completeness, accuracy, format, reliability, credibility, and readability. *The Journal of Rheumatology, 36*, 41–49.

Thompson, A. (2004). Moving beyond the rhetoric of citizen involvement: Strategies for enablement. *Eurohealth, 9*(4), 5–8.

Thurmond, V. A., & Boyle, D. K. (2002). An integrative review of patients' perceptions regarding telehealth used in their health care. *The Online Journal of Knowledge Synthesis for Nursing, E9*(1), 12–32.

Timperio, A., & Crawford, D. A. (2004). Public definitions of success in weight management. *Nutrition & Dietetics, 61*, 215–220.

Tingle, J. (1995). The legal accountability of the nurse . In Watson, R. (Ed.), *Accountability in Nursing Practice* (pp. 163–176). London: Chapman and Hall.

Tirri, K., & Nevgi, A. (2000). *In search of a Good Virtual Teacher.* Annual European Conference on Educational Research, Edinburgh, United Kingdom. Retrieved from http://www.eric.ed.gov/ERICDocs/data/ericdocs2sql/content_storage_01/0000019b/80/16/b6/9f.pdf

Townend, J. N. (2007). Guidelines on guidelines. *Lancet, 370*, 740. doi:10.1016/S0140-6736(07)61376-2

Trivers, R. L. (1971). The Evolution of Reciprocal Altruism. *The Quarterly Review of Biology, 46*, 35–57. doi:10.1086/406755

Troster, J., Henshaw, J., & Buss, E. (1993). *Filtering for quality.* Paper presented at the Proceedings of the 1993 conference of the Centre for Advanced Studies on Collaborative research: software engineering.

Truman, B. I., Smith-Akin, C. K., & Hinman, A. R. (2000). Developing the Guide to Community Preventive Services--overview and rationale. The Task Force on Community Preventive Services. *American Journal of Preventive Medicine, 18*(1), 18–26. doi:10.1016/S0749-3797(99)00124-5

Tu, S. W., & Musen, M. A. (1999). *A flexible approach to guideline modeling* (pp. 420–424). Proc. AMIA Symp.

Tudiver, F., Rose, D., Banks, B., & Pfortmiller, D. (2004). Reliability and Validity Testing of an Evidence-Based Medicine OSCE Station. *Society of Teachers in Family Medicine meeting*, Toronto, May 14, 2004. Date Submitted: May 22, 2008. Retrieved March 22, 2009 from http://www.stfm.org/fmhub/fm2009/February/Fred89.pdf

Tufte, E. (2001). *The visual display of quantitative information*. Cheshire, CT: Graphics Press.

Tulu, B., Chatterjee, S., & Laxminarayan, S. (2005). *A Taxonomy of Telemedicine Efforts with Respect to Applications, Infrastructure, Delivery Tools, Type of Setting and Purpose*. Paper presented at the 38th Annual Hawaii International Conference on System Sciences.

UEMS. 2007.19 – Bratislava Declaration on eMedicine. (2009, February 25). Retrieved June 17, 2009, from http://admin.uems.net/uploadedfiles/893.pdf.

Underhill, C., & Mkeown, L. (2008). Getting a second opinion: health information and the Internet. *Health Reports*, *19*, 65–69.

US Department of Health and Human Services. (1999). Managing the Risk from Medical Product Use, Creating a Risk Management Framework. Retrieved from http://www.fda.gov/downloads/Safety/SafetyofSpecificProducts/UCM180520.pdf

Vacata, V., Jahns-Streubel, G., Baldus, M., & Wood, W. G. (2007). Practical solution for control of the pre-analytical phase in decentralized clinical laboratories for meeting the requirements of the medical laboratory accreditation standard DIN EN ISO 15189. *Clinical Laboratory*, *53*, 211–215.

Valenčík, R. (2003). *Theory of a productive consumption (Teorie produktivní spotřeby)*. Praha, Czech Republic: Vysoká škola finanční a správní o.p.s.

Van Bemmel, J. H. (1984). The structure of medical informatics. *Medical Informatics*, *9*, 175–180. doi:10.3109/14639238409015187

Van Bemmel, J. H., & Musen, M. A. (Eds.). (1997). *Handbook of Medical Informatics*. Heidelberg, Germany: Springer.

Van Halteren, A., Konstantas, D., Bults, R., Wac, K., Dokovsky, N., & Koprinkov, G. (2004). MobiHealth: Ambulant Patient Monitoring Over Next Generation Public Wireless Networks . In Demiris, G. (Ed.), *E-Health: Current Status and Future Trends* (*Vol. 106*). Amsterdam: IOS Press.

Van Moore, A., Allen, B., & Campbell, S. C. (2005). Report of the ACR task force on international teleradiology. *Journal of the American College of Radiology*, *2*(2), 121–125. doi:10.1016/j.jacr.2004.08.003

Vanhecke, T., Barnes, M., Zimmerman, J., & Shoichet, S. (2006). *PubMed vs. HighWire Press: A head-to-head comparison of two medical literature search engines*. Computers in Biology and Medicine.

Varkey, P., Reller, K., & Resar, R. (2007, June). Basics of Quality Improvement in Health Care. [from Academic Search Complete database.]. *Mayo Clinic Proceedings*, *82*(6), 735–739. Retrieved September 30, 2009. doi:10.4065/82.6.735

Varlamis, I., & Apostolakis, I. (2007). *Self supportive web communities in the service of patients*. In Proceecings of IADIS International Conference on Web Based Communities (pp 133-140). Salamanca, Spain.

Veillard, J., Champagne, F., & Klazinga, N., & al. (2005). A performance assessment framework for hospitals: the WHO regional office for Europe PATH Project. *International Journal for Quality in Health Care*, *17*(6), 487–496. doi:10.1093/intqhc/mzi072

Vergados, D. D. (2007). Simulation and Modeling Bandwidth Control in Wireless Healthcare Information Systems. *Simulation*, *83*(4), 347–364. doi:10.1177/0037549707083114

Vincent, C., Taylor-Adams, S., & Stanhope, N. (1998). Framework for analysing risk and safety in clinical medicine. *British Medical Journal*, *316*, 1154–1157.

VirRAD - The Virtual Radiopharmacy - a Mindful Learning Environment (2007). Retrieved from http:// community.virrad.eu.org/.

Vitacca, M., Mazzu, M., & Scalvini, S. (2009). Socio-technical and organizational challenges to wider e-Health implementation. *Chronic Respiratory Disease*, *6*(2), 91–97. doi:10.1177/1479972309102805

Voicu, L. C., Schuldt, H., Breitbart, Y., & Schek, H. J. (2009). *Replicated Data Management in the Grid: The Re:GRIDiT Approach.* Paper presented at the 1st ACM workshop on Data grids for eScience.

Volckaert, B., Thysebaert, P., De Leenheer, M., De Turck, F., Dhoedt, B., & Demeester, P. (2004). Grid computing: the next network challenge! *Journal of the Communications Network*, *3*, 159–165.

Vygotsky, L. (1934). *Thought and language*. MIT Press.

Wac, K., van Halteren, A., & Konstantas, D. (2006). *QoS-Predictions Service: Infrastructural Support for Proactive QoS- and Context-Aware Mobile Services (Position Paper) On the Move to Meaningful Internet Systems 2006: OTM 2006 Workshops*. Berlin: Springer Berlin / Heidelberg.

Wac, K. (2005). *Towards QoS-awareness of Context-aware Mobile Applications and Services.* Paper presented at the On the Move to Meaningful Internet Systems 2005: OTM Workshops, Ph.D. Student Symposium.

Wachter, R. (2004). The End Of The Beginning: Patient Safety Five Years After 'To Err Is Human'. *Health Affairs*, 23534–23545.

Wagner, V., Dullaart, A., Bock, A. K., & Zweck, A. (2006). The emerging nanomedicine landscape. *Nature Biotechnology*, *24*(10), 1211–1217. doi:10.1038/nbt1006-1211

Wail, M. O., & Taleb-Bendiab, A. (2006). *Service Oriented Architecture for E-health Support Services Based on Grid Computing Over.* Paper presented at the IEEE International Conference on Services Computing.

Walker, R., Dieter, M., Panko, W., & Valenta, A. (2003). What it will take to create new Internet initiatives in health care. *Journal of Medical Systems*, *27*, 95–103. doi:10.1023/A:1021065330652

Wallace, S., Wyatt, J., & Taylor, P. (1998). Telemedicine in the NHS for the millennium and beyond. *Postgraduate Medical Journal*, *74*(878), 721–728. doi:10.1136/pgmj.74.878.721

Walston, S. L., & Bogue, R. J. (1999). The effects of reengineering: Fad or competitive factor? *Journal of Healthcare Management*, *44*(6), 456–474.

Walther, J. B., Pingree, S., Hawkins, R. P., & Buller, D. B. (2005). Attributes of interactive online health information systems. *Journal of Medical Internet Research*, *7*(3). doi:10.2196/jmir.7.3.e33

Wang, R. Y. (1998). A product perspective on Total Data Quality Management. *Communications of the ACM*, *41*(2), 58–65. doi:10.1145/269012.269022

Ward, J. P., Gordon, J., Field, M. J., & Lehmann, H. P. (2001). Communication and information technology in medical education. *Lancet*, *357*, 792–796. doi:10.1016/S0140-6736(00)04173-8

Warner, J. P., King, M., Blizard, R., McClenahan, Z., & Tang, S. (2000). Patient-held shared care records for individuals with mental illness. Randomised controlled evaluation. *The British Journal of Psychiatry*, *177*, 319–324. doi:10.1192/bjp.177.4.319

Weinberger, M., Murray, M. D., Marrero, D. G., Brewer, N., Lykens, M., & Harris, L. E. (2002). Issues in conducting randomized controlled trials of health services research interventions in nonacademic practice settings: the case of retail pharmacies. *Health Services Research*, *37*(4), 1067–1077. doi:10.1034/j.1600-0560.2002.66.x

Weiner, J., Kfuri, T., Chan, K., & Fowles, J. (2007). "e-Iatrogenesis": The Most Critical Unintended Consequence of CPOE and other HIT. *Journal of the American Medical Informatics Association*, *14*(3), 387–388. doi:10.1197/jamia.M2338

Weissleder, R., & Mahmood, U. (2001). Molecular imaging . *Radiology, 219*, 316–333.

Welschen, L. M., Bloemendal, E., Nijpels, G., Dekker, J. M., Heine, R. J., Stalman, W. A., & Bouter, L. M. (2005). Self-monitoring of blood glucose in patients with type 2 diabetes who are not using insulin. *Cochrane.Database. of Systematic.Reviews., (2),* CD005060.

Wenger, E. (2004). Communities of practice and social learning systems . In Starkey, K., Tempest, S., & McKinlay, A. (Eds.), *How organizations learn: Managing the search for knowledge* (2nd ed., pp. 238–258). London: Thomson Learning.

Wentling, T., Waight, C., Gallaher, J., La Fleur, J., Wang, C., & Kanfer, A. (2000). *E-Learning: A Review of Literature.* University of Illinois National Center for Supercomputer Applications, Urbana- Champaign, IL Retrieved January 30, 2009 from http://learning.ncsa.uiuc.edu/papers/elearnlit.pdf.

Westbrook, J. I., Georgiou, A., & Rob, M. I. (2008). Computerized order entry systems: sustained impact on laboratory efficiency and mortality rates? *Studies in Health Technology and Informatics*, *136*, 345–350.

WHO. (2009). *Environmental health.* Retrieved July 21, 2009, from http://www.who.int/topics/environmental_health/en/

WHO. (2009). *International Classification of Diseases (ICD).* Retrieved July 21, 2009, from http://www.who.int/classifications/icd/en/

Wikipedia. (2007a). *Information retrieval.* Retrieved from http://en.wikipedia.org/wiki/Information_retrieval.

Wikipedia. (2007b). *Wikipedia.* Retrieved from http://en.wikipedia.org/wiki/Wikipedia.

Wilkins, M., Pasquali, C., Appel, R., Ou, K., Golaz, O., & Sanchez, J. C. (1996). From Proteins to Proteomes: Large Scale Protein Identification by Two-Dimensional Electrophoresis and Arnino Acid Analysis. *Nature Biotechnology*, *14*(1), 61–65. doi:10.1038/nbt0196-61

Wilkins, M. R., Appel, R. D., Van Eyk, J. E., Chung, M. C., Gorg, A., & Hecker, M. (2006). Guidelines for the next 10 years of proteomics. *Proteomics*, *6*(1), 4–8. doi:10.1002/pmic.200500856

Williams, J., Cheung, W., Chetwynd, N., Cohen, D., El-Sharkawi, S., & Finlay, I. (2001). Pragmatic randomised trial to evaluate the use of patient held records for the continuing care of patients with cancer. *Quality in Health Care*, *10*(3), 159–165. doi:10.1136/qhc.0100159..

Williams, S. (2006). The Effectiveness of Distance Education in Allied Health Science Programs: A Meta-Analysis of Outcomes. *American Journal of Distance Education*, *20*(3), 127–141. doi:10.1207/s15389286ajde2003_2

Williams, M. B., Krupinski, E. A., & Strauss, K. J. (2007). Digital radiography image quality: image acquisition. *Journal of the American College of Radiology*, *4*(6), 371–388. doi:10.1016/j.jacr.2007.02.002

Wilson, P. (2005). *E-health - Building on Strength to Provide Better Healthcare Anytime Anywhere.* Paper presented at the eHealth 2005 Conference, Tromsø, Norway.

Winograd, T., & Flores, F. (1987). *Understanding computers and cognition: A new foundation for design.* Boston, MA: Addison-Wesley Publishing Company.

Wofford, J., Smith, E., & Miller, D. (2005). The multimedia computer for office-based patient education: a systematic review. *Patient Education and Counseling*, *59*(2), 148–157. doi:10.1016/j.pec.2004.10.011

Wong, H. J., Legnini, M. W., & Whitmore, H. H. (2000). The diffusion of decision support systems in healthcare: Are we there yet? *Journal of Healthcare Management*, *45*(4), 240–253.

World Health Organization. (2007). *People-Centred Health Care: A Policy Framework.* Geneva: World Health Organization.

Wyatt, J. (1997). Commentary: Measuring quality and impact of the world wide web. *British Medical Journal*, *314*, 1879–1881.

Xu, C., Smith, A. C., Scuffham, P. A., & Wootton, R. (2008). A cost minimisation analysis of telepaediatric otolaryngology service. *BMC Health Services Research*, *8*, 30. doi:10.1186/1472-6963-8-30

Yusof, M. M., Paul, R. J., & Stergioulas, L. K. (2006). *Towards a Framework for Health Information Systems Evaluation.* Paper presented at the 39th Annual Hawaii International Conference on System Sciences.

Zuckerman, A., & Coile, R. (2003). *Competing on Excellence: Healthcare Strategies for a Consumer-Driven Market.* Chicago, IL: Health Administration Press.

Zvárová, J., Dostálová, T., Hanzlíček, P., Teuberová, Z., Nagy, M., & Pieš, M. (2008). Electronic health record for forensic dentistry. *Methods of Information in Medicine*, *47*, 8–13.

Zvárová, J., Hanzlíček, P., Nagy, M., Přečková, P., Zvára, K., & Seidl, L. (2009). Biomedical Informatics Research for Individualized Life-Long Shared Healthcare. *Biocybernetis and Biomedical Engineering*, *29*(2), 31–41.

Zvárová, J., Veselý, A., & Vajda, I. (2009). Data, Information and Knowledge . In Berka, P., Rauch, J., & Zighed, D. A. (Eds.), *Data Mining and Medical Knowledge Management: Cases and Applications* (pp. 1–36). Hershey, PA: Medical Information Science.

About the Contributors

Anastasius Moumtzoglou is an Executive Board Member of the European Society for Quality in HealthCare (ESQH), and President of the Hellenic Society for Quality & Safety in HealthCare (HSQSH). He holds B.A in Economics (National & Kapodistrian University of Athens), MA in Health Services Management (National School of Public Health), MA in Macroeconomics (The University of Liverpool), and Ph.D. in Economics (National & Kapodistrian University of Athens), He works for 'P. & A. Kyriakou' Children's Hospital and teaches the module of quality at the graduate and postgraduate level. He has written three books, which are the only ones in the Greek references. He has also served as a scientific coordinator and researcher in Greek and European research programs. In 2004, he was declared "Person of Quality in Healthcare", with respect to Greece. His research interests include healthcare management, quality, knowledge management, pensions, and the dualism of the labor market.

Anastasia N. Kastania received her B.Sc. in Mathematics and her Ph.D degree in Medical Informatics from the National & Kapodistrian University of Athens, Greece. She works in the Athens University of Economics and Business, Greece since 1987. Research productivity is summarized in various articles (monographs or in collaboration with other researchers) in international journals, international conferences proceedings, international book series and international books chapters. She has more than twenty years teaching experience in University programs and she is the writer of many didactic books. She also has ten years experience as Researcher in National and European Research Projects. Research interests are telemedicine and e-health, e-learning, bioinformatics, tele-epidemiology, mathematical modeling and statistics, web engineering, quality engineering and reliability engineering.

* * *

Aleš Bourek (born 1957, Brno, Czech Republic) comes from a family of musicians. He is a medical doctor active since 1980 in the area of assisted reproduction. From 1990 he is also involved in activities relating to healthcare systems and health informatics and lectures these subjects at the Masaryk University and abroad. He works on national and international projects, is on the board of several medical journals and organizations, collaborates with ESQH, EFQM, WHO, World Bank and DG SANCO and favors non-presciptive methods of management. He is married to a hematologist, has two children, enjoys outdoor activities in extreme environments, the company of many exceptional friends, linguistics and systems thinking. His general view is that he is not a complete idiot (he is aware that some parts are still missing).

Aliki Stathopoulou received her bachelor degree from the Department of Biology, University of Crete, in 1994 and her PhD from the Medical School, University of Crete, in 2002. From 2002-2006 she worked as a Postdoctoral Researcher in the Laboratory of Clinical Chemistry, University of Athens. From 2003 to 2004 and from 2005 to 2007 she was employed as an Assistant Researcher in the Laboratory of Clinical Biochemistry and Molecular Biology, University General Hospital "ATTIKON", University of Athens. From 2006 she has been a Case officer of the Hellenic Accreditation System S.A. (ESYD S.A.), in the department of accreditation of clinical, chemical, biological and related testing laboratories. Since 2006, she has been appointed as the ESYD's delegate for the European co-operation for Accreditation Healthcare Working Group. She is a member of the Greek Society of Clinical Chemistry-Clinical Biochemistry and the Greek Society of Biologists. She has 15 papers of original scientific work published in Scientific Journals and 50 abstracts published in proceedings of conferences.

Amar Gupta is Tom Brown Endowed chair of management and technology; professor of entrepreneurship, management information systems, management of organizations, and computer science at the University of Arizona since 2004. Earlier, he was with the MIT Sloan School of Management (1979-2004); for half of this 25-year period, he served as the founding co-director of the Productivity from Information Technology (PROFIT) initiative. He has published over 100 papers, and serves as associate editor of ACM Transactions on Internet Technology and the Information Resources Management Journal. At the University of Arizona, Professor Gupta is the chief architect of new multi-degree graduate programs that involve concurrent study of management, entrepreneurship, and one specific technical or scientific domain. He has nurtured the development of several key technologies that are in widespread use today, and is currently focusing on the area of the 24-Hour Knowledge Factory.

Anne E. Burdick, MD, MPH, Associate Dean for Telemedicine and Clinical Outreach and Professor of Dermatology at the University of Miami, is expanding the Miller School of Medicine's clinical and educational telehealth services in the US and internationally. A graduate of New York University School of Medicine and Columbia University School of Public Health, she has over 15 years of telehealth experience. As a charter member of the American Telemedicine Association, she founded the ATA's Special Interest Group on Teledermatology and now serves as the Standards and Guidelines Committee Vice-Chair. Dr. Burdick is on the Editorial Board of the *Telemedicine Journal and e-Health.* She chaired the American Academy of Dermatology Telemedicine Task Force and received its 2007 Program in Innovative Continuing Medical Innovation Award for monthly interactive lectures by dermatologists to academic centers, hospitals, and remote medical sites in Latin America, Alaska, and Hawaii using videoconferencing.

Åsa Smedberg is a lecturer and researcher at the Department of Computer and Systems Sciences (DSV), Stockholm University, Sweden. She has a PhD degree in Computer and Systems Sciences. Her field of research is e-health communities for continuous learning, and her studies focus on communication patterns in e-health communities for people interested in changing their lifestyle. This involves discourse analyses of online conversations as well as analyses of contents of postings. The studies also include comparisons with Ask the Expert systems in which medical professionals answer questions from people. Åsa Smedberg is the author of a series of international publications. She is a program committee member of the IARIA conferences ICDS and e-Telemedicine. She is a member of the Editorial Board of the "International Journal on Advances in Internet Technology", IARIA journals, and a member of the IARIA fellowship program. She is also a committee member of the IADIS International conference on e-Health.

Christopher L. Pate is currently serving as the Dean of Health Sciences at St. Philip's College, San Antonio, Texas. Dr. Pate has nearly 25 years of military healthcare experience and nearly a decade of faculty experience at the graduate level. He has taught at the U.S. Army-Baylor Graduate Program in Health and Business Administration, Webster University, the University of Phoenix, and Trinity University. He is a 1994 graduate of Syracuse University (MPA) and a 2001 graduate of Penn State University (Ph.D). His areas of interest include decision making, use of quantitative methods in healthcare settings, and health disparities research.

Sisira Edirippulige is the coordinator of undergraduate and postgraduate e-Healthcare programs at the University of Queensland Centre for Online Health, Brisbane, Australia. He is also responsible for coordinating professional development courses at the Centre. Dr Edirippulige's research interests include the development, promotion ad integration of telehealth education and telemedicine applications into healthcare sector. Before joining the University of Queensland Dr Edirippulige help teaching positions at Kobe Gakuin University in Japan and the University of Auckland, New Zealand. He has extensive experience in higher education and development studies working in number of countries including Russia, Sri Lanka, South Africa, Japan and New Zealand.

Anthony Smith is the Senior Research Fellow and the Deputy Director of the Centre for Online Health at the University of Queensland. He completed a doctoral degree in the field of medicine in 2004 examining the feasibility and cost-effectiveness of a novel telepaediatric service in Queensland. His Principal role in the Centre for Online Health includes the management, coordination and evaluation of telepaediatric services. Dr Smith has made a substantial contribution to the literature on telepaediatrics publishing articles in peer-reviewed journal and book chapters on the subject. Dr Smith assists with the supervision of a broad range of telemedicine projects and teaching programs in the Centre for Online Health and also provides consultancy services to other university departments and external organizations.

Asen Atanasov is a founder and first president of MARC Institute – Bulgaria. MARC is an abbreviation of Medical Audit and Resource Control and the Institute is an associate member of the European Society for Quality in HealthCare (ESQH). Dr. Atanasov holds MD degree (Medical University Plovdiv), specializations in internal medicine (Medical University Sofia), rheumatology (MU Sofia BG and Instituto de Doencas Reumaticas de Sao Paulo Brasil) and PhD degree in immunology and cardiology (MU Sofia). Currently he is an Assistant Professor and Senior Lecturer in Medical University, Plovdiv, Department of Internal Medicine and Clinic of Rheumatology and Head of the Department of Internal Medicine and Rheumatology of the private Trimontium Hospital in Plovdiv. He has written 8 medical educational books and had publications in EULAR, Noninvasive Cardiology and in domestic scientific issues. His research interests include quality and healthcare management, medical audit and quality in rheumatology and cardiology.

Elizabeth Krupinski is a Professor at the University of Arizona in Radiology (Vice Chair of Research) and Psychology where she has been since 1992. She received her BA from Cornell University and PhD from Temple University, both in Experimental Psychology. Her main interests are medical image perception, observer performance, and human factors issues. She is Associate Director of Evaluation for the Arizona Telemedicine Program. She has published extensively in Radiology and Telemedicine, and has presented at conferences both nationally and internationally. She is President of the Medical Image Perception Society and serves on Editorial Boards of numerous journals in both radiology and telemedicine. She serves regularly on review panels for the NIH, DoD, FDA and TATRC. She is a Past-President of the American Telemedicine Association and Chair of the Society for Imaging Informatics in Medicine. In 2008, Dr. Krupinski was elected to the first American Telemedicine Association College of Fellows.

Emilio FCO. Ignacio Garcia is Graduate of Nursing from the University of Cadiz, with Master in Sciences of Nursing and Public Health from the University of Puerto Rico, Licentiate of Social Anthropology and Culture, a Diploma of Advanced Studies and a Doctorate in Public Health. He has participated in research projects quality management in sanitary in health care and education funded by national and international research agencies.

Rui Loureiro is a Pharmacist with a specialization in Industrial Pharmacy and postgraduate studies in Quality Management and Industrial Engineering, being a funding member of the Portuguese Society for Quality & Safety in HealthCare (APQS). He works for the National Authority of Medicines and Health Products (INFARMED, I.P.) and lectures the topic of Healthcare Quality Management, Faculty of Pharmacy, University of Lisbon at the graduate and postgraduate level. He has written one book, on medical devices regulatory, classification and quality. He has published more than 20 works on quality in healthcare, and he is an ISO 9001 auditor.

Susana Lorenzo is a medical doctor from the Complutense University in Madrid, with Diploma on Quality Assurance from Barcelona University, a Master degree in Public Health Policy Administration from the University of Michigan, and a Doctorate in Medicine. Dr. Lorenzo is a senior quality assurance expert with more than 12 years of experience as senior manager for a health care system in Spain, and as an international consultant in health quality of care. She has extensive experience in consulting on quality of care and has transferred the knowledge on using tools to improve the quality of care in Spain and around Europe. During the last 15 years Dr. Lorenzo has been teaching professionals on health management at numerous Universities, Schools of public health, local and state government Departments of Health, and Hospitals. Dr. Lorenzo is Editor of the Spanish Journal for Quality in Healthcare and past President of the Spanish Society for Quality in Health Care.

Suzana Parente is a Medical Doctor, anesthesiologist and intensivist and an Executive Board Member of the European Society for Quality in HealthCare (ESQH), and President of the Portuguese Society for Quality & Safety in HealthCare (APQS). She is also a member of the quality assurance and quality improvement committee of the European Society of Anesthesia as well as a member of the quality group of the Portuguese society of anesthesia. Previous founder and President of the Quality Council of the Portuguese Medical Association. She works at the S. Francisco Xavier Hospital in Lisbon (central hospital with university facilities) and teaches modules of quality and risk management at the graduate and postgraduate level. She is also director of the Quality Department of western Lisbon hospital trust. She has published more than 20 works on quality in healthcare, and she is an ISO 9001 auditor.

Vasileios G. Stamatopoulos after receiving a degree in Electrical and Computer Engineering from National Technical University of Athens, he was awarded an M.Sc. and a Ph.D. in Bioengineering from University of Strathclyde in Glasgow, where he also worked as a Research Assistant in the area of Experimental Neurophysiology and Neuroprosthetic control. From 2003 to 2006 he was a Project Manager and Research Fellow at the Royal Brompton & Harefield NHS Trust in London. From 2006 to 2008 he worked at the Biomedical Research Foundation of the Academy of Athens, as a Research Fellow in the Bioinformatics and Medical Informatics Team. From 2007-2009 he worked as an Adjunct Lecturer at the University of Central Greece, Department of Biomedical Informatics, and also at the Technological Educational Institutions of Chalkida and Lamia. He is currently employed with the Foundation for Research and Technology Hellas and the Hellenic Bio Cluster as a Technology Transfer Consultant.

Gilberto Llinás Santacreu is a medical doctor, with a Master in Primary Care Medicine, and a Doctorate in Medicine. Honorary collaborating professor of the Department of Clinical Medicine of the Miguel Hernández University of Elche (from 2001). Research fellow of the Miguel Hernández University. Educational contribution as professor in diverse courses, master and seminars. Co-author of 14 publications in books and national and international scientific journals, related fundamentally with styles of professional practice of the doctor of primary care, quality of hospital care and medical web pages. Collaborating investigator in 5 projects of competitive investigation financed by national agencies or covenants of I+D.

Nina Antoniotti has been Marshfield Clinic's TeleHealth Director since 1997. She has pioneered efforts in TeleHealth development, developed guidelines for TeleHealth standards, and presented at TeleHealth conferences on integration, business plan development, clinical services, evaluation, HIPAA, and needs assessments. She has a Diploma in Nursing (1976), a Bachelor in Management and Labor Relations (1988), an MBA (1992), and PhD in Organizational Systems (2002). She is Chair of the American Telemedicine Association Standards and Guidelines Committee, is past-chair of the ATA Policy Committee and current member, is a past ATA Board Member, and is past Vice-President of the Board of the Center for Telemedicine Law. In 2007, she received the ATA President's Award for Individual Achievement in the advancement of Telemedicine. In 2008, she was elected to the first ATA College of Fellows for her distinguished and unfailing contributions to the betterment of telemedicine to ATA and also worldwide.

George S. Athanasiou was born in Athens, Greece. He received a 5 years degree from Technical University of Crete on Electronic and Computer engineering in 2008, with grade of 8.51 out of 10 (Excellent) and honors by the Rector's Council for his proficiency. Since 2008 he has been working towards a PhD degree at the VLSI Design Laboratory of the Department of Electrical and Computer Engineering, University of Patras. He has earned three scholarships for his academic proficiency, two from the Technical University of Crete and one from the State Scholarships Foundation of Greece. His area of research includes VLSI Design for FPGA and ASIC, Cryptography (Algorithms and Architectures), High Level Synthesis, Hardware-Software Co-design, Compilation Techniques for embedded systems and Collective Intelligence with focus on VLCs. He has 3 Journal Publications (2 published – 1 submitted), 2 Conference Publications and 2 Book Chapters.

Igor Crk is a doctoral student at the department of computer science, University of Arizona. He has a BA in computer science and mathematics from Carthage College and a MS in computer science from the University of Arizona. His current research interests are in operating systems, networks, machine learning and energy management.

Ing. Karel Zvára has been actively researching in fields of the electronic health record, clinical guidelines and information exchange in healthcare for the last ten years. He is director of SME EuroMISE s.r.o. focused on research and complex services in the field of information technologies, especially in healthcare. He received the MSc. degree (Ing.) at the University of Finance and Administration, Prague, Czech Republic in 2008. Currently he is studying in doctoral programme of biomedical informatics at Charles University in Prague, Czech Republic. The topic of his Ph.D. thesis is the information extraction from medical texts.

Ioannis Apostolakis was born in Chania of Crete and studied Mathematics in the University of Athens. He has a MSc in Informatics, Operational Research and Education issues and also a PhD in Health Informatics. He had Post Doctoral studies in Medical Informatics issues. He had been for several years scientific researcher in the Department of clinical therapeutics in the University of Athens. He has research and educational activities in issues of Health Informatics and Education. He is working as Visiting Professor at National School of Public Health. More information is available at http://www.iapostolakis.gr

Ioannis Sitaras received his bachelor degree from the from the Faculty of Chemistry-National and Kapodistrian University of Athens in 1995, his Master of Science Diploma in Environmental Science on 1998 and his PhD thesis for Environmental Chemistry in 2005. He has a working experience on research projects, environmental studies and he was also employed as a Customer Engineer for analytical instrumentation (1998-2005). Since 2005 he has been a Case officer of the Hellenic Accreditation System S.A. (ESYD S.A.), in the department of accreditation of chemical, biological and clinical related testing laboratories. Since 2005, he has been appointed as the ESYD's delegate for the European co-operation for Accreditation Laboratory Committee (EA/LC). He is Chairman of the Scientific Committee for the Environmental Chemistry and member of the Scientific Committee of Analytical Chemistry of the Association of Greek Chemists. He is also member of the Scientific Committee of the Hellaslab (Greek Association of Labs). He has participated with oral presentations in 14 congresses and seminars and he has authored 6 articles in scientific journals for analytical chemistry, environmental chemistry and metrology.

Iraklis Varlamis is a lecturer at the Department of Informatics and Telematics of Harokopio University of Athens. He received his Ph.D. in Computer Science from Athens University of Economics and Business, Greece. From 1999–2004, he was member of the DB-NET (http://www.db-net.aueb.gr/) research group (Head: Asst. Prof. Vazirgiannis) and since 2005 he is collaborating with the WIM (http://wim.aueb.gr) research group (Head: Asst. Prof. Vassalos). His research interests focus in the area of data-mining and especially in the use of semantics in web mining. He has published several articles in international journals and conferences, concerning web document clustering, the use of semantics in web link analysis and web usage mining, the design and implementation aspects of virtual communities etc. More information is available at http://www.dit.hua.gr/~varlamis/

Jan Mainz is a MD, Ph.D. and Professor of Quality Improvement at University of Southern Denmark, the medical director in the Center for Quality Improvement and Accreditation in Psychiatry in the Northern Jutland Region, Denmark. He is the chairman of the Steering Group of the Nordic Minister Council Working Group of Quality Measurement, and chairman of the Indicator Group, Nordic Minister Council Working Group of Quality Measurement and he is also the Danish Representative at OECD Health Care Quality Indicators Project. Jan Mainz is a co-worker and a steering group member of the Office for Quality indicators, European Society for Quality in Health Care. Jan Mainz is a former executive director of the Danish National Indicator Project, the former Head of department for quality improvement at the Danish Institute for Quality and Accreditation in Healthcare. He is also a former President of The Danish Society for Quality in Health Care and former President of the European Society for Quality in Health Care. He is author and co-author of numerous publications on quality in health care and patient safety.

Jose J. Mira Solves holds a PhD in Psychology; Specialist in Clinical Psychology. At the time being he is Professor of the University Miguel Hernández –where is also a Principal Delegate for the Quality Program-, and clinical psychologist (conducting clinical assistance at Agencia Valenciana de Salud. Departament 17). Member of the Technical Commission of Accreditation of Research Institutes of Instituto de Salud Carlos III, Spanish Ministry of Health and Consumer Affairs. Previously: Residents' tutor in clinical Psychology. Coordinator of Communitary Psychiatry and Psychology in Alcoi and Mental Health in Alicante. Researcher of the Research Unit of the Hospital General Universitario (Alicante). Associate Professor at the University of Alicante and at the Miguel Hernández University. Director of the Quality Management and Control Service in the University Miguel Hernández.

Joyce E. Turner-Ferrier is the Simulation Coordinator for the St. Philip's College Health Sciences Division in San Antonio, Texas. She has over 25 years in nursing practice serving as Assistant Hospital Administrator, Director of Clinical Services, and Director of Nurses for seven healthcare institutions in California, Louisiana, New Mexico, and Texas in military and civilian settings. Her nursing expertise encompasses healthcare administration, long term care, psychiatric, maternal-child and women's health, medical-surgical, and clinical skills training simulation. She has taught in both vocational and registered nursing programs in the private and public sectors. She is also a commissioned officer in the United States Army Nurse Corps (Reserve). Mrs. Turner-Ferrier graduated from the Louisiana State University Medical Center School of Nursing (1983, ASN), the University of Texas at El Paso (1993, BSN), and Webster University at Fort Sam Houston, Texas (1997, MAHSM) and is currently pursuing her doctorate in education (EDD).

George E. Karagiannis is currently working as European Research Manager in the R&D Department of the Royal Brompton & Harefield NHS Foundation Trust, London, UK. His duties also include managing the registration and R&D approval procedures of the non-commercially funded projects ensuring that all research activities comply with the national research governance and ethics frameworks. He has significant experience in project management and research in a multinational and multidisciplinary environment. Since 2002 he has managed and conducted research in number of projects both within the UK and internationally, including the EU funded PROactive, EVINCI, eurIPFnet, Clinicip, iWebCare, PharmacoV, pEHR, Panaceia-iTV, eOpenDay and Iremma projects. He has published in eHealth related peer reviewed journals and has been an invited speaker at main scientific conferences. He is a full Member of the UK's Chartered Management Institute.

Periklis Valsamos works for the Greek Ministry of Health and Social Solidarity. He has graduated from the department of Computer Science and Telecommunications of university of Athens. He also holds a MSc. in Advanced Information Systems from the same department. Mr. Valsamos has graduated also from the Greek National School of Public Administration with a specialization in healthcare organizations management. He also holds a MBA from National Technical University of Athens. His main scientific interests are located in the areas of e-health and e-government.

Nikolaos Maris holds a 5 years degree from Technical University of Crete on Electronic and Computer Engineering with grade of 8.42 out of 10. He has earned 2 scholarships for his academic proficiency, one from the Technical University of Crete and one from the State Scholarships Foundation of Greece. His area of research includes Knowledge Representation(KR) and Collective Intelligence(CI). His 2 publications on the KR field deal with temporal reasoning on the web 3.0, whereas his 3 publications on the CI field focus on how the healthcare domain can benefit from the establishment of virtual learning communities.

O.Ferrer-Roca Born in Barcelona, studied Medicine in the Central University of Barcelona from 1966-1972 with Honors. Got the PhD with "Cariotyping and tissue culture of tumors" in 1974 with Honors. Specialized in Pathology in 1974 being trained in Paris, Milwakee-USA and London. Working as pathologist in the Clinic Hospital of Barcelona since 1972 got the Assistance Professorship in Pathology in 1974 and the Chair of Pathology of the University of La Laguna in 1982. Commercialized a pathology image analysis system TEXCAN ® ™ specialized in visual textural analysis of the cell chromatin and DNA and immunohistochemical quantification. Founded the CATAI association in 1993, being the president since then. Got the UNESCO Chair of Telemedicine in 1999 for the University of La Laguna. Since 1996 train on Telemedicine the students of medicine and Computer Science, creating the European Master of Telemedicine and Bioengineering applied to Telemedicine in 2004, at distance. Editor of 12 books and 317 Publications is the author of the first textbook of Telemedicine Handbook of Telemedicine. Amsterdam: IOS-Press, 1998, containing the Ontology of Telemedicine".

Paola Di Giacomo was born in Italy, on March 7th, 1974. On July 16th, 1998, she received with top marks the Italian Doctor Degree in 'Computer Engineering' at the University of Rome 'La Sapienza'. In 2004 it was conferred to her the PhD degree in 'Bioengineering' at the University of Bologna. In 2005 she received with top marks the Italian Doctor Degree in 'Economics' at the University of Bologna. The same year (2005) she received the Master of 'Head of Quality, Health and Environment' at the 'Bocconi' School of Business Administration (SDA) of the 'Bocconi' University in Milan. At the end of 2000 she joined Ericsson Company (Rome) where she is responsible for 'Quality, Health and Environment' for the Market Unit of South East Europe. Since 2004, Paola Di Giacomo is Assistant Professor at the Department of Informatics, Faculty of Medicine, of the University of Udine.

Paul D. Bartels is a MD, and a specialist in chemical pathology. He is Director of The Danish National Indicator Project and head of Department of Clinical Quality and Patient Safety, Central Denmark Region, also he is the head of the ESQH-Office for Quality Indicators, Aarhus and a board member of the ESQH. Paul D. Bartels is a representative of Denmark in the Patient Safety Sub group of the OECD Health Care Quality Indicators Project. Paul D. Bartels is a former Medical Director of Randers Central Hospital and a former senior lecturer in chemical pathology, University of Aarhus and former chairman of the Danish Committee for Quality Assurance in Chemical Pathology. He is a lecturer and author and co-author of numerous publications on quality and patient safety in health care.

Jana Zvárová graduated at Charles University in 1965. She has published internationally since 1969 on biomedical informatics and biomedical statistics issues. She received Ph.D. degree from Charles University in 1978 and DrSc. degree from Academy of Sciences CR in 1999. She passed habilitation (Associated Professor) in 1991 and was nominated as Prof. (Full Professor) at Charles University in 1999. She is the principal researcher at the Institute of Computer Science AS CR, head of the Department of Medical Informatics and the director of the Center of Biomedical Informatics. She has been the representative of the Czech Republic in the International Medical Informatics Association and European Federation for Medical Informatics. She has been a member of the national and international editorial boards and served as the expert for EC and Czech governmental institutions. She published more then 200 of papers and was awarded several prizes for outstanding results of research.

Bryan R. M. Manning is currently a Visiting Professor in Compunetics within the School of Informatics at the University of Westminster, London, where he leads the development of this new interdisciplinary subject, originating from the creation of the International Council for Medical and Care Compunetics some seven years ago. This topic focuses on the problems of technology-enabled change and brings together the psychology of change management from business psychology; process optimisation, risk assessment, and benefits realisation methods from management science; data acquisition, analysis, indexing and communication techniques from knowledge management science; and finally the appropriate use of enabling information technologies to support health and social care service provision.

Raymond Woosley is the founding president and chairman of the Board of The Critical Path Institute (C-Path). Dr. Woosley is also the director of the Arizona Center for Education and Research on Therapeutics that is funded by a grant to C-Path from the Agency for Healthcare Research and Quality. Prior to founding C-Path, Dr. Woosley was vice president for The University of Arizona (UA) Health Sciences Center and dean of the UA College of Medicine. He was associate dean for clinical research and chair of the Department of Pharmacology at Georgetown University School of Medicine. Dr. Woosley was a professor at Vanderbilt University Medical School and was one of the first scientists at Meyer Laboratories, now GlaxoSmithKline. Dr. Woosley earned his PhD in pharmacology from the University of Louisville, his MD from the University of Miami and completed post-doctoral training in pharmacology, internal medicine and clinical pharmacology. His research has been published in over 265 peer-reviewed publications and 50 book chapters.

Shiu-chung "Shoey" Au, holds an MD from SUNY Upstate Medical Unversity in Syracuse, NY, and a Masters and Bachelors of Computer Science from MIT. She is a lecturer, author, and co-author of publications on patient safety and quality in health care. His Master's thesis work, performed under Dr. Amar Gupta, is entitled *Technical and Strategic Issues in Implementing Internet2 in Brazil.* His corporate experiences include working for the Children's Hospital Boston's Informatics Program, where he helped develop the AEGIS automated epidemiological surveillance program. For Xpogen Inc., he developed the core Relevance Networks DNA microarray analysis tool. He has also developing prototype imaging devices and production .NET web applications for financial service and product companies. His professional interests include medical and bioinformatics software and consulting, and medical device development.

Solvejg Kristensen is a Master of Health Science from the University of Aarhus in Denmark. She is a chief consultant and the office manager of the Office for Quality Indicators of ESQH. Solvejg Kristensen is a researcher and task leader participating in EU co-funded project like: SimPatIE, EUNetPaS and DUQuE. She is a representative of Denmark in the Patient Safety Sub group of the OECD Health Care Quality Indicators Project. Solvejg Kristensen has a background as quality manager and regional risk manager of the Central Jutland Region. She is a lecturer, author, and co-author of publications on patient safety and quality in health care.

Sophia Kossida received her BSc in Biology from the University of Crete in Greece in 1995. She spent a year in Trinity College of Dublin, in Ireland within the Genetics Department, where she worked on the genome of Saccharomyces cerevisiae. She was awarded her DPhil in 1998 from Oxford University, UK. She worked on sequence analysis of viral genomes and deciphered their evolutionary history. She carried out a post-doc at Harvard University, USA at the Molecular & Cellular Biology Department. She was employed as Senior Scientist within the Target Discovery Group of Lion Bioscience Research Inc. in Cambridge, MA, USA where she worked on the human genome mining project. She was appointed Director of Bioinformatics of Endocube, a company focusing on endothelial cells in Toulouse, France. She joined Novartis in Switzerland as Lab head within the Functional Genomics Group. She joined BRF in July 2004 as tenure track research Bioinformatician.

Stavros Archondakis (MD, PhD) is certified pathologist, director of Cytopathology Department of 401 Athens Army Hospital. He has graduated from Thessaloniki Medical School and National Military Medical School in 1996. Since 2007, he is appointed member of the greek national technical committee of the Hellenic Accreditation System (ESYD) for the accreditation of medical laboratories according to ISO 15189:2007. He speaks English and French. He is member of Hellenic Society of Clinical Cytopathology, Society of Medical Studies and Society for Quality Management in the Health Sector. He is the author of 29 medical books, some of them awarded by the Greek Anticancer Society. He has participated with posters and oral presentations in more than 200 congresses and seminars, he has authored more than 25 articles in greek and foreign medical journals. He possesses more than 800 hours of teaching experience in medical and paramedical schools.

Surendra Sarnikar is an Assistant Professor in Information Systems at the College of Business and Information Systems, Dakota State University. He holds a Bachelors degree in Engineering from Osmania University, India, and a PhD in Management Information Systems from the University of Arizona. He teaches design research and knowledge management at the Dakota State University and has published several conference and Journal publications in the area of knowledge management systems, information retrieval and healthcare information systems.

Index

D

E

F

G

H

I

J

K

L

M

N

O

P

Q

R

S

Y

Breinigsville, PA USA
20 October 2010
247684BV00004B/1/P

9 781616 928438